Quick Find Guide

MW00344231

1 Ergonomics and Periodontal Instrumentation

2 Clinician Position in Relation to the Treatment Area

3 Instrument Grasp

4 Use of Dental Mouth Mirror

5 Finger Rests in the Anterior Sextants

6 Finger Rests in Mandibular Posterior Sextants

7 Finger Rests in Maxillary Posterior Sextants

8 Instrument Design and Classification

9 Technique Essentials: Movement and Orientation to Tooth Surface

10 Technique Essentials: Adaptation

11 Technique Essentials: Instrumentation Strokes

12 Periodontal Probes and Basic Probing Technique

13 Explorers

14 Technique Essentials: Supragingival Calculus Removal

15 Sickle Scalers

16 Technique Essentials: Subgingival Calculus Removal

17 Universal Curets

18 Advanced Probing Techniques

19 Area-Specific Curets

20 Specialized Periodontal Instruments

21 Advanced Techniques for Root Instrumentation

22 Fictitious Patient Cases: Communication and Planning for Success

23 Concepts for Instrument Sharpening

24 Instrument Sharpening Techniques

25 Pain Control During Periodontal Instrumentation

26 Powered Instrument Design and Function

27 Air Polishing for Biofilm Management

Appendix: Problem Identification: Difficulties in Instrumentation

Online @ thePoint

1B. Getting Ready for Instrumentation: Mathematical Principles & Anatomical Descriptors

20B. Dental Implants

21B. Alternate Clock Positions

26B. Cosmetic Polishing Procedures

27B. Set-Up of Air Polishing Devices

Glossary

REVISED REPRINT

Fundamentals of Periodontal Instrumentation & Advanced Root Instrumentation

EIGHTH EDITION

Jill S. Gehrig, RDH, MA

Dean Emeritus, Division of Allied Health & Public Service Education
Asheville-Buncombe Technical Community College
Asheville, North Carolina

Rebecca Sroda, RDH, MS

Dean, Health Sciences
South Florida State College
Avon Park, Florida

Darlene Saccuzzo, CDA, RDH, BASDH

Professor, Dental Education
South Florida State College
Avon Park, Florida

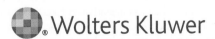

Philadelphia • Baltimore • New York • London
Buenos Aires • Hong Kong • Sydney • Tokyo

Acquisitions Editor: Jonathan Joyce
Product Development Editor: John Larkin
Editorial Assistant: Tish Rogers
Marketing Manager: Leah Thomson
Production Project Manager: David Saltzberg
Design Coordinator: Joan Wendt
Manufacturing Coordinator: Margie Orzech
Prepress Vendor: Aptara, Inc.

Eighth Edition Revised Reprint

9 8 7 6 5 4 3

Printed in the United States

Library of Congress Cataloging-in-Publication Data

Names: Gehrig, Jill S. (Jill Shiffer), author. | Sroda, Rebecca, author. |
   Saccuzzo, Darlene, author.
Title: Fundamentals of periodontal instrumentation & advanced root
   instrumentation / Jill S. Gehrig, Rebecca Sroda, Darlene Saccuzzo.
Other titles: Fundamentals of periodontal instrumentation and advanced root instrumentation
Description: Eighth edition, revised reprint. | Philadelphia : Wolters
   Kluwer, [2019] | Includes bibliographical references and index.
Identifiers: LCCN 2018024561 | ISBN 9781975117504
Subjects: | MESH: Dental Prophylaxis–instrumentation | Dental
   Prophylaxis–methods | Root Planing–instrumentation | Root
   Planing–methods
Classification: LCC RK681 | NLM WU 113 | DDC 617.6/01–dc23
LC record available at https://lccn.loc.gov/2018024561

Contributors

Christine Dominick, CDA, RDH, MEd
Associate Professor
Forsyth School of Dental Hygiene
Massachusetts College of Pharmacy and
  Health Sciences
Boston, Massachusetts

Richard Foster, DMD
Dental Director
Guilford Technical Community College
Jamestown, North Carolina

Cynthia Biron Leisica, RDH, EMT, MS
President, DH Meth-Ed, Inc.
Dental Hygiene Methodology
Tallahassee, Florida

Sharon Logue, RDH, MPH
Virginia Department of Health
Dental Health Program
Richmond, Virginia

Robin B. Matloff, RDH, BSDH, JD
Professor, Dental Hygiene Program
Mount Ida College
Newton, Massachusetts

Kimberly Nason, MSDH
Instructor, Dental Education Program
South Florida State College
Avon Park, Florida

Lydia T. Pierce, LPT
Physical Medicine and Rehabilitation
Asheville, North Carolina

Bobby A. Sconyers, BA, CDA
Professor, Dental Education
South Florida State College
Avon Park, Florida

Cherie M. Stevens, PhD
Professor, Computer Science
South Florida State College
Avon Park, Florida

Donald E. Willmann, DDS, MS
Professor Emeritus, Department of
  Periodontics
University of Texas Health Science Center
  at San Antonio
San Antonio, Texas

Reviewers

Denise Avrutik
LynnAnn Bryan
Michelle Ezzell
Jane Gray
Connie Grossman

Joyce Hudson
Susan Jenkins
Mark Kacerik
Michelle Klenk
Connie Preiser

Pamela Quinn
Shawna Rohner
Rebecca Smith
Dawn Smith
Debbie Zuern

Preface for Course Instructors

Fundamentals of Periodontal Instrumentation & Advanced Root Instrumentation, Eighth Edition is an instructional guide to periodontal instrumentation that takes students from the basic skills—patient positioning, intraoral finger rests, and basic instrumentation—all the way to advanced techniques—assessment of periodontal patients and instrumentation of the root branches of multirooted teeth, root concavities, and furcation areas. The foremost instructional goal of *Fundamentals* is to make it easy for students to learn and faculty to teach instrumentation. The eighth edition retains the features that have made it the market-leading textbook on periodontal instrumentation and adds new features and content organization designed to facilitate learning and teaching.

ONLINE INSTRUCTOR TEACHING RESOURCES

The online Faculty Resource section has a collection of instructional aids for use in teaching instrumentation. These resources are located online at thePoint website (http://thePoint.lww.com/GehrigFundamentals8e).

1. **PowerPoint Slides.** The PowerPoint slides were designed so as to be user-friendly for wide variety of software versions and equipment.
   - The PowerPoint presentations may be customized by saving the slides to your computer hard drive and using the formatting features of your slide presentation software.
   - Special effects, such as progressive disclosure, may be added to the slide presentations using the custom animation features of your slide presentation software. In addition, individual slides may be deleted and new instructor-created slides added to the presentations.
2. **Test Bank.** The test bank questions can be used for quizzes, combined to make up unit tests, or combined to create midterm and final examinations.
3. **Instructor Guide.** The instructor guide includes:
   - Suggestions for leading classroom discussions.
   - A list of phrases that facilitate the teaching of instrumentation.
   - Teaching tips for instruction, as well as, sources for periodontal typodonts.
   - Guidelines for introduction of alternate and advanced techniques.
4. **Module Evaluation Forms.** Evaluation forms for instructor grading are now located online in two formats.
   - Evaluations for Computerized Grading. These forms are designed to allow the instructor to enter grades and comments directly on a computer.
   - Evaluations for Paper Grading. These forms are designed to be printed out and used for "paper and pen" manual grading. Paper forms include evaluation forms for each module.

CONTENT ORGANIZATION

From an instructional viewpoint, it is important to note that *each major instrument classification is addressed in a stand-alone module*—sickle scalers, universal curets, and area-specific curets. Each stand-alone module provides complete step-by-step instruction in the use of an instrument classification. For example, the module on universal curets provides complete instruction on the use of universal curets. This chapter does not rely on the student having studied the previous module on sickle scalers before beginning the universal curet module. This stand-alone module structure means that it is not necessary to cover the instrument modules in any particular order or even to include all of the modules. If sickle scalers, for example, are not part of the school's instrument kit, this module does not need to be included in the course outline.

TEXTBOOK FEATURES

1. Module outlines. Each chapter begins with a module outline that provides an overview of content and makes it easier to locate material within the module. The outline provides the reader with an organizational framework with which to approach new material.
2. Learning objectives assist students in recognizing and studying important concepts in each chapter.
3. Step-by-step format. The clear, step-by-step self-instructional format allows the learner to work independently—fostering student autonomy and decision-making skills. The learner is free to work at his or her own pace spending more time on a skill that he or she finds difficult and moving on when a skill comes easily. The self-instructional format relieves the instructor from the task of endlessly repeating basic information, and frees him or her to demonstrate instrumentation techniques, observe student practice, and facilitate the process of skill acquisition.
4. Key terms are listed at the start of each module. One of the most challenging tasks for any student is learning a whole new dental vocabulary and gaining the confidence to use new terms with accuracy and ease. The key terms list assists students in this task by identifying important terminology and facilitating the study and review of terminology in each instructional module.
5. Study aids—boxes, tables, and flow charts—visually highlight and reinforce important content and permit quick reference during technique practice and at-home review.
6. Critical thinking activities—in the *Practical Focus* sections of the book—encourage students to apply concepts to clinical situations, facilitate classroom discussion, and promote the development of student problem-solving skills.
7. Case-based patient experiences allow students to apply instrumentation concepts to patient cases.
8. The glossary of instrumentation terms provides quick access to instrumentation terminology.
9. Student self-evaluation checklists guide practice, promote self-assessment skills, and provide benchmarks for faculty evaluation of skill attainment. Use of the student self-evaluation portion of the evaluation forms should be encouraged. The self-evaluation process helps students to develop the ability to assess their own level of competence rather than relying on instructor confirmation of skill attainment.

ONLINE CONTENT

In addition to the Student and Instructor Resources, the following resources are located online at thePoint website (http://thePoint.lww.com/GehrigFundamentals8e).

- 1B. Getting Ready for Instrumentation: Mathematical Principles & Anatomical Descriptors
- 20B. Instrumentation of Dental Implants
- 21B. Alternate Clock Positions
- 26B. Cosmetic Polishing Procedures
- 27B. Set-Up of Hu-Friedy/EMS Air Flow Polishing Devices

I appreciate the enthusiastic comments and suggestions from educators and students about previous editions of *Fundamentals,* and welcome continued input. Mastering the psychomotor skill of periodontal instrumentation is a very challenging process. It is my sincere hope that this textbook will help students to acquire the psychomotor skills that—combined with clinical experience—will lead to excellence in periodontal instrumentation.

Jill S. Gehrig, RDH, MA

Acknowledgments

It is gratifying to be members of a profession that includes so many individuals who strive for excellence in teaching. We are most grateful to all of the outstanding educators who shared their comments and suggestions for improving this edition. We thank all who generously gave their time, ideas, and resources, and gratefully acknowledge the special contributions of the following individuals:

- Charles D. Whitehead and Holly R. Fischer, MFA, the highly skilled medical illustrators, who created all the wonderful illustrations for the book.
- Kevin Dietz, a colleague and friend for his vision and guidance for this book.
- And finally, and with great thanks, my wonderful team at Lippincott Williams and Wilkins, without whose guidance and support this book would not have been possible: Jonathan Joyce, John Larkin, and Jennifer Clements.

Jill S. Gehrig, Rebecca Sroda, and Darlene Saccuzzo

Contents

Module 1 **ERGONOMICS AND PERIODONTAL INSTRUMENTATION** **1**
Jill S. Gehrig, Rebecca Sroda, and Darlene Saccuzzo

Ergonomic Risk Factors Associated with Periodontal Instrumentation 3
Foundational Skills for Periodontal Instrumentation 9
Ergonomic Dos and Don'ts for Seated Posture 11
Application of Ergonomic Principles: Seated Posture 14
Application of Ergonomic Principles: Positioning the Patient 19
Application of Ergonomic Principles: Adjusting the Overhead Light and
Instrument Tray 23
Application of Ergonomic Principles: Adjusting the Patient to Facilitate
Clinician Posture 25
Ancillary Equipment 28
Skill Application 36

Module 2 **CLINICIAN POSITION IN RELATION TO THE
TREATMENT AREA** **39**
Jill S. Gehrig, Rebecca Sroda, and Darlene Saccuzzo

Clock Positions for Instrumentation 41
Positioning for the RIGHT-Handed Clinician 43
Positioning for the LEFT-Handed Clinician 54
Modified Positioning: Working from a Standing Position 65
Skill Application 66

Module 3 **INSTRUMENT GRASP** **69**
Jill S. Gehrig, Rebecca Sroda, and Darlene Saccuzzo

Grasp for Periodontal Instrumentation 71
Grasp Variations 76
Predisposing Conditions for Hand Injuries 78
Exercises for Improved Hand Strength 82
Skill Application 86

Module 4   **USE OF THE DENTAL MOUTH MIRROR 89**
Jill S. Gehrig, Rebecca Sroda, and Darlene Saccuzzo

Fundamentals of Mirror Use 91
Is Achieving Direct Vision Really Best? 96
Technique Practice: RIGHT-Handed Clinician 98
Technique Practice: LEFT-Handed Clinician 103
Skill Application 109

Module 5   **FINGER RESTS IN THE ANTERIOR SEXTANTS 110**
Jill S. Gehrig, Rebecca Sroda, and Darlene Saccuzzo

The Intraoral Fulcrum 112
Wrist Position for Instrumentation 114
Technique Practice: RIGHT-Handed Clinician 118
Technique Practice: LEFT-Handed Clinician 131
Skill Application 145

Module 6   **FINGER RESTS IN MANDIBULAR POSTERIOR SEXTANTS 147**
Jill S. Gehrig, Rebecca Sroda, and Darlene Saccuzzo

Building Blocks for Posterior Sextants 149
Technique Practice: RIGHT-Handed Clinician 151
Technique Practice: LEFT-Handed Clinician 158
Skill Application 166

Module 7   **FINGER RESTS IN MAXILLARY POSTERIOR SEXTANTS 169**
Jill S. Gehrig, Rebecca Sroda, and Darlene Saccuzzo

Building Blocks for Posterior Sextants 171
Technique Practice: RIGHT-Handed Clinician 173
Technique Practice: LEFT-Handed Clinician 180
Preventive Strategies: Stretches 187
Skill Application 190

Module 8   **INSTRUMENT DESIGN AND CLASSIFICATION 193**
Jill S. Gehrig, Rebecca Sroda, and Darlene Saccuzzo

Design Characteristics of Instrument Handle 195
Design Characteristics of Instrument Shank 198
Design Characteristics of Instrument Working-End 202
Introduction to Instrument Classification 207
Skill Application 210

Module 9   **TECHNIQUE ESSENTIALS: MOVEMENT AND ORIENTATION TO TOOTH SURFACE 213**
Jill S. Gehrig, Rebecca Sroda, and Darlene Saccuzzo

Learning Periodontal Instrumentation 215
Moving the Instrument's Working-End 219
Rolling the Instrument Handle 223

Pivoting on the Fulcrum   224
Orientation of Instrument to Tooth Surface   225
Skill Application   231

Module 10   **TECHNIQUE ESSENTIALS: ADAPTATION   232**
Jill S. Gehrig, Rebecca Sroda, and Darlene Saccuzzo

Adaptation of the Working-End   234
Ergonomics of the Handle Roll for Adaptation   237
Selecting the Correct Working-End   240
Skill Application   243

Module 11   **TECHNIQUE ESSENTIALS: INSTRUMENTATION STROKES   246**
Jill S. Gehrig, Rebecca Sroda, and Darlene Saccuzzo

The Instrumentation Stroke   248
Use of Pressure During Instrumentation   253
Skill Application   258

Module 12   **PERIODONTAL PROBES AND BASIC PROBING
TECHNIQUE   260**
Jill S. Gehrig, Robin Matloff, Rebecca Sroda, and Darlene Saccuzzo

The Periodontal Probe   262
Assessing Tissue Health   266
Reading and Recording Depth Measurements   269
Probing Technique   272
Informed Consent for Periodontal Instrumentation   281
Skill Application   284

Module 13   **EXPLORERS   286**
Jill S. Gehrig, Rebecca Sroda, and Darlene Saccuzzo

Explorers   288
Technique Practice—Anterior Teeth   293
Technique Practice—Posterior Teeth   300
Technique Alerts   307
Detection of Dental Calculus Deposits   309
Detection of Dental Caries   314
Skill Application   318

Module 14   **TECHNIQUE ESSENTIALS: SUPRAGINGIVAL CALCULUS
REMOVAL   321**
Jill S. Gehrig, Rebecca Sroda, and Darlene Saccuzzo

Supragingival Calculus Deposits   323
Relationship of the Instrument Face to the Tooth Surface   324
Application of Force for Calculus Removal   327
Stroke Pattern for Supragingival Calculus Removal   329
Skill Application   332

Module 15   **SICKLE SCALERS   333**
Jill S. Gehrig, Rebecca Sroda, and Darlene Saccuzzo

Sickle Scalers   335
Calculus Removal Concepts   338
Technique Practice—Anterior Teeth   341
Maintaining Adaptation to Proximal Surfaces   345
Technique Practice—Posterior Teeth   349
Technique Practice—Primary Teeth   356
Skill Application   359

Module 16   **TECHNIQUE ESSENTIALS: SUBGINGIVAL CALCULUS REMOVAL   362**
Jill S. Gehrig, Rebecca Sroda, and Darlene Saccuzzo

The Sense of Touch for Subgingival Instrumentation   364
Inserting a Curet Beneath the Gingival Margin   366
The Theory Behind Subgingival Instrumentation   372
Systematic Pattern for Subgingival Calculus Removal   375
Production of a Calculus Removal Stroke   378
Skill Application   384

Module 17   **UNIVERSAL CURETS   385**
Jill S. Gehrig, Rebecca Sroda, and Darlene Saccuzzo

Universal Curets   387
Calculus Removal Concepts   390
Technique Practice—Posterior Teeth   392
Technique Alert—Lower Shank Position   403
Technique Practice—Anterior Teeth   405
Technique Alert—Horizontal Strokes   410
Skill Application   412

Module 18   **ADVANCED PROBING TECHNIQUES   415**
Jill S. Gehrig, Rebecca Sroda, Darlene Saccuzzo and Christine Dominick

The Periodontal Attachment System   417
Assessments with Calibrated Probes   420
Assessments that Require Calculations   427
Assessments with Furcation Probes   432
Skill Application   444

Module 19   **AREA-SPECIFIC CURETS   450**
Jill S. Gehrig, Rebecca Sroda, and Darlene Saccuzzo

Area-Specific Curets   452
Technique Practice—Anterior Teeth   459
Technique Practice—Posterior Teeth   463
Instrumentation Techniques on Root Surfaces   474
Production of a Root Debridement Stroke   477

Design Overview: Scalers and Curets   479
Skill Application   481

Module 20   **SPECIALIZED PERIODONTAL INSTRUMENTS   487**
Jill S. Gehrig, Rebecca Sroda, and Darlene Saccuzzo

Periodontal Files   489
Modified Langer Curets   497
Modified Gracey Curets for Advanced Root Instrumentation   499
Quétin, O'Hehir, DeMarco Curets and Diamond-Coated Instruments   507
Subgingival Dental Endoscope   513
Skill Application   516

Module 21   **ADVANCED TECHNIQUES FOR ROOT INSTRUMENTATION   518**
Jill S. Gehrig, Cynthia Biron Leisica, Rebecca Sroda, and Darlene Saccuzzo

Anatomical Features that Complicate Instrumentation of Root Surfaces   521
Introduction to Root Instrumentation   529
Advanced Intraoral Techniques for Root Instrumentation   533
Advanced Extraoral Fulcruming Techniques   536
Technique Practice: Extraoral Finger Rests for Right-Handed Clinicians   542
Technique Practice: Horizontal Strokes for Right-Handed Clinicians   549
Technique Practice: Extraoral Finger Rests for Left-Handed Clinicians   552
Technique Practice: Horizontal Strokes for
   Left-Handed Clinicians   559
Skill Application   563

Module 22   **FICTITIOUS PATIENT CASES: COMMUNICATION AND
PLANNING FOR SUCCESS   564**
Jill S. Gehrig, Rebecca Sroda, Darlene Saccuzzo

Understanding and Explaining Instrumentation   566
Planning for Calculus Removal   571
Practical Focus—Fictitious Patient Cases   574

Module 23   **CONCEPTS FOR INSTRUMENT SHARPENING   592**
Jill S. Gehrig, Rebecca Sroda, and Darlene Saccuzzo

Introduction to Sharpening Concepts   594
Preserving Working-End Design   599
Planning for Instrument Maintenance   604
Sharpening Armamentarium   605
Skill Application   609

Module 24   **INSTRUMENT SHARPENING TECHNIQUES   610**
Jill S. Gehrig, Rebecca Sroda, and Darlene Saccuzzo

Removing Metal to Restore a Sharp Cutting Edge   612
The Moving *Instrument* Technique   616
The Moving *Stone* Technique   624
Evaluating Sharpness   636

Sharpening a Periodontal File   637
Skill Application   639

Module 25   **PAIN CONTROL DURING PERIODONTAL INSTRUMENTATION   640**

Donald E. Willmann

Pain Control During Dental Hygiene Care   642
Strategies to Allay the Fear of Pain During Periodontal Instrumentation   644
Using Local Anesthesia for Pain Control During Periodontal
    Instrumentation   647

Module 26   **POWERED INSTRUMENT DESIGN AND FUNCTION   657**

Jill S. Gehrig, Rebecca Sroda, and Darlene Saccuzzo

Introduction to Powered Instrumentation   660
Powered Working-End Design   676
Adaptation—Orientation of Working-End to Tooth   682
Use of "Universal" Magneto & Piezo Working-Ends   685
Use of Curved, Paired Magneto Working-Ends   687
Use of Curved, Paired Piezo Working-Ends   693
Instrumentation Challenges   697
Technique Hints for Powered Instrumentation   701
Set-Up of an Ultrasonic Unit   705
Skill Application   708

Module 27   **AIR POLISHING FOR BIOFILM MANAGEMENT AND STAIN REMOVAL   715**

Jill S. Gehrig, Rebecca Sroda, and Darlene Saccuzzo

The Significance of Biofilm Management   717
Methods of Biofilm Management   718
Clinical Evidence for Subgingival Air Polishing   726
Supragingival Polishing: Using a Standard Nozzle and Conventional
    Sodium Bicarbonate Powder   727
Subgingival Polishing Using a Standard Metal Nozzle and Glycine-Based
    Powder   729
Subgingival Polishing Using a Flexible Plastic Tip and Glycine-Based
    Powder   732
Posttreatment Precautions and Instructions   738
Skill Application   739

Appendix   **PROBLEM IDENTIFICATION: DIFFICULTIES IN INSTRUMENTATION   743**

Jill S.Gehrig

ONLINE CONTENT (http://thepoint.lww.com/GehrigFundamentals8e)

Module 1B   **GETTING READY FOR INSTRUMENTATION: MATHEMATICAL PRINCIPLES AND ANATOMIC DESCRIPTORS**
Jill S. Gehrig, Rebecca Sroda, and Darlene Saccuzzo

Module 20B   **DEBRIDEMENT OF DENTAL IMPLANTS**
Jill S. Gehrig, Rebecca Sroda, and Darlene Saccuzzo

Module 21B   **ALTERNATE CLOCK POSITIONS**
Cynthia Biron Leisica

Module 26B   **COSMETIC POLISHING PROCEDURES**
Jill S. Gehrig, Rebecca Sroda, and Darlene Saccuzzo

Module 27B   **SET-UP OF AIR POLISHING DEVICES**
Jill S. Gehrig, Rebecca Sroda, and Darlene Saccuzzo

STUDENT AND INSTRUCTOR RESOURCES
Sharon Logue, Rebecca Sroda, and Jill S. Gehrig, Rebecca Sroda, and Darlene Saccuzzo

Glossary

Index   *751*

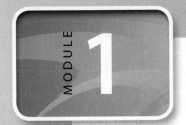

MODULE 1

Ergonomics and Periodontal Instrumentation

Module Overview

This module introduces the principles of positioning for periodontal instrumentation. Correct positioning techniques help to (1) prevent clinician discomfort and injury, (2) permit a clear view of the tooth being worked on, (3) allow easy access to the teeth during instrumentation, and (4) facilitate efficient treatment of the patient. **Prior to beginning this module, readers should review the online resource: *Getting Ready for Instrumentation: Mathematical Principles and Anatomical Descriptors.***

Module Outline

Section 1   **Ergonomic Risk Factors Associated with Periodontal Instrumentation**   **3**
What is Ergonomics and Why Should Hygienists Care?
Ergonomic Hazards for Dental Hygienists
Musculoskeletal Problems Common in Dental Hygienists

Section 2   **Foundational Skills for Periodontal Instrumentation**   **9**

Section 3   **Ergonomic Dos and Don'ts for Seated Posture**   **11**
Neutral Position for the Clinician

Section 4   **Application of Ergonomic Principles: Seated Posture**   **14**
Skill Building. Neutral Seated Position for the Clinician, p. 14
Skill Building. The Masking Tape Trick, p. 17
Important Elements of the Seated Position

Section 5   **Application of Ergonomic Principles: Positioning the Patient**   **19**
Supine and Semi-Supine Patient Position
Patient Head Position
Patient Head Adjustment for Optimal Visibility

Section 6   **Application of Ergonomic Principles: Adjusting the Overhead Light and Instrument Tray**   **23**
Positioning the Overhead Dental Light
Positioning the Instrument Tray

Section 7 **Application of Ergonomic Principles: Adjusting the Patient to Facilitate Clinician Posture** **25**
Skill Building. Establishing the Height of the Patient Chair, p. 27

Section 8 **Ancillary Equipment** **28**
Dental Headlights: Coaxial Illumination
Magnification Loupes

Section 9 **Skill Application** **36**
Practical Focus: Selecting a Clinician Stool
Online Module Skill Evaluations
Student Self-Evaluation Module 1: Position

Access the online module, *Getting Ready for Instrumentation: Mathematical Principles and Anatomical Descriptors.*
This module can be viewed at http://thepoint.lww.com/GehrigFundamentals8e

Key Terms

Ergonomics
Musculoskeletal
  disorder
Posture
Neutral posture
Static posture
Force

Repetitive task
Supine position
Semi-supine position
Chin-up position
Chin-down position
Coaxial illumination
  sources

Dental headlights
Magnification loupes
Working distance
Angle of declination
Depth of field
Field of view
Blind zone

Learning Objectives

- Define the term ergonomics and discuss how ergonomic principles are helpful in the practice of dental hygiene.

- Define the term musculoskeletal disorder (MSD) and discuss the significance of MSDs in the practice of dental hygiene.

- Name four ergonomic hazards for dental hygienists.

- Develop an understanding and appreciation for ergonomic guidelines to minimize the exposure of dental hygienists to musculoskeletal stress.

- Identify musculoskeletal disorders commonly experienced by dental health professionals, their causes and prevention.

- Discuss and demonstrate the elements of neutral seated posture for the clinician.

- Demonstrate correct patient position relative to the clinician and positioning of dental equipment so that it enhances neutral clinician posture.

- State the reason why it is important that the top of the patient's head is even with top edge of the chair headrest. Demonstrate how to correctly position a short individual and a child in the dental chair so that (1) the patient is comfortable and (2) the clinician has good vision and access to the oral cavity.

- In the preclinical or clinical setting, self-evaluate to identify the use of incorrect ergonomic principles and demonstrate how to correct the problem(s).

Section 1
Ergonomic Risk Factors Associated with Periodontal Instrumentation

WHAT IS ERGONOMICS AND WHY SHOULD HYGIENISTS CARE?

1. Ergonomics is an applied science concerned with the 'fit' between people and their technological tools and environments (1).
   A. In application, ergonomics is a discipline focused on making products and tasks comfortable and efficient for the user.
      1. A primary ergonomic principle is that equipment—such as computer keyboards and workstations—should be designed to fit the user instead of forcing the user to fit the equipment.
      2. Ergonomics is the science of making things efficient. Efficiency is quite simply making something easier to do.
   B. Poor Ergonomic Working Conditions and Working Practices. When the fit between an individual and his or her tools and working environment is less than optimal studies show that worker comfort, productivity, and workplace safety all suffer (1). For dental hygienists the work environment includes the dental office layout, dental equipment, and instruments.
2. Musculoskeletal Stresses and the Dental Professional. The dental literature indicates that both dentists and hygienists are exposed to ergonomic risk factors that often lead to discomfort, pain, and even disability.
   A. A musculoskeletal disorder (MSD) is a condition where parts of the musculoskeletal system—muscles, tendons, nerves—are injured over time.
      1. MSDs occur when too much stress is exerted on a body part resulting in pain. When a body part is overused repeatedly the constant stress causes damage.
      2. Almost all occupations require workers to use their arms and hands. Therefore, most MSDs affect the hands, wrists, elbows, neck, and shoulders.
   B. Prevalence of Musculoskeletal Problems in Dental Professionals
      1. Many studies have investigated the prevalence of MSDs among dental professionals. A systemic review on this topic found that the prevalence of MSDs ranged as high as 64% to 93% (2).
      2. Despite this high prevalence, there is a lack of evidence regarding the efficacy of preventive measure for MSDs for the dental hygiene profession (3). A complete understanding of the progression of MSDs in dental hygienists is still far from being realized, due to the lack of longitudinal studies and standardized research techniques (3–5).
   C. Causes of Musculoskeletal Pain in Dental Professionals
      1. The literature indicates that the causes of MSDs among periodontists and dental hygienists include excessive use of small hand muscles, forceful repetitive motions while maintaining muscles in same position during application of force, tight grips, and a fixed work position (maintaining the body in one position for extended periods) (2–13).
      2. The result is injury to the muscles, nerves, and tendon sheaths of the back, shoulders, neck, arms, elbows, wrists, and hands that can cause loss of strength, impairment of motor control, tingling, numbness, or pain.

3. Given the high incidence of musculoskeletal pain, it is important for clinicians to understand the causes of MSDs and to take actions to prevent them.
D. Ergonomic Guidelines in Dentistry
   1. It is important that dental hygiene students complete instructional modules on ergonomic principles during their education and training (3,5).
   2. Research shows that among practicing hygienists, education on patient and clinician positioning can help reduce the risk of MSDs (4,14,15).
   3. It is possible to define ergonomic guidelines to minimize exposure of dental healthcare providers to musculoskeletal stress.

ERGONOMIC HAZARDS FOR DENTAL HYGIENISTS

Four significant ergonomic hazards during periodontal instrumentation are (1) awkward clinician posture, static (fixed) working position, the force placed on a body part, and (4) repetitive movements. Figure 1-1 summarizes these hazards that can lead to musculoskeletal injury.

1. **Awkward Postures.** Posture is a term for the position of various parts of the body during an activity.
   A. For most joints, ideal or neutral posture means that the joint is being used near the middle of its full range of motion.
   B. The further a joint moves away from neutral posture, the more strain is placed on the muscles, tendons, and ligaments around the joint (37). For example, if an individual stands with his or her arms outstretched in front of the body, the elbow and shoulder joints are at their range of motion. If the individual pulls or lifts repeatedly in this outstretched position—versus held close to the body—there is a high risk of injury.
   C. The literature confirms the presence of awkward postures specifically in the neck, shoulders, back, wrist, and hand for dental hygienists. Awkward postures often are adopted due to improper adjustment of the clinician's chair, improper patient position in relation to the clinician, and poor work techniques.
   D. When dental hygienists use their bodies in awkward positions, the muscles must generate higher forces to accomplish a task than when muscles are used in a neutral position (38).
   E. A common awkward posture in dental hygienists is wrist flexion, which results in stress to neurovascular structures and ligaments. Poor wrist positioning can diminish grip strength (39). Figure 1-2 shows the reduction in strength that occurs as the wrist deviates further away from its neutral posture (37).

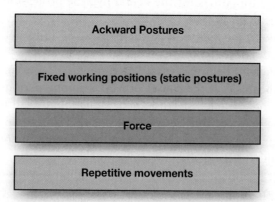

Figure 1-1. Ergonomic Hazards for Dental Hygienists. The dental hygienist has a high risk of musculoskeletal injury when awkward postures, static postures, and repetitive motions are combined with forceful movements (42–45).

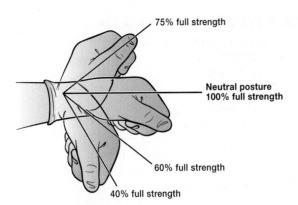

75% full strength

Neutral posture
100% full strength

60% full strength

40% full strength

Figure 1-2. Effect of Poor Positioning on Wrist Strength. This illustration shows the reduction in strength that occurs as the wrist deviates away from its neutral position (37).

2. **Static Postures**
   A. A static posture is defined as a fixed working position (maintaining the body in one position for an extended period of time) (1). The human body was not designed to maintain the same body position—prolonged static posture—hour after hour, day after day. In a static position, tensed muscles compress the blood vessels and reduce blood flow decreasing the oxygen and energy supply to the muscles. Waste products from the muscles accumulate causing muscle fatigue and eventually pain (1).
   B. Dental clinicians have been observed statically holding postures that require greater than 50% of the body's musculature to contract (37).
   C. Static gripping of instrument handles for durations exceeding 20 minutes is common during periodontal instrumentation (40).

3. **Force**
   A. Force refers to the amount of effort created by the muscles, as well as, the amount of pressure placed on a body part.
   B. Holding a small instrument for a prolonged period of time is an example of a gripping task requiring high force application. This task is commonly performed with a pinch grip where the fingers are on one side of the object and the thumb is on the other. This form of gripping is undesirable, as it requires a much greater force application than holding an object in the palm of the hand.
   C. Researchers suggest that excessive use of a pinch grip is the greatest contributing risk factor in the development of MSDs among dental hygienists (40,41).

4. **Repetitive Movements**
   A. Silverstein (42), in an article in the British Journal of Industrial Medicine, defined a repetitive task as a task that involves the same fundamental movement for more than 50% of the work cycle. Periodontal instrumentation would certainly be categorized as a repetitive task under this definition.
   B. The human body was not designed to engage in fine hand movements hour after hour, day after day. The risk of developing an MSD increases when the same or similar parts of the body are used continuously, with few breaks or changes for rest (37).
   C. Periodontal instrumentation requires excessive upper-body immobility while the tendons and muscles of the forearms, hands, and fingers overwork. Three critical components to consider with repetitive motions include:
      1. Frequency: how many times an action is repeated; such as how many instruments are gripped by one hand throughout the day.
      2. Duration: how long an action is performed; such as the length of time sitting in a static posture during the workday.
      3. Recovery time: periods of rest that break a repetitive cycle, such as time spent doing muscle stretches between patients.

MUSCULOSKELETAL PROBLEMS COMMON IN DENTAL HYGIENISTS

MSDs commonly experienced by dental hygienists and periodontists are illustrated in Figures 1-3 to 1-10.

Figure 1-3. Thoracic Outlet Syndrome

1. Definition

A painful disorder of the fingers, hand, and/ or wrist due to the compression of the brachial nerve plexus and vessels between the neck and shoulder

2. Causes

Tilting the head forward, hunching the shoulders forward, and continuously reaching overhead

3. Symptoms

Numbness, tingling, and/or pain in the fingers, hand, or wrist

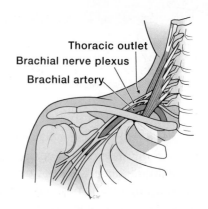

Figure 1-4. Rotator Cuff Tendinitis

1. Definition

A painful inflammation of the muscle tendons in the shoulder region

2. Causes

Holding the elbow above waist level and holding the upper arm away from the body

3 . Symptoms

Severe pain and impaired function of the shoulder joint

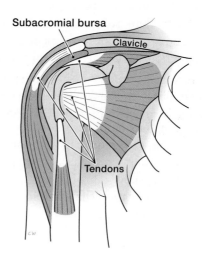

Figure 1-5. Pronator Syndrome

1. Definition

A painful disorder of the wrist and hand caused by compression of the median nerve between the two heads of the pronator teres muscle

2. Causes

Holding the lower arm away from the body

3. Symptoms

Similar to those of carpal tunnel syndrome

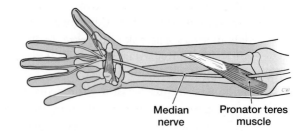

Figure 1-6. Extensor Wad Strain

1. Definition
A painful disorder of the fingers due to injury of the extensor muscles of the thumb and fingers

2. Causes
Extending the fingers independently of each other

3. Symptoms
Numbness, pain, and loss of strength in the fingers

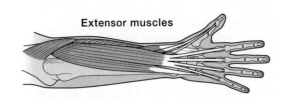

Extensor muscles

Figure 1-7. Carpal Tunnel Syndrome (CTS)

1. Definition
A painful disorder of the wrist and hand caused by compression of the median nerve within the carpal tunnel of the wrist

2. Causes
The nerve fibers of the median nerve originate in the spinal cord in the neck; therefore, poor posture can cause symptoms of CTS. Other causes include repeatedly bending the hand up, down, or from side-to-side at the wrist and continuously pinch-gripping an instrument without resting the muscles

3. Symptoms
Numbness, pain, tingling in the thumb, index, and middle fingers

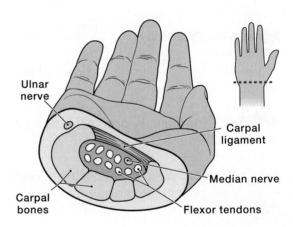

Ulnar nerve

Carpal ligament

Median nerve

Carpal bones

Flexor tendons

Figure 1-8. Ulnar Nerve Entrapment

1. Definition
A painful disorder of the lower arm and wrist caused by compression of the ulnar nerve of the arm as it passes through the wrist

2. Causes
Bending the hand up, down, or from side-to-side at the wrist and holding the little finger a full span away from the hand

3. Symptoms
Numbness, tingling, and/or loss of strength in the lower arm or wrist

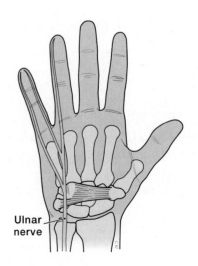

Ulnar nerve

Figure 1-9. Tenosynovitis

1. Definition

A painful inflammation of the tendons on the side of the wrist and at the base of the thumb

2. Causes

Hand twisting, forceful gripping, bending the hand back or to the side

3. Symptoms

Pain on the side of the wrist and the base of the thumb; sometimes movement of the wrist yields a crackling noise

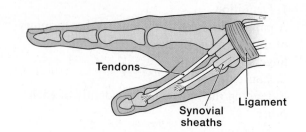

Figure 1-10. Tendinitis

1. Definition

A painful inflammation of the tendons of the wrist resulting from strain

2. Causes

Repeatedly extending the hand up or down at the wrist

3. Symptoms

Pain in the wrist, especially on the outer edges of the hand, rather than through the center of the wrist

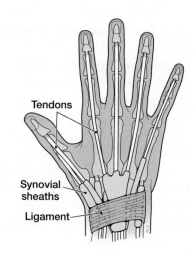

Section 2
Foundational Skills for Periodontal Instrumentation

Periodontal instrumentation is a complex psychomotor skill that involves the precise execution of many individual component skills. Swinging a golf club is an everyday example of a complex psychomotor skill that involves many component skills, for example, proper stance, grip on the club handle, position of the golfer's head, and movement to swing the golf club.

1. Foundational Building Blocks of Periodontal Instrumentation. Many building blocks—individual skill components—are involved in periodontal instrumentation. These building blocks are discussed below and illustrated in Figure 1-11.
   A. Building Block 1: Position. The building block of "positioning" entails the proper use of equipment, as well as, positioning the patient and clinician.
   B. Building Block 2: Instrument Grasp. This building block involves the way in which the clinician holds a periodontal instrument.
   C. Building Block 3: Mirror Use. A dental mirror allows a clinician to view tooth surfaces or other oral structures that are obscured from direct viewing.
   D. Building Block 4: Finger Rests. This building block entails the manner in which the clinician stabilizes his or her hand in the oral cavity during periodontal instrumentation.
   E. Building Block 5: Stroke Production. This building block refers to the manner in which the working-end of a periodontal instrument is moved against the tooth surface. Stroke production is a complex skill that involves several smaller component skills—activation, adaptation, and angulation—that are discussed later in this book.

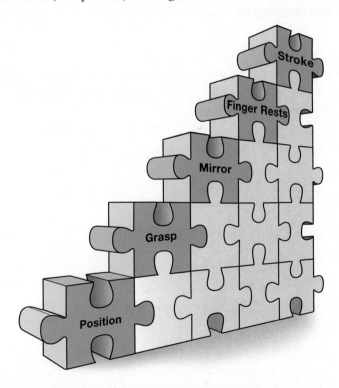

Figure 1-11. Building Blocks for Periodontal Instrumentation. Successful periodontal instrumentation requires the mastery the individual skill components of position, grasp, mirror use, finger rests, and stroke production.

2. Significance of the Building Blocks for Periodontal Instrumentation
   A. Precise Performance.
      1. Precise, accurate performance of the building blocks is essential if periodontal instrumentation is to be effective, efficient, safe for the patient, and comfortable for the clinician.
      2. Research on psychomotor skill acquisition indicates that a high level of mastery in the performance of skill building blocks is essential to successful mastery of periodontal instrumentation.
         a. The building block skills are the foundation that "supports" successful periodontal instrumentation.
         b. These skills should be mastered one-by-one.
         c. *Each skill should be overlearned until it can be performed easily and without hesitation. It is impossible to devote too much time to the practice of these building block skills.*
         d. If the building block skills are mastered, then the use of any periodontal instrument will be relatively easy to learn. The building block skills are the same no matter which periodontal instrument is used.
   B. Faulty Performance. Incorrect performance of even one of the building blocks means that at the very least periodontal instrumentation will be inefficient. Most likely faulty performance results in ineffective calculus removal, unnecessary discomfort for the patient, and musculoskeletal stress to the clinician.
3. Sequencing of Building Block Skills
   A. The modules (chapters) in this book are sequenced to allow beginning clinicians to practice the building blocks to periodontal instrumentation one-by-one.
   B. *Each building block should be practiced until it is easy to perform from memory before attempting the next building block in the skill sequence.*

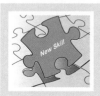

BUILDING BLOCK SKILLS. The puzzle piece shown here appears throughout the book to alert clinicians to the individual skill components of periodontal instrumentation.

Section 3
Ergonomic Dos and Don'ts for Seated Posture

NEUTRAL POSITION FOR THE CLINICIAN

1. Ergonomic Do's and Don'ts
   A. Ergonomic Don'ts
      1. When a dental hygienist alters his or her body position or equipment in a manner that is uncomfortable or painful just to "get the job done," musculoskeletal stress is the result.
      2. A mindset that it is acceptable to assume an uncomfortable position "just for 15 minutes while performing periodontal instrumentation on these two teeth" is destined to lead to MSDs.
      3. Pain and injury results when the body's natural spinal curves are not maintained in a seated position.
   B. Ergonomic Do's
      1. *For a healthy and productive career, first, the dental hygienist assumes a neutral, balanced body position and then alters the patient's chair and dental equipment to complete periodontal instrumentation.*
      2. Good posture requires the seated dental hygienist to use a neutral spine position that maintains the natural curves of the spine (Fig. 1-12).
2. Neutral Body Position
   A. Spine Basics: The Curves of a Healthy Back
      1. The spine is made up of three segments: the cervical, thoracic, and lumbar sections.
      2. The spine has three natural curves that form an S-shape (46). When the three natural curves are properly aligned, the ears, shoulders, and hips are in a straight line.
         a. When viewed from the side, the cervical and lumbar segments have a slight inward curve (lordosis).
         b. When viewed from the side, the thoracic segment of the spine has a gentle outward curve (kyphosis).
   B. Neutral Body Position for the Clinician. Figures 1-13 to 1-19 illustrate the characteristics of neutral body position for the clinician.

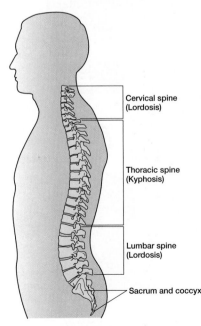

Cervical spine
(Lordosis)

Thoracic spine
(Kyphosis)

Lumbar spine
(Lordosis)

Sacrum and coccyx

Figure 1-12. Three Curves of a Healthy Back. The spine has three natural curves: cervical, thoracic, and lumbar curves. The cervical and lumbar segments have a gentle inward curve. The thoracic segment has a slight outward curve.

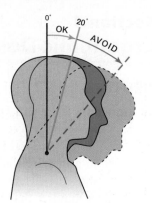

Figure 1-13. Neutral Neck Position
Goal:
- Head tilt of 0 to 20 degrees
- The line from eyes to the treatment area should be as near to vertical as possible

Avoid:
- Head tipped too far forward
- Head tilted to one side

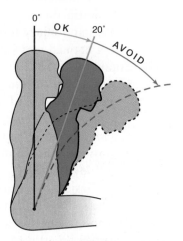

Figure 1-14. Neutral Back Position
Goal:
- Lean forward slightly from the hips (hinge at hips)
- Trunk flexion of 0 to 20 degrees

Avoid:
- Over flexion of the spine (curved back)

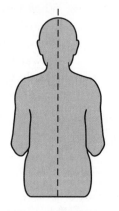

Figure 1-15. Neutral Torso Position
Goal:
- Torso in line with long axis of the body

Avoid:
- Leaning torso to one side
- Twisting the torso

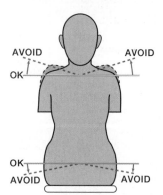

Figure 1-16. Neutral Shoulder Position
Goal:
- Shoulders in horizontal line
- Weight evenly balanced when seated

Avoid:
- Shoulders lifted up toward ears
- Shoulders hunched forward
- Sitting with weight on one hip

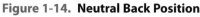

Figure 1-17. **Neutral Upper Arm Position**

Goal:

- Upper arms hang parallel to the long axis of torso
- Elbows at waist level held slightly away from body

Avoid:

- Greater than 20 degrees of elbow abduction away from the body
- Elbows held above waist level

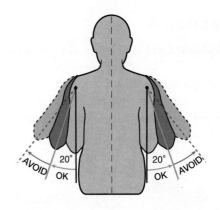

Figure 1-18. **Neutral Forearm Position**

Goal:

- Held parallel to the floor
- Raised or lowered, if necessary, by pivoting at the elbow joint

Avoid:

- Angle between forearm and upper arm of less than 60 degrees

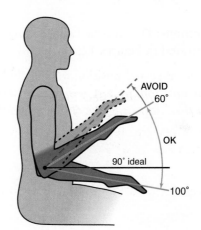

Figure 1-19. **Neutral Hand Position**

Goal:

- Little finger-side of palm is slightly lower than thumb-side of palm
- Wrist aligned with forearm

Avoid:

- Thumb-side of palm rotated down so that palm is parallel to floor
- Hand and wrist bent up or down

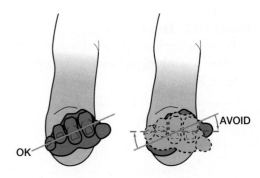

Section 4
Application of Ergonomic Principles: Seated Posture

Ergonomic principles can reduce the risk of developing an MSD by reducing muscle forces during periodontal instrumentation. Attention to the principles for neutral seated clinician posture can minimize the amount of physical stress that occurs during instrumentation.

SKILL BUILDING
Neutral Seated Posture for the Clinician

Directions: Practice the neutral clinician posture by following the steps 1 to 9 as illustrated in Figures 1-20 to 1-28.

The ideal seated position for the clinician is called the **neutral seated position**. *Adjust the clinician stool first. A common mistake clinicians make is positioning the patient first and then adjusting the clinician stool to accommodate the patient.*

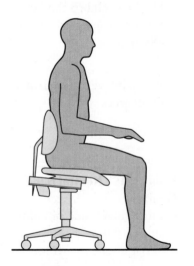

Figure 1-20. Step 1.
- Position the buttocks all the way back in the chair. Distribute the body's weight evenly on both hips.

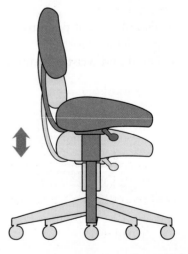

Figure 1-21. Step 2.
- Adjust seat height so the feet rest flat on the floor. Establish a "wide base of support" with feet on floor at least shoulder-width apart and in front of the hips (19).
- Legs should not dangle or be crossed at the knees or ankles. Dangling legs or crossing them puts pressure on the back of the thighs and restricts blood flow.

Figure 1-22. Step 3.
- Adjust the seat tilt so that the back is about an inch higher than the front (hips slightly higher than the knees) (16,17,19,20,22–24).
- The seat tilt helps to maintain the natural lower curve of the spine and relaxes the bend of the knees. The seat tilt should only be about 5 degrees; overtilting it can cause too much low back curve.
- Note: Chairs without a tilt feature can be retrofitted with an ergonomic wedge-shaped cushion.

Figure 1-23. Step 4.
- With buttocks seated all the way back in the chair, adjust the lumbar depth by moving the backrest closer or farther from the seat pan until the backrest nestles against the lower back.
- The unsupported lower back tends to straighten rather than maintain a healthy curve (21,24).

Figure 1-24. Step 5. Adjust the lumbar height by moving the backrest up or down until it nestles in the natural lumbar curve of the lower back. This helps to support the natural curve of the spine (21).

Figure 1-25. Step 6.
- Raise the tailbone up to establish correct spinal curves. All three normal back curves should be present while sitting.
- Studies of the seated body show that the position of the pelvis determines the shape of the spine (23).

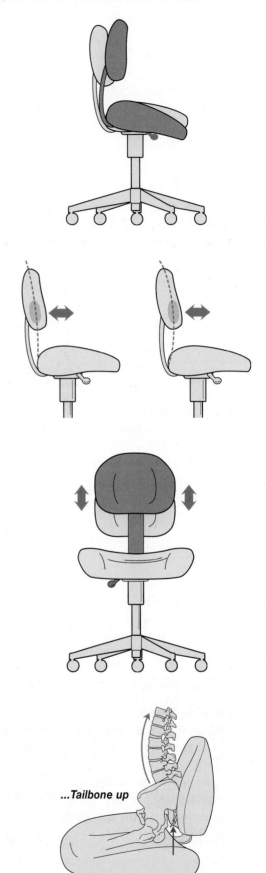

...Tailbone up

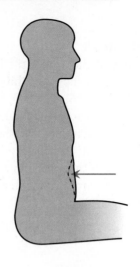

Figure 1-26. Step 7.
- Stabilize the low back curve by pulling the stomach muscles toward the spine (25).

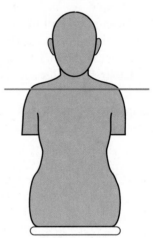

Figure 1-27. Step 8.
- Relax your shoulders so that they are down and back (16).
- If your stool has armrests, adjust the height of each arm so the arms are supported. This helps take the weight off the shoulders.

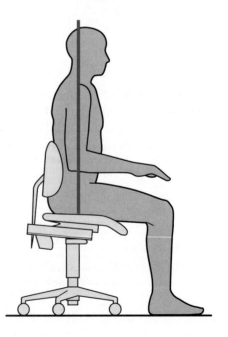

Figure 1-28. Step 9.
- Position the upper arms parallel to the long axis of the torso with elbows held near the body.
- Maintain a trunk position such that an imaginary straight line can be drawn connecting from the ear, shoulder, and hips (19).

SKILL BUILDING
The Masking Tape Trick

An easy way to monitor back position while practicing instrumentation in a preclinical setting is to use the "masking tape trick." While sitting with your back in a neutral position, have a friend apply a strip of masking tape down the center of your back, along your spinal column. Figure 1-29 shows how the masking tape will appear when a clinician is seated in neutral position. If a clinician bends forward, out of neutral position, the masking tape breaks as shown in Figure 1-30.

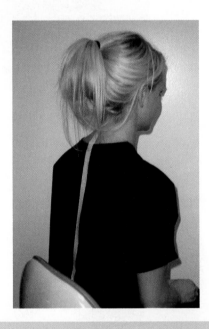

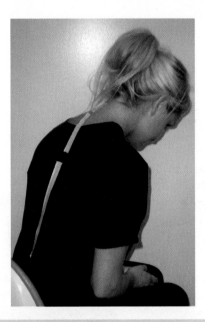

Figure 1-29. Correct Position—Neutral Back Position. Maintain a neutral back position while practicing positioning or periodontal instrumentation and the strip of masking tape remains intact and straight. (Photo courtesy of Dr. Richard Foster, Guilford Technical Community College, Jamestown, NC.)

Figure 1-30. Incorrect Position—Rounded Back Position. The masking tape strip will tear if you bend over, rounding your back while practicing positioning or periodontal instrumentation. Torn masking tape will alert you to problems with your seated position. (Photo courtesy of Dr. Richard Foster, Guilford Technical Community College, Jamestown, NC.)

IMPORTANT ELEMENTS OF THE SEATED POSITION

Figures 1-31 and 1-32 depict important elements of the seated clinician position.

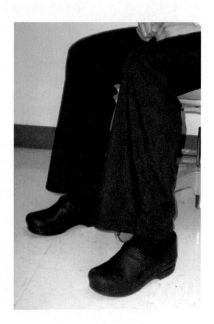

Figure 1-31. Correct Feet Position. The feet should be positioned to create a "wide base of support" for the seated clinician. That is, the feet should be flat on the floor about a shoulder's width apart for ideal balance while seated.

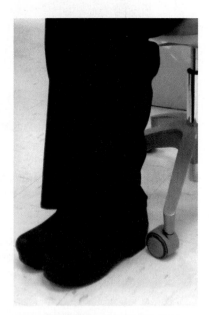
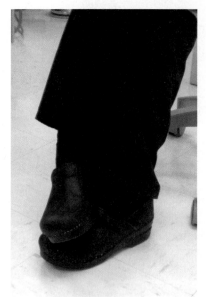

Figure 1-32. Incorrect Feet Position for Seated Clinician
A. Narrow Base of Support. A narrow base of support with the feet together or tucked under the chair interferes with the clinician's balance and can limit his or her range of motion during instrumentation.
B. Crossed Legs. Crossing the legs at the knees or ankles restricts blood flow to the legs and feet. In addition, this position places more weight on one side of the hip and interferes with the clinician's balance during periodontal instrumentation. (Photos courtesy of Dr. Richard Foster, Guilford Technical Community College, Jamestown, NC.)

Section 5
Application of Ergonomic Principles: Positioning the Patient

SUPINE AND SEMI-SUPINE PATIENT POSITION

The recommended patient position for dental treatment is with the patient lying on his or her back. For maxillary treatment areas, the back of the dental chair is nearly parallel to the floor in a supine position (Table 1-1, Fig. 1-33). For mandibular treatment areas, the back of the dental chair is slightly upright in a semi-supine position (Table 1-2, Fig. 1-34).

TABLE 1-1. POSITION FOR MAXILLARY TREATMENT AREAS

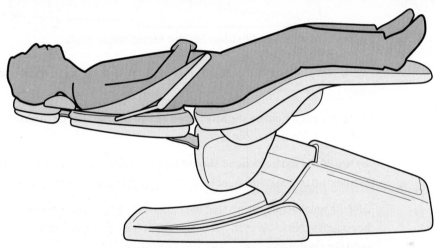

Figure 1-33. Patient Position for the Maxillary Arch.

Body	The patient's **feet should be even with or slightly higher than the tip of his or her nose**.
Chair Back	The chair back should be nearly **parallel to the floor** for maxillary treatment areas.
Head	The **top of the patient's head should be even with the upper edge of the headrest**. If necessary, ask the patient to slide up in the chair to assume this position.
Headrest	Adjust the headrest so that the patient's head is in a **chin-up position**, with the patient's nose and chin level. Patient head position is discussed in more detail later in this chapter.

TABLE 1-2. POSITION FOR MANDIBULAR TREATMENT AREAS

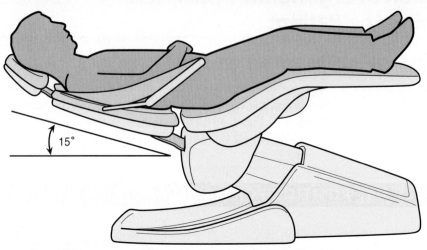

Figure 1-34. Patient Position for the Mandibular Arch.

Body	The patient's **feet should be even with or slightly higher than the tip of his or her nose**.
Chair Back	The chair back should be **slightly raised above the parallel position** at a 15- to 20-degree angle to the floor (24)
Head	The **top of the patient's head should be even with the upper edge of the head-rest**. If necessary, ask the patient to slide up in the chair to assume this position.
Headrest	Raise the headrest slightly so that the patient's head is in a **chin-down position**, with the patient's chin lower than the nose. Patient head position is discussed in greater detail later in this chapter.

PATIENT HEAD POSITION

The patient's head position is an important factor in determining whether the clinician can see and access the teeth in a treatment area.

*   Unfortunately, a clinician may ignore this important aspect of patient positioning, contorting his or her body into an uncomfortable position instead of asking the patient to change head positions. Working in this manner not only causes stress on the musculoskeletal system, but also makes it difficult to see the treatment area.
*   Remember that the patient is only in the chair for a limited period of time while the clinician spends hours at chairside day after day. The patient should be asked to adjust his or her head position to provide the clinician with the best view of the treatment area.
*   The patient's head should be positioned at the upper edge of the headrest. This position permits maximal visibility and access to the oral cavity. Figure 1-35A and B depicts correct patient head position for an adult and a young child. Incorrect head position is shown in Figure 1-36.

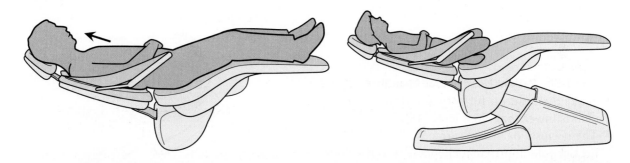

Figure 1-35. Correct Position.
A. Adult Patient. Once the patient chair is in a supine or semi-supine position, ask the patient to slide up until his or her head is even with the top edge of the headrest.
B. Young Child. Asking a young child to bend the knees and cross the legs may be helpful in keeping him or her from sliding down in the chair.

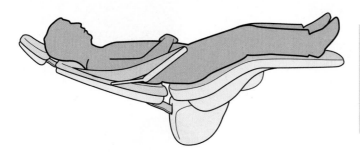

Figure 1-36. Incorrect Position. The patient may slide down in the chair when the patient chair is reclined. If patient's head is not even with the upper edge of the headrest, access and visibility of the oral cavity is restricted.

PATIENT HEAD ADJUSTMENT FOR OPTIMAL VISIBILITY

Once the patient is comfortably lying in a reclined position, the next objective is to ask the patient to adjust his of her head position to attain an optimal view of the treatment area. The patient can (1) tilt the head up or down, (2) rotate the head toward or away from the clinician, and (3) bend the head to the side (Figs. 1-37 to 1-40). *Articulating (adjustable) headrests facilitate adjustment of the patient's head.* Cervical rolls can be used with nonarticulating headrests to maintain patient head position.

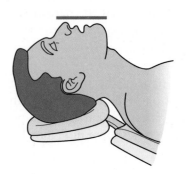

Figure 1-37. Patient Head Tilt for Maxillary Arch.
- Angle the headrest up into the back of the patient's head (occipital area) so that the nose and chin are approximately level (48).
- The upper arch needs to be angled backward past the vertical plane.
- This patient head position is known as the chin-up position.

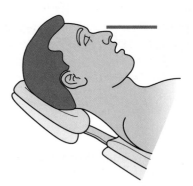

Figure 1-38. Patient Head Tilt for Mandibular Arch.
- Angle the headrest forward and down, so that the chin is lower than nose level (48).
- The occlusal or incisal surfaces of the treatment area should approximately parallel to the floor.
- This patient head position is known as the chin-down position.

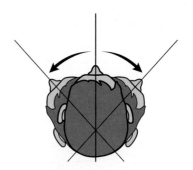

Figure 1-39. Patient Head Rotation for Both Arches.
- Ask the patient to rotate his or her head for easy access to the treatment area.
- Positions include turning toward the clinician, looking straight ahead, and turning slightly away from the clinician.

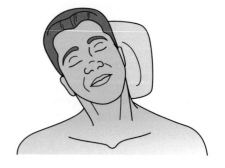

Figure 1-40. Bending the Head to the Side.
- If the patient chair has a flat, nonarticulated headrest, it is helpful to ask the patient to side-bend the head toward the clinician and then turn his or her head for the treatment area.
- This technique can position the oral cavity 2 to 3 in closer to the clinician and enhance viewing of the treatment area.

Section 6
Application of Ergonomic Principles: Adjusting the Overhead Light and Instrument Tray

POSITIONING THE OVERHEAD DENTAL LIGHT

Ideally, the overhead dental light is positioned so that the light beam is parallel to the clinician's line of sight (22,24,49).

- For mandibular treatment areas, the overhead dental light is positioned so that the light beam is approximately perpendicular to the floor (Fig. 1-41).
- For maxillary treatment areas, it usually is not possible to direct the light beam identically to the clinician's line of sight. For maxillary areas, it often is necessary to move the dental light above the patient's neck and angle the light beam into the mouth (Fig. 1-42). It is significant to note that dental hygienists whose overhead dental lights are positioned farther away from their sight lines (toward the patient's waist) are more likely to experience lower back pain (22,24,49).
- It is necessary to make tiny adjustments to the light throughout periodontal instrumentation—seldom is the light positioned for an arch and left in the identical position until moving to the opposite arch. As the clinician works around a dental arch and as the patient looks toward or away from the clinician, the dental light requires minor adjustments.

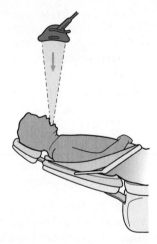

Figure 1-41. Light Position for Mandibular Arch.
- For the mandibular treatment areas, the overhead dental unit light is positioned directly over the oral cavity.
- Position the light at **arm's length within** comfortable reach. Avoid positioning the light close to the patient's head.
- The patient is in a chin-down head position.
- The light beam is directed approximately perpendicular to the floor.

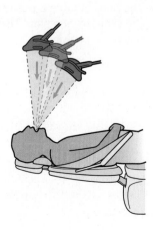

Figure 1-42. Light Position for Maxillary Arch.
- The maxillary treatment areas, the position of the overhead dental unit light ranges from being directly over the oral cavity to a position over the patient's neck.
- Position the light **at arm's length** within comfortable reach.
- Ideally, the light beam always would be perpendicular to the floor, but this is not always possible using an overhead dental light. This is why a coaxial illumination source is ideal. Coaxial illumination is discussed later in this chapter.
- The patient is in a chin-up position.
- The direction of the light beam ranges from perpendicular to the floor to a 60- to 90-degree angle to the floor.

POSITIONING THE INSTRUMENT TRAY

The instrument tray should be positioned within easy reach of the clinician's dominant hand as shown in Figure 1-43. Incorrect positioning of the instrument tray as depicted in Figure 1-44 places unnecessary stress on the clinician.

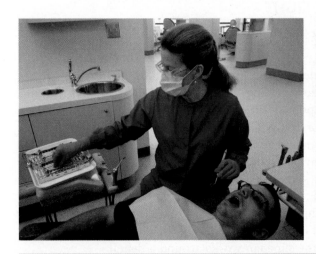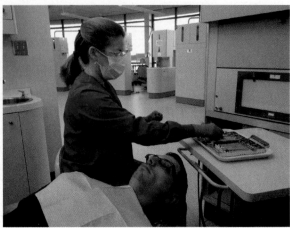

Figure 1-43. Correct Positioning of the Instrument Tray.
A. Front/Side Delivery. Instrument tray positioned correctly for front or side delivery within easy reach of the clinician's dominant hand.
B. Rear Delivery. Instrument tray positioned correctly for rear delivery within easy reach of the clinician's dominant hand.

Figure 1-44. Incorrect Positioning of Instrument Tray. A combination of positioning errors is demonstrated in this photo.

- The patient's oral cavity is positioned too high at midsternum level, instead of at the clinician's waist-level.
- The bracket table is positioned too far from the clinician. She would have to stretch to reach the instrument.

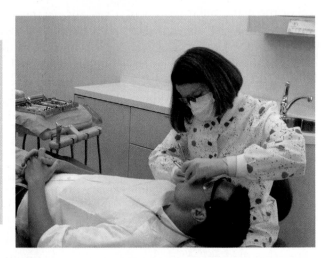

Section 7
Application of Ergonomic Principles: Adjusting the Patient to Facilitate Clinician Posture

A major component in avoiding fatigue and injury is proper positioning of the patient and dental equipment in relation to the seated clinician.

- While working, the clinician must be able to gain access to the patient's mouth and the dental unit without bending, stretching, or holding his or her elbows above waist level.
- *The neutral seated position is established first, and then everything else—the patient chair, the patient's head, the dental unit light, and other dental equipment are adjusted to facilitate maintenance of the neutral seated position.*
- Box 1-1 (Fig. 1-45) provides an overview of the relationship of the patient chair to the seated clinician while Figures 1-46 and 1-47 demonstrate correct and incorrect positioning.

Box 1-1   **Overview: Patient Chair Position Relative to the Seated Clinician**

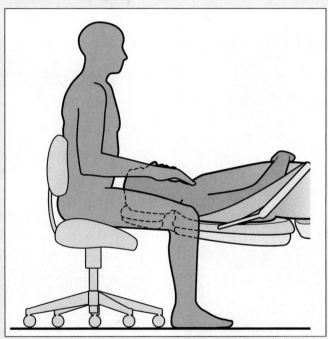

Figure 1-45

- Clinician assumes a neutral seated position.
- The clinician establishes a "wide base of support" with feet on floor at least shoulder-width apart and in front of the hips.
- The patient chair is lowered until the tip of the patient's nose is below the clinician's waist.
- The clinician should position his or her stool close to the patient to enhance vision of the treatment area and to minimize forward bending.
- Whenever possible, the clinician should straddle the headrest to facilitate neutral position.

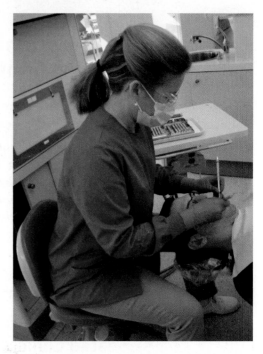

Figure 1-46. Correct Positioning. Here the patient chair and patient's head are positioned at the correct height in relation to the clinician. Note that the clinician holds her upper arms parallel to her torso, her arms are not raised, and her shoulders are relaxed.

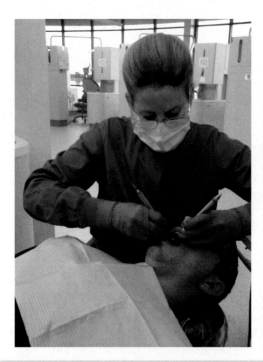

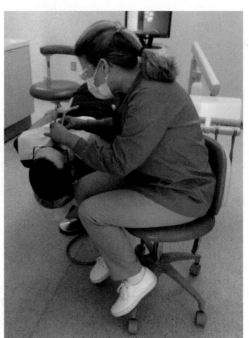

Figure 1-47. Incorrect Positioning—Patient Too High.

A. Note how this clinician must hold her elbows up in a stressful position in order to reach the mouth because she has positioned the patient's chair too high. This error is often due to the misconception that the clinician sees better if the patient is closer to the clinician's eyes. Actually, the reverse is true; the clinician has improved vision of the mouth when the patient is in a lower position.

B. In this example, the patient is positioned too high for the clinician. As a result, the clinician's chair is raised so the clinician can reach the mouth. The high chair position causes her to rest her feet on the rungs of the chair because she cannot touch the floor with the soles of her shoes.

SKILL BUILDING
Establishing the Height of the Patient Chair

Directions: Follow steps 1 to 5 below to practice establishing the correct height of the patient chair in relation to the seated clinician (Fig. 1-48).

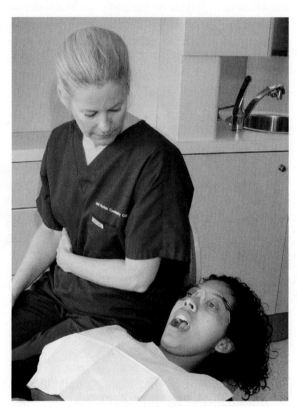

1. Assume a neutral seated position. Sit next to the patient with the forearms crossed at your waist with your hand at the side at waist, not at your midsection (Fig. 1-48).
2. Position the patient chair for the treatment area (maxillary: supine; mandibular: semi-supine).
3. Position the patient's head for the treatment area (chin-up or chin-down).
4. The patient's open mouth should be *below* the point of the clinician's elbow.
5. In this position, the clinician will be able to reach the treatment area without raising his or her elbows above waist level.

Figure 1-48

Section 8
Ancillary Equipment

Ancillary equipment that may be helpful to the clinician during periodontal instrumentation includes a coaxial illumination source and magnification loupes.

DENTAL HEADLIGHTS: COAXIAL ILLUMINATION

Adequate light must be present for human eyes to function effectively. In many instances, the clinician's hands or instruments block the light from the overhead dental light causing the clinician to crane the neck and assume a poor working posture. Instead of using the overhead dental light for illumination, many clinicians use a light source attached to a headband or mounted to magnification loupes (Fig. 1-49).

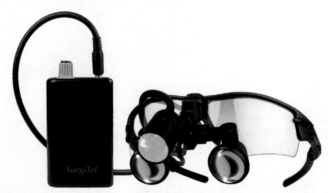

Figure 1-49. CoAxial Illumination Source. A headlight mounted to eyeglass frames. Note also that magnification loupes are mounted to the lenses of the glasses. The battery power source for headlight is shown on the left-hand side of this photo. (Courtesy of SurgiTel/General Scientific Corporation.)

1. Coaxial Illumination
   - Coaxial illumination sources are spectacle-mounted or headband-mounted miniature lights that provide a beam of light that is parallel to the clinician's sight line (Figs. 1-50 to 1-52). In everyday terms, coaxial illumination sources are called dental headlights.
2. Advantages of Dental Headlights
   - Coaxial illumination provides a light source that is parallel to the clinician's line of vision that eliminates shadows produced by hands and instruments. Dental headlights provide the clinician with shadow-free light and facilitate improved posture (50).
   - Dental professionals spend many hours per year adjusting traditional overhead dental lights. Dental headlights improve productivity because time is not wasted adjusting a traditional overhead dental light (50).
   - Recently, Dr. Janet Harrison researched ocular hazards from dental headlights (51). Although most manufacturers advertise that their devices emit "white" light, some dental headlights have a strong blue-light component versus the green-light component. Blue light is highly energized and is close in the color spectrum to ultraviolet light. The hazards of retinal damage with the use of high-intensity blue lights have been well-documented. There is limited research regarding the possible ocular hazards of usage of high-intensity illuminating devices. Another unexamined component is the effect of high-intensity light reflective glare and magnification back to the practitioner's eyes due to the use of water during dental procedures.

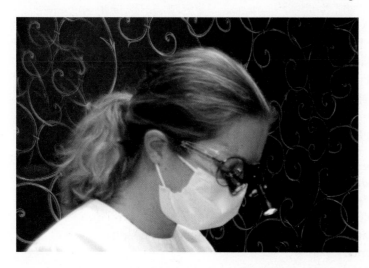

Figure 1-50. Dental Headlight. A dental hygienist wearing a spectacle-mounted dental headlight.

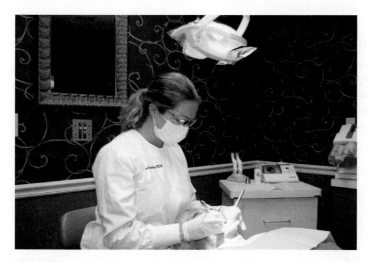

Figure 1-51. Illumination with an Overhead Light. Often, it is difficult to position an overhead light to achieve good illumination of the maxillary arch. Note that the hygienist's head is blocking the light beams.

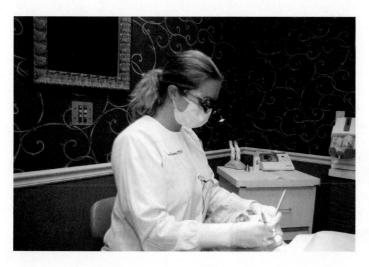

Figure 1-52. Coaxial Illumination. The dental headlight provides a beam of light that is parallel to the clinician's line of sight. The headlight provides good illumination of maxillary and mandibular treatment areas. And, there is no need to reach up to adjust an overhead light!

MAGNIFICATION LOUPES

1. Magnification Loupes: Ergonomically Helpful or Harmful? Magnification through surgical telescopes—known as magnification loupes—may be a technological aid during periodontal instrumentation (Fig. 1-53).
   A. Research Evidence Concerning Magnification Loupes
      1. While the use of loupes is often promoted as an ergonomic intervention, there is little published research to support this claim (8).
         a. A study by Hayes et al. (8) suggests that wearing loupes has both positive and negative effects on upper extremity MSDs among dental hygienists (22,50,53). *Additional research is needed to assess the long-term effects of loupes wear, over an extended period of time.*
         b. A study by Hoerler et al. (52) shows no statistically significant data to support the use of magnification loupes to enhance indirect vision skills among dental hygiene students.
      2. Magnification may reduce the tendency to lean forward in an attempt to obtain a better view of the treatment area and therefore, reduce musculoskeletal strain to the clinician's neck, back, and shoulder muscles.
   B. Problems Associated with Loupes
      1. As with most equipment, how the loupes are used determines whether this equipment is beneficial in reducing musculoskeletal strain (Fig. 1-54). *A poorly fitted or incorrectly used magnification system is more likely to exacerbate musculoskeletal problems than to solve them* (54–57). It is important to make sure that the magnification system is properly fitted to the clinician.
      2. According to Chang (55), President and Chief Scientist of SurgiTel/General Scientific Group, "Many clinicians think loupes solve ergonomic problems, but loupes can create ergonomic problems. The key is to find loupes that meet their ergonomic requirements."
         a. Loupes with improper working distances and declination angles can actually cause chronic neck and upper back pain (55,57–59).
         b. Misalignment of the two oculars can cause eyestrain, double vision, and headaches. Clinicians should try loupes before they buy and ensure the loupes are custom-fit.

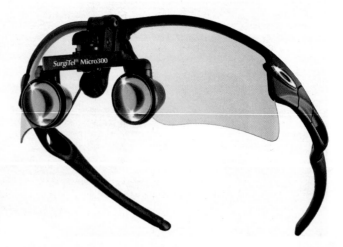

Figure 1-53. Flip-Up Style. Flip-up styles have the magnification telescopes attached to the eyeglasses by a hinged bracket. The bracket allows the clinician to obtain nonmagnified vision by rotating the telescopes above the eyewear. (Courtesy of SurgiTel/General Scientific Corporation.)

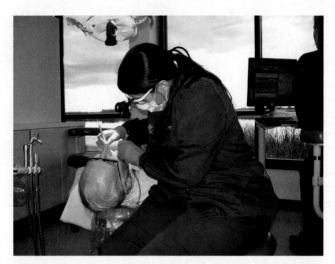

Figure 1-54. Loupes and Posture. As, this clinician's poor position clearly demonstrates, there is no "magic, easy fix" for maintaining neutral posture. As with most equipment, how the loupes are used determines whether this equipment is beneficial in reducing musculoskeletal strain.

2. Magnification Loupes for Periodontal Instrumentation
    A. **Ergonomic Criteria for Loupes Selection.** Three essential considerations when selecting loupes are working distance, declination angle, depth of field, and frame size and weight (55,59).
        1. Working distance is the distance measured from the eyes to the teeth being treated. If the working distance measured for the loupes is too short, the clinician needs to assume a head-forward or hunching posture to see the treatment area.
        2. Angle of declination is the angle between the temple piece of the spectacle-mounted magnification system and the actual line of sight chosen by the clinician (Fig. 1-55).
            a. Each clinician has a unique optimal declination angle determined by the individual's most balanced seated position (55,59).
            b. If the declination angle of the loupes is too small, the clinician will have to tip the head forward or use a hunching posture to view the treatment area through the loupes. If the declination angle is too great, the clinician will have to tilt the head backward in order to view the treatment area through the loupes.
        3. **Depth of Field.** Depth of field is the distance range within which the object being viewed remains in sharp focus.
            a. Adequate depth of field allows the clinician to move his or her head without the treatment area going out of focus.
            b. Inadequate depth of field may cause the clinician to assume an awkward head position in order to clearly view the treatment area.
        4. Sizes and Weight of Spectacle Frame
            a. Large frames that sit low on the cheek allow better placement of the telescopes than narrow, oval frames. In general, the lower the telescopes are in relation to the clinician's pupils, the better the declination angle.
            b. The dental professional may wear magnification loupes for many hours each day. It is important, therefore, that the frames be as light and comfortable as possible.

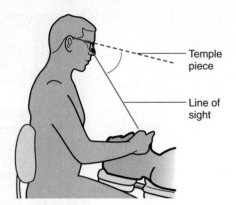

Temple piece

Line of sight

Figure 1-55. Declination Angle. The declination angle is the angle formed between the temple piece of spectacle-mounted magnification system and the clinician's actual line of sight.

3. Important Considerations for Preclinical Periodontal Instrumentation
   A. Limitations on What Can Be Seen with Magnification
      1. Limited Field of Vision with Magnification. The field of view is the total size of the object that can be viewed through the loupes. The most popular magnification strengths for periodontal instrumentation are 2.0×, 2.5×, and 2.6× (55). The lowest level of magnification required should be selected. Lower magnification levels increase the depth of field and minimize the blind zone.
      2. Blind Zone with Magnification. The blind zone is an area of vision between the unmagnified peripheral field of vision and the magnified center of the field of vision.
         a. The blind zone presents the most difficulty when an instrument is being moved into or out of the magnified field of view. Injury to the patient or the clinician is a possibility as the instrument is moved through the blind spot. Most clinicians simply move the loupes aside until a stable fulcrum has been established with the instrument.
         b. The lowest magnification should be selected to minimize the size of the blind zone.
   B. Criteria for Use of Magnification Loupes in Preclinical Setting
      1. Ability for Student Self-Assessment
         a. When learning the skills of clinician position, patient position, clock positions, mirror use, and finger rests it is vital that the student clinician is able to continuously self-assess the positioning of his or her body, arms, hands, and fingers.
         b. *Self-assessment of these skills during the learning process means that the student clinician must have a visual field that includes the patient's head and the clinician's arms, hands, and fingers as well as the oral cavity.*
         c. Figure 1-56 shows the minimum field of vision needed by the student clinician while practicing and mastering the fundamental skills of patient position, clock positions, mirror use, and finger rests.
         d. Magnification loupes limit the clinician's field of vision to the oral cavity (60). Figure 1-57 shows the clinician's field of vision using with 2.5× magnification loupes. Once a clinician has mastered the fundamental skills of patient position, clock positions, mirror use, and finger rests, the loupes provide a field of vision that is adequate for instrumentation.
         e. *This magnified field of vision, however, is too restrictive to permit self-evaluation of skills when acquiring the fundamental preclinical skills of positioning and finger rests.*

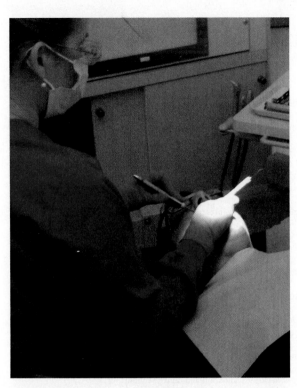

Figure 1-56. Field of Vision without Loupes. When learning and mastering the fundamental skills of positioning, mirror use, and finger rests, the student clinician needs a field of vision that allows him or her to continuously self-evaluate these skills.

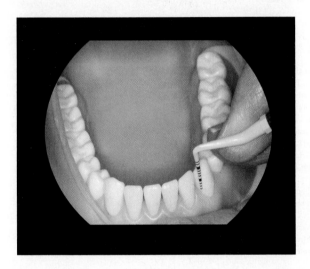

Figure 1-57. Limited Field of Vision with Loupes. When wearing magnification loupes, the clinician's field of vision is limited to the oral cavity. This field of vision is too restrictive when practicing and perfecting the fundamental skills of positioning, mirror use, and finger rests (Box 1-2).

Box 1-2   No Magnification, Please

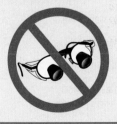

Magnification loupes should not be worn when practicing and perfecting certain fundamental skills of periodontal instrumentation. The limited field of vision created by magnification loupes make it impossible for student clinicians to self-evaluate fundamental skills such as positioning, grasp, and finger rests. Self-assessment of these skills requires an unlimited field of vision.

References

1. Kroemer KH. Fitting the human: introduction to ergonomics. 6th ed. Boca Raton, FL: CRC Press; 2009. xix, 437.

2. Hayes MJ, Smith DR, Cockrell D. Prevalence and correlates of musculoskeletal disorders among Australian dental hygiene students. *Int J Dent Hyg.* 2009;7(3):176–181.

3. Hayes MJ, Smith DR, Taylor JA. Musculoskeletal disorders in a 3 year longitudinal cohort of dental hygiene students. *J Dent Hyg.* 2014;88(1):36–41.

4. Hayes MJ, Taylor JA, Smith DR. Predictors of work-related musculoskeletal disorders among dental hygienists. *Int J Dent Hyg.* 2012;10(4):265–269.

5. Khan SA, Chew KY. Effect of working characteristics and taught ergonomics on the prevalence of musculoskeletal disorders amongst dental students. *BMC Musculoskelet Disord.* 2013;14:118.

6. Graham C. Ergonomics in dentistry, Part 1. *Dent Today.* 2002;21(4):98–103.

7. Hayes M, Cockrell D, Smith DR. A systematic review of musculoskeletal disorders among dental professionals. *Int J Dent Hyg.* 2009;7(3):159–165.

8. Hayes MJ, Osmotherly PG, Taylor JA, Smith DR, Ho A. The effect of wearing loupes on upper extremity musculoskeletal disorders among dental hygienists. *Int J Dent Hyg.* 2014;12(3):174–179.

9. Hayes MJ, Smith DR, Cockrell D. An international review of musculoskeletal disorders in the dental hygiene profession. *Int Dent J.* 2010;60(5):343–352.

10. Hayes MJ, Smith DR, Taylor JA. Musculoskeletal disorders and symptom severity among Australian dental hygienists. *BMC Res Notes.* 2013;6:250.

11. Kanteshwari K, Sridhar R, Mishra AK, Shirahatti R, Maru R, Bhusari P. Correlation of awareness and practice of working postures with prevalence of musculoskeletal disorders among dental professionals. *Gen Dent.* 2011;59(6):476–483; quiz 84–85.

12. Lindfors P, von Thiele U, Lundberg U. Work characteristics and upper extremity disorders in female dental health workers. *J Occup Health.* 2006;48(3):192–197.

13. Puriene A, Janulyte V, Musteikyte M, Bendinskaite R. General health of dentists. Literature review. *Stomatologija.* 2007;9(1):10–20.

14. Beach JC, DeBiase CB. Assessment of ergonomic education in dental hygiene curricula. *J Dent Educ.* 1998;62(6):421–425.

15. Morse T, Bruneau H, Dussetschleger J. Musculoskeletal disorders of the neck and shoulder in the dental professions. *Work.* 2010;35(4):419–429.

16. Andersson GB, Murphy RW, Ortengren R, Nachemson AL. The influence of backrest inclination and lumbar support on lumbar lordosis. *Spine (Phila Pa 1976).* 1979;4(1):52–58.

17. Dylia J, Forrest JL. Training to sit, starting with structure. *Access.* 2006;20(5):42–44.

18. Dylia J, Forrest JL. Training to sit, starting with structure part II. *Access.* 2006;20(8):19–23.

19. Dylla J, Forrest JL. Fit to sit–strategies to maximize function and minimize occupational pain. *J Mich Dent Assoc.* 2008;90(5):38–45.

20. Mandal AC. Balanced sitting posture on forward sloping seat. 2008. Epub March 17, 2008. Available online at http://www.acmandal.com on. Accessed October 6, 2015.

21. Rucker L. Musculoskeletal health status in B.C. dentist and dental hygienists: Evaluation the preventive impact of surgical ergonomics training and surgical magnification. Workers' Compensation Board of British Columbia. 2001.

22. Rucker LM, Sunell S. Ergonomic risk factors associated with clinical dentistry. *J Calif Dent Assoc.* 2002;30(2):139–148.

23. Schoberth H. Correct workplace sitting, scientific studies, results and solutions. Der Arbeitssitz in Industriellen Produktionsbereich. Dortmund, Germany: Schriftenreihe Arbeitsschutz; 1970.

24. Valachi B, Valachi K. Preventing musculoskeletal disorders in clinical dentistry: strategies to address the mechanisms leading to musculoskeletal disorders. *J Am Dent Assoc.* 2003;134(12):1604–1612.

25. Akesson I, Johnsson B, Rylander L, Moritz U, Skerfving S. Musculoskeletal disorders among female dental personnel–clinical examination and a 5-year follow-up study of symptoms. *Int Arch Occup Environ Health.* 1999;72(6):395–403.

26. Anton D, Rosecrance J, Merlino L, Cook T. Prevalence of musculoskeletal symptoms and carpal tunnel syndrome among dental hygienists. *Am J Ind Med.* 2002;42(3):248–257.

27. Barry RM, Woodall WR, Mahan JM. Postural changes in dental hygienists. Four-year longitudinal study. *J Dent Hyg.* 1992;66(3):147–150.

28. de Carvalho MV, Soriano EP, de Franca Caldas A Jr, Campello RI, de Miranda HF, Cavalcanti FI. Work-related musculoskel-etal disorders among Brazilian dental students. *J Dent Educ.* 2009;73(5):624–630.

29. Melis M, Abou-Atme YS, Cottogno L, Pittau R. Upper body musculoskeletal symptoms in Sardinian dental students. *J Can Dent Assoc.* 2004;70(5):306–310.

30. Michalak-Turcotte C. Controlling dental hygiene work-related musculoskeletal disorders: the ergonomic process. *J Dent Hyg.* 2000;74(1):41–48.

31. Morse T, Bruneau H, Michalak-Turcotte C, et al. Musculoskeletal disorders of the neck and shoulder in dental hygienists and dental hygiene students. *J Dent Hyg.* 2007;81(1):10.

32. Rising DW, Bennett BC, Hursh K, Plesh O. Reports of body pain in a dental student population. *J Am Dent Assoc.* 2005; 136(1):81–86.

33. Samotoi A, Moffat SM, Thomson WM. Musculoskeletal symptoms in New Zealand dental therapists: prevalence and associ-ated disability. *N Z Dent J.* 2008;104(2):49–53; quiz 65.

34. Thornton LJ, Barr AE, Stuart-Buttle C, et al. Perceived musculoskeletal symptoms among dental students in the clinic work environment. *Ergonomics.* 2008;51(4):573–586.

35. Warren N. Causes of musculoskeletal disorders in dental hygienists and dental hygiene students: a study of combined biome-chanical and psychosocial risk factors. *Work.* 2010;35(4):441–454.

36. Yamalik N. Musculoskeletal disorders (MSDs) and dental practice Part 2. Risk factors for dentistry, magnitude of the prob-lem, prevention, and dental ergonomics. *Int Dent J.* 2007;57(1):45–54.

37. Occupational Health and Safety Council of Ontario (OHSCO). Occupational Health and Safety Council of Ontario's MSD Prevention Series. Part 1: MSD Prevention Guideline for Ontario. 2007. www.osach.ca/misc_pdf/MSDGuideline.pdf. Accessed November 23, 2015.

38. Levangie PK, Norkin CC. *Joint Structure and Function : A Comprehensive Analysis.* 4th ed. Philadelphia, PA: F.A. Davis Co.; 2005. xix, 588.

39. Wyoming AgrAbility. What to look for when selecting or modifying hand tools to provide a better fit for the user. http://www.uwyo.edu/agrability/fact_sheets/what_to_look_for_in_hand_tools.pdf. Accessed October 6, 2015.

40. Sanders MJ, Turcotte CA. Ergonomic strategies for dental professionals. *Work.* 1997;8(1):55–72.

41. Sanders MA, Turcotte CM. Strategies to reduce work-related musculoskeletal disorders in dental hygienists: two case studies. *J Hand Ther.* 2002;15(4):363–374.

42. Silverstein BA, Fine LJ, Armstrong TJ. Occupational factors and carpal tunnel syndrome. *Am J Ind Med.* 1987;11(3): 343–358.

43. Kilbom S, Armstrong T, Buckle P, et al. Musculoskeletal disorders: work-related risk factors and prevention. *Int J Occup Environ Health.* 1996;2(3):239–246.

44. Latko WA, Armstrong TJ, Foulke JA, Herrin GD, Rabourn RA, Ulin SS. Development and evaluation of an observational method for assessing repetition in hand tasks. *Am Ind Hyg Assoc J.* 1997;58(4):278–285.

45. Silverstein BA, Fine LJ, Armstrong TJ. Hand wrist cumulative trauma disorders in industry. *Br J Ind Med.* 1986;43(11): 779–784.

46. Surgeons AAoO. Spine basics: spinal curves. American Academy of Orthopedic Surgeons.

47. Valachi B, Valachi K. Mechanisms leading to musculoskeletal disorders in dentistry. *J Am Dent Assoc.* 2003;134(10): 1344–1350.

48. Martin MM, Adhern D, Gotcher J, et al. In introduction to ergonomics: Risk factors, MSDs, Approaches and Interventions. Chicago, Illinois: American Dental Association; 2004.

49. Rucker LM, Sunell S. "Dental Clinical Ergonomics Module" materials, 22 modules. www.dentistry.ubc.ca/ergo, 2006-date. Accessed October 6, 2015.

50. Branson BG, Bray KK, Gadbury-Amyot C, et al. Effect of magnification lenses on student operator posture. *J Dent Educ.* 2004;68(3):384–389.

51. Stamatacos C, Harrison JL. The possible ocular hazards of LED dental illumination applications. *J Mich Dent Assoc.* 2014;96(4):34–39.

52. Hoerler SB, Branson BG, High AM, Mitchell TV. Effects of dental magnification lenses on indirect vision: a pilot study. *J Dent Hyg.* 2012;86(4):323–330.

53. Maillet JP, Millar AM, Burke JM, Maillet MA, Maillet WA, Neish NR. Effect of magnification loupes on dental hygiene student posture. *J Dent Educ.* 2008;72(1):33–44.

54. Alexopoulos EC, Stathi IC, Charizani F. Prevalence of musculoskeletal disorders in dentists. *BMC Musculoskelet Disord.* 2004;5:16.

55. Chang BJ. Ergonomic benefits of surgical telescope systems: selection guidelines. *J Calif Dent Assoc.* 2002;30(2):161–169.

56. Donaldson ME, Knight GW, Guenzel PJ. The effect of magnification on student performance in pediatric operative dentistry. *J Dent Educ.* 1998;62(11):905–910.

57. Rucker LM. Surgical Magnification: Posture Maker or Posture Breaker?, In: Ergonomics and the Dental Care Worker, Murphy DC, ed. Chapter 8, Washington, DC: American Public Health Association, pp. 191–216, 1998.

58. Chaffin DB. Localized muscle fatigue–definition and measurement. *J Occup Med.* 1973;15(4):346–354.

59. Rucker LM, Beattie C, McGregor C, Sunell S, Ito Y. Declination angle and its role in selecting surgical telescopes. *J Am Dent Assoc.* 1999;130(7):1096–1100.

60. Barbieri S. Magnification for the dental hygienist. *Dimen Dent Hyg.* 2006;4(11):28, 30–31.

Section 9
Skill Application

PRACTICAL FOCUS
Selecting A Clinician Stool

Dental professionals spend long hours sitting. Clinician stools cannot be a "one size fits all" design. Dentists and dental hygienists come in all sizes: tall or short with a delicate or round physique. A dental hygienist who is 6′4″ in height certainly needs a different chair than a dental hygienist who is 5′1″ in height. A stool that is adjusted correctly for clinician A may be uncomfortable for clinician B. Just as each driver of the family car must change the position of the driver's seat and mirrors, *each clinician should adjust the stool height and seat back to conform to his or her own body proportions and height.* Properly designed clinician seating is the foundation for a healthy neutral sitting position (18,19,22,47). Table 1-3 provides evaluation criteria for assessment of clinician seating.

TABLE 1-3. ERGONOMIC SEATING EVALUATION FORM	
Evaluation Criteria	**Scale:** **U = Unacceptable** **A = Average** **E = Excellent**
A. Legs 　1. Five legs for stability 　2. Large casters for easy movement	
B. Stool Adjustments 　1. Stool seat height, backrest, and seat pan adjust independently to allow for comfortable seating. 　2. Stool seat height, backrest, and seat pan adjust easily while in a seated position. 　3. Seat height easily adjusts to accommodate both tall and short clinicians (range of 14–20 in). 　4. Seat pan tilts slightly so that the seat back is an inch or so higher than the front.	
C. Seat Comfort 　1. Seat pan depth is comfortable and supportive. Seat pan is large enough to support the clinician's thighs and buttocks. 　2. Front edge of the seat pan has a waterfall shape (rounded front edge). 　3. When the clinician is seated with his or her back against the backrest, the seat pan does not impinge on the back of the clinician's knees, but allows a couple of inches between the edge and the back of the knee.	
D. Backrest Comfort 　1. The backrest adjusts in a vertical direction—up and down—to provide support to the lumbar region of the back for both short and tall clinicians. 　2. The backrest adjusts in a horizontal direction—closer or farther away from the seat—to provide lumbar support.	

ONLINE MODULE SKILL EVALUATIONS

 Module Skill Evaluations for instructor use can be downloaded at http://thepoint.lww.com/GehrigFundamentals8e

Module skill evaluations may be downloaded for use on a computer (Fig. 1-58) or printed out as paper copies.

- These computerized module evaluations automatically tabulate the percentage grade for each module evaluation.
- The computerized evaluation forms may be customized to meet each individual dental hygiene program's needs by adding or deleting criteria.
- In addition to the individual module evaluation forms, a summative evaluation form for use as a psychomotor final examination is available on The Point website.
- For details see the Instructor Resources section of the online materials at thePoint website accessed at http://thepoint.lww.com/GehrigFundamentals8e

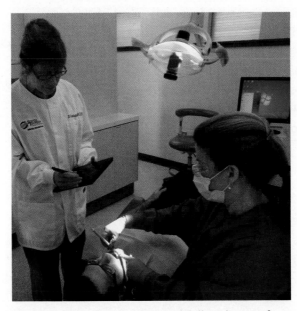

Figure 1-58. Computerized Skill Evaluation Forms. Skill Evaluation forms downloaded from thePoint website may be used on a computer during the preclinical evaluation process.

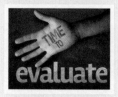

Student Self-Evaluation Module 1: Position

Student: _____

Date: _____

DIRECTIONS: Self-evaluate your skill level in each treatment area as: **S** (satisfactory) or **U** (unsatisfactory).

Positioning/Ergonomics	Self Evaluation
Adjusts clinician chair correctly	
Reclines patient chair and assures that patient's head is even with top of headrest	
Positions instrument table within easy reach for front, side, or rear delivery as appropriate for operatory configuration	
Positions unit light at arm's length or dons dental headlight and adjusts it for use	
Positions backrest of patient chair for the specified dental arch	
Adjusts height of patient chair so that clinician's elbows remain at waist level when the clinician's fingers are touching the teeth in treatment area	
Maintains neutral seated position	

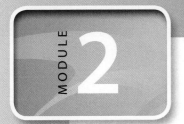

MODULE 2

Clinician Position in Relation to the Treatment Area

Module Overview

The manner in which the seated clinician is positioned in relation to a treatment area is known as the clock position. This module introduces the traditional clock positions for periodontal instrumentation.

Module Outline

Section 1   **Clock Positions for Instrumentation**   **41**

Section 2   **Positioning for the RIGHT-Handed Clinician**   **43**
Skill Building. Clock Positions for the RIGHT-Handed Clinician, p. 43
Flow Chart: Sequence for Practicing Patient/Clinician Position
Use of Textbook during Skill Practice
Quick Start Guide to the Anterior Sextants, p. 47
Skill Building. Clock Positions for the Anterior Surfaces Toward, p. 48
Skill Building. Clock Positions for the Anterior Surfaces Away, p. 49
Quick Start Guide to the Posterior Sextants, p. 50
Skill Building. Clock Positions for the Posterior Sextants, Aspects
    Facing Toward the Clinician, p. 51
Skill Building. Clock Positions for the Posterior Sextants, Aspects
    Facing Away From the Clinician, p. 52
Reference Sheet: Position for the RIGHT-Handed Clinician

Section 3   **Positioning for the LEFT-Handed Clinician**   **54**
Skill Building. Clock Positions for the LEFT-Handed Clinician, p. 54
Flow Chart: Sequence for Practicing Patient/Clinician Position
Use of Textbook During Skill Practice
Quick Start Guide to the Anterior Sextants, p. 58
Skill Building. Clock Positions for the Anterior Surfaces Toward, p. 59
Skill Building. Clock Positions for the Anterior Surfaces Away, p. 60
Quick Start Guide to the Posterior Sextants, p. 61
Skill Building. Clock Positions for the Posterior Sextants, Aspects
    Facing Toward the Clinician, p. 62
Skill Building. Clock Positions for the Posterior Sextants, Aspects
    Facing Away from the Clinician, p. 63
Reference Sheet: Position for the LEFT-Handed Clinician

Section 4   **Modified Positioning: Working from a
Standing Position**   **65**

Skill Application

Practical Focus. Assessing Patient and Clinician Position
Student Self Evaluation Module 2: Positioning and Clock Positions

Online resources for this module:

- Clock Positions for Anterior Teeth (right- and left-handed versions)
- Clock Positions for Posterior Teeth (right- and left-handed versions)

Available at: http://thepoint.lww.com/GehrigFundamentals8e

Key Terms

Clock positions
Anterior surfaces toward
  the clinician

Anterior surfaces away from
  the clinician
Posterior aspects facing
  toward the clinician

Posterior aspects facing away
  from the clinician

Learning Objectives

- Demonstrate and maintain neutral seated posture for each of the mandibular and maxillary treatment areas.
- Demonstrate correct patient position relative to the clinician.
- Demonstrate, from memory, the clock position(s) for each of the mandibular and maxillary treatment areas.
- Demonstrate standing clinician position for the mandibular treatment areas.
- Recognize incorrect position and describe or demonstrate how to correct the problem.

RIGHT- AND LEFT-HANDED SECTIONS IN THIS MODULE

- Beginning with Section 2, the sections in this module are customized for right-handed and left-handed clinicians.

- Having two different versions of the content in the Module sometimes can be annoying or confusing. For example, a left-handed clinician finds it time consuming to bypass all the right-handed pages to locate the left-handed version. Sometimes readers turn to the wrong version and become confused.

- For ease of use—and avoidance of confusion—if you are right-handed, it is recommended that you either (1) tear the left-handed pages from the book or (2) staple these pages together. If you are left-handed, use the same approach with the right-handed pages.

Section 1
Clock Positions for Instrumentation

1. **Range of Clinician Positions.** During periodontal instrumentation the seated clinician moves around the patient to maintain neutral body posture.
   A. Goal of Positioning. *Correct positioning of the seated clinician in relation to the treatment area (1) facilitates neutral posture of the clinician's head, arms, wrists, and hands and (2) provides optimal vision of the tooth surfaces.*
   B. Clock Positions
      1. Instrumentation of the various treatment areas may be accomplished from a range of clinician positions in relation to the patient's head (Fig. 2-1).
      2. Using an analog clock face as a guide—with the patient's head being at 12 o'clock and the feet being at 6 o'clock—is a common method of identifying the clinician's position in relation to the patient (Fig. 2-2).
      3. The positions that the clinician assumes in relation to the patient's head are known as "clock positions".
2. **Range of Patient Head Positions.** *In addition to assuming an optimal clock position, it is important to ask the patient to assume a head position that facilitates neutral arm, wrist, and hand position for the clinician* (Fig. 2-3).

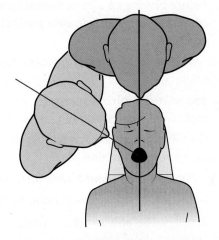

Figure 2-1. Movement Around the Patient.
- The seated clinician can assume a range of positions around the patient during periodontal instrumentation.
- This illustration shows two examples of possible seated positions in relation to the patient.

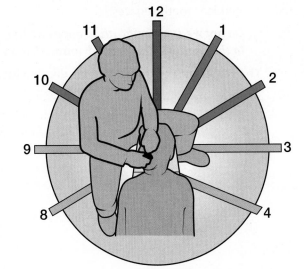

Figure 2-2. Clinician Clock Positions.
- Clinician clock positions are identified using the face of an analog clock as the guide (Box 2-1).
- The patient's head is at the 12 o'clock position and the feet are at the 6 o'clock position.
- Right-handed clinicians sit from 8 to 1 o'clock; left-handed from 11 to 4 o'clock.

Figure 2-3. Patient Head Positions.

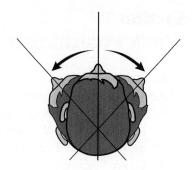

- The patient's head should be positioned to facilitate neutral arm, wrist, and hand posture for the clinician. The patient's head may be straight or turned toward or away from the clinician.
- The clinician should request that the patient position the head to facilitate visibility and access to the treatment area. The patient is in the dental chair only for 45 to 60 minutes, while the clinician works at chairside throughout an 8-hour day.

| Box 2-1 | Directions for Sections 2 and 3 of this Module |

1. The next two sections of this Module contain instructions for practicing the traditional clock positions for each treatment area of the mouth.

2. *For this module, you should concentrate on mastering your positioning for each treatment area.*

   - ***Work without dental instruments and just concentrate on learning positioning.***

   - ***Before picking up a periodontal instrument you should master the large motor skills of positioning yourself, your patient, and the dental equipment to facilitate neutral position.***

3. As you practice each clock position, position your arms and hands as described in this module.

   - You will use both of your hands for periodontal instrumentation, the periodontal instrument is held in your dominant hand and the mirror is held in your nondominant hand.

   - For this module, practice placing the fingertips of your hands as shown in the illustration for each clock position.

      ○ ***Place your dominant hand on the teeth in the treatment area.***

      ○ ***Rest your nondominant hand on the patient's cheek or chin.***

4. You will not be able to obtain a clear view of all tooth surfaces as you practice positioning in this module. In Modules 4 to 7, you will learn to use a dental mouth mirror to view these "hidden" tooth surfaces.

5. ***Do not wear magnification loupes when practicing and perfecting your positioning skills in this module. You need an unrestricted visual field for self-evaluation.***

The remainder of this module is divided into right- and left-handed sections.

Section 2
Positioning for the RIGHT-Handed Clinician

SKILL BUILDING
Clock Positions for the RIGHT-Handed Clinician

Directions: Practice each clock position by following the criteria outlined below.

8 o'clock Positions (To the Front of the Patient)

- **Torso Position.** Sit facing the patient with your hip in line with the patient's upper arm.
- **Leg Position.** Your thighs should rest against the side of the patient chair.
- **Arm Positions.** To reach the patient's mouth, hold your arms slightly away from your sides. Hold your lower right arm over the patient's chest. NOTE: Do not rest your arm on the patient's head or chest.
- **Line of Vision.** Your line of vision is straight ahead, into the patient's mouth.

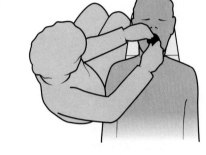

Ergonomic Considerations: Use of the 8 o'clock position should be limited since it is difficult to maintain neutral arm and torso posture in this clock position. The goal is to minimize postural abnormalities whenever possible.

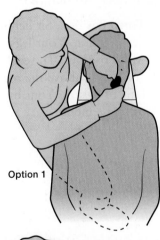

Option 1

9 o'clock Position (To the Side of the Patient)

- **Torso Position.** Sit facing the side of the patient's head. The midline of your torso is even with the patient's mouth.
- **Leg Position.** Your legs may be in either of two acceptable positions: (1) straddling the patient chair or (2) underneath the *headrest* of the patient chair—not under the chair back. Neutral position is best achieved by straddling the chair; however, you should use the alternative position if you find straddling uncomfortable.
- **Arm Positions.** To reach the patient's mouth, hold the lower half of your right arm in approximate alignment with the patient's shoulder. Hold your left hand and wrist over the region of the patient's right eye.
- **Line of Vision.** Your line of vision is straight down into the mouth.

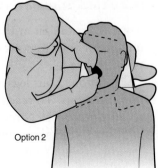

Option 2

RIGHT-HANDED CLINICIAN

10 to 11 o'clock Position (Near Corner of Headrest)

- **Torso Position.** Sit at the top right corner of the headrest; the midline of your torso is even with the temple region of the patient's head.
- **Leg Position.** Your legs should straddle the corner of the headrest.
- **Arm Positions.** To reach the patient's mouth, hold your right hand directly across the corner of the patient's mouth. Hold your left hand and wrist above the patient's nose and forehead.
- **Line of Vision.** Your line of vision is straight down into the mouth.

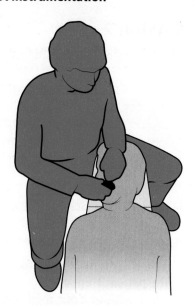

12 o'clock Position (Behind the Patient)

- **Torso Position.** Sit behind the patient's head.
- **Leg Position.** Your legs should straddle the headrest.
- **Arm Positions.** To reach the patient's mouth, hold your wrists and hands above the region of the patient's ears and cheeks.
- **Line of Vision.** Your line of vision is straight down into the patient's mouth.

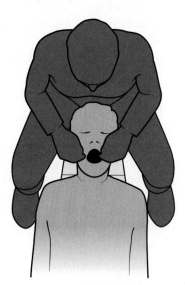

1 to 2 o'clock Position (Near Corner of Headrest)

- **Torso Position.** Sit at the top left corner of the headrest; the midline of your torso is even with the temple region of the patient's head.
- **Leg Position.** Your legs should straddle the corner of the headrest.
- **Arm Positions.** To reach the patient's mouth, hold your left hand directly across the corner of the patient's mouth. Hold your right hand and wrist above the patient's nose and forehead.
- **Line of Vision.** Your line of vision is straight down into the mouth.

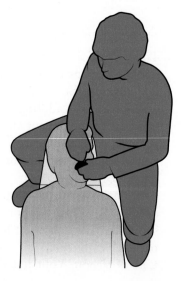

FLOW CHART: SEQUENCE FOR PRACTICING PATIENT/CLINICIAN POSITION

For successful periodontal instrumentation, it is important to proceed in a step-by-step manner. A useful saying to help you remember the step-by-step approach is *"Me, My Patient, My Light, My Non-dominant hand, My Dominant hand"* (Fig. 2-4).

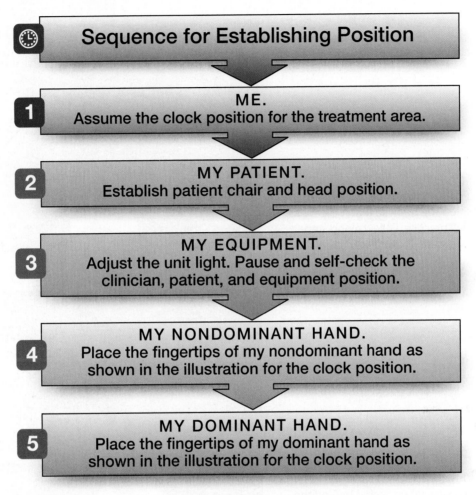

Sequence for Establishing Position

1 ME.
Assume the clock position for the treatment area.

2 MY PATIENT.
Establish patient chair and head position.

3 MY EQUIPMENT.
Adjust the unit light. Pause and self-check the clinician, patient, and equipment position.

4 MY NONDOMINANT HAND.
Place the fingertips of my nondominant hand as shown in the illustration for the clock position.

5 MY DOMINANT HAND.
Place the fingertips of my dominant hand as shown in the illustration for the clock position.

Figure 2-4. Sequence for Establishing Position.

RIGHT-HANDED CLINICIAN

USE OF TEXTBOOK DURING SKILL PRACTICE

The Skill Building sections of each module are designed to lead the reader step-by-step through each skill practice. It is important to position the textbook for ease of viewing throughout each skill practice (Figs. 2-5 and 2-6).

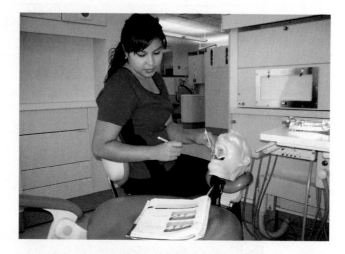

Figure 2-5. Position the Book for Ease of Viewing. Position the book so that it is easy to view during skill practice. Follow along step-by-step with the steps shown in the book.

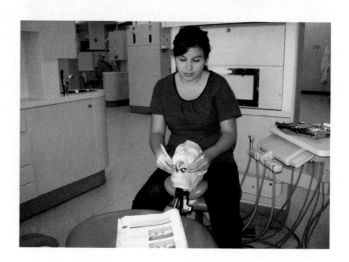

Figure 2-6. Book Position When Working Behind the Patient. Position the book so that it is easy to view when seated behind the patient.

RIGHT-HANDED CLINICIAN

QUICK START GUIDE TO THE ANTERIOR SEXTANTS

Directions: There is no need to waste time memorizing the clock position for each treatment area. The clock positions are easy to remember if you learn to recognize the positioning pattern for the anterior teeth (Figs. 2-7 and 2-8). *For periodontal instrumentation of the anterior teeth, each tooth is divided in half at the midline.*

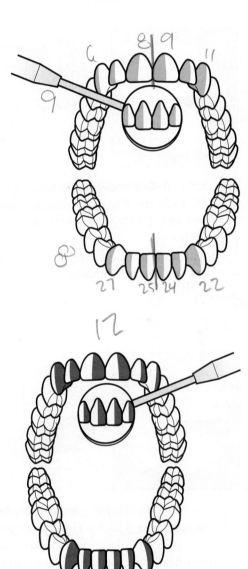

Figure 2-7. Anterior _Surfaces Toward_ the Right-Handed Clinician.

- The anterior tooth surfaces shaded in yellow on this drawing are called the anterior surfaces toward the clinician.
- The clock position for the anterior surfaces toward the clinician ranges from 8 to 9 o'clock.

Figure 2-8. Anterior _Surfaces Away_ from the Right-Handed Clinician.

- The anterior surfaces shaded in purple on this drawing are called the anterior surfaces away from the clinician.
- The clock position for anterior surfaces away from the clinician ranges from 11 to 1 o'clock.

RIGHT-HANDED CLINICIAN

SKILL BUILDING
Clock Positions for the Anterior Surfaces Toward

Directions: Practice the recommended clinician clock and patient head positions for the anterior "SURFACES TOWARD" by following the illustrations shown below in Figures 2-9 and 2-10.

RIGHT-HANDED CLINICIAN

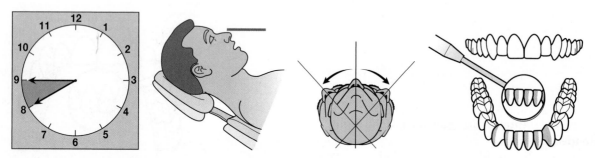

Figure 2-9. A–D: Mandibular Anterior Surfaces, TOWARD.
• Clinician in the 8 to 9 o'clock position.
• Patient chin DOWN; place the mandibular occlusal plane as parallel to the floor as possible.
• Patient head position ranges from neutral to turned to the right or left to facilitate vision of the tooth surfaces.

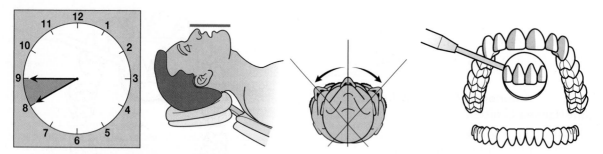

Figure 2-10. A–D: Maxillary Anterior Surfaces, TOWARD.
• Clinician in the 8 to 9 o'clock position.
• Patient chin UP; place the maxillary occlusal plane perpendicular to the floor.
• Patient head position ranges from neutral to turned to the right or left to facilitate vision of the tooth surfaces.

SKILL BUILDING
Clock Positions for the Anterior Surfaces Away

Directions: Practice the recommended clinician clock and patient head positions for the anterior "SURFACES AWAY" by following the illustrations shown below in Figures 2-11 and 2-12.

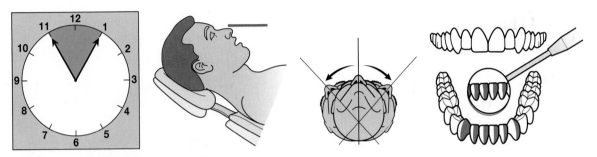

Figure 2-11. A–D: Mandibular Anterior Surfaces, AWAY.
- Clinician in the 11 to 1 o'clock position.
- Patient chin DOWN; place the mandibular occlusal plane as parallel to the floor as possible.
- Patient head position ranges from a neutral position to turning the head to the right or left to facilitate vision of the tooth surfaces.

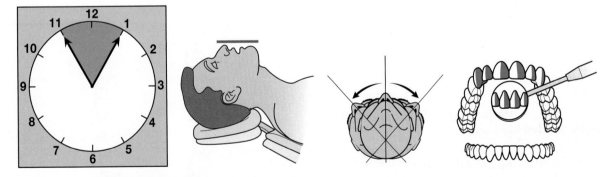

Figure 2-12. A–D: Maxillary Anterior Surfaces, AWAY.
- Clinician in the 11 to 1 o'clock position.
- Patient chin UP; place the maxillary occlusal plane perpendicular to the floor.
- Patient head position ranges a neutral position to turning the head to the right or left to facilitate vision of the tooth surfaces.

RIGHT-HANDED CLINICIAN

QUICK START GUIDE TO THE POSTERIOR SEXTANTS

Directions: There is no need to waste time memorizing the clock position for each posterior treatment area. The clock positions are easy to remember if you learn to recognize the positioning pattern for the posterior sextants (Figs. 2-13 and 2-14). *For periodontal instrumentation each posterior sextant is divided into two aspects: the (1) facial aspect and (2) lingual aspect of the sextant.*

Figure 2-13. Posterior _Aspects Facing Toward_ the Right-Handed Clinician.

- The posterior surfaces shaded in yellow on this drawing are called the posterior aspects facing toward the clinician.
- The clock position for posterior aspects toward the clinician is 9 o'clock.

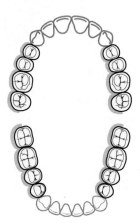

Figure 2-14. Posterior _Aspects Facing Away_ from the Right-Handed Clinician.

- The posterior surfaces shaded in blue on this drawing are called the posterior aspects facing away from the clinician.
- The clock position for posterior aspects away from the clinician ranges from 10 to 11 o'clock.

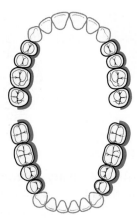

SKILL BUILDING
Clock Positions for the Posterior Sextants, Aspects Facing Toward the Clinician

Directions: Practice the recommended clinician clock and patient head positions for the posterior sextants "FACING TOWARD" the clinician by following the illustrations shown below in Figures 2-15 and 2-16.

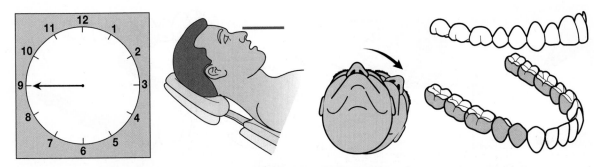

Figure 2-15. A–D: Mandibular Posterior Aspects Facing TOWARD.
- Clinician in the 9 o'clock position.
- Chin DOWN; place the mandibular occlusal plan as parallel to the floor as possible.
- Patient head position ranges from a neutral position to turning the head slightly away from the clinician.

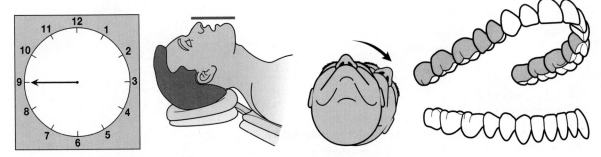

Figure 2-16. A–D: Maxillary Posterior Aspects Facing TOWARD.
- Clinician in the 9:00 o'clock position.
- Chin UP; place the maxillary occlusal plane perpendicular to the floor.
- Patient head position ranges from a neutral position to turning the head slightly away from the clinician.

RIGHT-HANDED CLINICIAN

SKILL BUILDING
Clock Positions for the Posterior Sextants, Aspects Facing Away From the Clinician

Directions: Practice the recommended clinician clock and patient head positions for the posterior sextants "FACING AWAY FROM" the clinician by following the illustrations shown below in Figures 2-17 and 2-18.

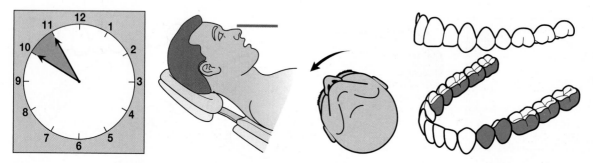

Figure 2-17. A–D: Mandibular Posterior Aspects Facing AWAY.
- Clinician seated in the 10 to 11 o'clock position.
- Chin DOWN; place the mandibular occlusal plan as parallel to the floor as possible.
- Patient head position is turned toward the clinician.

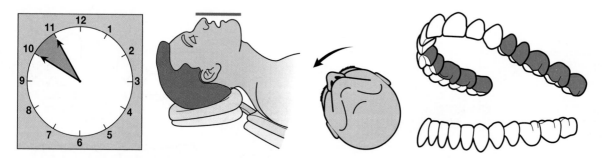

Figure 2-18. A–D: Maxillary Posterior Aspects Facing AWAY.
- Clinician seated in the 10 to 11 o'clock position.
- Chin UP; place the maxillary occlusal plane perpendicular to the floor.
- Patient head position is turned toward the clinician.

RIGHT-HANDED CLINICIAN

REFERENCE SHEET: POSITION FOR THE RIGHT-HANDED CLINICIAN

Table 2-1 summarizes the clock positions for the right-handed clinician. Photocopy this page and use it for quick reference as you practice your positioning skills. Place the photocopied reference sheet in a plastic page protector for longer use.

TABLE 2-1. CLOCK POSITIONS—POSITIONING SUMMARY

Treatment Area	Clock Position	Patient Head Position
Mandibular arch—Anterior surfaces toward	8–9	Chin-down; neutral to turned right or left
Maxillary arch—Anterior surfaces toward	8–9	Chin-up; neutral to turned right or left
Mandibular arch—Anterior surfaces away	11–1	Chin-down; neutral to turned right or left
Maxillary arch—Anterior surfaces away	11–1	Chin-up; neutral to turned right or left
Mandibular arch—Posterior aspects toward	9	Chin-down; neutral
Maxillary arch—Posterior aspects toward	9	Chin-up: neutral to turned slightly away
Mandibular arch—Posterior aspects away	10–11	Chin-down: toward
Maxillary arch—Posterior aspects away	10–11	Chin-up; toward

RIGHT-Handed Clinicians: This ends Section 2 for the RIGHT-Handed clinician. Please turn to Section 4. Working from a Standing Position.

Section 3
Positioning for the LEFT-Handed Clinician

SKILL BUILDING
Clock Positions for the LEFT-Handed Clinician

Directions: Practice each clock position by following the criteria outlined below.

3 to 4 o'clock Position (To the Front of the Patient)

- **Torso Position.** Sit facing the patient with your hip in line with the patient's upper arm.
- **Leg Position.** Your thighs should rest against the side of the patient chair.
- **Arm Positions.** To reach the patient's mouth, hold your arms slightly away from your sides. Hold your lower left arm over the patient's chest. The side of your right hand rests in the area of the patient's right cheekbone and upper lip. NOTE: Do not rest your arm on the patient's head or chest.
- **Line of Vision.** Your line of vision is straight ahead, into the patient's mouth.

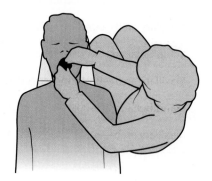

Ergonomic Considerations: Use of the 4 o'clock position should be limited since it is difficult to maintain neutral arm and torso posture in this clock position. The goal is to minimize postural abnormalities whenever possible.

3 o'clock Position (To the Side)

- **Torso Position.** Sit facing the side of the patient's head. The midline of your torso is even with the patient's mouth.
- **Leg Position.** Your legs may be in either of two acceptable positions: (1) straddling the patient chair or (2) underneath the *headrest* of the patient chair. Neutral position is best achieved by straddling the chair, however you should use the alternative position if you find straddling uncomfortable.
- **Arm Positions.** To reach the patient's mouth, hold the lower half of your left arm in approximate alignment with the patient's shoulder. Hold your right hand and wrist over the region of patient's left eye.
- **Hand Positions.** Rest your right hand in the area of the patient's left cheekbone. Rest the fingertips of your left hand on the premolar teeth of the mandibular left posterior sextant.
- **Line of Vision.** Your line of vision is straight down into the mouth.

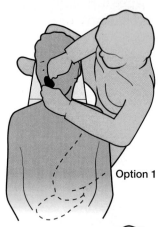

Option 1

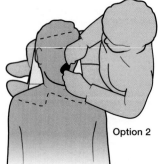

Option 2

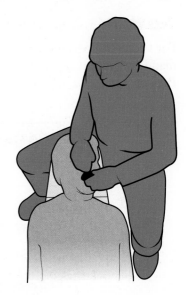

1 to 2 o'clock Position (Near Corner of Headrest)

- **Torso Position.** Sit at the top left corner of the headrest; the midline of your torso is even with the temple region of the patient's head.
- **Leg Position.** Your legs should straddle the corner of the headrest.
- **Arm Positions.** To reach the patient's mouth, hold your left hand directly across the corner of the patient's mouth. Hold your right hand and wrist above the patient's nose and forehead.
- **Line of Vision.** Your line of vision is straight down into the mouth.

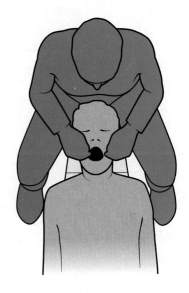

12 o'clock Position (Directly behind Patient)

- **Torso Position.** Sit directly behind the patient's head; you may sit anywhere from the left corner of the headrest to directly behind the headrest.
- **Leg Position.** Your legs should straddle the headrest.
- **Arm Positions.** To reach the patient's mouth, hold your wrists and hands above the region of the patient's ears and cheeks.
- **Line of Vision.** Your line of vision is straight down into the patient's mouth.

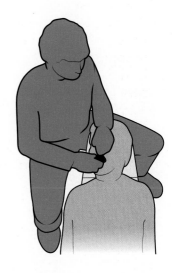

10 to 11 o'clock Position (Near Corner of Headrest)

- **Torso Position.** Sit at the top right corner of the headrest; the midline of your torso is even with the temple region of the patient's head.
- **Leg Position.** Your legs should straddle the corner of the headrest.
- **Arm Positions.** To reach the patient's mouth, hold your right hand directly across the corner of the patient's mouth. Hold your left hand and wrist above the patient's nose and forehead.
- **Line of Vision.** Your line of vision is straight down into the mouth.

LEFT-HANDED CLINICIAN

FLOW CHART: SEQUENCE FOR PRACTICING PATIENT/CLINICIAN POSITION

For successful periodontal instrumentation, it is important to proceed in a step-by-step manner. A useful saying to help you remember the step-by-step approach is *"Me, My Patient, My Light, My Non-dominant hand, My Dominant hand"* (Fig. 2-19).

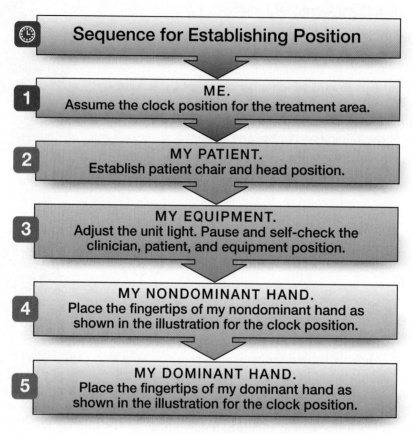

Figure 2-19. **Sequence for Establishing Position.**

LEFT-HANDED CLINICIAN

USE OF TEXTBOOK DURING SKILL PRACTICE

The Skill Building sections of each module are designed to lead the reader step-by-step through each skill practice. It is important to position the textbook for ease of viewing throughout each skill practice (Figs. 2-20 and 2-21).

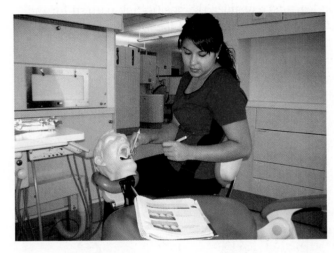

Figure 2-20. Position the Book for Ease of Viewing. Position the book so that it is easy to view during skill practice. Follow along step-by-step with the steps shown in the book.

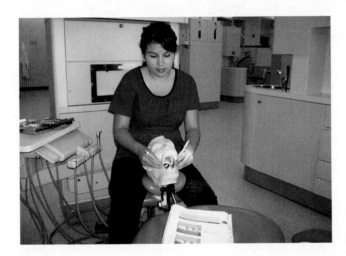

Figure 2-21. Book Position When Working Behind the Patient. Position the book so that it is easy to view when seated behind the patient.

LEFT-HANDED CLINICIAN

QUICK START GUIDE TO THE ANTERIOR SEXTANTS

Directions: There is no need to waste time memorizing the clock position for each treatment area. The clock positions are easy to remember if you learn to recognize the positioning pattern for the anterior teeth (Figs. 2-22 and 2-23). *For periodontal instrumentation of the anterior teeth, each tooth is divided in half at the midline.*

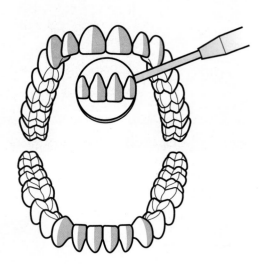

Figure 2-22. **Anterior _Surfaces Toward_ the Left-Handed Clinician.**

- The anterior tooth surfaces shaded in yellow on this drawing are called the anterior surfaces toward the clinician.
- The clock position for the anterior surfaces toward the clinician ranges from 3 to 4 o'clock.

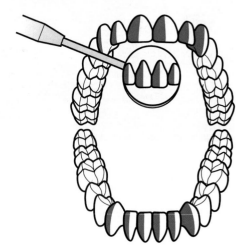

Figure 2-23. **Anterior _Surfaces Away_ from the Left-Handed Clinician.**

- The anterior surfaces shaded in purple on this drawing are called the anterior surfaces away from the clinician.
- The clock position for the anterior surfaces away from the clinician ranges from 11 to 1 o'clock.

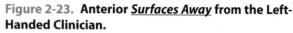

LEFT-HANDED CLINICIAN

SKILL BUILDING
Clock Positions for the Anterior Surfaces Toward

Directions: Practice the recommended clinician clock and patient head positions for the anterior "SURFACES TOWARD" by following the illustrations shown below in Figures 2-24 and 2-25.

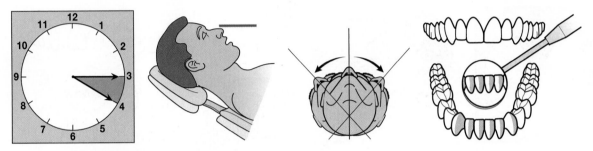

Figure 2-24. A–D: Mandibular Anterior Surfaces, TOWARD.
- Clinician seated in the 3 to 4 o'clock position.
- Patient chin DOWN; place the mandibular occlusal plane as parallel to the floor as possible.
- Patient head position ranges from neutral to turned to the right or left to facilitate vision of the tooth surfaces.

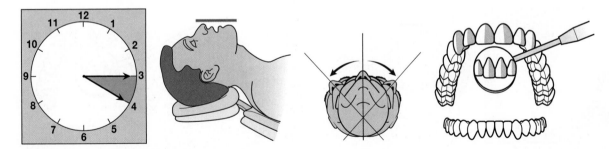

Figure 2-25. A–D: Maxillary Anterior Surfaces, TOWARD.
- Clinician in the 3 to 4 o'clock position.
- Patient chin UP; place the maxillary occlusal plane perpendicular to the floor.
- Patient head position ranges from neutral to turned to the right or left to facilitate vision of the tooth surfaces.

LEFT-HANDED CLINICIAN

SKILL BUILDING
Clock Positions for the Anterior Surfaces Away

Directions: Practice the recommended clinician clock and patient head positions for the anterior "SURFACES AWAY" by following the illustrations shown below in Figures 2-26 and 2-27.

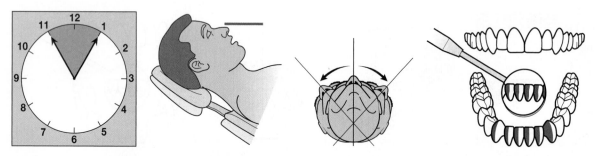

Figure 2-26. A–D: Mandibular Anterior Surfaces, AWAY.
- Clinician seated in the 11 to 1 o'clock position.
- Patient chin DOWN; place the mandibular occlusal plane as parallel to the floor as possible.
- Patient head position ranges from a neutral position to turning the head to the right or left to facilitate vision of the tooth surfaces.

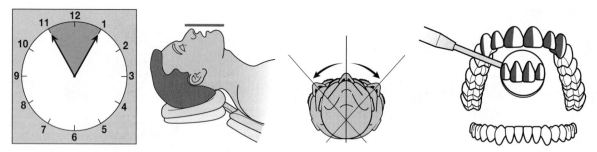

Figure 2-27. A–D: Maxillary Anterior Surfaces, AWAY.
- Clinician seated in the 11 to 1 o'clock position.
- Patient chin UP; place the maxillary occlusal plane perpendicular to the floor.
- Patient head position ranges from a neutral position to turning the head to the right or left to facilitate vision of the tooth surfaces.

LEFT-HANDED CLINICIAN

QUICK START GUIDE TO THE POSTERIOR SEXTANTS

Directions: There is no need to waste time memorizing the clock position for each posterior treatment area. The clock positions are easy to remember if you learn to recognize the positioning pattern for the posterior sextants (Figs. 2-28 and 2-29). *For periodontal instrumentation each posterior sextant is divided into two aspects: the (1) facial aspect and (2) lingual aspect of the sextant.*

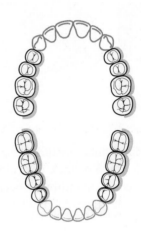

Figure 2-28. **Posterior _Aspects Facing Toward_ the Left-Handed Clinician.**

- The posterior surfaces shaded in yellow on this drawing are called the posterior aspects facing toward the clinician.
- The clock position for the posterior aspects toward the clinician is 3 o'clock.

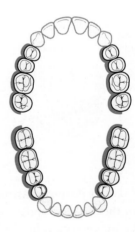

Figure 2-29. **Posterior _Aspects Facing Away_ from the Left-Handed Clinician.**

- The posterior surfaces shaded in blue on this drawing are called the posterior aspects facing away from the clinician.
- The clock position for posterior aspects away from the clinician ranges from 1 to 2 o'clock.

LEFT-HANDED CLINICIAN

Directions: Practice the recommended clinician clock and patient head positions for the posterior sextants "FACING TOWARD" the clinician by following the illustrations shown below in Figures 2-30 and 2-31.

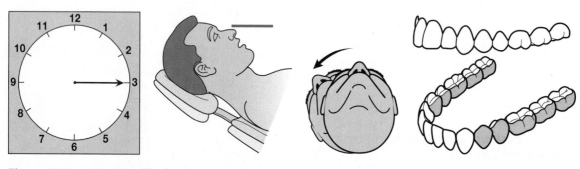

Figure 2-30. A–D: Mandibular Posterior Aspects Facing TOWARD.
- Clinician seated in the 3 o'clock position.
- Chin DOWN; place the mandibular occlusal plane as parallel to the floor as possible.
- Patient head position ranges from a neutral position to turning the head slightly away from the clinician.

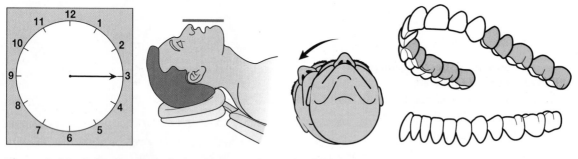

Figure 2-31. A–D: Maxillary Posterior Aspects Facing TOWARD.
- Clinician seated in the 3 o'clock position.
- Chin UP; place the maxillary occlusal plane perpendicular to the floor.
- Patient head position ranges from a neutral position to turning the head slightly away from the clinician.

LEFT-HANDED CLINICIAN

SKILL BUILDING
Clock Positions for the Posterior Sextants, Aspects Facing Away From the Clinician

Directions: Practice the recommended clinician clock and patient head positions for the posterior sextants "FACING AWAY FROM" the clinician by following the illustrations shown below in Figures 2-32 and 2-33.

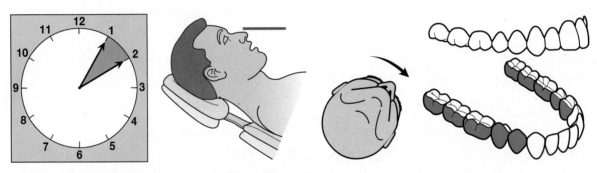

Figure 2-32. Mandibular Posterior Aspects Facing AWAY.
- Clinician seated in the 1 to 2 o'clock position.
- Chin DOWN; place the mandibular occlusal plane as parallel to the floor as possible.
- Patient head position is turned toward the clinician.

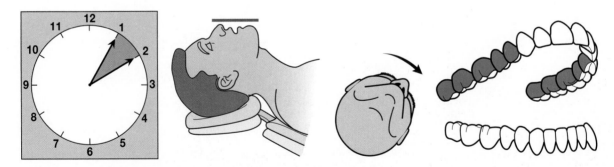

Figure 2-33. Maxillary Posterior Aspects Facing AWAY.
- Clinician seated in the 1 to 2 o'clock position.
- Chin UP; place the maxillary occlusal plane perpendicular to the floor.
- Patient head position is turned toward the clinician.

LEFT-HANDED CLINICIAN

REFERENCE SHEET: POSITION FOR THE LEFT-HANDED CLINICIAN

Table 2-2 summarizes the clock positions for the left-handed clinician. Photocopy this page and use it for quick reference as you practice your positioning skills. Place the photocopied reference sheet in a plastic page protector for longer use.

TABLE 2-2. CLOCK POSITIONS—POSITIONING SUMMARY

Treatment Area	Clock Position	Patient Head Position
Mandibular arch—Anterior surfaces toward	3–4	Chin-down; neutral to turned right or left
Maxillary arch—Anterior surfaces toward	3–4	Chin-up: neutral to turned right or left
Mandibular arch—Anterior surfaces away	11–1	Chin-down; neutral to turned right or left
Maxillary arch—Anterior surfaces away	11–1	Chin-up: neutral to turned right or left
Mandibular arch—Posterior aspects toward	3	Chin-down; neutral
Maxillary arch—Posterior aspects toward	3	Chin-up: neutral to turned slightly away
Mandibular arch—Posterior aspects away	1–2	Chin-down; toward
Maxillary arch—Posterior aspects away	1–2	Chin-up; toward

Section 4
Modified Positioning: Working from a Standing Position

At times, it may be helpful for the clinician to use a standing, rather than a seated position, for periodontal instrumentation. A standing position can be used when there is difficulty accessing the treatment area, when the patient cannot be placed in a supine position due to medical or physical contraindications, or when working on mandibular treatment areas (Figs. 2-34 and 2-35).

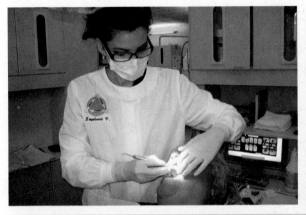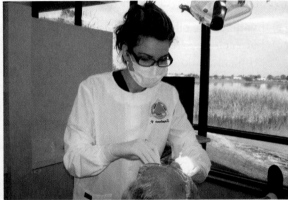

Figure 2-34. A–B: Correct Standing Clinician Position.
- A standing clinician position can be used to facilitate access to a treatment area or when a supine position is contraindicated for a patient due to medical or physical limitations.
- Notice that the clinician's shoulders are relaxed, the elbow of her dominant hand is a waist level, her torso is in neutral position, and she is not leaning over the patient.

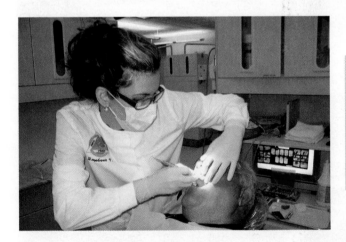

Figure 2-35. Incorrect Standing Clinician Position.
- This is an example of incorrect standing position.
- Note that the clinician's shoulders are hunched, her torso is tilted and twisted, and her elbows are raised.

Section 5
Skill Application

PRACTICAL FOCUS
Assessing Patient and Clinician Position

Evaluate the photographs shown in Figures 2-36 to 2-43:

(1) Evaluate the clinician, patient, and equipment position in each photograph.
(2) For each incorrect positioning element describe (a) what the problem is, (2) how the problem could be corrected, and (c) the musculoskeletal problems that could result from each positioning problem.

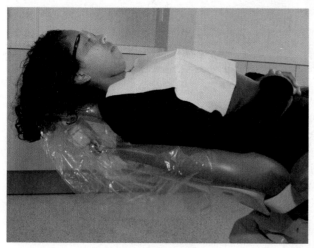

Figure 2-36. Photo 1

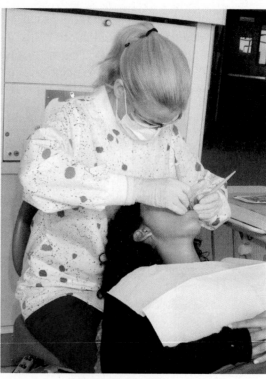

Figure 2-38. Photo 3

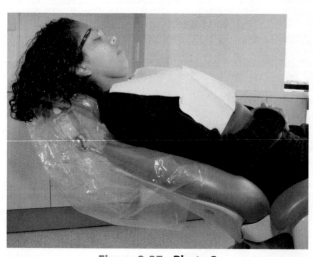

Figure 2-37. Photo 2

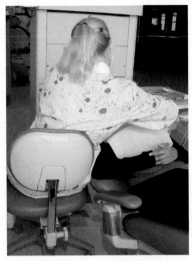

Figure 2-39. **Photo 4**

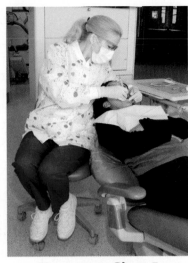

Figure 2-40. **Photo 5**

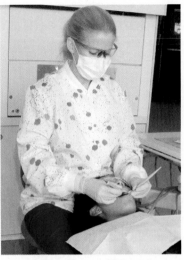

Figure 2-41. **Photo 6**

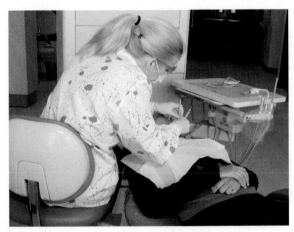

Figure 2-42. **Photo 7**

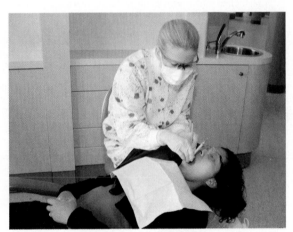

Figure 2-43. **Photo 8**

Student Self Evaluation Module 2: Positioning and Clock Positions

Student: _____

Date: _____

Area 1 = anterior sextant, facial aspect
Area 2 = anterior sextant, lingual aspect
Area 3 = right posterior sextant, facial aspect
Area 4 = right posterior sextant, lingual aspect
Area 5 = left posterior sextant, facial aspect
Area 6 = left posterior sextant, lingual aspect

DIRECTIONS: Self-evaluate your skill level in each treatment area as: **S** (satisfactory) or **U** (unsatisfactory).

Criteria: Mandibular Arch						
Positioning/Ergonomics	**Area 1**	**Area 2**	**Area 3**	**Area 4**	**Area 5**	**Area 6**
Adjusts clinician chair correctly						
Reclines patient chair and assures that patient's head is even with top of headrest						
Positions instrument tray within easy reach for front, side, or rear delivery as appropriate for operatory configuration						
Positions unit light at arm's length or dons dental headlight and adjusts it for use						
Assumes the recommended clock position						
Positions backrest of patient chair for the specified arch and adjusts height of patient chair so that clinician's elbows remain at waist level when accessing the specified treatment area						
Asks patient to assume the head position that facilitates the clinician's view of the specified treatment area						
Maintains neutral position						
Directs light to illuminate the specified treatment area						
Criteria: Maxillary Arch						
Positioning/Ergonomics	**Area 1**	**Area 2**	**Area 3**	**Area 4**	**Area 5**	**Area 6**
Adjusts clinician chair correctly						
Reclines patient chair and assures that patient's head is even with top of headrest						
Positions instrument tray within easy reach for front, side, or rear delivery as appropriate for operatory configuration						
Positions unit light at arm's length or dons dental headlight and adjusts it for use						
Assumes the recommended clock position						
Positions backrest of patient chair for the specified arch and adjusts height of patient chair so that clinician's elbows remain at waist level when accessing the specified treatment area						
Asks patient to assume the head position that facilitates the clinician's view of the specified treatment area						
Maintains neutral position						
Directs light to illuminate the specified treatment area						

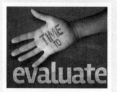

NOTE TO COURSE INSTRUCTORS: Module Evaluation forms—in both computerized and paper formats—are available online at: http://thepoint.lww.com/GehrigFundamentals8e

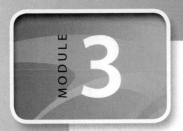
Instrument Grasp

Module Overview

Module 3 introduces the modified pen grasp for holding a periodontal instrument. The correct instrument grasp—called the modified pen grasp—allows precise control of the working-end of a periodontal instrument, permits a wide range of movement, and facilitates good tactile conduction (allows the clinician to feel rough areas on the tooth).

Module Outline

Section 1   **Grasp for Periodontal Instrumentation**   **71**
The Modified Pen Grasp
Parts of the Periodontal Instrument
Finger Identification for the Instrument Grasp
Skill-Building. Modified Pen Grasp: RIGHT-Handed Clinician, p. 73
Skill-Building. Modified Pen Grasp: LEFT-Handed Clinician, p. 74
Fine-Tuning Your Grasp

Section 2   **Grasp Variations**   **76**
Impact of Finger Length on the Grasp
Proper Glove Fit for Periodontal Instrumentation

Section 3   **Predisposing Conditions for Hand Injuries**   **78**
Joint Hypermobility in the Hand
Arthritis
Muscle Strength
Fingernail Length

Section 4   **Exercises for Improved Hand Strength**   **82**

Section 5   **Skill Application**   **86**
Practical Focus: Evaluation of Modified Pen Grasp and Glove Fit
Student Self Evaluation Module 3: Instrument Grasp

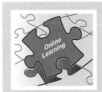

Online resources for this module: Instrument Grasp
Available at: http://thepoint.lww.com/GehrigFundamentals8e

Key Terms

Modified pen grasp
Handle

Shank
Working-end

Joint hypermobility

Learning Objectives

- Given a variety of periodontal instruments, identify the parts of each instrument.

- Identify the fingers of the hand as thumb, index, middle, ring, and little fingers.

- Understand the relationship among correct finger position in the modified pen grasp, the prevention of musculoskeletal problems, and the control of a periodontal instrument during instrumentation.

- Demonstrate the modified pen grasp using precise finger placement on the handle of a periodontal instrument:

  o Finger pads of thumb and index finger opposite one another on the handle

  o Thumb and index finger NOT overlapping each other on the handle

  o Pad of middle finger rests lightly on the shank

  o Pad of middle finger touches the ring finger

  o Thumb, index, and middle fingers in a neutral joint position

  o Ring finger is straight and supports weight of the hand

- Describe the function each finger serves in the modified pen grasp.

- Define joint hypermobility and describe how hyperextended joints in the modified pen grasp can affect periodontal instrumentation.

- Recognize incorrect finger position in the modified pen grasp and describe how to correct the problem(s).

- Select the correct glove size for your own hands and explain how the glove size selected meets the criteria for proper glove fit.

- Understand the relationship between proper glove fit and the prevention of musculoskeletal problems in the hands.

- Perform exercises for improved hand strength.

Section 1
Grasp for Periodontal Instrumentation

THE MODIFIED PEN GRASP

The modified pen grasp—as shown in Figure 3-1—is the recommended method for holding a periodontal instrument (1,2). The modified pen grasp facilitates precise control of the instrument as it moves over the tooth, allows the clinician to detect rough areas on the tooth surface, and lessens musculoskeletal stress to the clinician's fingers during periodontal instrumentation.

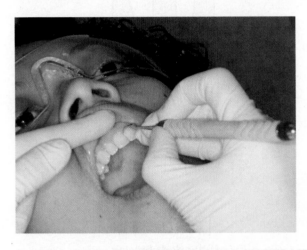

Figure 3-1. The Modified Pen Grasp. The right-handed clinician pictured here is using a modified pen grasp to hold a periodontal instrument.

PARTS OF THE PERIODONTAL INSTRUMENT

In order to master the modified pen grasp, the preclinical student must be able to identify the parts of a periodontal instrument (Fig. 3-2).

- Handle—the part of a periodontal instrument used for holding the instrument.
- Shank—a rod-shaped length of metal located between the handle and the working-end of a dental instrument. The shank generally is circular, smooth, and much smaller in diameter than the handle. The shank may be straight or it may be bent in one or more places.
- Working-End—the part of a dental instrument that does the work of the instrument. The working-end begins where the instrument shank ends. On a periodontal instrument the working-end may be shaped or flattened on some of its surfaces. The working-end could appear wire-like, look like a tiny ruler, or even be a small mirror. A single instrument may have one or two working-ends.

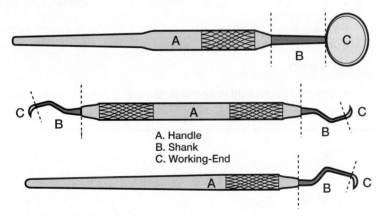

Figure 3-2. Parts of a Periodontal Instrument. The parts of a periodontal instrument are (**A**) the handle, (**B**) the shank, and (**C**) the working-end.

FINGER IDENTIFICATION FOR THE INSTRUMENT GRASP

The correct instrument grasp requires precise finger placement on the instrument (2–4). Figure 3-3 shows how the fingers of the hand are identified for purposes of the modified pen grasp. Table 3-1 outlines the placement and function of each finger in the instrument grasp.

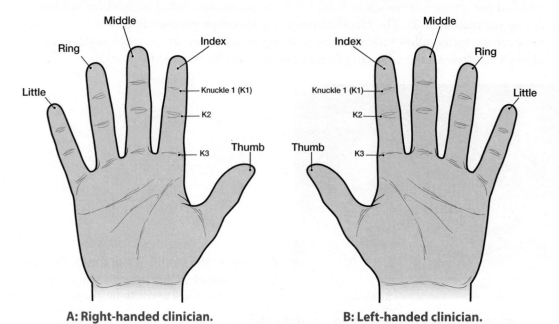

A: Right-handed clinician. **B: Left-handed clinician.**

Figure 3-3. Finger Identification and Placement in Modified Pen Grasp. A: Right-handed clinician. **B:** Left-handed clinician.

TABLE 3-1. FINGER PLACEMENT AND FUNCTION

Digit(s)	Placement	Function
Index and Thumb	• On the instrument handle	• Hold the instrument
Middle Finger	• Rests lightly against the shank	• Helps to guide the working-end • Feels vibrations transmitted from the working-end to the shank (5)
Ring Finger	• On oral structure; often a tooth surface • Advances ahead of the other fingers in the grasp	• Stabilizes and supports the hand for control and strength
Little Finger	• Near ring finger, held in a natural, relaxed manner	• Has no function in the grasp

SKILL BUILDING
Modified Pen Grasp: RIGHT-Handed Clinician

The correct grasp allows the clinician to achieve precise control of the working-end during instrumentation and reduce musculoskeletal stress to the hands and fingers (2–4,6).

Directions: Practice the modified pen grasp for the right-handed clinician by referring to the criteria labeled in Figure 3-4. Left-handed clinicians should refer to Figure 3-5.

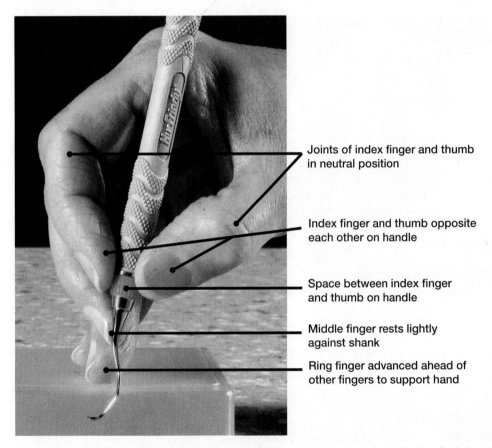

Joints of index finger and thumb in neutral position

Index finger and thumb opposite each other on handle

Space between index finger and thumb on handle

Middle finger rests lightly against shank

Ring finger advanced ahead of other fingers to support hand

Figure 3-4. Modified Pen Grasp for Right-Handed Clinician. A side view of a right-handed clinician holding a periodontal instrument in a modified pen grasp.

RIGHT-HANDED CLINICIAN

SKILL BUILDING
Modified Pen Grasp: LEFT-Handed Clinician

The correct grasp allows the clinician to achieve precise control of the working-end during instrumentation and reduce musculoskeletal stress to the hands and fingers (2–4,6).

Directions: Practice the modified pen grasp for the left-handed clinician by referring to the criteria labeled in Figure 3-5.

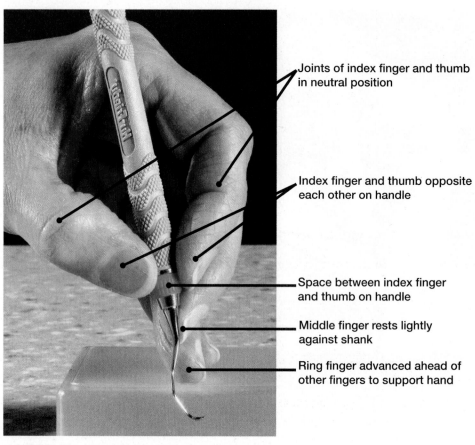

Joints of index finger and thumb in neutral position

Index finger and thumb opposite each other on handle

Space between index finger and thumb on handle

Middle finger rests lightly against shank

Ring finger advanced ahead of other fingers to support hand

Figure 3-5. Modified Pen Grasp for Left-Handed Clinician. A side view of a left-handed clinician holding a periodontal instrument in a modified pen grasp.

LEFT-HANDED CLINICIAN

FINE-TUNING YOUR GRASP

Precise finger placement in the modified pen grasp is critical to successful instrumentation (Table 3-2). Note the finger placement for a modified pen grasp differs from that used when writing.

TABLE 3-2. SUMMARY SHEET: CORRECT FINGER PLACEMENT

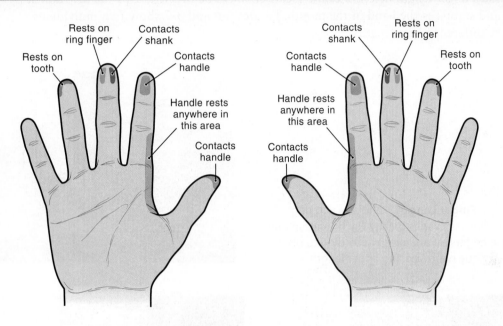

Digit	Recommended Position
Thumb and Index Finger	• The finger pads rest opposite each other at or near the junction of the handle and the shank (2). • The fingers do NOT overlap; there is a tiny space between them (2). • The fingers hold the handle in a relaxed manner. If your fingers are blanched, you are holding too tightly. • The instrument handle rests against the hand anywhere between the second and third knuckles.
Middle Finger	• One side of the finger pad rests lightly on the instrument shank. The other side of the finger pad rests against (or slightly overlaps) the ring finger. • Not used to hold the instrument. You should be able to lift your middle finger off of the shank without dropping the instrument. If you drop the instrument, then you are incorrectly using the middle finger to help hold the instrument.
Ring Finger	• Fingertip of the ring finger—not the pad—balances firmly on a tooth to support the weight of the hand and a periodontal instrument. • When grasping a dental mirror, the ring finger may rest on a tooth or against the patient's lip or cheek area. • The ring finger of the dominant hand advances ahead of the other fingers in the grasp. It is held upright and rigid to act as a strong support beam for the hand. The finger should not feel tense, but it should not be held limply against a tooth. Fingernail length must not impede the ability to keep the ring finger upright and rigid.
Little Finger	• The little finger is held in a relaxed manner close to the ring finger.

Section 2
Grasp Variations

IMPACT OF FINGER LENGTH ON THE GRASP

A clinician's finger length determines the location where he or she grasps the instrument handle and stabilizes the hand in the mouth. Figures 3-6 and 3-7 show two individuals with very different finger lengths.

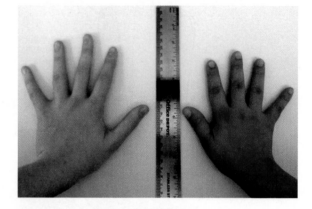

Figure 3-6. Finger Length. Hand size and finger length of clinicians varies greatly. Each clinician must adjust the finger rest and grasp according to his or her own unique hand size and finger length.

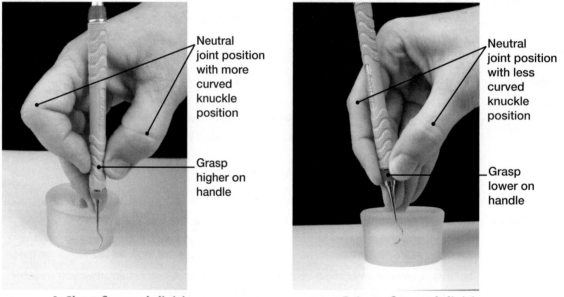

Neutral joint position with more curved knuckle position

Grasp higher on handle

Neutral joint position with less curved knuckle position

Grasp lower on handle

A: Short-fingered clinician.

B: Long-fingered clinician.

Figure 3-7. Variations in Modified Pen Grasp. The exact position of the fingers in the modified pen grasp will vary slightly among clinicians. A clinician with shorter fingers will tend to hold the knuckles of the index finger and thumb in a more curved—knuckles up—position and grasp the instrument higher on the handle. A clinician with longer fingers might hold the knuckles of the index finger and thumb in a less curved—knuckles flat—position and grasp the instrument nearer to the junction of the handle and the shank. **A:** Short-fingered clinician. **B:** Long-fingered clinician.

PROPER GLOVE FIT FOR PERIODONTAL INSTRUMENTATION

Proper glove fit is important in avoiding muscle strain during instrumentation. Gloves should be loose fitting across the palm and wrist areas of the hand (Fig. 3-8).

- Surgical glove-induced injury is a type of musculoskeletal disorder that is caused by improperly fitting gloves. Symptoms include numbness, tingling or pain in the wrist, hand, and/or fingers. This disorder is caused by wearing gloves that are too tight or by wearing ambidextrous gloves (Fig. 3-9).
- It is best to wear right- and left-fitted gloves rather than ambidextrous gloves that are designed to fit either hand. Ambidextrous gloves do not fit as well as fitted gloves, causing them to exert greater force on the hands. Tight ambidextrous gloves can produce significant and debilitating hand pain (7). Over time, this force could contribute to vascular constriction, nerve compression, muscle fatigue, and hand pain (7–9).
- Tactile sensitivity—touch perception—is enhanced when wearing thin gloves with a good fit in the fingertip area (10). Thin gloves may improve dexterity when performing tasks that require fine motor control, such as periodontal instrumentation.
- Nitrile gloves provide more grip friction than latex gloves when grasping periodontal instruments in the wet environment of the oral cavity (11). Gloves are available with texture on the fingertip area of the glove; texturing may help increase friction in the pinch grip.

Select a glove size that is loose fitting across the palm of the hand and wrist. Try gloves from several manufacturers to find the brand that fits best. Clinicians with long fingers need to find a brand that accommodates their finger length. Conversely, clinicians with shorter fingers should find a brand of gloves with fingers that do not hang over the fingertips.

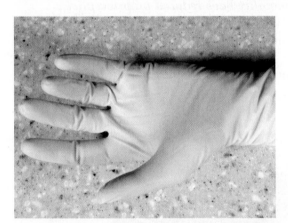

Figure 3-8. Correct Glove Fit. Gloves should be loose fitting across the palm and wrist areas of the hand. The index finger of your opposite hand should slip easily under the wrist area of the gloved hand.

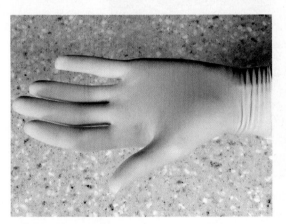

Figure 3-9. Incorrect Glove Fit. Gloves that are tight fitting across the palm and/or wrist area of your hand can cause muscle strain during periodontal instrumentation.

Section 3
Predisposing Conditions for Hand Injuries

Physical conditions can be predisposing factors to hand pain and injury during periodontal instrumentation.

JOINT HYPERMOBILITY IN THE HAND

1. Joint Hypermobility
   a. Many people have flexible or loose joints. Their joints move farther and more easily than most people's joints. The medical term for joints that move too far is joint hypermobility or joint laxity. Figure 3-10 shows an individual with joint hypermobility.
   b. The term *double-jointed* often is used to describe hypermobility, however the name is a misnomer as the individual with hypermobility does not actually have two separate joints where others have just one (12).
   c. Experts estimate that 4% to 13% of normal children have hypermobile joints or joints that can move beyond the normal range of motion (13,14).
2. Hypermobility and Proprioception
   a. If everything is working properly, an individual can close his eyes and easily touch his nose. This act is possible because he can sense his body, as well as its position and movement through space. This ability is called **proprioception.**
      1. Proprioception includes the sense of position and movement of our limbs and trunk, the sense of effort, the sense of force, and the sense of heaviness.
      2. Proprioception works because of sensory receptors within muscles and joints.
   b. *Studies show that individuals with joint hypermobility have reduced proprioceptive sensitivity in the joints of the hands* (15,16).
      1. Decreased proprioceptive sensitivity may require greater power—tighter gripping—to hold something that is small or narrow.
      2. Muscles of the hand frequently are stressed in an attempt to compensate for joint instability (17,18).

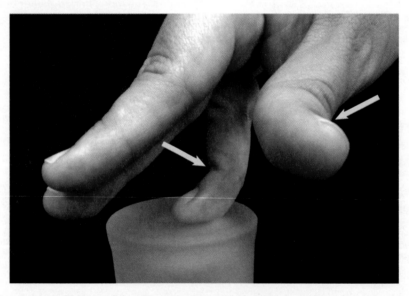

Figure 3-10. Joint Hypermobility of the Fingers. The individual pictured here has joint hypermobility allowing her to bend her fingers beyond the normal range of movement.

3. **Periodontal Instrumentation and Hypermobility.** Clinicians may not know they have joint hypermobility as this condition usually is not disfiguring (19). It is important for the dental hygienist to recognize joint hypermobility because this condition may cause problems during periodontal instrumentation:

   a. Increased flexibility in the finger joints make the hands less stable and the muscles have to work a lot harder when using the hands to grip and manipulate objects (18).

   b. *An individual with hypermobility must learn to grasp an instrument without having the joint of the thumb or index finger hyperextend with the joint "collapsed inward".*

      1. Since proprioceptive sensitivity may be reduced, the individual should take care not to grip the instrument handle with too much force.

      2. Retraining of the clinician's grasp may be helpful. *The use of a Lycra or silicon sleeve, such as a Silipos sleeve, can assist with proprioceptive retraining while grasping the instrument handle* (Fig. 3-11A–D) (20).

   c. In addition, performing periodontal instrumentation with the joints in a hyperextended position may cause injury to a hypermobile joint by overstretching it (21).

4. **Interventions**

   1. An orthopedic hand specialist should evaluate a clinician who experiences pain or weakness due to joint hypermobility. Physical therapy, as well as joint stabilizing devices that can be worn under surgical gloves, may be helpful (22). Brandfonbrener (23) comments that the use of ring splints helps to prevent joint hyperextension and to retrain proprioceptivity (perception) of finger position.

   2. Depending upon the extent of joint hypermobility and the number of fingers involved, a clinician may need to modify the finger placement in the grasp.

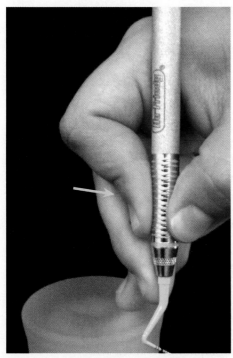

Figure 3-11. A: Joint Hypermobility in Grasp. Note how this clinician's index finger is hyperextended in the grasp. This hyperextension places stress on the joint.

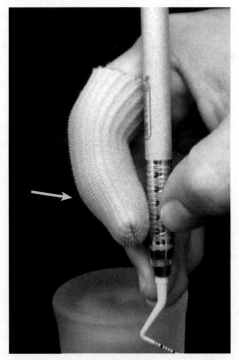

Figure 3-11. B: Grasp with Silicone Sleeve. The same clinician as pictured in **A** grasps an instrument while wearing a silicone sleeve.

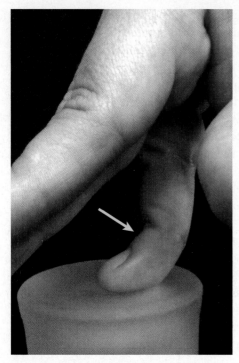

Figure 3-11. C: Joint Hyperextension of Ring Finger. When the clinician pictured here attempts to establish a finger rest with her ring finger, the joint hyperextends resulting in stress on the joint.

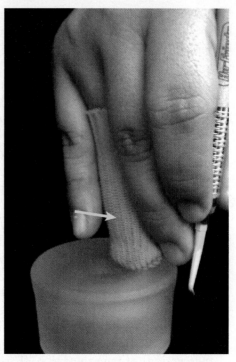

Figure 3-11. D: Finger Rest with Silicone Sleeve. The silicone sleeve is helpful to the clinician in training the joint of her ring finger. The silicone sleeve may be worn under surgical gloves during instrumentation.

ARTHRITIS

A condition less commonly seen in dental hygiene students is arthritis of the hands.

- Arthritis may cause the hygienist to reduce work hours or leave the profession. An orthopedic hand specialist or a rheumatologist can diagnose the type and severity of arthritis and recommend treatment and physical therapy.
- Employing ergonomic principles during periodontal instrumentation—especially those relating to grasp, grip force, and relaxation of grip force between strokes—can make a difference in whether the hygienist with arthritis can practice dental hygiene (19).

MUSCLE STRENGTH

Although anyone can have weak hands, hand weakness is most common in female clinicians with petite hands (24). The research literature indicates that hand size and optimal grip is correlated in women, but not in men, with small hand size (25).

- Orthopedic hand specialists assess muscle strength with a hand-held dynamometry device (24). Figure 3-12 shows an example of one type of dynamometer.
- Weak hand strength in a female clinician may contribute to pain associated with periodontal instrumentation.
- Hand strengthening exercises are beneficial for all clinicians but essential for those with poor hand strength (26,27).

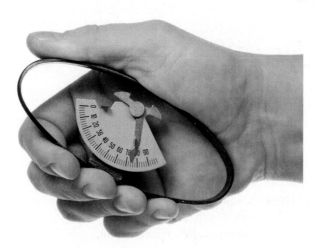

Figure 3-12. Dynamometer. A dynamometer is a device used to measure hand strength.

FINGERNAIL LENGTH

The research literature shows that long fingernails reduce hand strength and pinch force while performing psychomotor tasks.

- A study by Jansen et al. (28) tested the impact of fingernails not extending past the fingertips and with fingernails extending 2, 1, and 0.5 cm beyond the tip of the finger.
  - Analyses show that fingernails extending *any length beyond the fingertips* result in a decreased pinch grip strength.
  - Fingernails 1 or 2 cm in length result in decreased ability to manipulate the fingers and limited flexion of the finger joints, particularly the metacarpophalangeal joints.
- Longer fingernails also interfere with the clinician's ability to stabilize the dominant hand in the patient's mouth. Figure 3-13 depicts how long fingernails interfere with correct grasp and finger rest technique. Stabilization of the hand for periodontal instrumentation with a finger rest is discussed in Modules 5, 6, and 7.
- In addition to the ergonomic problems that long fingernails present, longer nails may pinch the soft tissues in the patient's oral cavity causing patient discomfort.

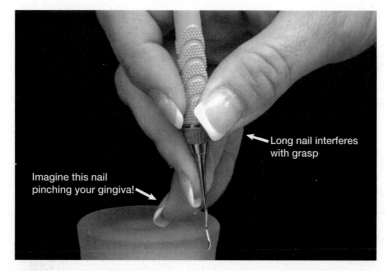

Figure 3-13. Long Fingernails and the Instrument Grasp. Fingernails that extend beyond the fingertips result in (1) reduced pinch grip strength, (2) decreased ability to manipulate the fingers, (3) decreased ability to stabilize the hand for periodontal instrumentation, and (4) patient discomfort during instrumentation.

Section 4
Exercises for Improved Hand Strength

Well-conditioned hand muscles have improved control and endurance, allow for freer wrist movement, and reduce the likelihood of injury. Skilled finger movement training improves the ability to control finger-force, hand steadiness, and multi-finger coordination (26,27). The hand exercises shown here will help to develop and maintain muscle strength for periodontal instrumentation.

Directions: These exercises use Power Putty, a silicone rubber material that resists both squeezing and stretching forces. For each exercise illustrated, squeeze or stretch the Power Putty for the suggested number of repetitions. The exercise set, for both hands doing all nine exercises, should take no more than 10 to 20 minutes. When exercising, maintain your hands at waist level.

> **CAUTION:** Not all exercise programs are suitable for everyone; discontinue any exercise that causes you discomfort and consult a medical expert. If you have or suspect that you may have a musculoskeletal injury, joint hypermobility, or arthritis, do not attempt these exercises without the permission of a physician. Any user assumes the risk of injury resulting from performing the exercises. The creators and authors disclaim any liabilities in connection with the exercises and advice herein.

1. **Full Grip (flexor muscles).** Squeeze putty with your fingers against the palm of your hand. Roll it over and around in your hand and repeat as rapidly and with as much strength as possible. Suggested Repetitions: 10

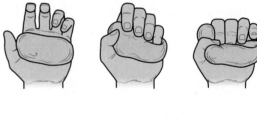

2. **All Finger Spread (extensor and abductor muscles).** Form putty into a thick pancake shape and place on a tabletop. Bunch fingertips together and place in putty. Spread fingers out as fast as possible. Suggested Repetitions: 3

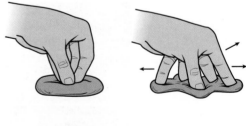

3. Fingers Dig (flexor muscles). Place putty in the palm of your hand and dig fingertips deep into the putty. Release the fingers, roll putty over and repeat. Suggested Repetitions: 10

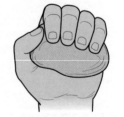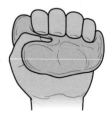

4. **Finger Extension (extensor muscles).** Close one finger into palm of hand. Wrap putty over tip of finger and hold loose ends with the other hand. As quickly as possible, extend finger to a fully opened position. Regulate difficulty by increasing or decreasing thickness of putty wrapped over the fingertip. Repeat with each finger. Suggested Repetitions: 3

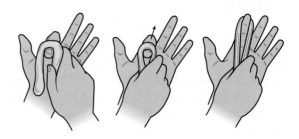

5. **Thumb Press (flexor muscles).** Form putty into a barrel shape and place in the palm of your hand. Press your thumb into the putty with as much force as you can. Reform putty and repeat. Suggested Repetitions: 5

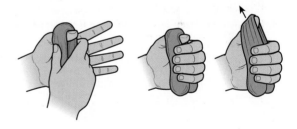

6. **Thumb Extension (extensor muscles).** Bend your thumb toward the palm of the hand; wrap putty over the thumb tip. Hold the loose ends down and extend the thumb open as quickly as possible. Regulate difficulty by increasing or decreasing the thickness of putty wrapped over tip of thumb. Suggested Repetitions: 3

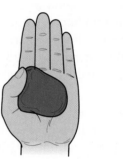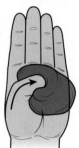

7. **Fingers Only (flexor muscles).** Lay putty across fingers and squeeze with fingertips only. Keep the palm of your hand flat and open. Rotate putty with thumb and repeat. Suggested Repetitions: 10

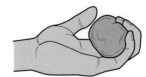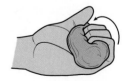

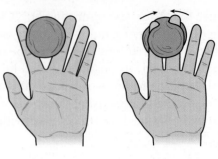

8. **Finger Scissors (adductor muscles).** Form putty into the shape of a ball and place between any two fingers. Squeeze fingers together in scissors-like motion. Repeat with each pair of fingers. Suggested Repetitions: 3

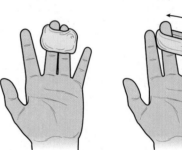

9. **Finger Splits (abductor muscles).** Mold putty around any two fingers while they are closed together. Spread fingers apart as quickly as possible. Repeat exercise with each pair of fingers. Suggested Repetitions: 3

Power Putty can be purchased in sport stores or directly from *SportsHealth*, 527 West Windsor Road, Glendale, California 91204 USA, 818-240-7170; http://www.powerputty.com

References

1. Canakci V, Orbak R, Tezel A, Canakci CF. Influence of different periodontal curette grips on the outcome of mechanical non-surgical therapy. *Int Dent J.* 2003;53(3):153–158.
2. Gentilucci M, Caselli L, Secchi C. Finger control in the tripod grasp. *Exp Brain Res.* 2003;149(3):351–360.
3. Baur B, Furholzer W, Jasper I, Marquardt C, Hermsdorfer J. Effects of modified pen grip and handwriting training on writer's cramp. *Arch Phys Med Rehabil.* 2009;90(5):867–875.
4. Scaramucci M. Getting a grasp. *Dimen Dent Hyg.* 2008;5(6):24–26.
5. Rucker LM, Gibson G, McGregor C. Getting the "feel" of it: the non-visual component of dimensional accuracy during operative tooth preparation. *J Can Dent Assoc.* 1990;56(10):937–941.
6. Chin DH, Jones NF. Repetitive motion hand disorders. *J Calif Dent Assoc.* 2002;30(2):149–160.
7. Christensen GJ. Operating gloves. The good and the bad. *J Am Dent Assoc.* 2001;132(10):1455–1457.
8. Hamann C, Werner RA, Franzblau A, Rodgers PA, Siew C, Gruninger S. Prevalence of carpal tunnel syndrome and median mononeuropathy among dentists. *J Am Dent Assoc.* 2001;132(2):163–170; quiz 223–224.

9. Powell BJ, Winkley GP, Brown JO, Etersque S. Evaluating the fit of ambidextrous and fitted gloves: implications for hand discomfort. *J Am Dent Assoc*. 1994;125(9):1235–1242.
10. Kopka A, Crawford JM, Broome IJ. Anaesthetists should wear gloves–touch sensitivity is improved with a new type of thin glove. *Acta Anaesthesiol Scand*. 2005;49(4):459–462.
11. Laroche C, Barr A, Dong H, Rempel D. Effect of dental tool surface texture and material on static friction with a wet gloved fingertip. *J Biomech*. 2007;40(3):697–701.
12. Pacey V, Tofts L, Wesley A, Collins F, Singh-Grewal D. Joint hypermobility syndrome: a review for clinicians. *J Paediatr Child Health*. 2015;51(4):373–380.
13. Biro F, Gewanter HL, Baum J. The hyper-mobility syndrome. *Pediatrics*. 1983;72(5):701–706.
14. Seckin U, Tur BS, Yilmaz O, Yagci I, Bodur H, Arasil T. The prevalence of joint hyper-mobility among high school students. *Rheumatol Int*. 2005;25(4):260–263.
15. Mullick G, Bhakuni DS, Shanmuganandan K, et al. Clinical profile of benign joint hyper-mobility syndrome from a tertiary care military hospital in India. *Int J Rheum Dis*. 2013;16(5):590–594.
16. Smith TO, Jerman E, Easton V, et al. Do people with benign joint hyper-mobility syndrome (BJHS) have reduced joint proprioception? A systematic review and meta-analysis. *Rheumatol Int*. 2013;33(11):2709–2716.
17. Brandfonbrener AG. The epidemiology and prevention of hand and wrist injuries in performing artists. *Hand Clin*. 1990;6(3):365–377.
18. Warrington J. Hand therapy for the musician: instrument-focused rehabilitation. *Hand Clin*. 2003;19(2):287–301, vii.
19. Leiseca CB. How not to overwork your hands. *RDH*. 2014;34(5):64–69.
20. Hakim A, Keer R, Grahame R. Hyper-mobility, fibromyalgia and chronic pain. Edinburgh; New York: Churchill Livingstone/Elsevier; 2010. xxi, 310.
21. Simpson MR. Benign joint hyper-mobility syndrome: evaluation, diagnosis, and management. *J Am Osteopath Assoc*. 2006;106(9):531–536.
22. Smith TO, Bacon H, Jerman E, et al. Physiotherapy and occupational therapy interventions for people with benign joint hyper-mobility syndrome: a systematic review of clinical trials. *Disabil Rehabil*. 2014;36(10):797–803.
23. Brandfonbrener AG. Musculoskeletal problems of instrumental musicians. *Hand Clin*. 2003;19(2):231–239, v–vi.
24. Stark T, Walker B, Phillips JK, Fejer R, Beck R. Hand-held dynamometry correlation with the gold standard isokinetic dynamometry: a systematic review. *PM R*. 2011;3(5):472–479.
25. Ruiz-Ruiz J, Mesa JL, Gutierrez A, Castillo MJ. Hand size influences optimal grip span in women but not in men. *J Hand Surg Am*. 2002;27(5):897–901.
26. Ranganathan VK, Siemionow V, Sahgal V, Liu JZ, Yue GH. Skilled finger movement exercise improves hand function. *J Gerontol A Biol Sci Med Sci*. 2001;56(8):M518–M522.
27. Shim JK, Hsu J, Karol S, Hurley BF. Strength training increases training-specific multifinger coordination in humans. *Motor Control*. 2008;12(4):311–329.
28. Jansen CW, Patterson R, Viegas SF. Effects of fingernail length on finger and hand performance. *J Hand Ther*. 2000;13(3):211–217.

Section 5
Skill Application

PRACTICAL FOCUS
Evaluation of Modified Pen Grasp and Glove Fit

Directions, Part 1: Evaluate the modified pen grasps pictured in Figures 3-14 to 3-22. Indicate if each grasp is correct or incorrect. For each incorrect grasp element describe (1) what is incorrect about the finger placement and (2) what problems might result from the incorrect finger placement.

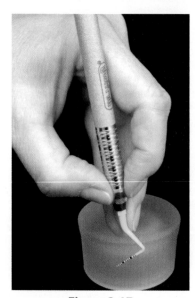

Figure 3-14

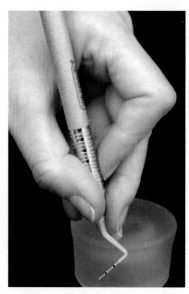

Figure 3-15

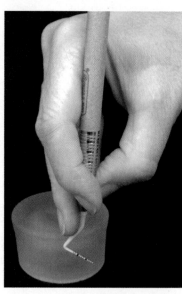

Figure 3-16

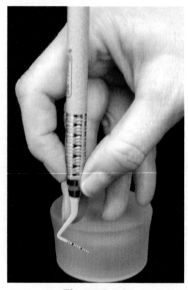

Figure 3-17

Figure 3-18

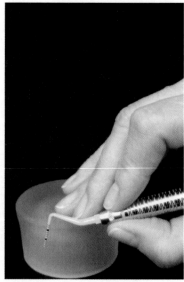

Figure 3-19

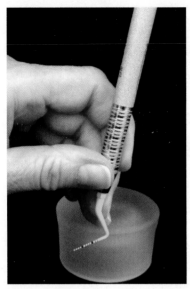

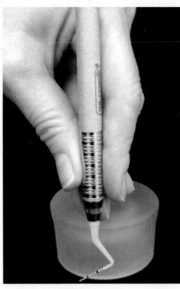

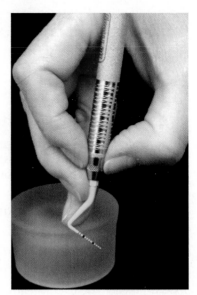

| Figure 3-20 | Figure 3-21 | Figure 3-22 |

Directions, Part 2: Examine the gloved hands pictured in Figure 3-23. Evaluate the glove fit for the right and left hands pictured below.

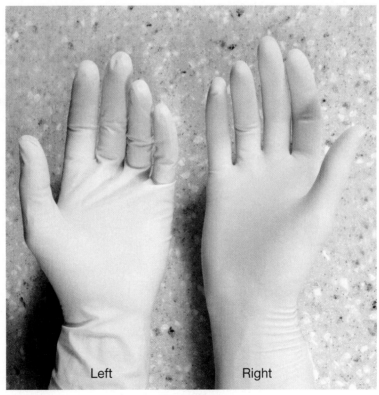

Figure 3-23

Student Self Evaluation Module 3: Instrument Grasp

Student: _____

Date: _____

1 = Grasp with mirror hand
2 = Grasp with instrument hand

DIRECTIONS: Self-evaluate your skill level as: **S** (satisfactory) or **U** (unsatisfactory)

Instrument Grasp: Dominant Hand	1	2
Identifies handle, shank, and working-end(s) of a mirror and periodontal instruments		
Describes the function each finger serves in the grasp		
Describes criteria for proper glove fit		
Grasps handle with tips of finger pads of index finger and thumb so that these fingers are opposite each other on the handle, but do NOT touch or overlap		
Rests pad of middle finger lightly on instrument shank; middle finger makes contact with ring finger		
Positions the thumb, index, and middle fingers in the neutral joint position; hyperextended joint position is avoided		
Holds ring finger straight so that it supports the weight of hand and instrument; ring finger position is "advanced ahead of" the other fingers in the grasp		
Keeps index, middle, ring and little fingers in contact; "like fingers inside a mitten"		
Maintains a relaxed grasp; fingers are NOT blanched in grasp		

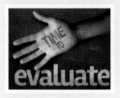

NOTE TO COURSE INSTRUCTORS: To download Module Evaluations for this textbook, go to http://thepoint.lww.com/GehrigFundamentals8e and log on to access the Instructor Resources for *Fundamentals of Periodontal Instrumentation and Advanced Root Instrumentation*.

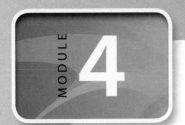

MODULE

4

Use of the Dental Mouth Mirror

Module Overview

This module describes techniques for using a dental mirror during periodontal instrumentation. Proper use of a dental mirror significantly increases the clinician's ability to maintain a neutral working posture. Content in this module includes the topics of (1) stabilization of the mirror in the patient's mouth, (2) functions of the mirror during periodontal instrumentation, (3) significance of indirect vision for neutral posture, and (4) transillumination of the anterior teeth.

A step-by-step technique practice for using a mirror in the anterior and posterior sextants is found in Sections 3 and 4.

Module Outline

Section 1 **Fundamentals of Mirror Use** **91**
Types of Dental Mirrors
Stabilization of the Dental Mirror for Use in the Mouth
Functions of the Dental Mirror
Skill Building. Transillumination of the Anterior Teeth, p. 94

Section 2 **Is Achieving Direct Vision Really Best?** **96**
The Dangerous Myth of Direct Vision
Mastery of Indirect Vision in the Preclinical Setting is Key

Section 3 **Technique Practice: RIGHT-Handed Clinician** **98**
Skill Building. Using the Mirror for Retraction, p. 98
Skill Building. Mirror Use: Maxillary Teeth, p. 99
Skill Building. Mirror Use: Mandibular Teeth, p. 101

Section 4 **Technique Practice: LEFT-Handed Clinician** **103**
Skill Building. Using the Mirror for Retraction, p. 103
Skill Building. Mirror Use: Maxillary Teeth, p. 104
Skill Building. Mirror Use: Mandibular Teeth, p. 106

Section 5 **Skill Application** **109**
Student Self Evaluation Module 4: Mirror Use

Key Terms

Extraoral fulcrum   Indirect vision   Indirect illumination
Intraoral fulcrum   Retraction   Transillumination

Learning Objectives

- Name and describe three common types of dental mirrors.

- Demonstrate the use of a mirror for indirect vision, retraction, indirect illumination, and transillumination.

- Maintain neutral seated posture while using the recommended clock position for each of the mandibular and maxillary treatment areas.

- While seated in the correct clock position with the patient's head correctly positioned, demonstrate optimum INDIRECT vision in each sextant of the mouth while maintaining neutral positioning.

RIGHT- AND LEFT-HANDED SECTIONS IN THIS MODULE

- Sections 3 and 4 of this module are customized for right-handed and left-handed clinicians.

- Having two different versions of the content in the Module sometimes can be annoying or confusing. For example, a left-handed clinician finds it time consuming to bypass all the right-handed pages to get to the left-handed version. Sometimes readers turn to the wrong version and become confused.

- For ease of use—and avoidance of confusion—if you are right-handed, it is recommended that you either (1) tear the left-handed pages from the book or (2) staple these pages together. If you are left-handed, use the same approach with the right-handed pages.

Section 1
Fundamentals of Mirror Use

TYPES OF DENTAL MIRRORS

A dental mirror is used to view tooth surfaces that cannot be seen using direct vision (Fig. 4-1). In Figure 4-1, a clinician uses the mirror to view the lingual surfaces of the maxillary anterior teeth. There are three common types of dental mirrors; the characteristics of each type of dental mirror are listed in Table 4-1.

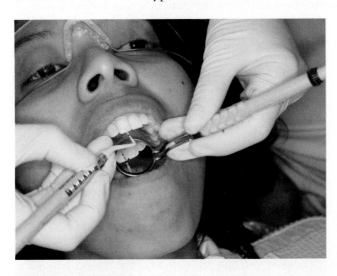

Figure 4-1. Dental Mirror or Mouth Mirror. The clinician pictured here uses the reflecting mirrored surface of a dental mirror to view the lingual surfaces of the maxillary anterior teeth. Note that the instrument's yellow working-end can be seen in the mirror.

TABLE 4-1. TYPES OF MIRROR SURFACES

Type	Characteristics
Front Surface	• Reflecting surface is on the front surface of the glass • Produces a clear mirror image with no distortion • Most commonly used type because of good image quality • Reflecting surface of mirror is easily scratched
Concave	• Reflecting surface is on the front surface of the mirror lens • Produces a magnified image (image is enlarged) • Magnification distorts the image
Plane (Flat Surface)	• Reflecting surface is on the back surface of the mirror lens • Produces a double image (ghost image) • Double image may be distracting

• In all cases, the mirror head is positioned with the reflecting surface exposed, so the clinician can easily use the mirror for indirect vision at any time during periodontal instrumentation.

• NEVER position the mirror head with the reflecting surface against the buccal mucosa or tongue (hiding the reflecting surface from view).

STABILIZATION OF THE DENTAL MIRROR FOR USE IN THE MOUTH

A Fulcrum provides stabilization of the clinician's hand during periodontal instrumentation.

- *During periodontal instrumentation, the clinician grasps a dental mirror in his or her nondominant hand.* Thus, a right-handed clinician holds the mirror with the left hand whereas a left-handed clinician uses the right hand to grasp the mirror.
- The ring and index fingers of the clinician's nondominant hand are used to stabilize the mirror in the mouth. The clinician may rest his or her fingers on the patient's chin or cheek or on a tooth surface to stabilize the mirror.
  - A stabilization point outside the patient's mouth—usually on the patient's chin or cheek—is termed an extraoral fulcrum.
  - An intraoral fulcrum is a stabilizing point for the hand on a tooth surface. An intraoral fulcrum is optional with a dental mirror, but recommended for use when using a periodontal instrument. Intraoral fulcrums are discussed in detail in upcoming chapters.
- Figure 4-2 depicts a right-handed clinician stabilizing the left-hand on the patient's cheek.

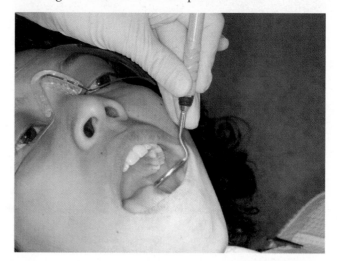

Figure 4-2. Extraoral Finger Rest. This right-handed clinician is seated in the 12:00 position. His ring finger rests on the patient's cheek to stabilize the mirror. An extraoral finger rest is used most commonly to stabilize the mouth mirror in the oral cavity.

FUNCTIONS OF THE DENTAL MIRROR

The dental mirror is used in four ways during periodontal instrumentation: (1) indirect vision, (2) retraction, (3) indirect illumination, and (4) transillumination. Figures 4-3 to 4-10 depict the functions of the mirror.

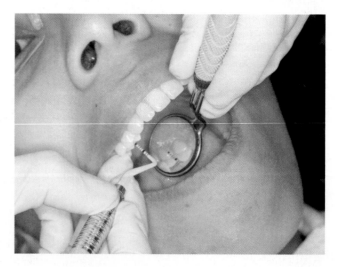

Figure 4-3. Indirect Vision. Indirect vision is the use of a dental mirror to view a tooth surface or intraoral structure that cannot be seen directly.

- The clinician pictured here uses the mirror to indirectly view the lingual surfaces of the maxillary right first premolar.
- Note that the working-end of the dental instrument is visible in the mirror's reflecting surface.

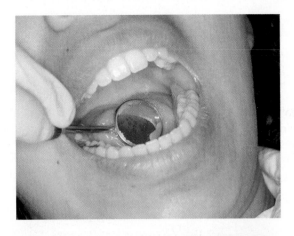

Figure 4-4. Retraction of Tongue. Retraction is the use of the mirror head to hold the patient's cheek, lip, or tongue so that the clinician can view tooth surfaces that are otherwise hidden from view by these soft tissue structures.

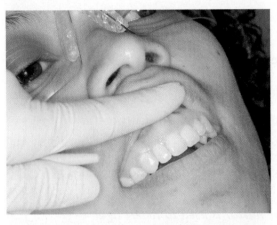

Figure 4-5. Retraction of the Lip. The index finger of the nondominant hand usually is used to retract the lip away from a facial aspect of anterior teeth. The patient will be more comfortable if a finger rather than the mirror is used for retraction of the lip.
- **Tip:** the mirror may be held in the palm of the hand when retracting with the finger. Palming the mirror avoids having to put down the mirror and pick it up again when moving on to another sextant.

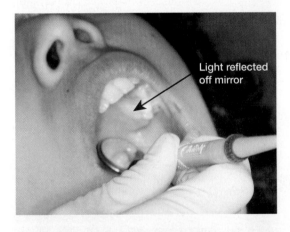

Light reflected off mirror

Figure 4-6. Indirect Illumination. Indirect illumination is the use of the mirror surface to reflect light onto a tooth surface in a dark area of the mouth.

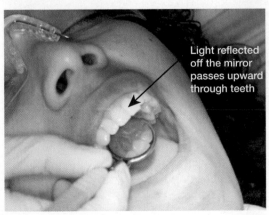

Light reflected off the mirror passes upward through teeth

Figure 4-7. Transillumination. Transillumination is the technique of directing light off of the mirror surface and through the anterior teeth. [*Trans* = through + *Illumination* = lighting up]. **A:** As light is reflected off the mirror surface, the light beams pass back through the teeth.

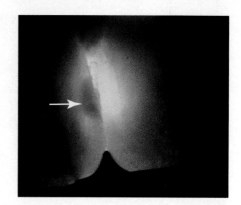

Figure 4-7. B: A light source directed through the proximal surfaces of this central and lateral incisor reveals a change in translucency just above the contact area, indicating the presence of class III caries.
● Follow the directions below to practice transillumination of the anterior teeth.

SKILL BUILDING
Transillumination of the Anterior Teeth

Directions: Practice the technique for transillumination by following the instructions in Figures 4-8 to 4-10.

The technique of transillumination reveals carious lesions (decay) as dark regions within the enamel of an interproximal surface of an anterior tooth.

● When employing the transillumination technique, *the mirror is used to reflect light through the anterior teeth.*
● Transillumination is effective only with anterior teeth because these teeth are thin enough to allow light to pass through.
● *A carious lesion or an anterior restoration of an anterior tooth appears as a shadow when an anterior tooth is transilluminated.*

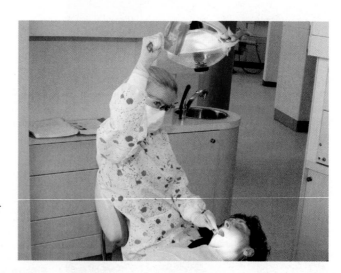

Figure 4-8. Light Position. Position the unit light directly over the oral cavity so that the *light beam is perpendicular to the facial surfaces* of the anterior teeth. The patient should be in a chin-down position.

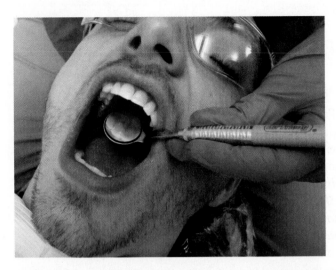

Figure 4-9. Position Mouth Mirror. *Position yourself in the 12:00.* Hold the mirror behind the central incisors so that the reflecting surface is parallel to the lingual surfaces. Figure 4-10 shows how the teeth should appear if you are using a correct technique.

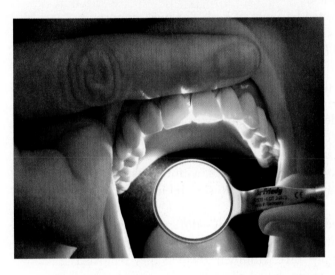

Figure 4-10. View Transilluminated Anterior Teeth. If you have correctly positioned the light and the mirror, the anterior teeth will appear to "glow." Note, during transillumination you are looking *directly at the teeth, NOT at the mirror's reflecting surface.*

Remember to Adjust the Patient's Head Position. When practicing the use of a dental mirror, remember to ask your patient to position his or her head straight, toward or away from you, as appropriate for the sextant that you are viewing with the mirror.

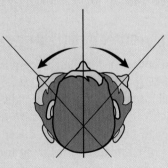

Section 2
Is Achieving Direct Vision Really Best?

THE DANGEROUS MYTH OF DIRECT VISION

1. **Visual Dominance as an Ergonomic Risk.** For the great majority of dental hygiene students and clinicians, the visual sense is the most dominant sense—the sense that they rely on more than any other. Being a visual learner is a great asset in many instances, but it can present problems during periodontal instrumentation.
   A. **The Visual Sense is Not Your Friend.** *Strangely one of the most important things that a dental hygienist should learn is that the sense of TOUCH is his or her greatest asset during periodontal instrumentation while the VISUAL sense is the greatest hinderance to effective instrumentation.* The belief that "nothing is better than direct vision" causes the clincian to assume awkward postures placing strain on the muscles of the head, neck, and back.
   B. **Most Calculus Deposits Should be Detected by Sense of Feel.** The most important aspect of periodontal instrumentation is removal of plaque biofilm and calculus deposits from the root surfaces *located beneath the gingival margin within periodontal pockets.*
      1. A refined ability to detect subgingival calculus through sensory perception—touch—is the efficient and expert manner for calculus removal.
      2. Clinicians who do NOT develop a delicate, refined ability to feel calculus must forever be condemned to remove calculus "by default." In other words, the clinician simply makes many, many strokes with the instrument's cutting edge until he or she removes the calculus. Unnecessary strokes, with the instrument, place stress on the clinician's hands and lead to musculoskeletal injury of the muscles and joints of the hand.
      3. Clinicians who have the ability to feel a calculus deposit—differentiating the deposit from the root surface—are able to make many fewer strokes with the instrument. Skilled clinicians only apply force with their grasp as they remove a calculus deposit. During calculus detection, skilled clinicians relax their hold on the instrumentation handle providing a rest period for the muscles and joints of their hand.
2. **Determination to Use Direct Vision as an Ergonomic Risk.** Achieving direct vision—not looking into the mirror—causes unnatural postures that result in muscle contractions. Static postures of the trapezius muscle have been noted as a specific problem in relation to neck and shoulder injury (1,2).

MASTERY OF INDIRECT VISION IN THE PRECLINICAL SETTING IS KEY

1. **Mastery of Indirect Vision is the Key.** If the clinician is unable to visualize the treatment area directly while maintaining a neutral posture, he or she must use indirect vision to prevent awkward body positioning, specially of the neck and back (3).
   A. Dental professionals who routinely use a mouth mirror for indirect vision have been shown to have fewer headaches and reduced neck/shoulder discomfort (4).
   B. Although most studies of training and utilizing indirect vision were conducted in the 1980s, the skill of indirect vision has not changed over the years (5,6).

2. **Learn Mirror Use First on the Maxillary Arch**
    A. *Boyd et al. found that when mirror use is taught first on the mandibular arch, student clinicians often "cheat" and use direct vision (and thus do not master indirect vision). These same student clinicians—who "cheated" on the mandibular arch—then continue to depend on direct vision as they move to the maxillary arch. Cheating by using direct vision results in early acquisition of poor postural habits* (5).
    B. With poor indirect vision skills, the student clinician's attention is so concentrated on being able to position the periodontal instrument on the tooth that he or she is unaware of awkard body position.
    C. Students who master indirect vision on the maxillary arch first build confidence in the use of indirect vision and are more likely to use neutral body posture. Mastery of indirect vision allows the clinician to work in neutral position for all treatment areas of the mouth (Box 4-1).

Box 4-1   **Mastery of Indirect Vision is a MUST**

- The mouth mirror is the most important, yet underutilized instrument within dental practice. Proper use of a mirror for indirect vision significantly increases the clinician's ability to maintain a neutral working posture (3).
- Students who master indirect vision on the maxillary arch first build confidence and are more likely to use neutral body posture (5).

Online video clip for this module: Introduction to Mirror Use
Available at: http://thepoint.lww.com/GehrigFundamentals8e

Section 3
Technique Practice: RIGHT-Handed Clinician

SKILL BUILDING
Using the Mirror for Retraction

Directions: Practice mirror use by referring to Figures 4-11 to 4-24 on the following pages.

Retracting the buccal mucosa away from the facial surfaces of the posterior teeth can be a challenging task, especially if your patient tenses his or her cheek muscles. It is a good idea to practice the retraction technique before attempting the posterior finger rests.

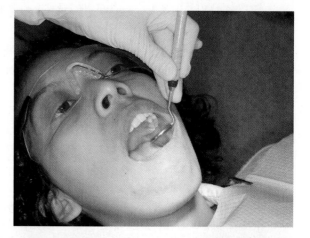

Figure 4-11. Step 1.
1. Assume a 10 to 11 o'clock position for the facial aspect of the mandibular left posteriors.
2. Grasp the mirror in your nondominant hand.
3. Place the mirror head between the dental arches with the reflecting surface parallel to the maxillary occlusal surfaces ("Frisbee-style").
4. Slide the mirror back until it is in line with the second molar.

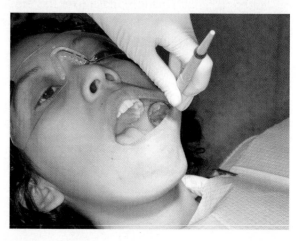

Figure 4-12. Step 2.
5. Position the mirror by turning the mirror handle until the mirror head is parallel to the buccal mucosa. The back of the mirror head rests against the buccal mucosa and the mirror's reflecting surface is facing the facial surfaces of the teeth.
6. Establish an extraoral finger rest on the side of the patient's cheek.
7. Use your arm muscles for retraction. Pulling with only your finger muscles is a difficult and tiring way to retract the check.

- Avoid hitting the mirror head against the patient's teeth or resting the outer rim of the mirror head against the patient's gingival tissues.

- Do not use the instrument shank for retraction. Retracting in this manner will be uncomfortable for your patient.

SKILL BUILDING
Mirror Use: Maxillary Teeth

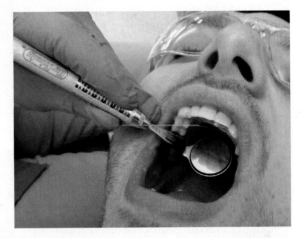

Figure 4-13. Maxillary Anteriors, Lingual Aspect: Surfaces Toward

- Sit in an 8 to 9 o'clock position.
- Grasp the mirror in your left hand and rest your ring and little fingers on the patient's right cheek or premolar teeth.
- Adjust the position of the mirror head to view the lingual surfaces in the mirrored surface.
- Swivel the mirror head so that the surfaces toward you are easily seen in the reflecting surface of the mirror.

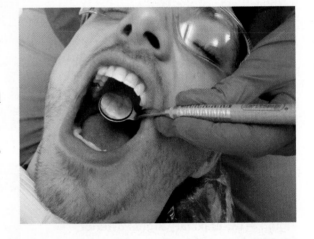

Figure 4-14. Maxillary Anteriors, Lingual Aspect: Surfaces Away

- Sit in the 11 to 1 o'clock position.
- Rest the ring and little fingers of your left hand either on the patient's left cheek or on the incisal edges of the maxillary anterior teeth.
- Note that the mirror head is NOT held near to the maxillary anteriors, rather it is positioned closer to the tongue.
- Swivel the mirror head so that the surfaces away from you are easily seen.

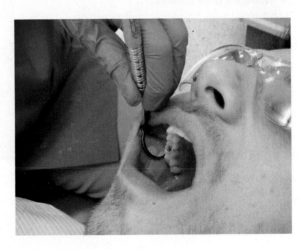

Figure 4-15. Maxillary Right Posterior Sextant, Facial Aspect

- Sit in a 9 o'clock position.
- Slide the mirror head between the dental arches and rest the ring and little fingers on right side of the patient's face. Retract the buccal mucosa with the mirror.
- Use the mirror for indirect vision, particularly to view the distal surfaces of the teeth. Swivel the mirror head, until you can easily view the distal surfaces in the reflecting surface.

Figure 4-16. Maxillary Left Posterior Sextant, Lingual Aspect
- Sit in a 9 o'clock position.
- Rest the ring and little fingers on the right side of the patient's face, near the corner of the mouth.
- Position the mirror head away from the teeth, closer to the tongue.
- Use the mirror for indirect vision, particularly to view the distal surfaces of the teeth. Swivel the mirror head, until you can easily view the distal surfaces in the reflecting surface.

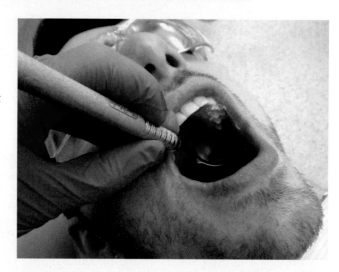

Figure 4-17. Maxillary Right Posterior Sextant, Facial Aspect
- Sit in the 10 to 11 o'clock position.
- Slide the mirror head between the dental arches; rest the ring and little fingers on the left side of the face.
- Use the mirror to retract the buccal mucosa away from the teeth.
- Swivel the mirror head until you can easily view the distal surfaces in the mirror. Swivel the mirror head until you can view the facial and mesial surfaces in the reflecting surface.

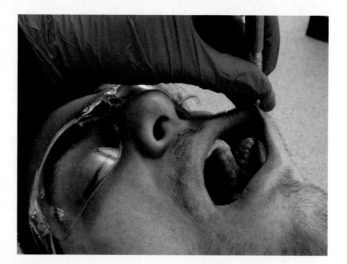

Figure 4-18. Maxillary Right Posterior Sextant, Lingual Aspect
- Sit in the 10 to 11 o'clock position.
- Rest the ring and little fingers on the left side of the patient's face, near the corner of the mouth.
- Position the mirror head near the tongue.
- Swivel the mirror head to view the distal surfaces in the mirror.
- Swivel the mirror head to view the lingual and mesial surfaces.

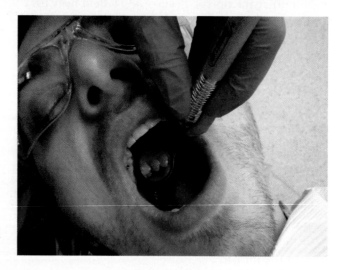

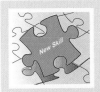

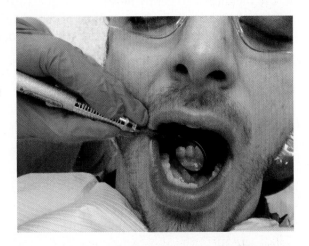

Figure 4-19. Mandibular Anteriors, Lingual Aspect: Surfaces Toward
- Sit in an 8 to 9 o'clock position.
- Rest your ring and little fingers on the right side of the patient's face near the corner of the mouth or on the premolar teeth.
- Use the mirror head to push the tongue back gently so that the lingual surfaces of the teeth can be seen in the mirror.

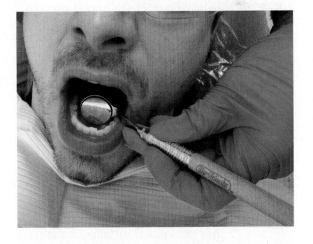

Figure 4-20. Mandibular Anteriors, Lingual Aspect: Surfaces Away
- Sit in the 11 to 1 o'clock position.
- Rest your ring and little fingers on the left side of the patient's face near the corner of the mouth or on the premolar teeth.
- Use the mirror head to push the tongue back gently so that the lingual surfaces of the teeth can be seen in the mirror.

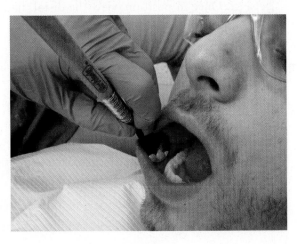

Figure 4-21. Mandibular Right Posterior Sextant, Facial Aspect
- Sit in the 9 o'clock position.
- Rest your fingers on the right side of the patient's face.
- Retract the buccal mucosa with the mirror. Use the mirror for indirect vision, particularly to view the distal surfaces of the teeth.

RIGHT-HANDED CLINICIAN

Figure 4-22. Mandibular Left Posterior Sextant, Lingual Aspect
- Sit in the 9 o'clock position.
- Rest your fingers on the right side of the patient's face.
- Use the mirror to gently move the tongue away from the teeth, toward the midline of the mouth. Use indirect vision to view the distal and lingual surfaces.
- Tip: Avoid pressing down against the floor of the mouth with the mirror head.

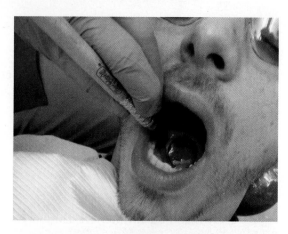

Figure 4-23. Mandibular Left Posterior Sextant, Facial Aspect
- Sit in the 10 to 11 o'clock position.
- Rest your fingers on the left side of the patient's face.
- Use the mirror to retract the buccal mucosa down and away from the teeth.
- View the distal, facial, and mesial surfaces in the mirror's reflecting surface.

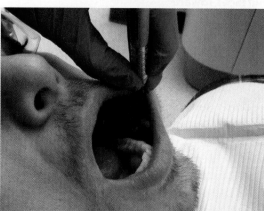

Figure 4-24. Mandibular Right Posterior Sextant, Lingual Aspect
- Sit in the 10 to 11 o'clock position.
- Rest your fingers on the left side of the patient's face.
- Use the mirror head to push the tongue back gently so that the lingual surfaces of the teeth can be seen. Once in position, view the distal, lingual, and mesial surfaces in the mirror's reflecting surface.

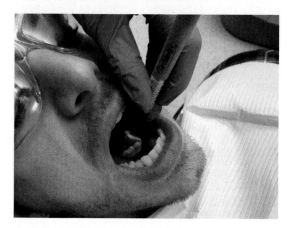

Box 4-2   **Techniques to Stop Fogging of Reflecting Surface**

Use one of the following techniques to stop fogging of the reflecting surface:
- Warm the reflecting surface against the patient's buccal mucosa.
- Ask patient to breathe through the nose.
- Wipe the reflecting surface with a commercial defogging solution.
- Wipe the reflecting surface with a gauze square moistened with mouthwash.

Section 4
Technique Practice: LEFT-Handed Clinician

SKILL BUILDING
Using the Mirror for Retraction

Directions: Practice mirror use by referring to Figures 4-25 to 4-38 on the following pages.

Retracting the buccal mucosa away from the facial surfaces of the posterior teeth can be a challenging task, especially if your patient tenses his or her cheek muscles. It is a good idea to practice the retraction technique before attempting the posterior finger rests.

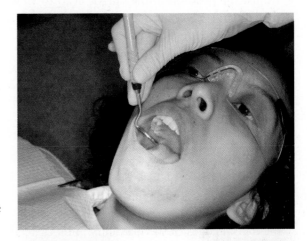

Figure 4-25. Step 1.
1. Assume a 1 to 2 o'clock position for the facial aspect of the mandibular right posteriors.
2. Grasp the mirror in your nondominant hand.
3. Place the mirror head between the dental arches with the reflecting surface parallel to the maxillary occlusal surfaces ("Frisbee-style").
4. Slide the mirror back until it is in line with the second molar.

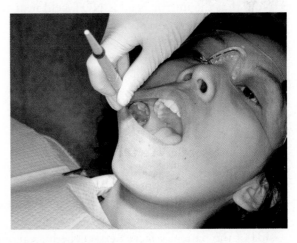

Figure 4-26. Step 2.
5. Position the mirror by turning the mirror handle until the mirror head is parallel to the buccal mucosa. The back of the mirror head is against the buccal mucosa and the mirror's reflecting surface is facing the facial surfaces of the teeth.
6. Establish an extraoral finger rest on the side of the patient's cheek.
7. Use your arm muscles for retraction. Pulling with only your finger muscles is a difficult and tiring way to retract the check.

- Avoid hitting the mirror head against the patient's teeth or resting the outer rim of the mirror head against the patient's gingival tissues.

- Do not use the instrument shank for retraction. Retracting in this manner will be uncomfortable for your patient.

SKILL BUILDING
Mirror Use: Maxillary Teeth

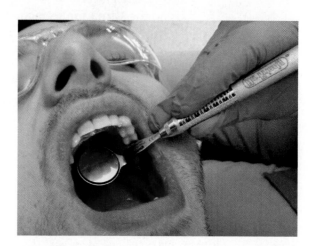

Figure 4-27. Maxillary Anteriors, Lingual Aspect: Surfaces Toward
- Sit in a 3 to 4 o'clock position.
- Grasp the mirror in your right hand and rest your ring and little fingers on the patient's left cheek or premolar teeth.
- Adjust the position of the mirror head to view the lingual surfaces in the mirrored surface.
- Swivel the mirror head so that the surfaces toward you are easily seen in the reflecting surface of the mirror.

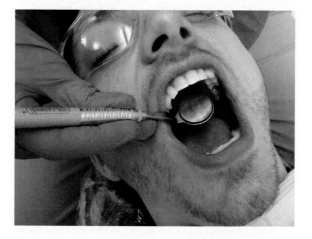

Figure 4-28. Maxillary Anteriors, Lingual Aspect: Surfaces Away
- Sit in the 11 to 1 o'clock position.
- Rest the ring and little fingers of your right hand either on the patient's right cheek or on the incisal edges of the maxillary anterior teeth.
- Note that the mirror head is NOT held near to the maxillary anteriors, rather it is positioned closer to the tongue.
- Swivel the mirror head so that the surfaces away from you are easily seen.

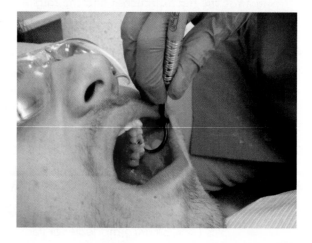

Figure 4-29. Maxillary Left Posterior Sextant, Facial Aspect
- Sit in the 3 o'clock position.
- Side the mirror head between the dental arches and rest the ring and little fingers on the left side of the patient's face. Retract the buccal mucosa with the mirror.
- Use the mirror for indirect vision, particularly to view the distal surfaces of the teeth. Swivel the mirror head, until you can easily view the distal surfaces in the reflecting surface.

Figure 4-30. Maxillary Right Posterior Sextant, Lingual Aspect

- Sit in the 3 o'clock position.
- Rest the ring and little fingers on the left side of the patient's mouth, near the corner of the mouth.
- Position the mirror head away from the teeth, closer to the tongue.
- Use the mirror for indirect vision, particularly to view the distal surfaces of the teeth. Swivel the mirror head until you can easily view the distal surfaces in the reflecting surface.

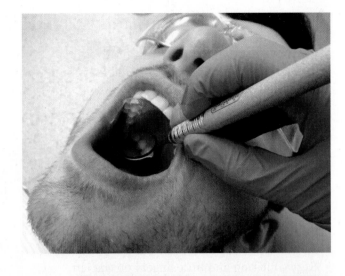

Figure 4-31. Maxillary Right Posterior Sextant, Facial Aspect

- Sit in the 1 to 2 o'clock position.
- Slide the mirror head between the dental arches; rest the ring and little fingers on the right side of the face.
- Use the mirror to retract the buccal mucosa away from the teeth.
- Swivel the mirror head until you can easily view the distal surfaces in the mirror. Swivel the mirror head until you can view the facial and mesial surfaces in the reflecting surface.

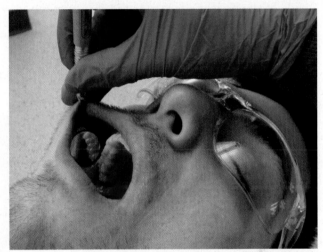

Figure 4-32. Maxillary Left Posterior Sextant, Lingual Aspect

- Sit in the 1 to 2 o'clock position.
- Rest the ring and little fingers on the right side of the patient's face, near the corner of the mouth.
- Position the mirror head near the tongue.
- Swivel the mirror head to view the distal surfaces in the mirror.
- Swivel the mirror head to view the lingual and mesial surfaces.

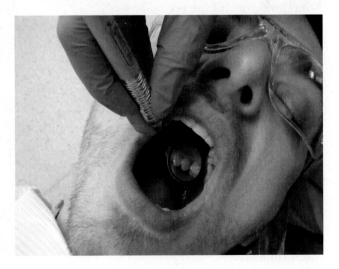

LEFT-HANDED CLINICIAN

SKILL BUILDING
Mirror Use: Mandibular Teeth

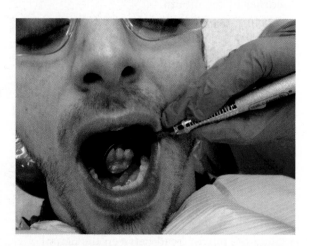

Figure 4-33. Mandibular Anteriors, Lingual Aspect: Surfaces Toward

- Sit in a 3 to 4 o'clock position.
- Rest your ring and little fingers on the left side of the patient's face near the corner of the mouth or on the premolar teeth.
- Use the mirror head to push the tongue away gently so the lingual surfaces of the anterior teeth can be seen in the mirror.

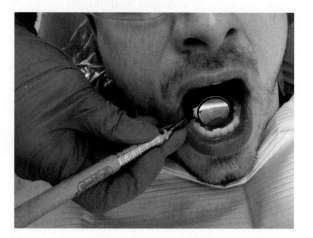

Figure 4-34. Mandibular Anteriors, Lingual Aspect: Surfaces Away

- Sit in a 11 to 1 o'clock position.
- Rest your ring and little fingers on the right side of the patient's face near the corner of the mouth or one of the premolar teeth.
- Use the mirror head to push the tongue back gently so that the lingual surfaces of the teeth can be seen in the mirror.

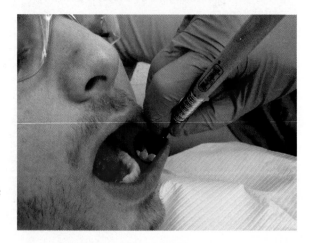

Figure 4-35. Mandibular Left Posterior Sextant, Facial Aspect

- Sit in the 3 o'clock position.
- Rest your fingers on the left side of the patient's face.
- Retract the buccal mucosa with the mirror. Use the mirror for indirect vision, particularly to view the distal surfaces of the teeth.

Figure 4-36. Mandibular Right Posterior Sextant, Lingual Aspect
- Sit in the 3 o'clock position.
- Rest your fingers on the left side of the patient's face.
- Use the mirror to gently move the tongue away from the teeth, toward the midline of the mouth. Use indirect vision to view the distal and lingual surfaces.
- Tip: Avoid pressing down against the floor of the mouth with the mirror head.

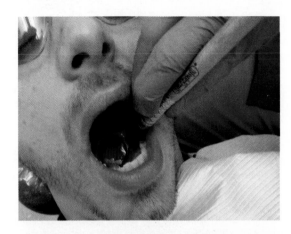

Figure 4-37. Mandibular Right Posterior Sextant, Facial Aspect
- Sit in the 1 to 2 o'clock position.
- Rest your fingers on the right side of the patient's face.
- Use the mirror to retract the buccal mucosa down and away from the teeth.
- View the distal, facial, and mesial surfaces in the mirror's reflecting surface.

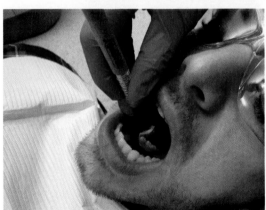

Figure 4-38. Mandibular Left Posterior Sextant, Lingual Aspect
- Sit in the 1 to 2 o'clock position.
- Rest your fingers on the right side of the patient's face.
- Use the mirror to gently move the tongue away from the teeth, so that the lingual surfaces of the teeth can be seen. Once in position, view the distal, lingual, and mesial surfaces in the mirror's reflecting surface.

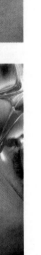

LEFT-HANDED CLINICIAN

Box 4-3 **Techniques to Stop Fogging of Reflecting Surface**

Use one of the following techniques to stop fogging of the reflecting surface:
- Warm the reflecting surface against the patient's buccal mucosa.
- Ask patient to breathe through the nose.
- Wipe the reflecting surface with a commercial defogging solution.
- Wipe the reflecting surface with a gauze square moistened with mouthwash.

References

1. Morse T, Bruneau H, Dussetschleger J. Musculoskeletal disorders of the neck and shoulder in the dental professions. *Work.* 2010;35(4):419–429.
2. Morse T, Bruneau H, Michalak-Turcotte C, et al. Musculoskeletal disorders of the neck and shoulder in dental hygienists and dental hygiene students. *J Dent Hyg.* 2007;81(1):10.
3. *Ergonomics and Dental Work.* Ontario, Canada: Occupational Health Clinics for Ontario Workers, Inc. (OHCOW); January 12, 2012. Available online at http://www.ohcow.on.ca/uploads/Resource/Workbooks/ERGONOMICS AND DENTAL WORK. pdf. Accessed October 9, 2015.
4. Diaz MJ, Sanchez E, Hidalgo JJ, Vega JM, Yanguas M. Assessment of a preclinical training system with indirect vision for dental education. *Eur J Dent Educ.* 2001;5(3):120–126.
5. Boyd MA, Rucker LM. Effects of immediate introduction of indirect vision on performance and posture. *J Dent Educ.* 1987;51(2):98–101.
6. Lundergan WP, Soderstrom EJ, Chambers DW. Tweezer dexterity aptitude of dental students. *J Dent Educ.* 2007;71(8): 1090–1097.

Section 5
Skill Application

STUDENT SELF EVALUATION MODULE 4: MIRROR USE

Student: _____

Date: _____

Area 1 = maxillary anteriors, lingual surfaces
Area 2 = maxillary left posteriors, facial aspect
Area 3 = maxillary right posteriors, facial aspect
Area 4 = maxillary right posteriors, lingual aspect

DIRECTIONS: Self-evaluate your skill level in each treatment area as: **S** (satisfactory) or **U** (unsatisfactory).

Criteria				
Positioning/Ergonomics	**Area 1**	**Area 2**	**Area 3**	**Area 4**
Adjusts clinician chair correctly				
Reclines patient chair and assures that patient's head is even with top of headrest				
Positions instrument tray within easy reach for front, side, or rear delivery as appropriate for operatory configuration				
Positions unit light at arm's length or dons dental headlight and adjusts it for use				
Assumes the recommended clock position				
Positions backrest of patient chair for the specified arch and adjusts height of patient chair so that clinician's elbows remain at waist level when accessing the specified treatment area				
Asks patient to assume the head position that facilitates the clinician's view of the specified treatment area.				
Maintains neutral position				
Directs light to illuminate the specified treatment area				
Mirror Use	**Area 1**	**Area 2**	**Area 3**	**Area 4**
Grasps the mirror handle in a modified pen grasp.				
Establishes an appropriate finger rest; ensures patient comfort.				
Positions the mirror head with the reflecting surface exposed (not against the buccal mucosa or tongue)	N/A			N/A
If appropriate, uses the mirror head to retract the mucosa.	N/A			N/A
Swivels the reflecting surface, first, to view the distal tooth surfaces, then to view the facial/lingual surfaces, and finally to view the mesial surfaces.				

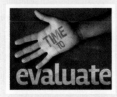

NOTE TO COURSE INSTRUCTORS: To download Module Evaluations for this textbook, go to http://thepoint.lww.com/GehrigFundamentals8e and log on to access the Instructor Resources for Fundamentals of Periodontal Instrumentation and Advanced Root Instrumentation.

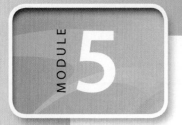

MODULE 5

Finger Rests in the Anterior Sextants

Module Overview

This module describes techniques for using intraoral finger rests in the anterior treatment areas. Content in this module includes the topics of fulcrums and finger rests, and recommended wrist position and hand placement during periodontal instrumentation. A step-by-step technique practice for using intraoral finger rests in the anterior treatment sextants is found in Sections 3 and 4.

Module Outline

Section 1 — **The Intraoral Fulcrum** — 112
Summary Sheet: Technique for Intraoral Fulcrum

Section 2 — **Wrist Position for Instrumentation** — 114
Neutral Wrist Position
Guidelines for Neutral Wrist Position
Building Blocks from Position to Finger Rests

Section 3 — **Technique Practice: RIGHT-Handed Clinician** — 118
Skill Building. Mandibular Anterior Teeth, Surfaces TOWARD, p. 118
Skill Building. Mandibular Anterior Teeth, Surfaces AWAY, p. 121
Skill Building. Maxillary Anterior Teeth, Surfaces TOWARD, p. 124
Skill Building. Maxillary Anterior Teeth, Surfaces AWAY, p. 127
Reference Sheet for Anterior Treatment Areas for the Right-Handed
    Clinician

Section 4 — **Technique Practice: LEFT-Handed Clinician** — 131
Skill Building. Mandibular Anterior Teeth, Surfaces TOWARD, p. 131
Skill Building. Mandibular Anterior Teeth, Surfaces AWAY, p. 134
Skill Building. Maxillary Anterior Teeth, Surfaces TOWARD, p. 137
Skill Building. Maxillary Anterior Teeth, Surfaces AWAY, p. 140
Reference Sheet for Anterior Treatment Areas for the Left-Handed
    Clinician

Section 5 — **Skill Application** — 145
Practical Focus: Evaluation of Position, Grasp, and Finger Rest
Student Self Evaluation Module 5: Mirror and Finger Rests in Anterior
    Sextants

Key Terms

Fulcrum
Support beam
Intraoral fulcrum

Extraoral fulcrum
Advanced fulcrum

Out of the line of fire
Neutral wrist position

Learning Objectives

- Position equipment so that it enhances neutral positioning.

- Maintain neutral seated position while using the recommended clock position for each of the mandibular and maxillary anterior treatment areas.

- While seated in the correct clock position for the treatment area, access the anterior teeth with optimum vision while maintaining neutral positioning.

- Demonstrate correct mirror use, grasp, and finger rest in each of the anterior sextants while maintaining neutral positioning of your wrist and finger joints.

- Demonstrate finger rests using precise finger placement on the handle of a periodontal instrument:

  o Finger pads of thumb and index finger opposite one another on handle

  o Thumb and index finger do not overlap each other on the handle

  o Pad of middle finger rests lightly on the shank

  o Thumb, index, and middle fingers in a neutral position

  o Ring finger is advanced ahead of the other fingers in the grasp, held straight and supporting the hand and instrument in the grasp

- Recognize incorrect mirror use, grasp, or finger rest and describe how to correct the problem(s).

- Understand the relationship between proper stabilization of the dominant hand during instrumentation and the prevention of (1) musculoskeletal problems in the clinician's hands and (2) injury to the patient.

- Understand the relationship between the large motor skills, such as positioning, and small motor skills, such as finger rests. Recognize the importance of initiating these skills in a step-by-step manner.

Online resource for this module: Establishing a Finger Rest
Available at: http://thepoint.lww.com/GehrigFundamentals8e

RIGHT- AND LEFT-HANDED SECTIONS IN THIS MODULE

- Sections 3 and 4 of this module are customized for right-handed and left-handed clinicians.

- For ease of use—and avoidance of confusion—if you are right-handed, it is recommended that you either (1) tear the left-handed pages from the book or (2) staple these pages together. If you are left-handed, use the same approach with the right-handed pages.

Section 1
The Intraoral Fulcrum

The fulcrum is a finger rest used to stabilize the clinician's hand during periodontal instrumentation. The fulcrum improves the precision of instrumentation strokes, prevents sudden movements that could injure the patient, and reduces muscle load to the clinician's hand (1–5).

1. Functions of the Fulcrum
   a. Serves as a "*support beam*" for the hand during instrumentation.
   b. Enables the hand and instrument to move as a unit as strokes are made against the tooth.
   c. Allows precise control of stroke pressure and length during periodontal instrumentation.
2. Types of Fulcrums
   a. Intraoral fulcrum—stabilization of the clinician's dominant hand by placing the pad of the ring finger on a tooth near to the tooth being instrumented. Figure 5-1 shows an example of right-handed clinician using an intraoral fulcrum for the facial aspects of the maxillary anterior teeth. Characteristics and techniques of the intraoral fulcrum are summarized in Box 5-1 and Table 5-1.
   b. Extraoral fulcrum—stabilization of the clinician's nondominant hand outside the patient's mouth, usually on the chin or cheek. An extraoral fulcrum may be used with a mirror. Extraoral fulcrums for use with a dental mirror are presented in Module 4.
   c. Advanced fulcrum—variations of an intraoral or extraoral finger rest used to gain access to root surfaces within periodontal pockets.

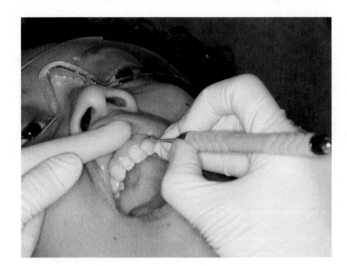

Figure 5-1. Intraoral Finger Rest. The right-handed clinician pictured here rests the pad of her ring finger on the incisal edge of a tooth adjacent to the tooth being instrumented. This intraoral finger rest stabilizes her hand and the instrument in the oral cavity.

Box 5-1 **Characteristics of Intraoral Fulcrum**

- Provides stable support for the hand
- Enables the hand and instrument to move as a unit
- Facilitates precise stroke length and pressure against the tooth surface
- Decreases the likelihood of injury to the patient or clinician if the patient moves unexpectedly during instrumentation

TABLE 5-1.   SUMMARY SHEET: TECHNIQUE FOR INTRAORAL FULCRUM

	Technique
Grasp	Hold the instrument in a precise modified pen grasp.
Fulcrum	Advance the ring finger ahead of the other fingers in the grasp. Keep ring finger straight, with the tip of the finger supporting the hand and instrument.
Location	Position the finger rest of the dominant hand near the tooth being instrumented. • Depending on the tooth being instrumented and length of your fingers, the finger rest may be one to four teeth away from the tooth on which you are working. • A finger rest is always established out of the line of fire. The phrase "out of the line of fire" refers to the concept that the finger rest is never established directly above the tooth surface being worked on. If the finger rest is on the tooth being worked on, it is possible that the clinician's finger will be injured by the sharp cutting edge. Staying out of the line of fire lessens the likelihood of instrument sticks.
Rest	Place the finger rest on the same arch as the tooth being instrumented. • Rest the fingertip of the fulcrum finger on the incisal edge of an anterior tooth or on the occlusofacial or occlusolingual line angle of a posterior tooth. • The teeth are saliva-covered, so you will be more likely to slip if you establish a finger rest directly on the facial or lingual surface. • Avoid resting on a mobile tooth or one with a large carious lesion.

Section 2
Wrist Position for Instrumentation

NEUTRAL WRIST POSITION

Neutral wrist position is the ideal positioning of the wrist while performing work activities and is associated with decreased risk of musculoskeletal injury (Box 5-2, Fig. 5-2) (6).

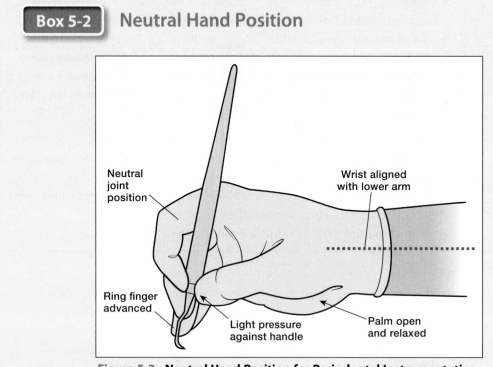

| Box 5-2 | Neutral Hand Position |

Figure 5-2. **Neutral Hand Position for Periodontal Instrumentation.**

- Wrist aligned with the long axis of the lower arm
- Little finger-side of the palm rotated slightly downward
- Palm open and relaxed
- Thumb, middle, and index fingers held in a neutral joint position (not hyperextended)
- Light finger pressure against the instrument handle
- Ring finger advanced ahead of other fingers in the grasp; held straight in a neutral joint position and not hyperextended

GUIDELINES FOR NEUTRAL WRIST POSITION

Keeping the wrist aligned with the long axis of the arm decreases musculoskeletal stresses on the wrist joint. Avoiding fully flexed or fully extended joint positions keeps the muscles used to control hand movements at more ideal muscle lengths for generating motions (7–9). Figures 5-3 to 5-6 show do's and don'ts for neutral wrist position.

Figure 5-3.
OK:
Wrist aligned with the long axis of the forearm

AVOID:
Bending the wrist and hand down towards the palm (flexion)

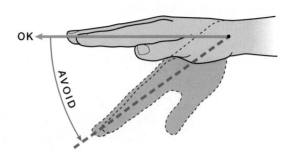

Figure 5-4.
OK:
Wrist in alignment with the forearm

AVOID:
Bending the wrist and hand up and back (extension)

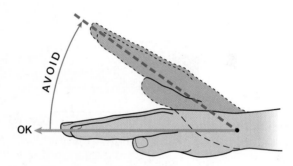

Figure 5-5.
OK:
Wrist aligned with long axis of forearm

AVOID:
Bending the wrist toward the thumb (radial deviation)

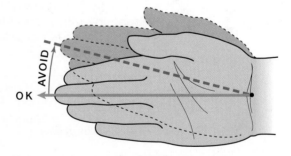

Figure 5-6.
OK:
Wrist in alignment with the long axis of the forearm

AVOID:
Bending the wrist toward the little finger (ulnar deviation)

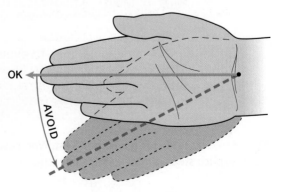

BUILDING BLOCKS FROM POSITION TO FINGER RESTS

Precise, accurate performance of the building block skills is essential if periodontal instrumentation is to be effective, efficient, safe for the patient, and comfortable the clinician.

- Research on psychomotor skill acquisition indicates that a high level of mastery in the performance of the skill building blocks is essential for successful mastery of periodontal instrumentation.
- The building block skills are the foundation that "supports" successful periodontal instrumentation.
- While practicing finger rests, it is important to complete each of the skills listed in Figure 5-7 in sequence. Follow the directions in Box 5-3 for technique practice.

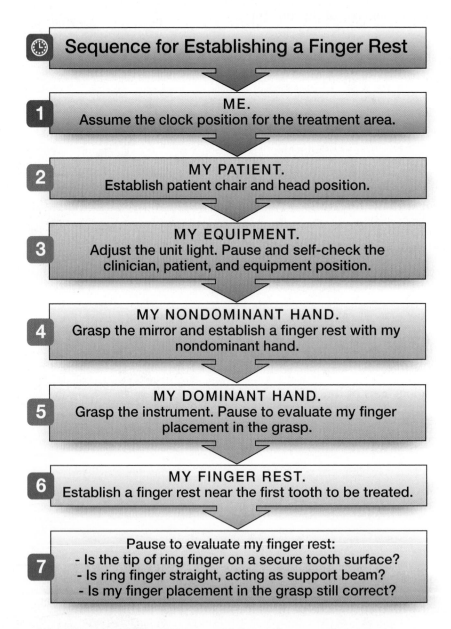

Sequence for Establishing a Finger Rest

1 ME.
Assume the clock position for the treatment area.

2 MY PATIENT.
Establish patient chair and head position.

3 MY EQUIPMENT.
Adjust the unit light. Pause and self-check the clinician, patient, and equipment position.

4 MY NONDOMINANT HAND.
Grasp the mirror and establish a finger rest with my nondominant hand.

5 MY DOMINANT HAND.
Grasp the instrument. Pause to evaluate my finger placement in the grasp.

6 MY FINGER REST.
Establish a finger rest near the first tooth to be treated.

7 Pause to evaluate my finger rest:
- Is the tip of ring finger on a secure tooth surface?
- Is ring finger straight, acting as support beam?
- Is my finger placement in the grasp still correct?

Figure 5-7. Establishing a Finger Rest. When establishing a finger rest it is important to proceed in the small, explicit steps outlined in this flow chart (10).

| Box 5-3 | Directions for Technique Practice |

1. The next two sections of this Module contain instructions for practicing finger rests for each anterior treatment area of the mouth.

2. The photographs in the Technique Practice sections depict the use of a mirror and finger rests in the anterior treatment areas. Some photographs were taken on a patient. *Others were taken using a manikin and without gloves so that you can easily see the finger placement in the grasp.*

3. The photographs provide a *general guideline* for finger rests; however, the location of your own finger rest depends on the size and length of your fingers. You may need to fulcrum closer to or farther from the tooth being treated than is shown in the photograph.

4. Focus your attention on mastering wrist position and the finger rests. Use the following instruments in this module:
   - **For your nondominant (mirror) hand**—Use a dental mirror.
   - **For your dominant (instrument) hand**
     (a) Remove the mirror head from one of your dental mirrors and use the mirror handle as if it were a periodontal instrument, or
     (b) Use a periodontal probe to represent the periodontal instrument in this module.

5. Do not wear magnification loupes when practicing and perfecting your positioning and finger rest skills in this module. You need an unrestricted visual field for self-evaluation.

6. Remove Figure 5-7 from your book and refer to it as you practice and self-evaluate your skills during the Technique Practice.

Section 3
Technique Practice: RIGHT-Handed Clinician

SKILL BUILDING
Mandibular Anterior Teeth, Surfaces TOWARD

Directions: Practice establishing a finger rest for the mandibular anterior teeth, surfaces toward, by referring to Figures 5-8 to 5-15. Refer to Box 5-4 for handle location.

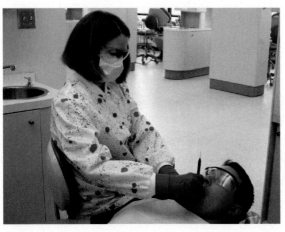

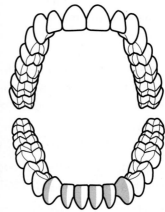

Figure 5-8. Clock Position for Mandibular Anterior Teeth, Surfaces Toward. The clinician's clock position for the mandibular anterior surfaces toward the clinician—facial and lingual aspects—is the 8:00 to 9:00 position. The patient should be in a chin-down head position.

| **Box 5-4** | **Handle Positions for Mandibular Anterior Teeth** |

1. Hold the hand in a palm-down position.
2. Rest the handle against the index finger somewhere in the green shaded area.

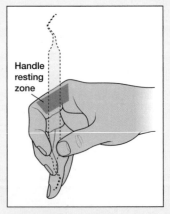

Figure 5-9. Handle Positions for Mandibular Treatment Areas.

Mandibular Anteriors, Facial Aspect: Surfaces Toward

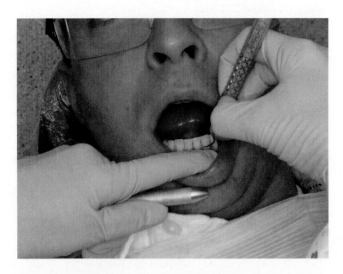

Figure 5-10. Retraction. Retract the lip with the index finger or thumb of your left hand.

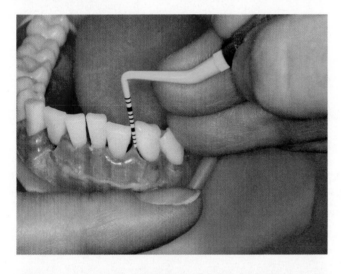

Figure 5-11. Task 1—Mesial Surface of the Left Canine.
- Finger rest on an occlusofacial line angle.
- Place the instrument tip on the mesial surface of the left canine.

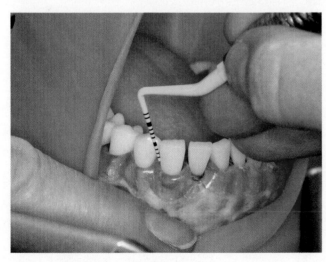

Figure 5-12. Task 2—Distal Surface of Right Canine.
- Finger rest on an incisal edge.
- Place the instrument tip on the distal surface of the right canine.

RIGHT-HANDED CLINICIAN

Mandibular Anteriors, Lingual Aspect: Surfaces Toward

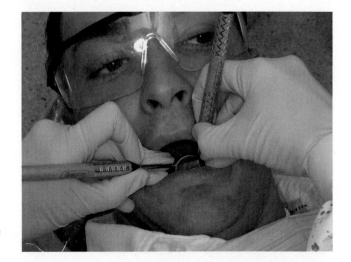

Figure 5-13. **Mirror.** Use the mirror head to push the tongue away gently so the lingual surfaces of the anterior teeth can be seen in the reflecting surface of the mirror.

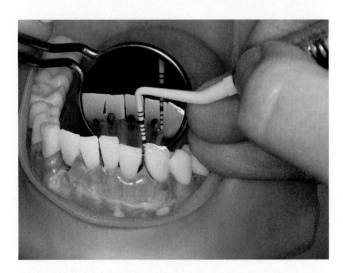

Figure 5-14. **Task 1—Mesial Surface of the Left Canine.**
- Finger rest on an occlusofacial line angle.
- Place the instrument tip on the mesial surface of the left canine.

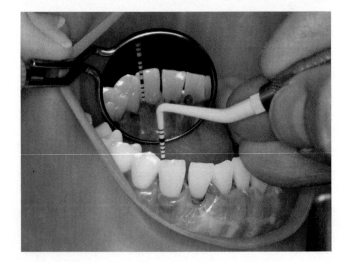

Figure 5-15. **Task 2—Distal Surface of the Right Canine.**
- Finger rest on an incisal edge.
- Place the instrument tip on the distal surface of the right canine.

SKILL BUILDING
Mandibular Anterior Teeth, Surfaces AWAY

Directions: Practice establishing a finger rest for the mandibular anterior teeth, surfaces toward, by referring to Figures 5-16 to 5-23. Refer to Box 5-5 for handle location.

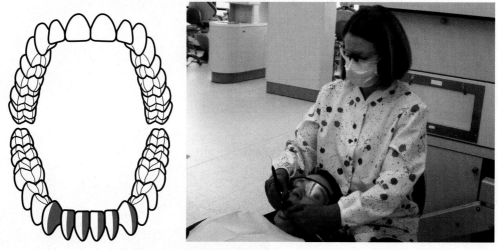

Figure 5-16. Clock Position for Mandibular Anterior Teeth, Surfaces Away. The clinician's clock position for the mandibular anterior surfaces away from the clinician—facial and lingual aspects—is the 11:00 to 1:00 position. The patient is in a chin-down head position.

Box 5-5 **Handle Positions for Mandibular Anterior Teeth**

1. Hold the hand in a palm-down position.
2. Rest the handle against the index finger somewhere in the green shaded area.

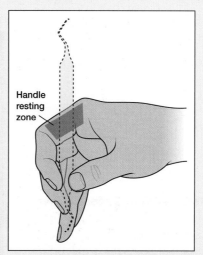

Handle resting zone

Figure 5-17. Handle Positions for Mandibular Treatment Areas.

RIGHT-HANDED CLINICIAN

Mandibular Anteriors, Facial Aspect: Surfaces Away

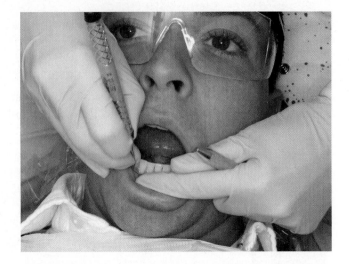

Figure 5-18. Retraction. Retract the lip with your index finger or thumb. Note that the clinician pictured is holding the mirror in the palm of her hand.

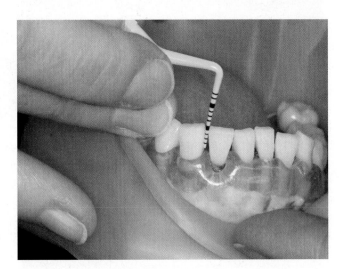

Figure 5-19. Task 1—Mesial Surface of the Right Canine.
- Finger rest on an occlusofacial line angle.
- Place the instrument tip on the mesial surface of the right canine.

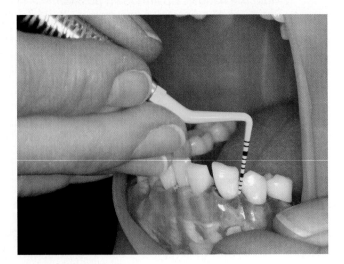

Figure 5-20. Task 2—Distal Surface of the Left Canine.
- Finger rest on an incisal edge.
- Place the instrument tip on the distal surface of the left canine.

Mandibular Anteriors, Lingual Aspect: Surfaces Away

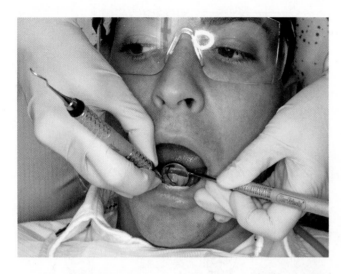

Figure 5-21. Mirror. Use the mirror head to push the tongue back gently so that the lingual surfaces of the teeth can be seen.

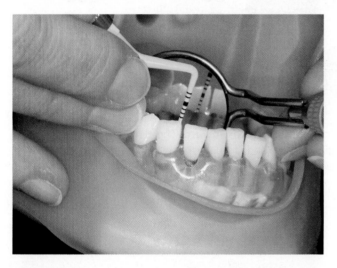

Figure 5-22. Task 1—Mesial Surface of the Right Canine.
- Finger rest on an occlusofacial line angle.
- Place the instrument tip on the mesial surface of the right canine.

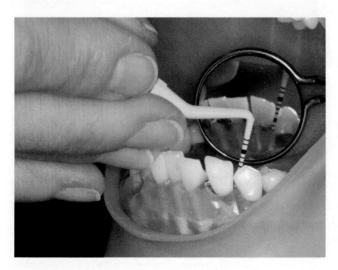

Figure 5-23. Task 2—Distal Surface of the Left Canine.
- Finger rest on an incisal edge.
- Place the instrument tip on the distal surface of the left canine.

RIGHT-HANDED CLINICIAN

SKILL BUILDING
Maxillary Anterior Teeth, Surfaces TOWARD

Directions: Practice establishing a finger rest for the maxillary anterior teeth, surfaces toward, by referring to Figures 5-24 to 5-31. Refer to Box 5-6 for handle location.

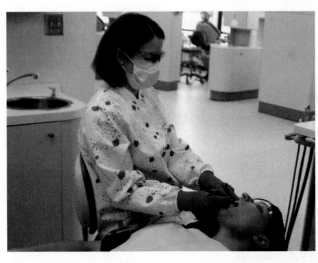

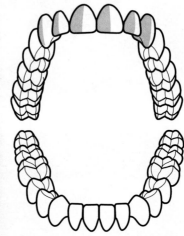

Figure 5-24. Clock Position for Maxillary Anterior Teeth, Surfaces Toward. The clinician's clock position for the maxillary anterior surfaces toward the clinician—facial and lingual aspects—is the 8:00 to 9:00 position. The patient should be in a chin-up head position.

Box 5-6 | Handle Positions for Maxillary Anterior Teeth

1. Hold the hand in a palm-up position.

2. Rest the handle against the index finger somewhere in the green shaded area.

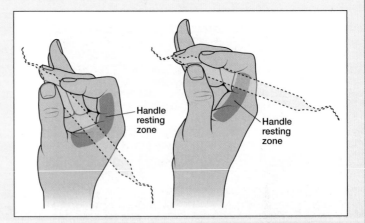

Figure 5-25. Handle Positions for Maxillary Treatment Areas.

Maxillary Anteriors, Facial Aspect: Surfaces Toward

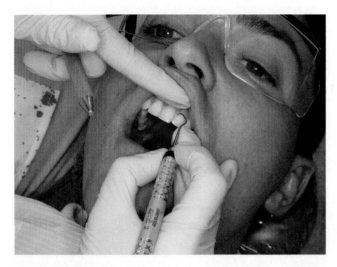

Figure 5-26. Retraction. Retract the lip with the index finger or thumb of your left hand.

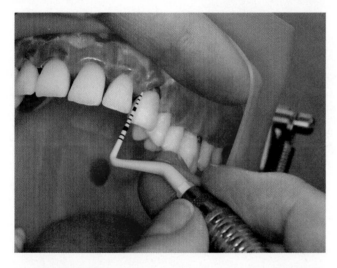

Figure 5-27. Task 1—Mesial Surface of the Left Canine.
- Finger rest on an occlusofacial line angle.
- Place the instrument tip on the mesial surface of the left canine.

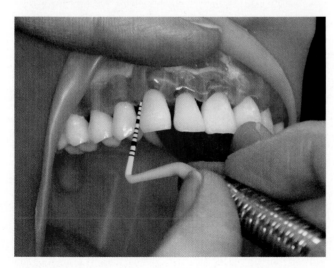

Figure 5-28. Task 2—Distal Surface of Right Canine.
- Finger rest on an incisal edge.
- Place the instrument tip on the distal surface of the right canine.

Maxillary Anteriors, Lingual Aspect: Surfaces Toward

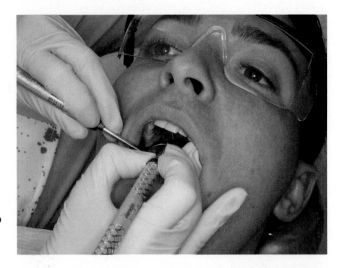

Figure 5-29. Mirror. Position the mirror head so the lingual surfaces of the anterior teeth can be seen in the reflecting surface of the mirror.

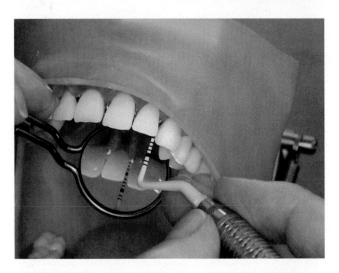

Figure 5-30. Task 1—Mesial Surface of the Left Canine.
- Finger rest on an occlusofacial line angle.
- Place the instrument tip on the mesial surface of the left canine.

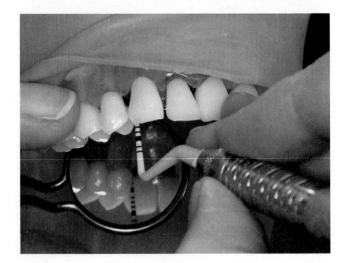

Figure 5-31. Task 2—Distal Surface of the Right Canine.
- Finger rest on an incisal edge.
- Place the instrument tip on the distal surface of the right canine.

SKILL BUILDING
Maxillary Anterior Teeth, Surfaces AWAY

Directions: Practice establishing a finger rest for the maxillary anterior teeth, surfaces toward, by referring to Figures 5-32 to 5-39. Refer to Box 5-7 for handle location.

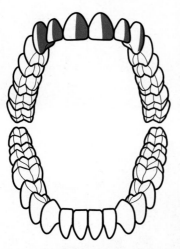

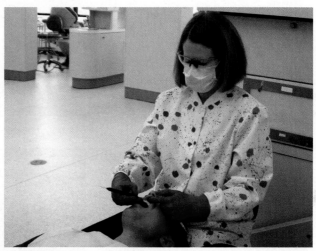

Figure 5-32. Clock Position for Maxillary Anterior Teeth, Surfaces Away. The clinician's clock position for the maxillary anterior surfaces away from the clinician—facial and lingual aspects—is the 11:00 to 1:00 position. The patient is in a chin-up head position.

RIGHT-HANDED CLINICIAN

Box 5-7 **Handle Positions for Maxillary Anterior Teeth**

1. Hold the hand in a palm-up position.

2. Rest the handle against the index finger somewhere in the green shaded area.

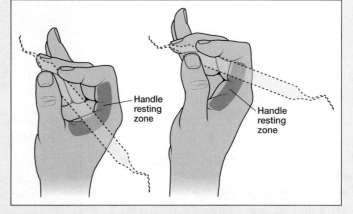

Handle resting zone

Handle resting zone

Figure 5-33. Handle Positions for Maxillary Treatment Areas.

Maxillary Anteriors, Facial Aspect: Surfaces Away

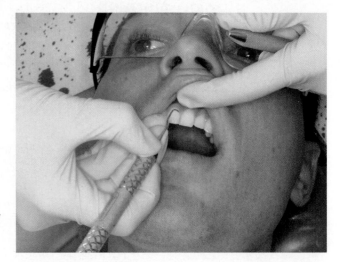

Figure 5-34. **Retraction.** Retract the lip with your index finger or thumb. **Technique hint:** your dominant hand is positioned correctly if you can see the underside of your middle and ring fingers.

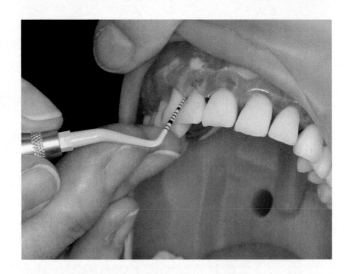

Figure 5-35. **Task 1—Mesial Surface of the Right Canine.**
- Finger rest on an occlusal surface.
- Place the instrument tip on the mesial surface of the right canine.

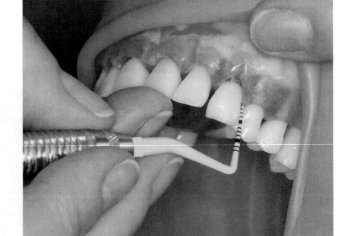

Figure 5-36. **Task 2—Distal Surface of the Left Canine.**
- Finger rest on an incisal edge.
- Place the instrument tip on the distal surface of the left canine.

Maxillary Anterior Sextant, Lingual Aspect: Surfaces Away

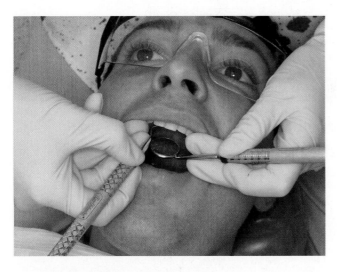

Figure 5-37. **Mirror.** Position the mirror head so that the lingual surfaces of the teeth can be seen. **Technique hint:** your dominant hand is positioned correctly if you can see the underside of your middle and ring fingers.

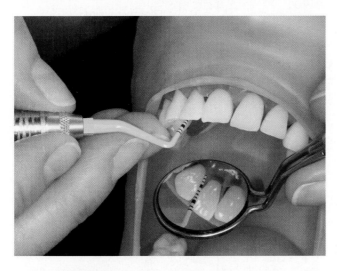

Figure 5-38. **Task 1—Mesial Surface of the Right Canine.**
- Finger rest on an occlusal surface.
- Place the instrument tip on the mesial surface of the right canine.

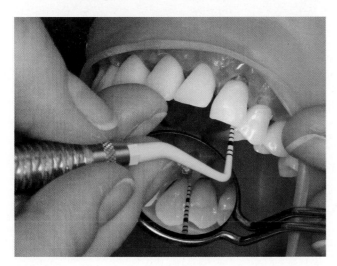

Figure 5-39. **Task 2—Distal Surface of the Left Canine.**
- Finger rest on an incisal edge.
- Place the instrument tip on the distal surface of the left canine.

RIGHT-HANDED CLINICIAN

REFERENCE SHEET FOR ANTERIOR TREATMENT AREAS FOR THE RIGHT-HANDED CLINICIAN

Photocopy this reference sheet in Table 5-2 and use it for quick reference as you practice your skills. Place the photocopied reference sheet in a plastic page protector for longer use.

TABLE 5-2. REFERENCE SHEET: ANTERIOR TREATMENT AREAS

Treatment Area	Clock Position	Patient's Head
Mandibular Teeth		
Facial Surfaces TOWARD	8:00–9:00	Slightly toward
Lingual Surfaces TOWARD		Chin DOWN
Facial Surfaces AWAY	11:00–1:00	
Lingual Surfaces AWAY		
Maxillary Teeth		
Facial Surfaces TOWARD	8:00–9:00	Slightly toward
Lingual Surfaces TOWARD		Chin UP
Facial Surfaces AWAY	11:00–1:00	
Lingual Surfaces AWAY		

RIGHT-HANDED CLINICIAN

Section 4
Technique Practice: LEFT-Handed Clinician

SKILL BUILDING
Mandibular Anterior Teeth, Surfaces TOWARD

Directions: Practice establishing a finger rest for the mandibular anterior teeth, surfaces toward, by referring to Figures 5-40 to 5-47 and Box 5-8.

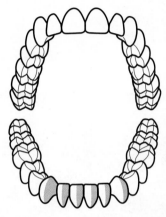 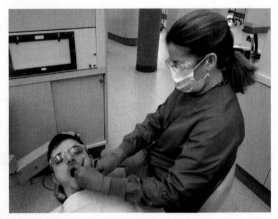

Figure 5-40. Clock Position for Mandibular Anterior Teeth, Surfaces Toward. The clinician's clock position for the mandibular anterior surfaces toward the clinician—facial and lingual aspects—is the 3:00 to 4:00 position. The patient should be in a chin-down head position.

Box 5-8 Handle Positions for Mandibular Anterior Teeth

1. Hold the hand in a palm-down position.
2. Rest the handle against the index finger somewhere in the green shaded area.

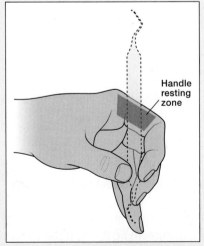

Handle resting zone

Figure 5-41. Handle Positions for Mandibular Treatment Areas.

Mandibular Anteriors, Facial Aspect: Surfaces Toward

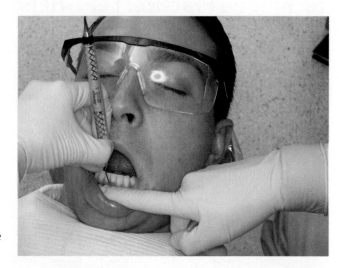

Figure 5-42. Retraction. Retract the lip with the index finger or thumb of your right hand.

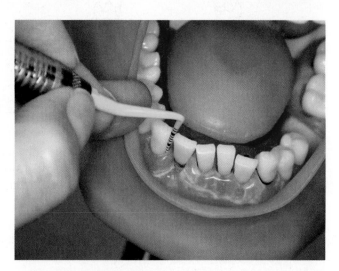

Figure 5-43. Task 1—Mesial Surface of the Right Canine.
- Finger rest on an occlusofacial line angle.
- Place the instrument tip on the mesial surface of the right canine.

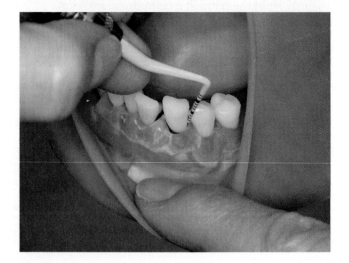

Figure 5-44. Task 2—Distal Surface of Left Canine.
- Finger rest on an incisal edge.
- Place the instrument tip on the distal surface of the left canine.

Mandibular Anteriors, Lingual Aspect: Surfaces Toward

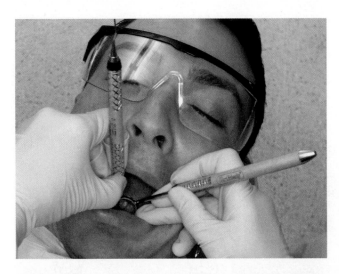

Figure 5-45. Mirror. Use the mirror head to push the tongue away gently so the lingual surfaces of the anterior teeth can be seen in the reflecting surface of the mirror.

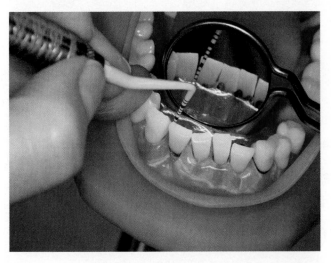

Figure 5-46. Task 1—Mesial Surface of the Right Canine.
- Finger rest on an occlusofacial line angle.
- Place the instrument tip on the mesial surface of the right canine.

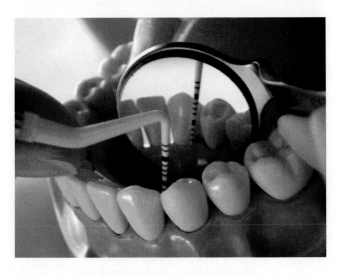

Figure 5-47. Task 2—Distal Surface of the Left Canine.
- Finger rest on an incisal edge.
- Place the instrument tip on the distal surface of the left canine.

LEFT-HANDED CLINICIAN

SKILL BUILDING
Mandibular Anterior Teeth, Surfaces AWAY

Directions: Practice establishing a finger rest for the mandibular anterior teeth, surfaces toward, by referring to Figures 5-48 to 5-55 and Box 5-9.

LEFT-HANDED CLINICIAN

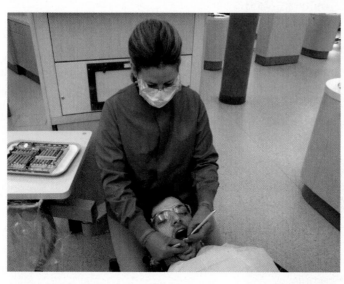

Figure 5-48. Clock Position for Mandibular Anterior Teeth, Surfaces Away. The clinician's clock position for the mandibular anterior surfaces away from the clinician—facial and lingual aspects—is the 11:00 to 1:00 position. The patient is in a chin-down head position.

Box 5-9 | **Handle Positions for Mandibular Anterior Teeth**

1. Hold the hand in a palm-down position.
2. Rest the handle against the index finger somewhere in the green shaded area.

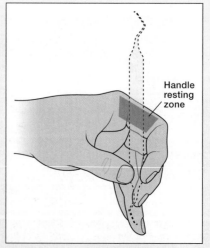

Handle resting zone

Figure 5-49. Handle Positions for Mandibular Treatment Areas.

Mandibular Anteriors, Facial Aspect: Surfaces Away

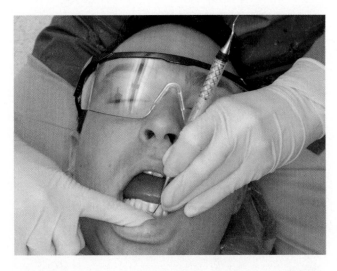

Figure 5-50. Retraction. Retract the lip with your index finger or thumb. Hold the mirror in your palm until it is needed for another treatment area.

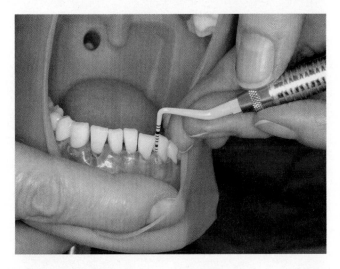

Figure 5-51. Task 1—Mesial Surface of the Left Canine.
- Finger rest on an occlusofacial line angle.
- Place the instrument tip on the mesial surface of the left canine.

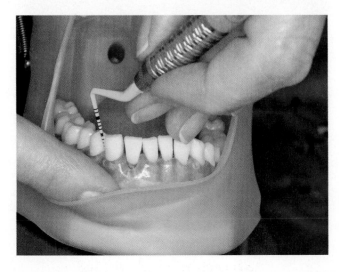

Figure 5-52. Task 2—Distal Surface of the Right Canine.
- Finger rest on an incisal edge.
- Place the instrument tip on the distal surface of the right canine.

Mandibular Anteriors, Lingual Aspect: Surfaces Away

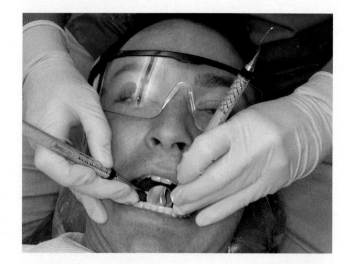

Figure 5-53. Mirror. Use the mirror head to push the tongue back gently so that the lingual surfaces of the teeth can be seen.

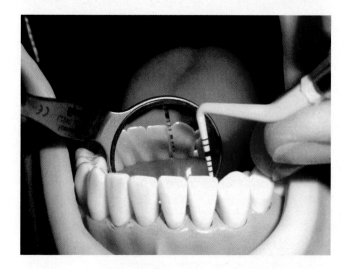

Figure 5-54. Task 1—Mesial Surface of the Left Canine.
- Finger rest on an occlusofacial line angle.
- Place the instrument tip on the mesial surface of the left canine.

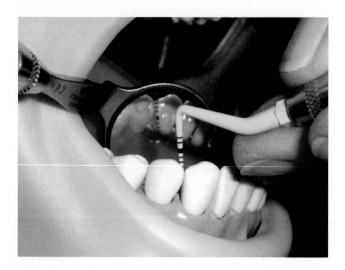

Figure 5-55. Task 2—Distal Surface of the Right Canine.
- Finger rest on an incisal edge.
- Place the instrument tip on the distal surface of the right canine.

SKILL BUILDING
Maxillary Anterior Teeth, Surfaces TOWARD

Directions: Practice establishing a finger rest for the maxillary anterior teeth, surfaces toward, by referring to Figures 5-56 to 5-63 and Box 5-10.

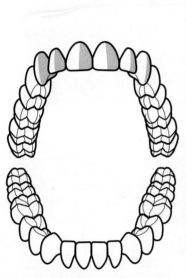
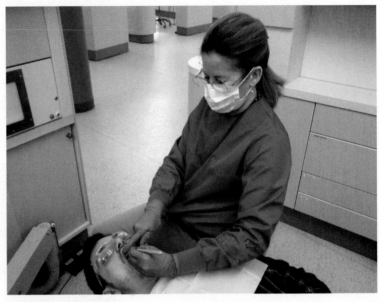

Figure 5-56. Clock Position for Maxillary Anterior Teeth, Surfaces Toward. The clinician's clock position for the maxillary anterior surfaces toward the clinician—facial and lingual aspects—is the 3:00 to 4:00 position. The patient should be in a chin-up head position.

Box 5-10 **Handle Positions for Maxillary Anterior Teeth**

1. Hold the hand in a palm-up position.

2. Rest the handle against the index finger somewhere in the green shaded area.

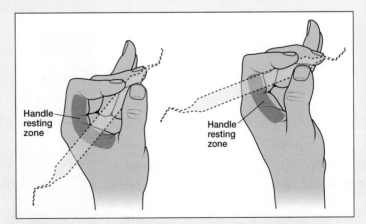

Handle resting zone

Handle resting zone

Figure 5-57. Handle Positions for Maxillary Treatment Areas.

Maxillary Anteriors, Facial Aspect: Surfaces Toward

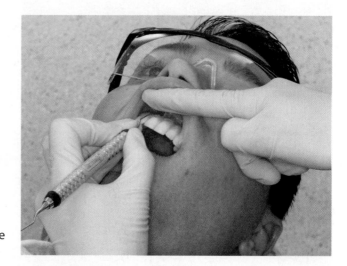

Figure 5-58. **Retraction.** Retract the lip with the index finger or thumb of your right hand.

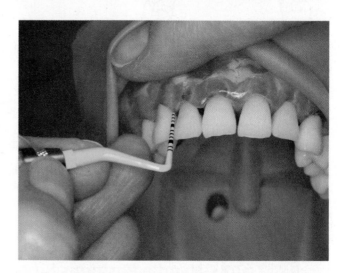

Figure 5-59. **Task 1—Mesial Surface of the Right Canine.**
- Finger rest on an occlusofacial line angle.
- Place the instrument tip on the mesial surface of the right canine.

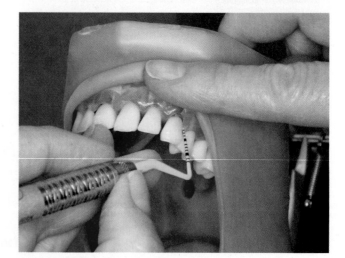

Figure 5-60. **Task 2—Distal Surface of Left Canine.**
- Finger rest on an incisal edge.
- Place the instrument tip on the distal surface of the left canine.

Maxillary Anteriors, Lingual Aspect: Surfaces Toward

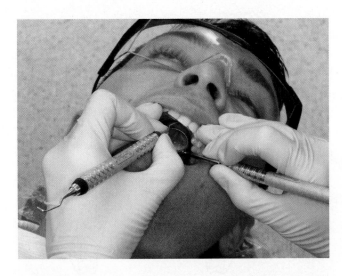

Figure 5-61. Mirror. Position the mirror head so the lingual surfaces of the anterior teeth can be seen in the reflecting surface of the mirror.

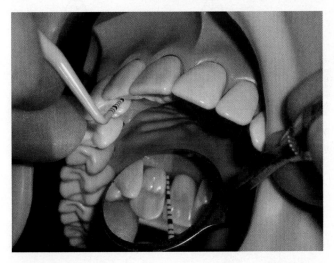

Figure 5-62. Task 1—Mesial Surface of the Right Canine.
- Finger rest on an occlusofacial line angle.
- Place the instrument tip on the mesial surface of the right canine.

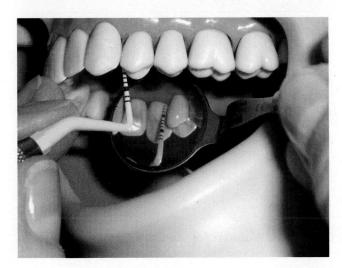

Figure 5-63. Task 2—Distal Surface of the Left Canine.
- Finger rest on an incisal edge.
- Place the instrument tip on the distal surface of the left canine.

SKILL BUILDING
Maxillary Anterior Teeth, Surfaces AWAY

Directions: Practice establishing a finger rest for the maxillary anterior teeth, surfaces away, by referring to Figures 5-64 to 5-71 and Box 5-11.

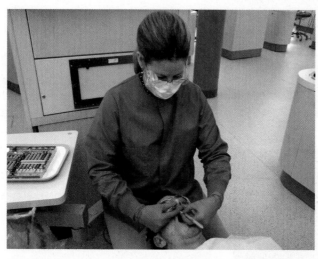

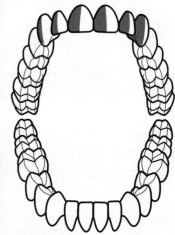

Figure 5-64. Clock Position for Maxillary Anterior Teeth, Surfaces Away. The clinician's clock position for the maxillary anterior surfaces away from the clinician—facial and lingual aspects—is the 11:00 to 1:00 position. The patient is in a chin-up head position.

Box 5-11 **Handle Positions for Maxillary Anterior Teeth**

1. Hold the hand in a palm-up position.

2. Rest the handle against the index finger somewhere in the green shaded area.

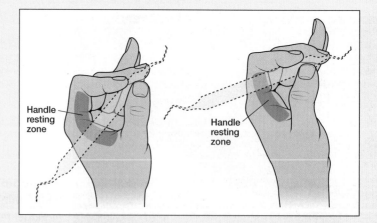

Handle resting zone

Handle resting zone

Figure 5-65. Handle Positions for Maxillary Treatment Areas.

Maxillary Anteriors, Facial Aspect: Surfaces Away

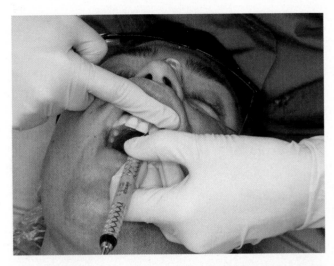

Figure 5-66. Retraction. Retract the lip with your index finger or thumb. **Technique hint:** your dominant hand is positioned correctly if you can see the underside of your middle and ring fingers.

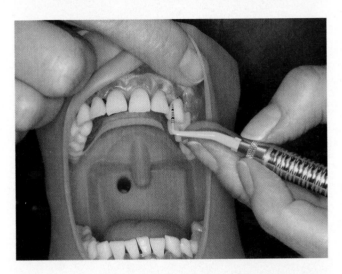

Figure 5-67. Task 1—Mesial Surface of the Left Canine.
- Finger rest on an occlusal surface.
- Place the instrument tip on the mesial surface of the left canine.

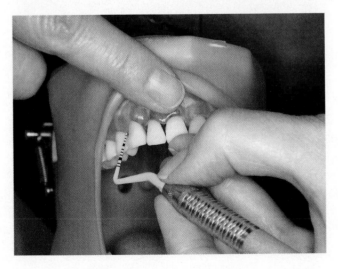

Figure 5-68. Task 2—Distal Surface of the Right Canine.
- Finger rest on an incisal edge.
- Place the instrument tip on the distal surface of the right canine.

LEFT-HANDED CLINICIAN

Maxillary Anteriors, Lingual Aspect: Surfaces Away

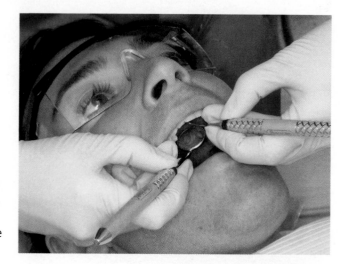

Figure 5-69. Mirror. Position the mirror head so that the lingual surfaces of the teeth can be seen. **Technique hint:** your dominant hand is positioned correctly if you can see the underside of your middle and ring fingers.

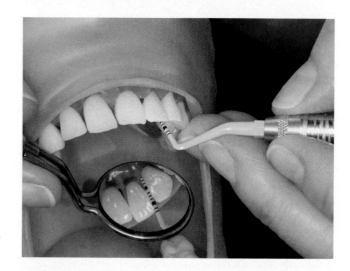

Figure 5-70. Task 1—Mesial Surface of the Left Canine.
- Finger rest on an occlusal surface.
- Place the instrument tip on the mesial surface of the left canine.

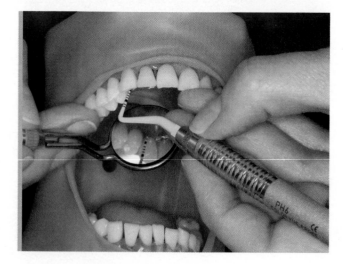

Figure 5-71. Task 2—Distal Surface of the Right Canine.
- Finger rest on an incisal edge.
- Place the instrument tip on the distal surface of the right canine.

REFERENCE SHEET FOR ANTERIOR TREATMENT AREAS FOR THE LEFT-HANDED CLINICIAN

Photocopy this reference sheet in Table 5-3 and use it for quick reference as you practice your skills. Place the photocopied reference sheet in a plastic page protector for longer use.

TABLE 5-3. REFERENCE SHEET: ANTERIOR TREATMENT AREAS

Treatment Area	Clock Position	Patient's Head
Mandibular Teeth		
Facial Surfaces TOWARD	4:00–3:00	
Lingual Surfaces TOWARD		Slightly toward
Facial Surfaces AWAY	11:00–1:00	Chin DOWN
Lingual Surfaces AWAY		
Maxillary Teeth		
Facial Surfaces TOWARD	4:00–3:00	
Lingual Surfaces TOWARD		Slightly toward
Facial Surfaces AWAY	11:00–1:00	Chin UP
Lingual Surfaces AWAY		

LEFT-HANDED CLINICIAN

References

1. Dong H, Barr A, Loomer P, Rempel D. The effects of finger rest positions on hand muscle load and pinch force in simulated dental hygiene work. *J Dent Educ.* 2005;69(4):453–460.

2. Dong H, Loomer P, Villanueva A, Rempel D. Pinch forces and instrument tip forces during periodontal scaling. *J Periodontol.* 2007;78(1):97–103.

3. Meador HL. The biocentric technique: a guide to avoiding occupational pain. *J Dent Hyg.* 1993;67(1):38–51.

4. Millar D. Reinforced periodontal instrumentation and ergonomics. The best practice to ensure optimal performance and career longevity. *CDHA.* 2009;24(3):8–16.

5. Scaramucci M. Getting a grasp. *Dimens Dent Hyg.* 2008;6(5):24–26.

6. Sugawara E. The study of wrist postures of musicians using the WristSystem (Greenleaf Medical System). *Work.* 1999;13(3):217–228.

7. Liskiewicz ST, Kerschbaum WE. Cumulative trauma disorders: an ergonomic approach for prevention. *J Dent Hyg.* 1997;71(4):162–167.

8. Loren GJ, Shoemaker SD, Burkholder TJ, Jacobson MD, Friden J, Lieber RL. Human wrist motors: biomechanical design and application to tendon transfers. *J Biomech.* 1996;29(3):331–342.

9. Michalak-Turcotte C. Controlling dental hygiene work-related musculoskeletal disorders: the ergonomic process. *J Dent Hyg.* 2000;74(1):41–48.

10. Hauser AM, Bowen DM. Primer on preclinical instruction and evaluation. *J Dent Educ.* 2009;73(3):390–398.

Section 5
Skill Application

PRACTICAL FOCUS
Evaluation of Position, Grasp, and Finger Rest

Evaluate the photographs shown in Figures 5-72 to 5-75 for position, grasp, and finger rest. For each incorrect element describe (a) how the problem could be corrected and (b) the musculoskeletal problems that could result from each positioning problem.

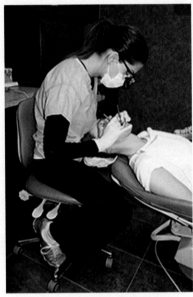

Figure 5-72. Photo 1.

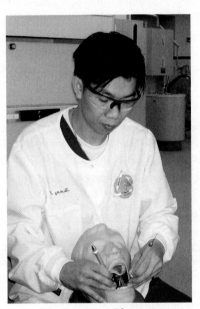

Figure 5-73. Photo 2.

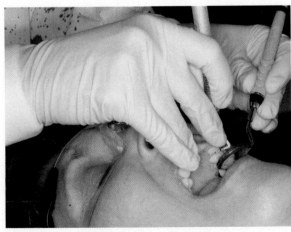

Figure 5-74. Photo 3.

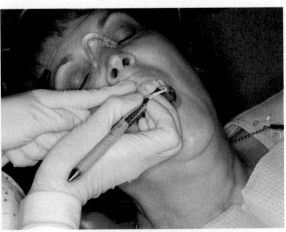

Figure 5-75. Photo 4.

Student Self Evaluation Module 5: Mirror and Finger Rests in Anterior Sextants

Student: _____

Date: _____

Area 1 = mandibular anteriors, facial aspect
Area 2 = mandibular anteriors, lingual aspect
Area 3 = maxillary anteriors, facial aspect
Area 4 = maxillary anteriors, lingual aspect

DIRECTIONS: Self-evaluate your skill level in each treatment area as: **S** (satisfactory) or **U** (unsatisfactory).

Criteria				
Positioning/Ergonomics	**Area 1**	**Area 2**	**Area 3**	**Area 4**
Adjusts clinician chair correctly				
Reclines patient chair and assures that patient's head is even with top of headrest				
Positions instrument tray within easy reach for front, side, or rear delivery as appropriate for operatory configuration				
Positions unit light at arm's length or dons dental headlight and adjusts it for use				
Assumes the recommended clock position				
Positions backrest of patient chair for the specified arch and adjusts height of patient chair so that clinician's elbows remain at waist level when accessing the specified treatment area				
Asks patient to assume the head position that facilitates the clinician's view of the specified treatment area				
Maintains neutral position				
Directs light to illuminate the specified treatment area				
Instrument Grasp: Dominant Hand	**Area 1**	**Area 2**	**Area 3**	**Area 4**
Grasps handle with tips of finger pads of index finger and thumb so that these fingers are opposite each other on the handle, but do NOT touch or overlap				
Rests pad of middle finger lightly on instrument shank; middle finger makes contact with ring finger				
Positions the thumb, index, and middle fingers in the "knuckles up" convex position; hyperextended joint position is avoided				
Holds ring finger straight so that it supports the weight of hand and instrument; ring finger position is "advanced ahead of" the other fingers in the grasp				
Keeps index, middle, ring, and little fingers in contact; "like fingers inside a mitten"				
Maintains a relaxed grasp; fingers are NOT blanched in grasp				
Finger Rest: Dominant Hand	**Area 1**	**Area 2**	**Area 3**	**Area 4**
Establishes secure finger rest that is appropriate for tooth to be treated				
Once finger rest is established, pauses to self-evaluate finger placement in the grasp, verbalizes to evaluator his/her self-assessment of grasp, and corrects finger placement if necessary				

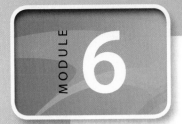

MODULE

6

Finger Rests in Mandibular Posterior Sextants

Module Overview

This module describes techniques for using a dental mirror and finger rests in the mandibular posterior treatment areas. The fulcrum improves the precision of instrumentation strokes, prevents sudden movements that could injure the patient, and reduces muscle load to the clinician's hand.

Module Outline

Section 1   **Building Blocks for Posterior Sextants**   **149**
Building Blocks from Position to Finger Rest
Impact of Finger Length on the Grasp and Finger Rest

Section 2   **Technique Practice: RIGHT-Handed Clinician**   **151**
Skill Building. Mandibular Posterior Sextants, Aspects Facing
     TOWARD the Clinician, p. 151
Skill Building. Mandibular Posterior Sextants, Aspects Facing
     AWAY From the Clinician, p. 154
Reference Sheet for Mandibular Posterior Sextants

Section 3   **Technique Practice: LEFT-Handed Clinician**   **158**
Skill Building. Mandibular Posterior Sextants, Aspects Facing
     TOWARD the Clinician, p. 158
Skill Building. Mandibular Posterior Sextants, Aspects Facing
     AWAY From the Clinician, p. 161
Reference Sheet for Mandibular Posterior Sextants

Section 4   **Skill Application**   **166**
Practical Focus
Student Self Evaluation Module 6: Mirror and Rests in Mandibular
     Posterior Sextants

Key Terms: Review these key terms found in Chapter 5

Neutral wrist position   Support beam   Extraoral fulcrum
Fulcrum   Finger rest   Intraoral fulcrum

Learning Objectives

- Position equipment so that it enhances neutral positioning.
- While seated in the correct clock position for the treatment area, access the mandibular posterior teeth with optimum vision while maintaining neutral positioning.
- Demonstrate correct mirror use, grasp, and finger rest in each of the mandibular posterior sextants while maintaining neutral positioning of your wrist.
- Demonstrate finger rests using precise finger placement on the handle of a periodontal instrument:
  - Finger pads of thumb and index finger opposite one another on handle
  - Thumb and index finger do not overlap each other on the handle
  - Pad of middle finger rests lightly on the shank
  - Thumb, index, and middle fingers in a neutral position
  - Ring finger is advanced ahead of the other fingers in the grasp, held straight and support the hand and instrument in the grasp
- Recognize incorrect mirror use, grasp, or finger rest and describe how to correct the problem(s).
- Understand the relationship between proper stabilization of the dominant hand during instrumentation and the prevention of (1) musculoskeletal problems in the clinician's hands and (2) injury to the patient.
- Understand the relationship between the large motor skills, such as positioning, and small motor skills, such as finger rests. Recognize the importance of initiating these skills in a step-by-step manner.

Online resource for this module: "Laying Down" vs. "Standing up" on Your Fulcrum.
Available at: http://thepoint.lww.com/GehrigFundamentals8e
Optional online content is available for this module (Module 6) and for Module 7. If assigned by the course instructor, the online module: *Alternate Clock Positions* can be viewed at http://thepoint.lww.com/GehrigFundamentals8e

RIGHT- AND LEFT-HANDED SECTIONS IN THIS MODULE

- Sections 2 and 3 of this module are customized for right-handed and left-handed clinicians.
- For ease of use—and avoidance of confusion—if you are right-handed, it is recommended that you either (1) tear the left-handed pages from the book or (2) staple these pages together. If you are left-handed, use the same approach with the right-handed pages.

Section 1
Building Blocks for Posterior Sextants

BUILDING BLOCKS FROM POSITION TO FINGER REST

An intraoral fulcrum acts as a "support beam" for clinician's dominant hand and allows precise control of the instrument's working-end during periodontal instrumentation (1–5).

- Precise, accurate performance of the building block skills is essential if periodontal instrumentation is to be effective, efficient, safe for the patient, and comfortable the clinician (6).
- While practicing finger rests, it is important to complete each of the skills listed in Figure 6-1 in sequence.

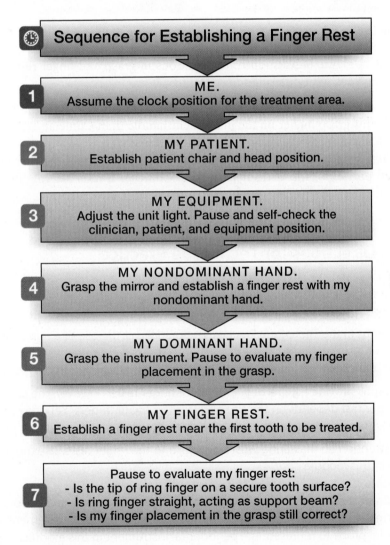

Sequence for Establishing a Finger Rest

1 ME.
Assume the clock position for the treatment area.

2 MY PATIENT.
Establish patient chair and head position.

3 MY EQUIPMENT.
Adjust the unit light. Pause and self-check the clinician, patient, and equipment position.

4 MY NONDOMINANT HAND.
Grasp the mirror and establish a finger rest with my nondominant hand.

5 MY DOMINANT HAND.
Grasp the instrument. Pause to evaluate my finger placement in the grasp.

6 MY FINGER REST.
Establish a finger rest near the first tooth to be treated.

7 Pause to evaluate my finger rest:
- Is the tip of ring finger on a secure tooth surface?
- Is ring finger straight, acting as support beam?
- Is my finger placement in the grasp still correct?

Figure 6-1. Establishing a Finger Rest. When establishing a finger rest it is important to proceed in the small, explicit steps outlined in this flow chart.

IMPACT OF FINGER LENGTH ON THE GRASP AND FINGER REST

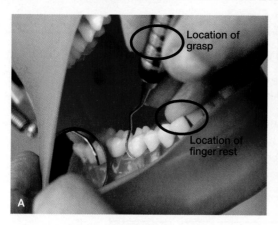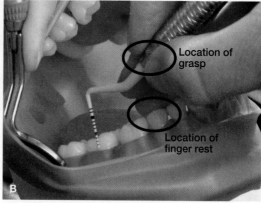

Figure 6-2. Variation in Grasp and Finger Rest Position According to Finger Length.

The two photographs in Figure 6-2 demonstrate variations in grasp and finger rest placement for two clinicians with differing finger lengths.

- **A: Clinician A: Long Finger Length (Photo on Left).** Note that clinician A—who has long fingers—establishes his grasp higher on the instrument handle than Clinician B (who has shorter fingers). Clinician A rests his ring finger on the canine.
- **B: Clinician B: Short Finger Length (Photo on Right).** Clinician B establishes her grasp low on the tapered portion of the instrument handle. Clinician B rests her ring finger on the second premolar.

Box 6-1   **Directions for Technique Practice**

1. The next two sections of this Module contain instructions for practicing finger rests for the mandibular posterior treatment areas of the mouth.

2. The photographs in the Technique Practice sections depict the use of a mirror and finger rests. Some photographs were taken on a patient. *Others were taken using a manikin and without gloves so that you can easily see the finger placement in the grasp.*

3. The photographs provide a *general guideline* for finger rests; however, the location of your own finger rest depends on the size and length of your fingers. You may need to fulcrum closer to or farther from the tooth being treated than is shown in the photograph.

4. Focus your attention on mastering wrist position, and the finger rests. Use the following instruments in this module:
   - **For your nondominant (mirror) hand**—Use a dental mirror.
   - **For your dominant (instrument) hand**—(a) Remove the mirror head from one of your dental mirrors and use the mirror handle as if it were a periodontal instrument, or (b) Use a periodontal probe to represent the periodontal instrument in this module.

5. Do not wear magnification loupes when practicing and perfecting your positioning and finger rest skills in this module. You need an unrestricted visual field for self-evaluation.

6. Remove Figure 6-1 from your book and refer to it as you practice and self-evaluate your skills during the Technique Practice.

Section 2
Technique Practice: RIGHT-Handed Clinician

SKILL BUILDING
Mandibular Posterior Sextants, Aspects Facing TOWARD the Clinician

Directions: Practice establishing a finger rest for the mandibular posterior aspects toward the clinician by referring to Figures 6-3 to 6-10 and Box 6-2.

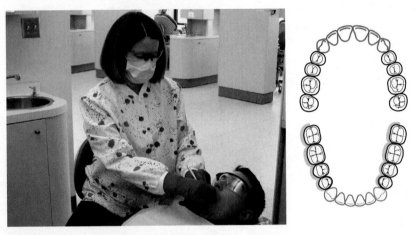

Figure 6-3. Clock Position for Mandibular Posterior Teeth, Aspects Facing Toward the Clinician. The clinician's clock position for the mandibular posterior aspects toward the clinician is the 9:00 position. The patient should be in a chin-down head position.

Box 6-2   Handle Positions for Mandibular Posterior Teeth

1. Hold the hand in a palm-down position.
2. Rest the handle against the index finger somewhere in the green shaded area.

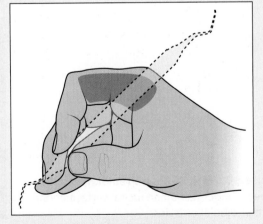

Figure 6-4. Handle Positions for Mandibular Posterior Treatment Areas.

Mandibular Right Posterior Sextant, Facial Aspect

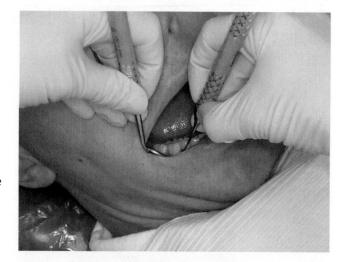

Figure 6-5. Mirror.
- Retract the buccal mucosa with the mirror. Use the mirror for indirect vision, particularly to view the distal surfaces of the teeth.
- Tip: Avoid resting the edge of the mirror head against the alveolar process.

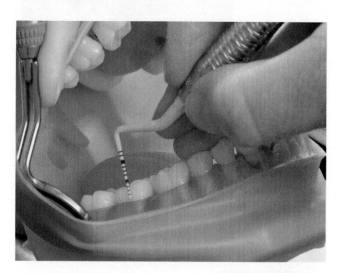

Figure 6-6. Task 1—Second Molar, Facial Aspect. Finger rest on an occlusal surface.

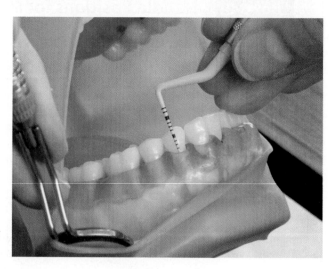

Figure 6-7. Task 2—First Premolar, Facial Aspect. Finger rest on an incisal surface of one of the mandibular anteriors.

Mandibular Left Posterior Sextant, Lingual Aspect

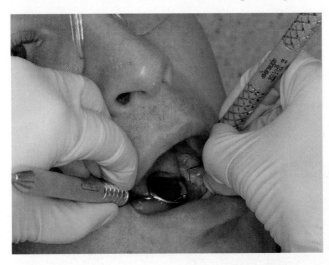

Figure 6-8. Mirror. Use the mirror to gently move the tongue away from the teeth, toward the midline of the mouth. Once in position, the mirror also is used for indirect vision of the tooth surfaces. Tip: Avoid pressing down against the floor of the mouth with the mirror head.

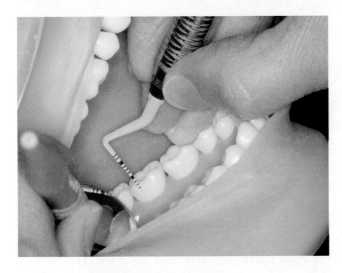

Figure 6-9. Task 1—Second Molar, Lingual Aspect. Finger rest on an occlusofacial line angle.

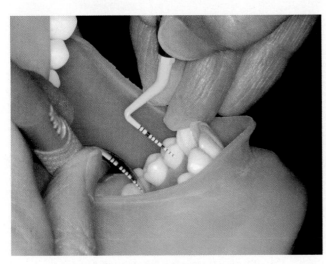

Figure 6-10. Task 2—First Premolar, Lingual Aspect. Finger rest on an incisal edge of one of the mandibular anterior teeth.

RIGHT-HANDED CLINICIAN

SKILL BUILDING
Mandibular Posterior Sextants, Aspects Facing AWAY From the Clinician

Directions: Practice establishing a finger rest for the mandibular posterior aspects facing away from the clinician by referring to Figures 6-11 to 6-18 and Box 6-3.

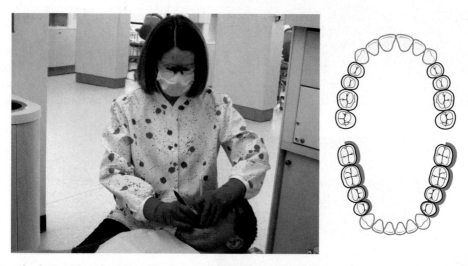

Figure 6-11. Clock Position for Mandibular Posterior Teeth, Aspects Facing Away From the Clinician.
The clinician's clock position for the mandibular posterior aspects facing away from the clinician is a 10:00 to 11:00 position. The patient should be in a chin-down head position.

| Box 6-3 | Handle Positions for Mandibular Posterior Teeth |

1. Hold the hand in a palm-down position.
2. Rest the handle against the index finger somewhere in the green shaded area.

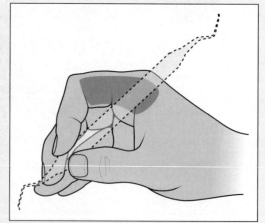

Figure 6-12. Handle Positions for Mandibular Posterior Treatment Areas.

RIGHT-HANDED CLINICIAN

Mandibular Left Posterior Sextant, Facial Aspect

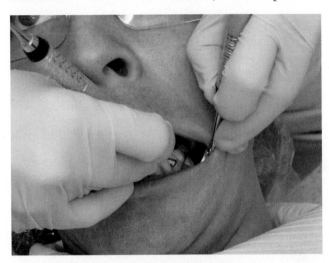

Figure 6-13. Retraction. Use the mirror to retract the buccal mucosa down and away from the teeth.

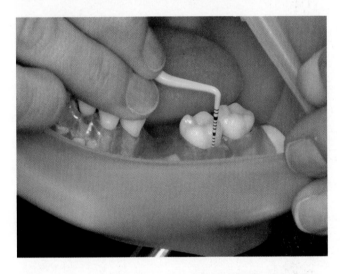

Figure 6-14. Task 1—Second Molar, Facial Aspect. Finger rest on an occlusofacial line angle.

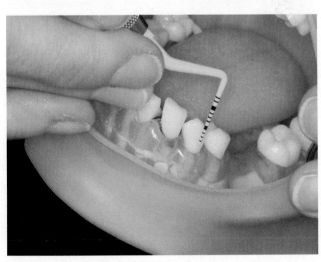

Figure 6-15. Task 2—First Premolar, Facial Aspect. Finger rest on an incisal edge of an anterior tooth.

Mandibular Right Posterior Sextant, Lingual Aspect

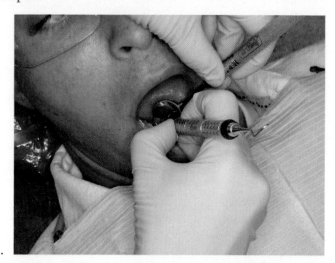

Figure 6-16. Mirror. Use the mirror head to push the tongue back gently so that the lingual surfaces of the teeth can be seen. Once in position, the mirror also is used for indirect vision.

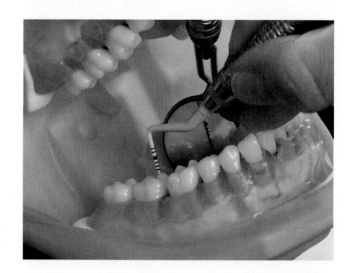

Figure 6-17. Task 1—Second Molar, Lingual Aspect. Finger rest on an occlusal surface.

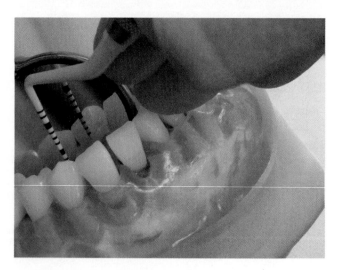

Figure 6-18. Task 2—First Premolar, Lingual Aspect. Finger rest on an incisal edge of an anterior tooth.

REFERENCE SHEET FOR MANDIBULAR POSTERIOR SEXTANTS

Photocopy this reference sheet and use it for quick reference as you practice your skills
(Table 6-1). Place the photocopied reference sheet in a plastic page protector for longer use.

TABLE 6-1. REFERENCE SHEET: MANDIBULAR POSTERIOR SEXTANTS

Treatment Area	Clock Position	Patient's Head
Posterior Aspects Facing Toward (Right Posterior, Facial Aspect) (Left Posterior, Lingual Aspect)	9:00	Straight or slightly away Chin DOWN
Posterior Aspects Facing Away (Right Posterior, Lingual Aspect) (Left Posterior, Facial Aspect)	10:00–11:00	Toward Chin DOWN

RIGHT-HANDED CLINICIAN

Section 3
Technique Practice: LEFT-Handed Clinician

SKILL BUILDING
Mandibular Posterior Sextants, Aspects Facing TOWARD the Clinician

Directions: Practice establishing a finger rest for the mandibular posterior aspects toward the clinician by referring to Figures 6-19 to 6-26 and Box 6-4.

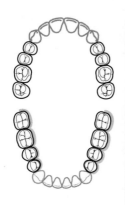
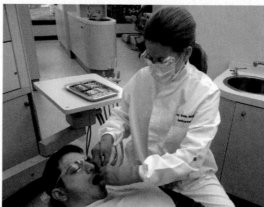

Figure 6-19. Clock Position for Mandibular Posterior Teeth, Aspects Facing Toward the Clinician. The clinician's clock position for the mandibular posterior aspects toward the clinician is the 3:00 position. The patient should be in a chin-down head position.

Box 6-4   Handle Positions for Mandibular Posterior Teeth

1. Hold the hand in a palm-down position.
2. Rest the handle against the index finger somewhere in the green shaded area.

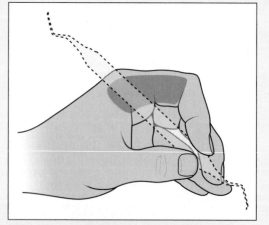

Figure 6-20. Handle Positions for Mandibular Posterior Treatment Areas.

Mandibular Left Posterior Sextant, Facial Aspect

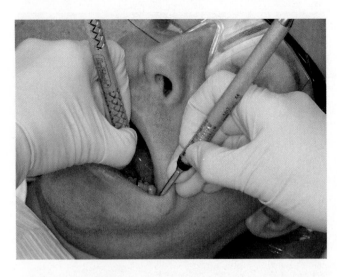

Figure 6-21. Mirror. Retract the buccal mucosa with the mirror. Use the mirror for indirect vision, particularly to view the distal surfaces of the teeth. Tip: Avoid resting the edge of the mirror head against the alveolar ridge.

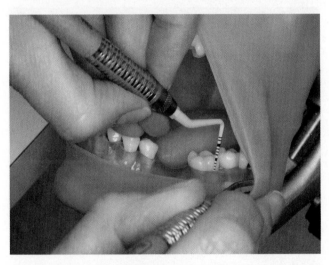

Figure 6-22. Task 1—Second Molar, Facial Aspect. Finger rest on an occlusal surface.

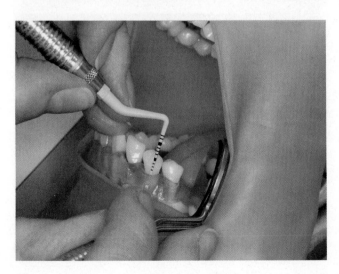

Figure 6-23. Task 2—First Premolar, Facial Aspect. Finger rest on an incisal surface of one of the mandibular anteriors.

LEFT-HANDED CLINICIAN

Mandibular Right Posterior Sextant, Lingual Aspect

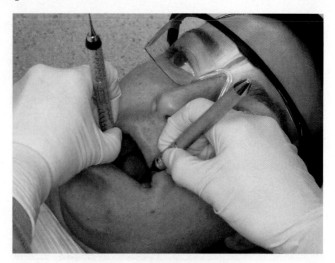

Figure 6-24. **Mirror.** Use the mirror to gently move the tongue away from the teeth, toward the midline of the mouth. Once in position, the mirror also is used for indirect vision of the tooth surfaces. Tip: Avoid pressing down against the floor of the mouth with the mirror head.

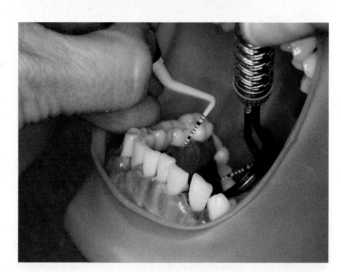

Figure 6-25. **Task 1—Second Molar, Lingual Aspect.** Finger rest on an occlusofacial line angle.

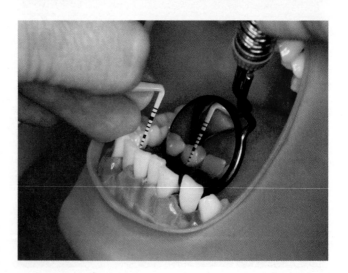

Figure 6-26. **Task 2—First Premolar, Lingual Aspect.** Finger rest on an incisal edge of one of the mandibular anterior teeth.

SKILL BUILDING
Mandibular Posterior Sextants, Aspects AWAY From the Clinician

Directions: Practice establishing a finger rest for the mandibular posterior aspects facing away from the clinician by referring to Figures 6-27 to 6-34 and Box 6-5.

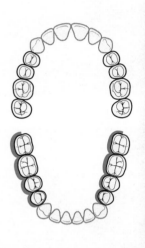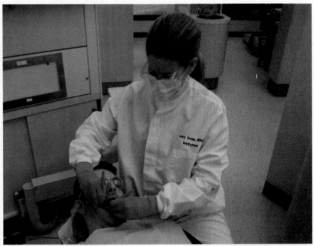

Figure 6-27. Clock Position for Mandibular Posterior Teeth, Aspects Facing Away From the Clinician. The clinician's clock position for the mandibular posterior aspects facing away from the clinician is a 1:00 to 2:00 position. The patient should be in a chin-down head position.

| Box 6-5 | Handle Positions for Mandibular Posterior Teeth |

1. Hold the hand in a palm-down position.
2. Rest the handle against the index finger somewhere in the green shaded area.

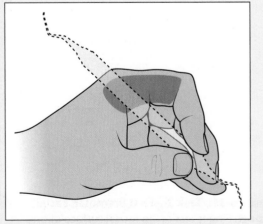

Figure 6-28. Handle Positions for Mandibular Posterior Treatment Areas.

Mandibular Right Posterior Sextant, Facial Aspect

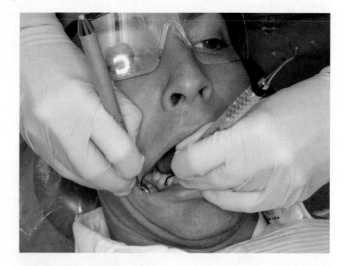

Figure 6-29. Retraction. Use the mirror to retract the buccal mucosa down and away from the teeth.

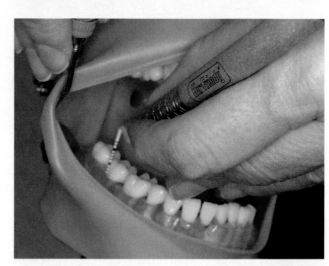

Figure 6-30. Task 1—Second Molar, Facial Aspect. Finger rest on an occlusofacial line angle.

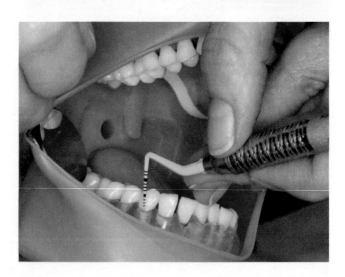

Figure 6-31. Task 2—First Premolar, Facial Aspect. Finger rest on an incisal surface of one of the mandibular anteriors.

Mandibular Left Posterior Sextant, Lingual Aspect

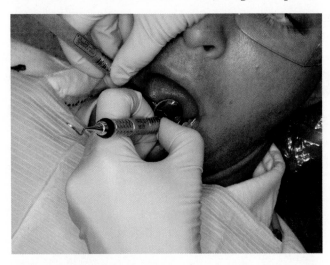

Figure 6-32. Mirror. Use the mirror head to push the tongue back gently so that the lingual surfaces of the teeth can be seen. Once in position, the mirror also is used for indirect vision.

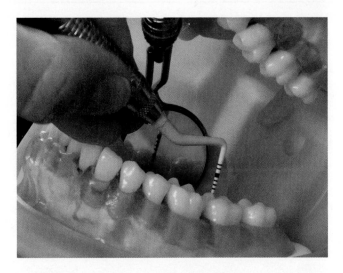

Figure 6-33. Task 1—Second Molar, Lingual Aspect. Finger rest on an occlusal surface.

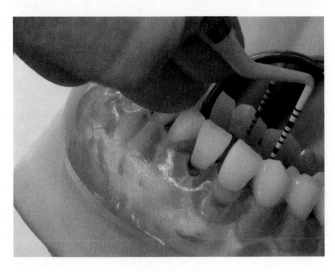

Figure 6-34. Task 2—First Premolar, Lingual Aspect. Finger rest on an incisal edge of an anterior tooth.

REFERENCE SHEET FOR MANDIBULAR POSTERIOR SEXTANTS

Photocopy this reference sheet and use it for quick reference as you practice your skills (Table 6-2). Place the photocopied reference sheet in a plastic page protector for longer use.

TABLE 6-2. REFERENCE SHEET: MANDIBULAR POSTERIOR SEXTANTS

Treatment Area	Clock Position	Patient's Head
Posterior Aspects Facing Toward (Left Posterior, Facial Aspect) (Right Posterior, Lingual Aspect)	3:00	Straight or slightly away Chin DOWN
Posterior Aspects Facing Away (Left Posterior, Lingual Aspect) (Right Posterior, Facial Aspect)	2:00–1:00	Toward Chin DOWN

LEFT-HANDED CLINICIAN

References

1. Dong H, Barr A, Loomer P, Rempel D. The effects of finger rest positions on hand muscle load and pinch force in simulated dental hygiene work. *J Dent Educ.* 2005;69(4):453–460.
2. Dong H, Loomer P, Villanueva A, Rempel D. Pinch forces and instrument tip forces during periodontal scaling. *J Periodontol.* 2007;78(1):97–103.
3. Meador HL. The biocentric technique: a guide to avoiding occupational pain. *J Dent Hyg.* 1993;67(1):38–51.
4. Millar D. Reinforced periodontal instrumentation and ergonomics. The best practice to ensure optimal performance and career longevity. *CDHA.* 2009;24(3):8–16.
5. Scaramucci M. Getting a grasp. *Dimens Dent Hyg.* 2008;6(5):24–26.
6. Hauser AM, Bowen DM. Primer on preclinical instruction and evaluation. *J Dent Educ.* 2009;73(3):390–398.

Suggested Readings

Leonard DM. The effectiveness of intervention strategies used to educate clients about prevention of upper extremity cumulative trauma disorders. *Work.* 2000;14(2):151–157.
Liskiewicz ST, Kerschbaum WE. Cumulative trauma disorders: an ergonomic approach for prevention. *J Dent Hyg.* 1997;71(4):162–167.
Marcoux BC, Krause V, Nieuwenhuijsen ER. Effectiveness of an educational intervention to increase knowledge and reduce use of risky behaviors associated with cumulative trauma in office workers. *Work.* 2000;14(2):127–135.
Michalak-Turcotte C. Controlling dental hygiene work-related musculoskeletal disorders: the ergonomic process. *J Dent Hyg.* 2000;74(1):41–48.
Sugawara E. The study of wrist postures of musicians using the WristSystem (Greenleaf Medical System). *Work.* 1999;13(3): 217–228.

Section 4
Skill Application

PRACTICAL FOCUS

HOW DOES POOR POSTURE AFFECT YOU?

To experience the importance of large motor skills for yourself, position your patient so that the tip of the patient's mouth is level with the mid-region of your chest (base of your sternum). Establish a finger rest in each of the mandibular treatment areas. What kind of muscle strain do you think you might experience if you were to work for several hours with the patient positioned in this manner? Unfortunately, many clinicians do not self-check their large motor skills (thinking these skills to be unimportant).

TECHNIQUE EVALUATION

Evaluate the photographs in Figures 6-35 to 6-37 for clinician and patient position, grasp, and finger rest. For each incorrect element describe (a) how the problem could be corrected and (b) the musculoskeletal problems that could result from each positioning problem.

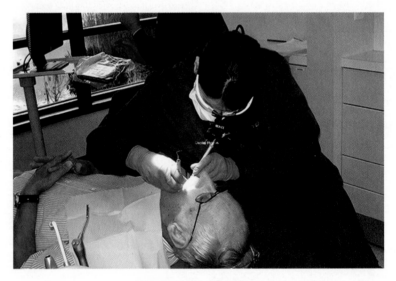

Figure 6-35. **Photo 1.**

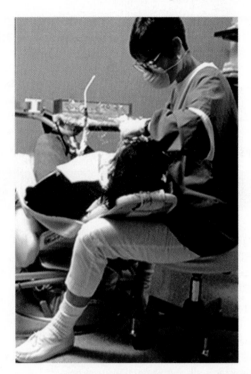

Figure 6-36. Photo 2.

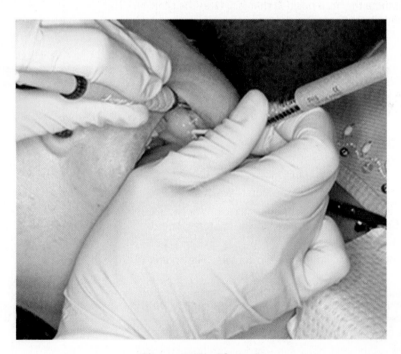

Figure 6-37. Photo 3.

Student Self Evaluation Module 6: Mirror and Rests in Mandibular Posterior Sextants

Student: _____

Date: _____

Area 1 = right posterior sextant, facial aspect
Area 2 = right posterior sextant, lingual aspect
Area 3 = left posterior sextant, facial aspect
Area 4 = left posterior sextant, lingual aspect

DIRECTIONS: Self-evaluate your skill level in each treatment area as: **S** (satisfactory) or **U** (unsatisfactory).

Criteria				
Positioning/Ergonomics	**Area 1**	**Area 2**	**Area 3**	**Area 4**
Adjusts clinician chair correctly				
Reclines patient chair and assures that patient's head is even with top of headrest				
Positions instrument tray within easy reach for front, side, or rear delivery as appropriate for operatory configuration				
Positions unit light at arm's length or dons dental headlight and adjusts it for use				
Assumes the recommended clock position				
Positions backrest of patient chair for the specified arch and adjusts height of patient chair so that clinician's elbows remain at waist level when accessing the specified treatment area				
Asks patient to assume the head position that facilitates the clinician's view of the specified treatment area				
Maintains neutral position				
Directs light to illuminate the specified treatment area				
Instrument Grasp: Dominant Hand	**Area 1**	**Area 2**	**Area 3**	**Area 4**
Grasps handle with tips of finger pads of index finger and thumb so that these fingers are opposite each other on the handle, but do NOT touch or overlap				
Rests pad of middle finger lightly on instrument shank; middle finger makes contact with ring finger				
Positions the thumb, index, and middle fingers in the "knuckles up" convex position; hyperextended joint position is avoided				
Holds ring finger straight so that it supports the weight of hand and instrument; ring finger position is "advanced ahead of" the other fingers in the grasp				
Keeps index, middle, ring and little fingers in contact; "like fingers inside a mitten"				
Maintains a relaxed grasp; fingers are NOT blanched in grasp				
Finger Rest: Dominant Hand	**Area 1**	**Area 2**	**Area 3**	**Area 4**
Establishes secure finger rest that is appropriate for tooth to be treated				
Once finger rest is established, pauses to self-evaluate finger placement in the grasp, verbalizes to evaluator his/her self-assessment of grasp, and corrects finger placement if necessary				

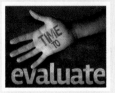

NOTE TO COURSE INSTRUCTORS: To download Module Evaluations for this textbook, go to http://thepoint.lww.com/GehrigFundamentals8e and log on to access the Instructor Resources for *Fundamentals of Periodontal Instrumentation and Advanced Root Instrumentation*.

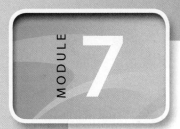

MODULE 7

Finger Rests in Maxillary Posterior Sextants

Module Overview

This module describes techniques for using a dental mirror and finger rests in the maxillary posterior treatment areas. The fulcrum reduces muscle load to the clinician's back, neck, arms, and hands; improves the precision of instrumentation strokes; and prevents loss of control of the instrument that could result in injury to the patient.

Module Outline

Section 1 **Building Blocks for Posterior Sextants** **171**
Building Blocks from Position to Finger Rest
Indirect Vision and Prevention of Musculoskeletal Strain

Section 2 **Technique Practice: RIGHT-Handed Clinician** **173**
Skill Building. Maxillary Posterior Sextants, Aspects Facing
   TOWARD the Clinician, p. 173
Skill Building. Maxillary Posterior Sextants, Aspects Facing
   AWAY From the Clinician, p. 176
Reference Sheet for Maxillary Posterior Sextants (Right-Handed Clinician)

Section 3 **Technique Practice: LEFT-Handed Clinician** **180**
Skill Building. Maxillary Posterior Sextants, Aspects Facing
   TOWARD the Clinician, p. 180
Skill Building. Maxillary Posterior Sextants, Aspects Facing
   AWAY From the Clinician, p. 183
Reference Sheet for Maxillary Posterior Sextants (Left-Handed Clinician)

Section 4 **Preventive Strategies: Stretches** **187**
Mini-Break Chairside Stretches
Hip-Hinge Technique Practice
After a Long Day: At Home Stretch

Section 5 **Skill Application** **190**
Practical Focus
Musculoskeletal Risk Assessment
Student Self Evaluation Module 7: Mirror and Rests in Maxillary Posterior Sextants

Key Terms: Review these key terms found in Chapter 5

Neutral wrist position   Support beam   Extraoral fulcrum
Fulcrum   Finger rest   Intraoral fulcrum

Learning Objectives

- Position equipment so that it enhances neutral positioning.
- While seated in the correct clock position for the treatment area, access the maxillary posterior teeth with optimum vision while maintaining neutral positioning.
- Demonstrate finger rests using precise finger placement on the handle of a periodontal instrument:
  - Finger pads of thumb and index finger opposite one another on handle
  - Thumb and index finger do not overlap each other on the handle
  - Pad of middle finger rests lightly on the shank
  - Thumb, index, and middle fingers in a neutral position
  - Ring finger is advanced ahead of the other fingers in the grasp, held straight and support the hand and instrument in the grasp
- Recognize incorrect mirror use, grasp, or finger rest and describe how to correct the problem(s).
- Understand the relationship between proper stabilization of the dominant hand during instrumentation and the prevention of (1) musculoskeletal problems in the clinician's hands and (2) injury to the patient.
- Understand the relationship between the large motor skills, such as positioning, and small motor skills, such as finger rests. Recognize the importance of initiating these skills in a step-by-step manner.
- Demonstrate exercises that lessen muscle imbalances through chairside stretching throughout the workday.

Optional online content is available for this module. If assigned by the course instructor, the online module: **Alternate Clock Positions** can be viewed at http://thepoint.lww.com/GehrigFundamentals8e

RIGHT- AND LEFT-HANDED SECTIONS IN THIS MODULE
- Sections 2 and 3 of this module are customized for right-handed and left-handed clinicians.
- For ease of use—and avoidance of confusion—if you are right-handed, it is recommended that you either (1) tear the left-handed pages from the book or (2) staple these pages together. If you are left-handed, use the same approach with the right-handed pages.

Section 1
Building Blocks for Posterior Sextants

BUILDING BLOCKS FROM POSITION TO FINGER REST

Precise, accurate performance of the building block skills is essential if periodontal instrumentation is to be effective, efficient, safe for the patient, and comfortable the clinician.

- Research on psychomotor skill acquisition indicates that a high level of mastery in the performance of skill building blocks is essential for successful mastery of periodontal instrumentation (1).
- The building block skills are the foundation that "supports" successful periodontal instrumentation.
- While practicing finger rests, it is important to complete each of the skills listed in Figure 7-1 in sequence.

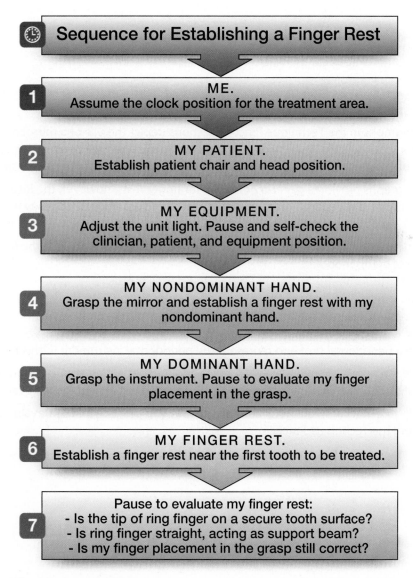

Sequence for Establishing a Finger Rest

1 ME.
Assume the clock position for the treatment area.

2 MY PATIENT.
Establish patient chair and head position.

3 MY EQUIPMENT.
Adjust the unit light. Pause and self-check the clinician, patient, and equipment position.

4 MY NONDOMINANT HAND.
Grasp the mirror and establish a finger rest with my nondominant hand.

5 MY DOMINANT HAND.
Grasp the instrument. Pause to evaluate my finger placement in the grasp.

6 MY FINGER REST.
Establish a finger rest near the first tooth to be treated.

7 Pause to evaluate my finger rest:
- Is the tip of ring finger on a secure tooth surface?
- Is ring finger straight, acting as support beam?
- Is my finger placement in the grasp still correct?

Figure 7-1. Establishing a Finger Rest. When establishing a finger rest it is important to proceed in the small, explicit steps outlined in this flow chart.

INDIRECT VISION AND PREVENTION OF MUSCULOSKELETAL STRAIN

Dental healthcare providers who routinely use a mirror for indirect vision have less pain in the neck, shoulders, or headaches than clinicians who used indirect vision less often (2). Clinicians who do not use a mirror for indirect vision tend to keep their heads bent to the side and rotated more than 15 degrees during patient treatment (3).

Experience the Difference for Yourself

1. Sit in the recommended clock position, and endeavor to view the lingual aspect of the maxillary right posterior sextant.
2. Without using a mirror, view these lingual surfaces. How does your body position change in order to view the lingual surfaces?
3. Now, view the lingual surfaces using indirect vision with a mirror. Compare your body position with and without the use of indirect vision.

Box 7-1 Directions for Technique Practice

1. The next two sections of this Module contain instructions for practicing finger rests for the maxillary posterior treatment areas of the mouth.

2. The photographs in the Technique Practice sections depict the use of a mirror and finger rests. Some photographs were taken on a patient. **Others were taken using a manikin and without gloves so that you can easily see the finger placement in the grasp.**

3. The photographs provide a **general guideline** for finger rests; however, the location of your own finger rest depends on the size and length of your fingers. You may need to fulcrum closer to or farther from the tooth being treated than is shown in the photograph.

4. Focus your attention on mastering wrist position, and the finger rests. Use the following instruments in this module:
   • **For your nondominant (mirror) hand**—Use a dental mirror.
   • **For your dominant (instrument) hand**
     (a) Remove the mirror head from one of your dental mirrors and use the mirror handle as if it were a periodontal instrument, or
     (b) Use a periodontal probe to represent the periodontal instrument in this module.

5. Do not wear magnification loupes when practicing and perfecting your positioning and finger rest skills in this module. You need an unrestricted visual field for self-evaluation.

6. Remove Figure 7-1 from your book and refer to it as you practice and self-evaluate your skills during the Technique Practice.

Section 2
Technique Practice: RIGHT-Handed Clinician

SKILL BUILDING
Maxillary Posterior Sextants, Aspects Facing TOWARD the Clinician

Directions: Practice establishing a finger rest for the maxillary posterior teeth, aspects facing toward, by referring to Figures 7-2 to 7-9 and Box 7-2.

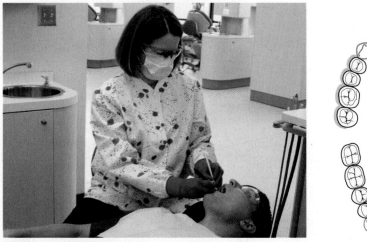

Figure 7-2. Clock Position for Maxillary Posterior Teeth, Aspects Facing Toward the Clinician. The clinician's clock position for the maxillary posterior aspects toward the clinician is the 9:00 position. The patient should be in a chin-up head position.

Box 7-2	Handle Positions for Maxillary Posterior Teeth

1. Hold the hand in a palm-up position.
2. Rest the handle against the index finger somewhere in the green shaded area.

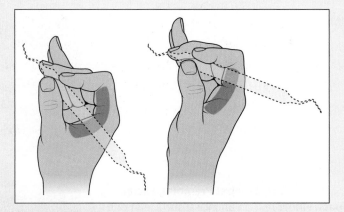

Figure 7-3. Handle Positions for Maxillary Posterior Treatment Areas.

Maxillary Right Posterior Sextant, Facial Aspect

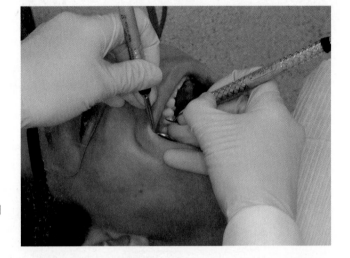

Figure 7-4. **Retraction.** Retract the buccal mucosa with the mirror. Use the mirror for indirect vision, particularly to view the distal surfaces of the teeth. Note the clinician pictured here is using an extraoral finger rest with the dental mirror.

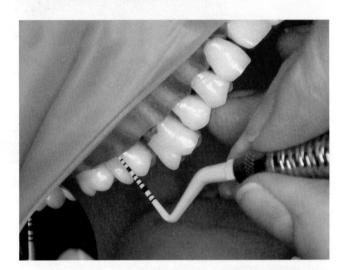

Figure 7-5. **Task 1—Second Molar, Facial Aspect.** Finger rest on an occlusal surface.

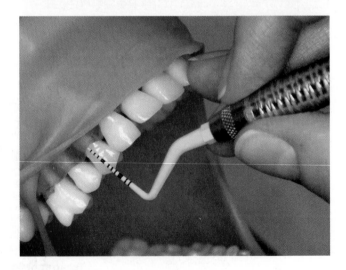

Figure 7-6. **Task 2—First Premolar, Facial Aspect.** Finger rest on an incisal surface of one of the maxillary anteriors.

Maxillary Left Posterior Sextant, Lingual Aspect

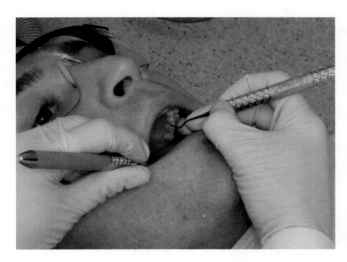

Figure 7-7. Mirror. Use the mirror to view the distal surfaces of the teeth.

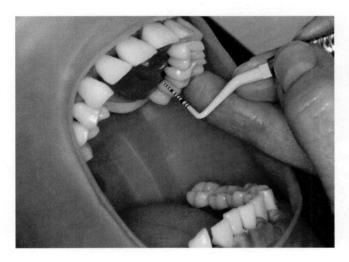

Figure 7-8. Task 1—Second Molar, Lingual Aspect. Finger rest on an occlusofacial line angle.

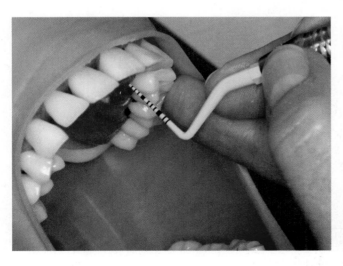

Figure 7-9. Task 2—First Premolar, Lingual Aspect. Finger rest on the occlusofacial line angle or an incisal edge.

RIGHT-HANDED CLINICIAN

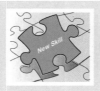

SKILL BUILDING
Maxillary Posterior Sextants, Aspects Facing AWAY From the Clinician

Directions: Practice establishing a finger rest for the maxillary posterior teeth, aspects facing away, by referring to Figures 7-10 to 7-17 and Box 7-3.

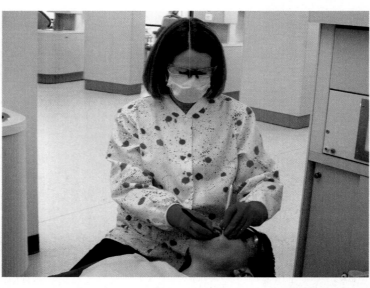

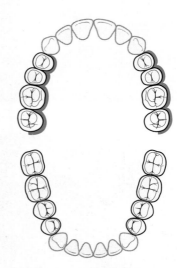

Figure 7-10. Clock Position for Maxillary Posterior Teeth, Aspects Facing Away From the Clinician. The clinician's clock position for the maxillary posterior aspects facing away from the clinician is a 10:00 to 11:00 position. The patient should be in a chin-up head position.

Box 7-3 **Handle Positions for Maxillary Posterior Teeth**

1. Hold the hand in a palm-up position.
2. Rest the handle against the index finger somewhere in the green shaded area.

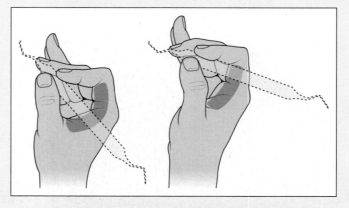

Figure 7-11. Handle Positions for Maxillary Posterior Treatment Areas.

Maxillary Left Posterior Sextant, Facial Aspect

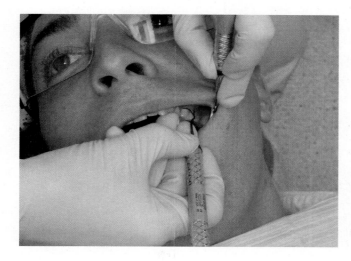

Figure 7-12. Mirror. Use the mirror to retract the buccal mucosa down and away from the teeth. Technique hint: your dominant hand is positioned correctly if you can see the underside of your middle and ring fingers.

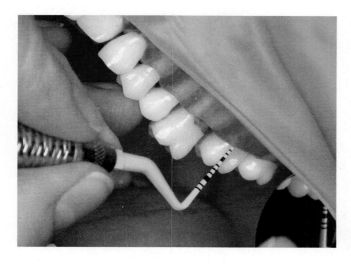

Figure 7-13. Task 1—Second Molar, Facial Aspect. Finger rest on an occlusal surface.

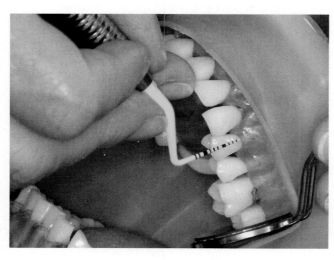

Figure 7-14. Task 2—First Premolar, Facial Aspect. Finger rest on an incisal edge of an anterior tooth.

RIGHT-HANDED CLINICIAN

Maxillary Right Posterior Sextant, Lingual Aspect

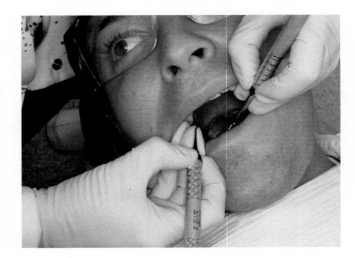

Figure 7-15. **Mirror.** Use the mirror for indirect vision.

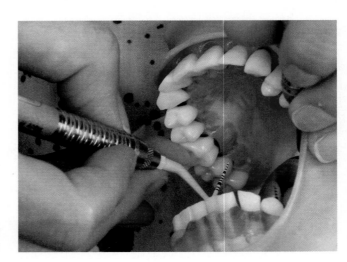

Figure 7-16. **Task 1—Second Molar, Lingual Aspect.** Finger rest on an occlusal surface.

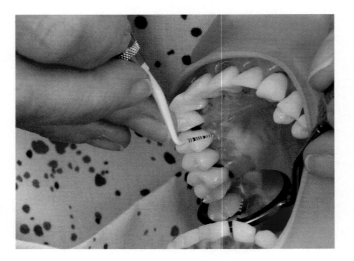

Figure 7-17. **Task 2—First Premolar, Lingual Aspect.** Finger rest on the occlusal surface or an incisal edge.

REFERENCE SHEET FOR MAXILLARY POSTERIOR SEXTANTS (RIGHT-HANDED CLINICIAN)

Photocopy this reference sheet (Table 7-1) and use it for quick reference as you practice your skills. Place the photocopied reference sheet in a plastic page protector for longer use.

TABLE 7-1. REFERENCE SHEET: MAXILLARY POSTERIOR SEXTANTS

Treatment Area	Clock Position	Patient's Head
Posterior Aspects Facing Toward Me (Right Posterior, Facial Aspect) (Left Posterior, Lingual Aspect)	9:00	Straight or slightly away Chin UP
Posterior Aspects Facing Away From Me (Right Posterior, Lingual Aspect) (Left Posterior, Facial Aspect)	10:00–11:00	Toward Chin UP

RIGHT-HANDED CLINICIAN

Section 3
Technique Practice: LEFT-Handed Clinician

SKILL BUILDING
Maxillary Posterior Sextants, Aspects Facing TOWARD the Clinician

Directions: Practice establishing a finger rest for the maxillary posterior teeth, aspects facing toward, by referring to Figures 7-18 to 7-25 and Box 7-4.

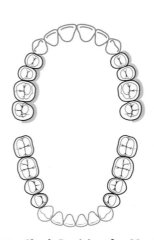

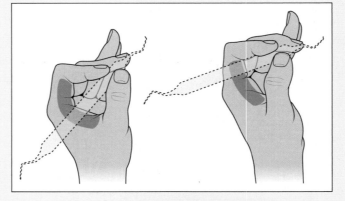

Figure 7-18. Clock Position for Maxillary Posterior Teeth, Aspects Facing Toward the Clinician. The clinician's clock position for the maxillary posterior aspects toward the clinician is the 3:00 position. The patient should be in a chin-up head position.

Box 7-4   Handle Positions for Maxillary Posterior Teeth

1. Hold the hand in a palm-up position.
2. Rest the handle against the index finger somewhere in the green shaded area.

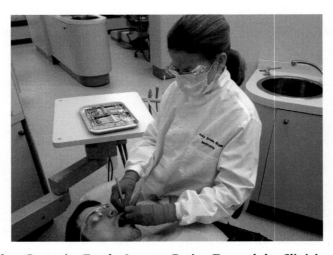

Figure 7-19. Handle Positions for Maxillary Posterior Treatment Areas.

Maxillary Left Posterior Sextant, Facial Aspect

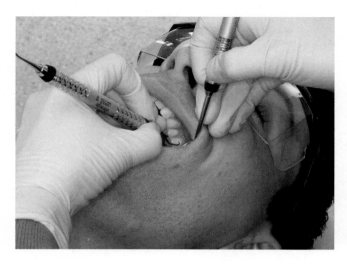

Figure 7-20. Mirror. Retract the buccal mucosa with the mirror. Use the mirror for indirect vision, particularly to view the distal surfaces of the teeth. Note the clinician pictured here is using an extraoral finger rest with the dental mirror.

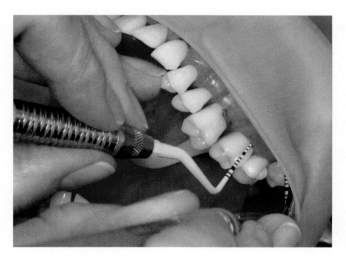

Figure 7-21. Task 1—Second Molar, Facial Aspect. Finger rest on an occlusal surface.

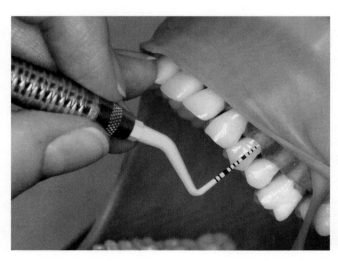

Figure 7-22. Task 2—First Premolar, Facial Aspect. Finger rest on an incisal surface of one of the maxillary anteriors.

LEFT-HANDED CLINICIAN

Maxillary Right Posterior Sextant, Lingual Aspect

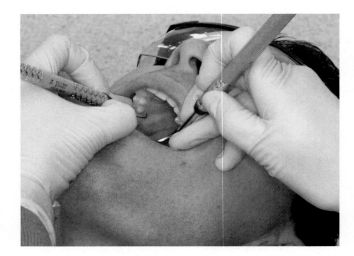

Figure 7-23. Mirror. Use the mirror to view the distal surfaces of the teeth.

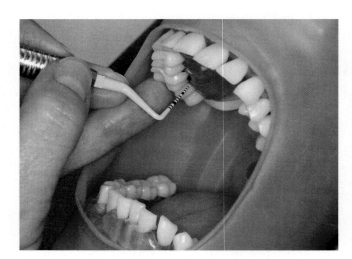

Figure 7-24. Task 1—Second Molar, Lingual Aspect. Finger rest on an occlusofacial line angle.

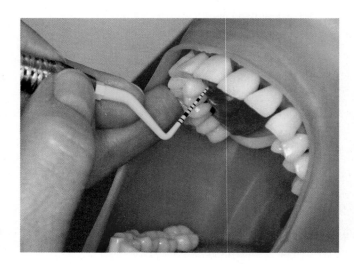

Figure 7-25. Task 2—First Premolar, Lingual Aspect. Finger rest on the occlusofacial line angle or an incisal edge.

SKILL BUILDING
Maxillary Posterior Sextants, Aspects Facing AWAY From the Clinician

Directions: Practice establishing a finger rest for the maxillary posterior teeth, aspects facing away, by referring to Figures 7-26 to 7-33 and Box 7-5.

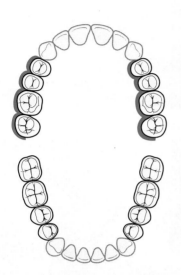

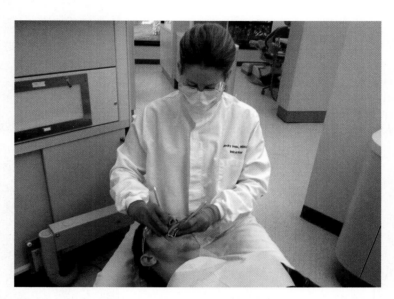

Figure 7-26. Clock Position for Maxillary Posterior Teeth, Aspects Facing Away From the Clinician. The clinician's clock position for the maxillary posterior aspects facing away from the clinician is a 1:00 to 2:00 position. The patient should be in a chin-up head position.

Box 7-5 | Handle Positions for Maxillary Posterior Teeth

1. Hold the hand in a palm-up position.
2. Rest the handle against the index finger somewhere in the green shaded area.

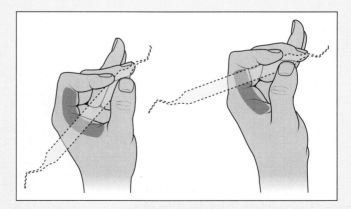

Figure 7-27. Handle Positions for Maxillary Posterior Treatment Areas.

Maxillary Right Posterior Sextant, Facial Aspect

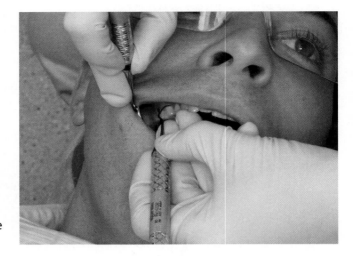

Figure 7-28. Mirror. Use the mirror to retract the buccal mucosa down and away from the teeth. Technique hint: your dominant hand is positioned correctly if you can see the underside of your middle and ring fingers.

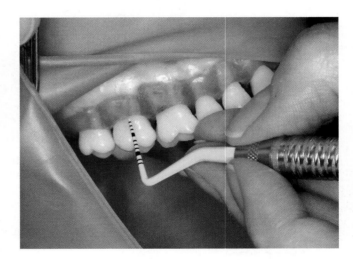

Figure 7-29. Task 1—Second Molar, Facial Aspect. Finger rest on an occlusal surface.

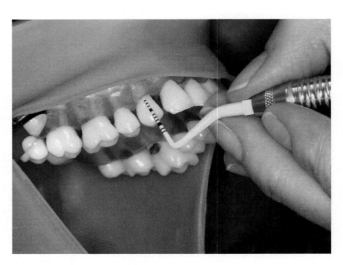

Figure 7-30. Task 2—First Premolar, Facial Aspect. Finger rest on an incisal edge of an anterior tooth.

Maxillary Left Posterior Sextant, Lingual Aspect

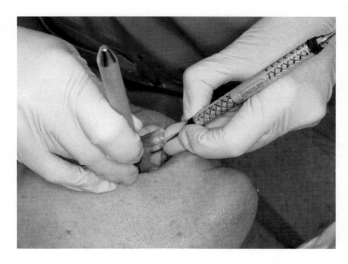

Figure 7-31. Mirror. Use the mirror for indirect vision.

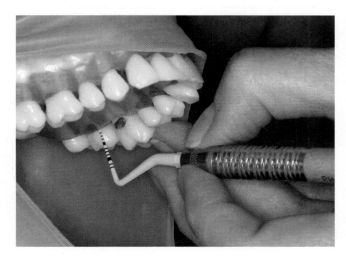

Figure 7-32. Task 1—Second Molar, Lingual Aspect. Finger rest on an occlusal surface.

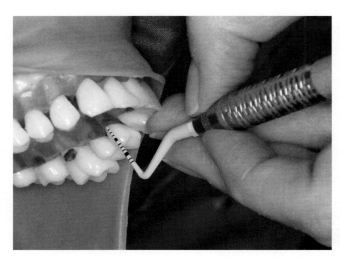

Figure 7-33. Task 2—First Premolar, Lingual Aspect. Finger rest on the occlusal surface or an incisal edge.

LEFT-HANDED CLINICIAN

REFERENCE SHEET FOR MAXILLARY POSTERIOR SEXTANTS (LEFT-HANDED CLINICIAN)

Photocopy this reference sheet and use it for quick reference as you practice your skills (Table 7-2). Place the photocopied reference sheet in a plastic page protector for longer use.

TABLE 7-2. REFERENCE SHEET: MAXILLARY POSTERIOR SEXTANTS		
Treatment Area	**Clock Position**	**Patient's Head**
Posterior Aspects Facing Toward Me (Left Posterior, Facial Aspect) (Right Posterior, Lingual Aspect)	3:00	Straight or slightly away Chin UP
Posterior Aspects Facing Away From Me (Left Posterior, Lingual Aspect) (Right Posterior, Facial Aspect)	2:00–1:00	Toward Chin UP

LEFT-HANDED CLINICIAN

Section 4
Preventive Strategies: Stretches

Stretching can promote dynamic movement that is important for muscle health, balance of forces, and blood flow. Dental professionals should perform stretches throughout the day, using the time between patients. Clinicians should hold stretches for 10 to 30 seconds, stretching muscle groups in the opposite direction of static positions (4,5).

1. Strong postural muscles of the trunk and shoulders stabilize the body in the neutral seated position, allowing the arms and hands to perform the exacting task of periodontal instrumentation.
2. Most dental hygienists sit for sustained periods of time in static positions that can cause muscle tension and stiffness. Over time unbalanced seated positions cause muscle imbalances—tightness in one muscle group and weakness in the opposing group—leading to musculoskeletal pain.
3. Performing stretching exercises offers numerous benefits (Boxes 7-6 and 7-7).
   a. Many authors recommend short work breaks and a routine of chairside stretching throughout the day between patients (1,6–10).
   b. A schedule of brief, yet frequent rest periods is more beneficial than lengthy infrequent stretching breaks. Chairside stretches should be performed every 30 to 60 minutes throughout the day.
4. Figure 7-34 shows stretches that can be performed at chairside. Place this guide in a plastic page protector for use in the preclinical/clinical setting.

Box 7-6 **Benefits of Stretching**

- Warms up muscles before beginning to work (9)
- Helps prevent muscle strains and spasms (9,11)
- Decreases muscle soreness and tender spots (9,12)
- Increases production of joint synovial fluid to reduce friction between joints during movement (1)
- Increases range of motion, which promotes increased flexibility (9,13,14)
- Increases coordination which enhances control of fine motor skills (9,15)
- Increases nutrient supply to the vertebral discs of the spine (9)
- Reduces stress and promotes relaxation (9,16,17)

Box 7-7 **How to Stretch Safely**

- Assume the starting position for the stretch.
- Breathe in deeply as you begin the stretch.
- Hold the stretch for about 10 seconds.
- Slowly release the stretch as you return to the starting position. Repeat the stretch if time allows.
- Never stretch in a painful range. If stretching increases your pain, stop immediately.

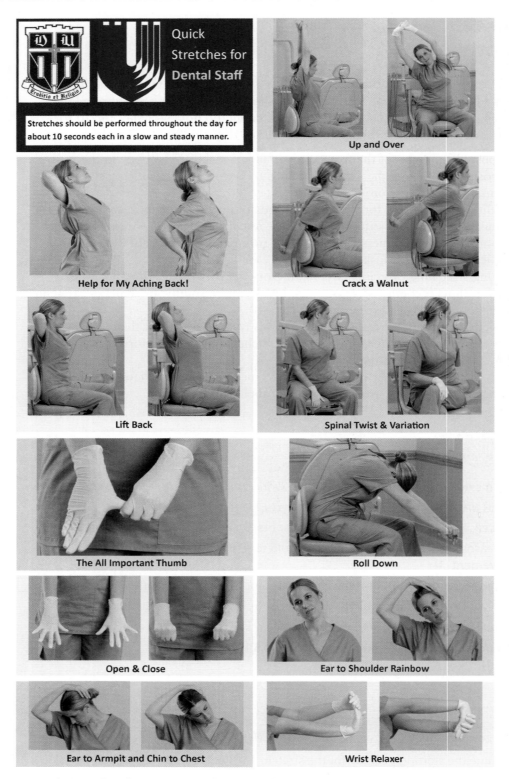

Figure 7-34. Quick Stretches for Dental Staff. Complements of Duke Ergonomics Program (919–668-ERGO) and Juli Kagan (18).

References

1. Hauser AM, Bowen DM. Primer on preclinical instruction and evaluation. *J Dent Educ.* 2009;73(3):390–398.
2. Rundcrantz BL, Johnsson B, Moritz U. Cervical pain and discomfort among dentists. Epidemiological, clinical and therapeutic aspects. Part 1. A survey of pain and discomfort. *Swed Dent J.* 1990;14(2):71–80.
3. Rundcrantz BL, Johnsson B, Moritz U. Occupational cervico-brachial disorders among dentists. Analysis of ergonomics and locomotor functions. *Swed Dent J.* 1991;15(3):105–115.
4. Sanders MJ. Ergonomics and the management of musculoskeletal disorders. 2nd ed. St. Louis, MO: Butterworth-Heinemann; 2004:556.
5. Sanders MA, Turcotte CM. Strategies to reduce work-related musculoskeletal disorders in dental hygienists: two case studies. *J Hand Ther.* 2002;15(4):363–374.
6. Andrews N, Vigoren G. Ergonomics : muscle fatigue, posture, magnification, and illumination. *Compend Contin Educ Dent.* 2002;23(3):261–266, 268, 270 passim; quiz 74.
7. Dylla J, Forrest J. Stretching and strengthening for balance and stability: Part 1. *Access.* 2006(11):38–43.
8. Tovoc T, Gutmann M. Making the principles of ergonomics work for you. *Dimens Dent Hyg.* 2005;3(1):16–18, 20–21.
9. Valachi B. Practice dentistry pain-free: evidence-based strategies to prevent pain and extend your career. Portland, OR: Posturedontics Press; 2008:239.
10. Wann O, Canull B. Ergonomics and dental hygienists. *Contemp Oral Hyg.* 2003;3(5):16–22.
11. Coppin RJ, Wicke DM, Little PS. Managing nocturnal leg cramps—calf-stretching exercises and cessation of quinine treatment: a factorial randomised controlled trial. *Br J Gen Pract.* 2005;55(512):186–191.
12. Rahnama N, Rahmani-Nia F, Ebrahim K. The isolated and combined effects of selected physical activity and ibuprofen on delayed-onset muscle soreness. *J Sports Sci.* 2005;23(8):843–850.
13. Decicco PV, Fisher MM. The effects of proprioceptive neuromuscular facilitation stretching on shoulder range of motion in overhand athletes. *J Sports Med Phys Fitness.* 2005;45(2):183–187.
14. Decoster LC, Cleland J, Altieri C, Russell P. The effects of hamstring stretching on range of motion: a systematic literature review. *J Orthop Sports Phys Ther.* 2005;35(6):377–387.
15. Lane JM, Nydick M. Osteoporosis: current modes of prevention and treatment. *J Am Acad Orthop Surg.* 1999;7(1):19–31.
16. Khasky AD, Smith JC. Stress, relaxation states, and creativity. *Percept Mot Skills.* 1999;88(2):409–416.
17. Parshad O. Role of yoga in stress management. *West Indian Med J.* 2004;53(3):191–194.
18. Kagan J. Mind your body: Pilates for the seated professional. 1st ed: Pleasant Ridge, MI: MindBody Publishing; 2007.

Section 5
Skill Application

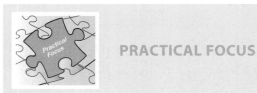

PRACTICAL FOCUS

MUSCULOSKELETAL RISK ASSESSMENT

Do you sometimes forget about neutral body position as you concentrate on the finger rests? Use this checklist to assess your habits. *A "YES" answer means that changes are indicated.*

TABLE 7-3. BODY BREAKERS RISK ASSESSMENT CHECKLIST

Structure	Incorrect Body Mechanics	YES	NO
Head	Tilted to one side?	☐	☐
	Tipped too far forward?	☐	☐
Shoulders	Lifted up toward ears?	☐	☐
	Tense?	☐	☐
	Hunched forward?	☐	☐
Upper Arms	Held more than 20 degrees away from body?	☐	☐
Elbows	Held above waist level?	☐	☐
Wrists	Hand bent up? down?	☐	☐
	Hand angled toward thumb? toward little finger?	☐	☐
	Thumb-side of palm tipped down?	☐	☐
Hands	Gloves too tight?	☐	☐
	Fingers blanched in grasp?	☐	☐
	Fingers tense?	☐	☐
Back	Rounded back?	☐	☐
Hips	Perched forward on seat?	☐	☐
	All weight on one hip?	☐	☐
Legs	Under back of patient's chair?	☐	☐
	Thighs "cut" by edge of chair seat?	☐	☐
	Legs crossed?	☐	☐
Feet	Dangling?	☐	☐
	Ankles crossed?	☐	☐

TECHNIQUE EVALUATION

Evaluate the photographs in Figures 7-35 and 7-36 for clinician and patient position, grasp, and finger rest. For each incorrect element describe (a) how the problem could be corrected and (b) the musculoskeletal problems that could result from each positioning problem.

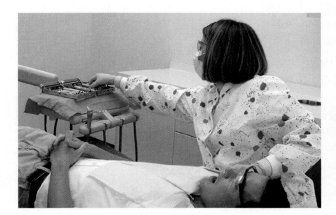

Figure 7-35. Photo 1.

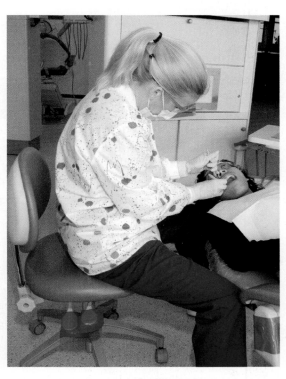

Figure 7-36. Photo 2.

PRACTICE FOR PRECISE INSTRUMENT CONTROL WITH INDIRECT VISION

This activity simulates the skills you will need to use when placing the instrument's working end on the various tooth surfaces while using indirect vision.

Materials and Equipment: Printed page from a textbook or magazine, a dental mirror, and a sharpened pencil.

- Lay the printed page flat on a desk or tabletop. Hold a dental mirror in your nondominant hand and position it on the page. Angle the mirror head so that you are able to see several letters reflected in the mirror. How do the letters appear?
- Still looking in the mirror, locate a letter "e" in one of the words. Grasp the pencil in a modified pen grasp and touch the pencil point to the "e" *on the paper.*
- Move the mirror to a different location on the paper. Looking in the mirror, select a letter and touch it with the pencil point.

Student Self Evaluation Module 7: Mirror and Rests in Maxillary Posterior Sextants

Student: _____

Date: _____

Area 1 = right posterior sextant, facial aspect
Area 2 = right posterior sextant, lingual aspect
Area 3 = left posterior sextant, facial aspect
Area 4 = left posterior sextant, lingual aspect

DIRECTIONS: Self-evaluate your skill level in each treatment area as: **S** (satisfactory) or **U** (unsatisfactory).

Criteria				
Positioning/Ergonomics	**Area 1**	**Area 2**	**Area 3**	**Area 4**
Adjusts clinician chair correctly				
Reclines patient chair and assures that patient's head is even with top of headrest				
Positions instrument tray within easy reach for front, side, or rear delivery as appropriate for operatory configuration				
Positions unit light at arm's length or dons dental headlight and adjusts it for use				
Assumes the recommended clock position				
Positions backrest of patient chair for the specified arch and adjusts height of patient chair so that clinician's elbows remain at waist level when accessing the specified treatment area				
Asks patient to assume the head position that facilitates the clinician's view of the specified treatment area				
Maintains neutral position				
Directs light to illuminate the specified treatment area				
Instrument Grasp: Dominant Hand	**Area 1**	**Area 2**	**Area 3**	**Area 4**
Grasps handle with tips of finger pads of index finger and thumb so that these fingers are opposite each other on the handle, but do NOT touch or overlap				
Rests pad of middle finger lightly on instrument shank; middle finger makes contact with ring finger				
Positions the thumb, index, and middle fingers in the "knuckles up" convex position; hyperextended joint position is avoided				
Holds ring finger straight so that it supports the weight of hand and instrument; ring finger position is "advanced ahead of" the other fingers in the grasp				
Keeps index, middle, ring, and little fingers in contact; "like fingers inside a mitten"				
Maintains a relaxed grasp; fingers are NOT blanched in grasp				
Finger Rest: Dominant Hand	**Area 1**	**Area 2**	**Area 3**	**Area 4**
Establishes secure finger rest that is appropriate for tooth to be treated				
Once finger rest is established, pauses to self-evaluate finger placement in the grasp, verbalizes to evaluator his/her self-assessment of grasp, and corrects finger placement if necessary				

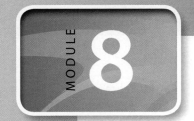

MODULE

8

Instrument Design and Classification

Module Overview

Module 8 introduces the various design characteristics of periodontal instruments. To select an appropriate instrument for a particular instrumentation task, the clinician must have a thorough understanding of the design features of the handles, shanks, and working-ends of periodontal instruments. With so many instruments currently on the market and new designs introduced regularly, it is impossible for any one clinician to recognize each instrument by name. Fortunately, a clinician who understands the principles of design and classification can easily determine the intended use of any unfamiliar instrument.

Module Outline

Section 1   **Design Characteristics of Instrument Handle**   **195**
The Significance of Handle Design

Section 2   **Design Characteristics of Instrument Shank**   **198**
Simple and Complex Shank Design
Application of Simple and Complex Shanks to the Teeth
Shank Flexibility and the Instrumentation Task
Functional and Lower Shank Identification

Section 3   **Design Characteristics of Instrument Working-End**   **202**
Single and Double-Ended Instruments
Design Name and Number
Working-End Identification
Parts of the Working-End
The Working-End in Cross Section

Section 4   **Introduction to Instrument Classification**   **207**

Section 5   **Skill Application**   **210**
Practical Focus
Skill Self Evaluation Module 8: Instrument Design and Classification

Key Terms

Knurling pattern
Balanced instrument
Simple shank design
Complex shank design
Rigid shank
Flexible shank
Visual information
Tactile sensitivity
Vibrations
Functional shank

Lower shank
Terminal shank
Extended lower shank
Unpaired working-ends
Paired working-ends
Design name
Design number
Face
Back
Lateral surfaces

Cutting edge
Toe of working-end
Tip of working-end
Cross section
Classifications
Periodontal probe
Explorer
Sickle scaler
Curet
Periodontal file

Learning Objectives

- Identify each working-end of a periodontal instrument by its design name and number.

- Recognize the design features of instrument handles and shanks, and discuss how these design features relate to the instrument's use.

- Describe the advantages and limitations of the various design features available for instrument handles and shanks.

- Given a variety of periodontal instruments, demonstrate the ability to select instruments with handle design characteristics that will reduce the pinch force required to grasp the instrument.

- Given a variety of periodontal instruments, sort the instruments into those with simple shank design and those with complex shank design.

- Given a variety of sickle scalers and curets, identify the face, back, lateral surfaces, cutting edges, and toe or tip on each working-end.

- Given a variety of periodontal instruments, determine the intended use of each instrument by evaluating its design features and classification.

- Given any instrument, identify where and how it may be used on the dentition (i.e., assessment or calculus removal, anterior/posterior teeth, supragingival or subgingival use).

Section 1
Design Characteristics of Instrument Handle

The design characteristics of periodontal instruments vary widely from manufacturer to manufacturer. Selecting instruments with ergonomic design is important in the prevention of musculoskeletal injury during instrumentation. The design characteristics of the handle, shank, and working-end should be considered when selecting instruments for periodontal instrumentation. Identification of the parts of a periodontal instrument is reviewed in Figure 8-1.

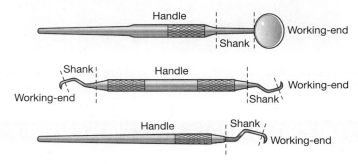

Figure 8-1. Parts of a Periodontal Instrument. The parts of a periodontal instrument are the handle, the shank, and the working-end.

THE SIGNIFICANCE OF HANDLE DESIGN

1. Effect of Handle Shape on Muscle Load and Pinch Force
   A. Carpal Tunnel Syndrome and Dental Hygiene
      1. Among all occupations in the United States, dental hygiene ranks the highest by the Bureau of Labor Statistics in the number of carpal tunnel syndromes cases (1).
      2. Risk factors for carpal tunnel syndrome in dental hygienists includes repetitive forceful pinching during periodontal instrumentation and sustained non-neutral wrist positions (2–6).
   B. Pinch Force in the Grasp
      1. The average pinch force exerted during periodontal instrumentation is 11% to 20% of the clinician's maximum pinch strength (7).
      2. Relaxing the fingers of the grasp between instrumentation strokes reduces the pinch force required during periodontal instrumentation.
   C. Variation in Handle Design
      1. The design characteristics of instrument handles vary greatly among instrument manufacturers. Ergonomically designed periodontal instruments may help reduce the prevalence of carpal tunnel syndrome among dental hygienists and periodontists (8,9).
      2. The weight and diameter of periodontal instrument handles has significant effects on the hand muscle load and pinch form of clinicians performing periodontal instrumentation (8,9). Figure 8-2 shows examples of different handle diameters and texture.

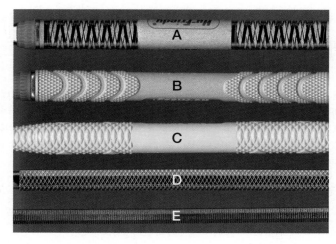

Figure 8-2. Handle Diameter and Texturing. The diameter and texturing of a handle varies greatly from manufacturer to manufacturer. Shown here are examples of the variations in design characteristics of instrument handles.

TABLE 8-1. HANDLE SELECTION CRITERIA

Recommended:	**Avoid:**
• Large handle diameter (10 mm)	• Small handle diameter (6 mm)
• Lightweight hollow handle (≥15 g)	• Heavy, solid metal handle
• Handle tapers near shank	• Nontapered handle
• Raised texturing	• No texturing or nonraised texturing

2. **Criteria for Selecting Instrument Handles.** In selecting an instrument handle, there are several characteristics to consider: (1) weight, (2) diameter, (3) taper, and (4) texture (8–14). Table 8-1 summarizes criteria for selecting instruments with ergonomic handle design.
   A. **Instrument Weight**
      1. An instrument that is lightweight—15 g or less—is optimal for periodontal instrumentation (8,9,13,14).
      2. Lightweight instruments place less stress on the muscles of the hand during periodontal instrumentation. Periodontal instruments with heavier weight handles are associated with greater muscle activity (8,9).
   B. **Handle Diameter and Taper**
      1. An instrument with a large diameter handle (10 mm) requires the least amount of pinch force while traditional smaller handle diameters (7 mm) are associated with greater pinch force and tend to cause muscle cramping (8,9,13,15).
      2. A round instrument handle, compared to a hexagon-shaped handle, reduces muscle force and compression (9,16).
      3. In order to minimize the effect of the pinch grasp, it may be helpful to select handles in a range of larger diameters; thus, providing some variety for the muscles of the fingers (10–12,14).
      4. Instrument handles that taper at the end of the handle where it is grasped may decrease pinch force by improving the coupling of the finger pads to the handle (reduced slipping of fingers) during instrumentation in the wet environment of the oral cavity (9). A taper to the instrument handle resulted in a 11% reduction of average pinch force compared to a non-tapered instrument handle (9).

5. Dong et al. (9) found that a lightweight instrument with a round and tapered shape and a large diameter (10 mm) handle requires the least pinch force during use.

C. **Handle Texture.** Another term for texturing is a **knurling pattern**. Texturing increases the static friction between the fingers and handle resulting in reduced pinch force in the grasp (17–20).

1. Handles with no texturing decrease control of the instrument in the wet environment of the oral cavity and increase muscle fatigue.

2. Handles with raised texturing are easier to hold in the wet oral environment, thus maximizing control of the instrument and reducing muscle fatigue (20).

3. **Instrument Balance.** A periodontal instrumented is said to be **balanced** when its working-ends are aligned with an imaginary line that runs vertically through the center of the handle lengthwise (the long axis of the handle). Figure 8-3 compares an instrument that is not balanced with a balanced instrument.

- During instrumentation, balance insures that finger pressure applied against the handle is transferred to the working-end resulting in pressure against the tooth.
- An instrument that is not balanced is more difficult to use and stresses the muscles of the hand and arm.
- An easy method for determining if an instrument is balanced is to place the instrument on a line of a lined writing tablet. Align the midline of the handle with a line on the paper; the instrument is balanced if the working-ends are centered on the line.

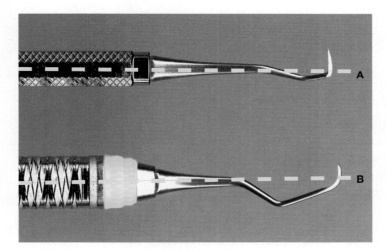

Figure 8-3. Instrument Balance. An instrument in which the working-end is aligned with the long axis of the handle is termed balanced. A balanced instrument assures that pressure applied with the fingers against the handle is transferred to the working-end. In the photograph above, instrument **A** is not balanced. Instrument **B** is balanced since the working-end is centered on a line running through the long axis of the handle.

Section 2
Design Characteristics of Instrument Shank

SIMPLE AND COMPLEX SHANK DESIGN

The shanks of most periodontal instruments are bent in one or more places to facilitate placement of the working-end against the tooth surface.

1. Simple shank design—a shank that is bent in one plane (front-to-back). Figure 8-4A shows a curet with a simple shank design. Application of an instrument with a simple shank is shown in Figure 8-5.
   a. Another term for a simple shank is a straight shank.
   b. Instruments with simple shanks are used primarily on anterior teeth.
2. Complex shank design—a shank that is bent in two planes (front-to-back and side-to-side) to facilitate instrumentation of posterior teeth. Figure 8-4B shows a curet with a complex shank design. Application of an instrument with a complex shank is illustrated in Figures 8-6 and 8-7.
   a. Another term for a complex shank is an angled or curved shank.
   b. The crowns of posterior teeth are rounded and overhang their roots. An instrument with a complex shank is needed to reach around a posterior crown and onto the root surface.

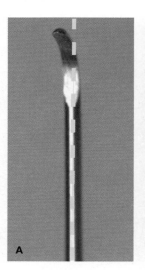 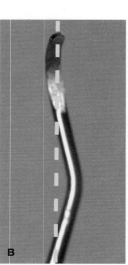

Figure 8-4. Simple and Complex Shank Design.

To determine whether the shank is simple or complex, hold the instrument so that the working-end tip or toe is facing you.
- Instrument A has a simple shank design.
- Instrument B has a complex shank design.

APPLICATION OF SIMPLE AND COMPLEX SHANKS TO THE TEETH

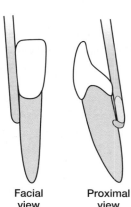

Figure 8-5. Simple Shank on an Anterior Tooth. The crowns of anterior teeth are wedge-shaped. A simple straight shank design is adequate to reach along the crown and onto the root surface.

Facial view   Proximal view

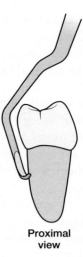

Figure 8-6. Complex Shank on a Lingual Surface. The illustration shows a mandibular molar when viewed from the mesial aspect. The drawing depicts the shank bends that allow the working-end to be placed on the lingual surface of the tooth root.

Front-to-back shank bends enable the working-end to reach around the crown and onto the lingual and facial surfaces of the root.

Proximal view

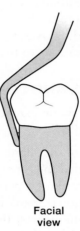

Figure 8-7. Complex Shank on a Proximal Surface. The illustration shows a mandibular molar when viewed from the facial aspect. The drawing depicts the shank bends that allow the working-end to be placed on the proximal surface of the tooth root.

Side-to-side shank bends enable the working-end to reach around the crown and onto proximal (mesial and distal) surfaces of the tooth.

Facial view

SHANK FLEXIBILITY AND THE INSTRUMENTATION TASK

An important characteristic of an instrument shank is its strength. To remove calculus deposits, the clinician applies pressure against the handle and shank to press the working-end against the tooth surface. The type and diameter of metal used in a shank determines its strength. Instrument shanks are classified as either rigid or flexible in design.

1. Rigid shank—an instrument shank that will withstand the pressure needed to remove heavy calculus deposits. A large calculus deposit can be removed more quickly and with less effort if the instrument has a rigid shank.
2. Flexible shank—an instrument shank that will not withstand the pressure needed to remove heavy calculus deposits but works well to remove small and medium-sized calculus deposits.
   a. When used against a heavy calculus deposit, a flexible shank will bend or flex as pressure is applied against the deposit.

b. Flexible shanks enhance the amount of tactile information transmitted to the clinician's fingers. For this reason, a flexible shank design is desirable for instruments—such as explorers—that are used to locate calculus deposits hidden beneath the gingival margin.
   1. Visual information is of limited use when using instruments beneath the gingival margin since the clinician cannot see the working-end hidden subgingivally.
   2. *Instead of using visual information, the clinician must rely on his or her sense of touch to locate the calculus deposits hidden beneath the gingival margin* (12).
   3. Tactile sensitivity is the clinician's ability to feel vibrations transmitted from the instrument working-end with his or her fingers as they rest on the shank and handle.
   4. Vibrations are created when the working-end quivers slightly as it moves over irregularities on the surface of the tooth.
      a) These vibrations are transmitted from the working-end, through the shank, and into the handle.
      b) The ability to feel vibrations through the instrument handle is similar in nature to the ability to feel sensations in the soles of the feet when roller blading over a gravel surface. The rollers encounter the gravel and transmit vibrations to the soles of the feet.

FUNCTIONAL AND LOWER SHANK IDENTIFICATION

The instrument shank extends from below the working-end to the junction of the instrument handle.

1. The portion of the shank that allows the working-end to be adapted to the tooth surface is called the functional shank. The dotted line on Figure 8-8 indicates the functional shank of a periodontal instrument.
   a. The functional shank begins below the working-end and extends to the last bend in the shank nearest the handle.
   b. Instruments with short functional shanks are used on the crowns of the teeth. For example, an instrument with a short functional shank might be used to remove supragingival calculus deposits from a tooth crown.
   c. Instruments with long functional shanks are used on both the crowns and roots of the teeth (Table 8-2). Instruments with long functional shanks might be used to detect calculus deposits beneath the gingival margin on the roots of the teeth.
2. The section of the functional shank that is nearest to the working-end is termed the lower shank. Another term for the lower shank is the terminal shank. On Figure 8-8, the blue shading indicates the lower shank of the instrument.
   a. *The ability to identify the lower shank is important because the lower shank provides an important visual clue for the clinician in selecting the correct working-end for the particular tooth surface to be instrumented.*
   b. A general rule for working-end selection is that the lower shank should be parallel to the tooth surface—distal, mesial, facial, or lingual—of the crown or root surface to be instrumented.
   c. The lower shank may be standard or extended in length (Fig. 8-9). An extended lower shank has a shank length that is 3 mm longer than that of a standard lower shank. Instruments designed for use in deep periodontal pockets have extended lower shanks.

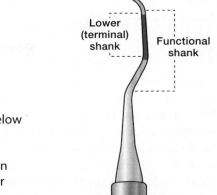

Figure 8-8. Functional and Lower Shanks.
- The functional shank, indicated by the dotted line, begins below the working-end and extends to the last bend in the shank nearest the handle.
- The lower shank, indicated by the blue shading, is the portion of the functional shank nearest to the working-end. The lower shank is important in selecting the correct working-end of an instrument.

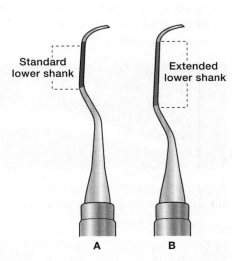

Figure 8-9. Standard and Extended Lower Shank Designs.
Some instruments, such as the Gracey curets, are available with either a standard or extended lower shank design.
- In the illustration, **A** represents a curet with a standard lower shank length.
- Illustration **B** shows the same instrument, but with an extended lower shank.
- The instrument with the extended shank is ideal for use in deep periodontal pockets or when using advanced fulcruming techniques.

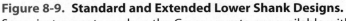

TABLE 8-2. SHANK DESIGN RELATED TO INSTRUMENT USE

Shank Design	Use
Simple shank with short functional length	**Supra**gingival use on anterior teeth
Simple shank with long functional length	**Sub**gingival use on anterior teeth
Complex shank with short functional length	**Supra**gingival use on posterior teeth
Complex shank with long functional length	**Sub**gingival use on posterior teeth

Section 3
Design Characteristics of Instrument Working-End

SINGLE AND DOUBLE-ENDED INSTRUMENTS

1. Periodontal instruments are available in single-ended and double-ended configurations. Figures 8-10 and 8-11 show examples of single-ended and double-ended instruments. Periodontal probes often are single-ended instruments. Curets frequently are found on double-ended instruments.

2. Some double-ended instruments have unpaired working-ends that are dissimilar. An example of a double-ended instrument with unpaired working-ends is an explorer and a probe combination. Figure 8-11A shows a double-ended instrument with unpaired, dissimilar working-ends; one end is a curet, the other a sickle scaler.

3. Many double-ended instruments have paired working-ends that are exact mirror images. An example of an instrument with paired working-ends is a Gracey 11/12 curet. Figure 8-11B shows a double-ended instrument with paired working-ends; these curets are mirror images.

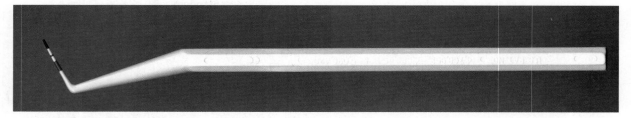

Figure 8-10. Single-Ended Instrument. This photo shows an example of a single-ended instrument. The single working-end is a periodontal probe.

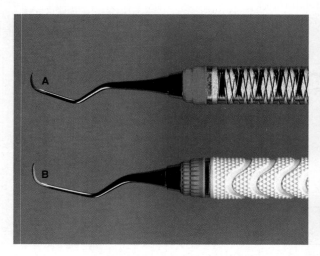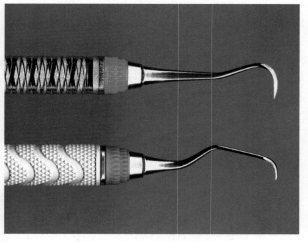

Figure 8-11. Double-Ended Instruments. Instrument A has unpaired, dissimilar working-ends. **Instrument B** has paired, mirror image working-ends.

DESIGN NAME AND NUMBER

A unique design name and number(s) identifies each individual periodontal instrument.

1. The design name identifies the school or individual originally responsible for the design or development of an instrument or group of instruments.
   - Instruments often are named after the designer or an academic institution.
   - A well-known example is the design name "Gracey". In the late 1930s, Dr. Clayton H. Gracey designed the 14 original single-ended instruments in this series that bears his name.
2. The design number is a number designation that when combined with the design name provides an exact identification of the working-end.
   - Using an instrument from the Gracey series of periodontal curets as an example— Gracey 11—"Gracey" is the design name and "11" is the design number that identifies a specific instrument in this instrument series.

WORKING-END IDENTIFICATION

The design name and number usually are stamped on the handle of a periodontal instrument. A double-ended instrument will have two design numbers, each number identifies a working-end of the instrument. For example, the original Gracey series of instruments includes seven double-ended instruments, such as, the Gracey 3/4, Gracey 5/6, Gracey 11/12, and Gracey 13/14. Figures 8-12 and 8-13 explain how to determine the correct design number on a double-ended instrument.

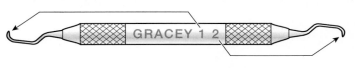

Figure 8-12. Design Name and Number Marked Along the Handle. In this example the name and numbers are marked across the long axis of the handle; each working-end is identified by the number closest to it.

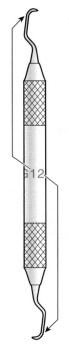

Figure 8-13. Design Name and Number Marked Around the Handle. In this example the name and numbers are marked around the handle; the first number (on the left) identifies the working-end at the top end of the handle and the second number identifies the working-end at the lower end of the handle.

PARTS OF THE WORKING-END

An instrument's function is determined, primarily, by the design of its working-end. Some instruments are used to assess the teeth or soft tissues; others are used to remove calculus deposits. To determine an instrument's use it is necessary to be able to identify the face, back, lateral surfaces, cutting edges, and toe or tip of the working-end (Figs. 8-14 to 8-17).

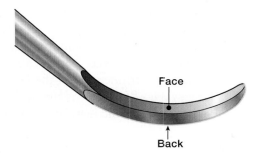

Figure 8-14. Face and Back of the Working-End. The surface shaded in purple on this illustration is the instrument **face**. The surface opposite the face—indicated by a gold line—is the instrument **back**.

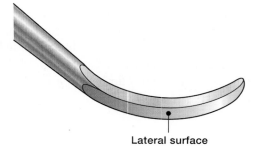

Figure 8-15. Lateral Surfaces of the Working-End. The surfaces of the working-end on either side of the face are called the **lateral surfaces** of the instrument. The green shading on this illustration indicates one lateral surface of the working-end.

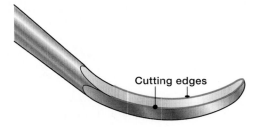

Figure 8-16. Cutting Edge of the Working-End. The **cutting edge** is a sharp area of the working-end formed where the face and lateral surfaces meet. The orange lines on this illustration indicate the cutting edges of the working-end.

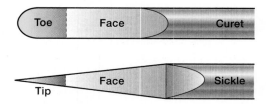

Figure 8-17. Toe or Tip of the Working-End. These illustrations show a curet and a sickle scaler from a birds-eye-view, looking directly down on the instrument face. The cutting edges of a curet meet to form a rounded surface called a **toe**. The cutting edges of a sickle scaler meet in a point called a **tip**.

THE WORKING-END IN CROSS SECTION

A cross section is a cut through something at an angle perpendicular to its long axis in order to view its interior structure. A well-known example is a cross section of a tree that shows its growth rings and tells its age.

- The cross section of a working-end determines whether it can be used subgingivally beneath the gingival margin or is restricted to supragingival use.
- At first, understanding cross sections may seem difficult, but looking at an everyday object pictured in Figure 8-18 should help to clarify understand this concept. Figures 8-19 to 8-21 illustrate periodontal instruments in cross section.

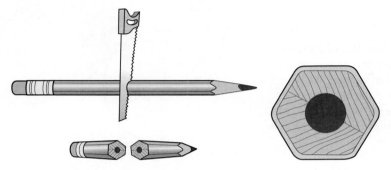

Figure 8-18. Creating a Cross Section of a Pencil. Imagine sawing a lead pencil into two parts by cutting it in the middle perpendicular to the long axis of the pencil. When the pencil has been cut, it is possible to view its shape in cross section. The pencil is hexagonal (six-sided) in cross section.

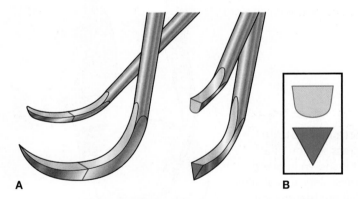

A   B

Figure 8-19. Instrument Working-Ends in Cross Section. A, In a similar manner to the pencil in Figure 8-18, imagine cutting the working-ends of periodontal instruments in half. **B,** After the cut is made, the cross sections of the working-ends are visible. The top instrument is semi-circular in cross section. The lower instrument is triangular in cross section.

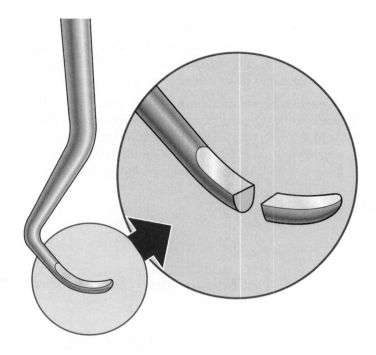

Figure 8-20. Cross Section of a Curet. The semi-circular cross section of a periodontal instrument is shown in yellow on this illustration. Curets are calculus removal instruments that are semicircular in cross section. The working-end of a curet has a rounded back and toe.

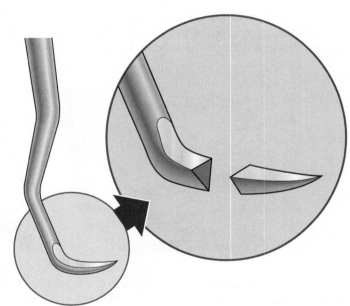

Figure 8-21. Cross Section of a Sickle Scaler. The triangular cross section of a periodontal instrument is shown in green on this illustration. Sickle scalers are calculus removal instruments that are triangular in cross section. The working-end of a sickle scaler has a pointed back and pointed tip.

Section 4
Introduction to Instrument Classification

Periodontal instruments are divided into types, or **classifications**, based on the specific design characteristics of the working-ends (Fig. 8-22). This section presents a basic introduction to instrument classification; detailed information about each of the different instrumentation classifications is presented in later modules.

- Nonsurgical, hand-activated periodontal instruments are classified as periodontal probes, explorers, sickle scalers, periodontal files, curets, hoes, or chisels. Commonly used instrument classifications are pictured in Figures 8-23 to 8-27.
- Hoes and chisels are periodontal hand instruments that are rarely used in modern periodontal instrumentation. Mechanized (powered) instruments have largely replaced the function of hoes and chisels for removing large, heavy calculus deposits.

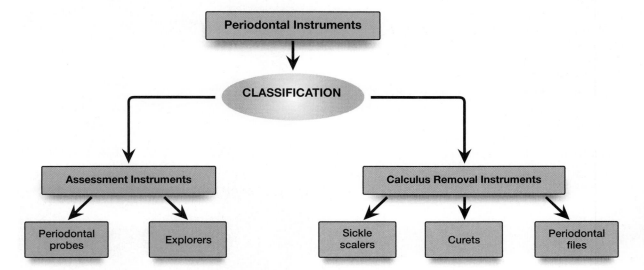

Figure 8-22. Classification of Hand-Activated Periodontal Instruments. Two major classifications of periodontal instruments are assessment instruments and calculus removal instruments.

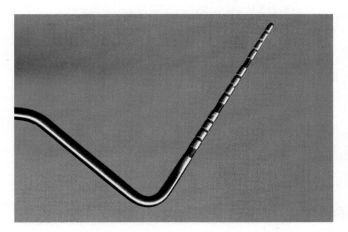

Figure 8-23. Periodontal Probe. The **periodontal probe** is a slender assessment instrument used to evaluate the health of the periodontal tissues. Probes have blunt, rod-shaped working-ends that are circular or rectangular in cross section.

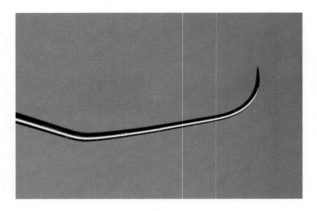

Figure 8-24. Explorer. An **explorer** is an assessment instrument used to locate calculus deposits, tooth surface irregularities, and defective margins on restorations. Explorers have flexible shanks and are circular in cross section.

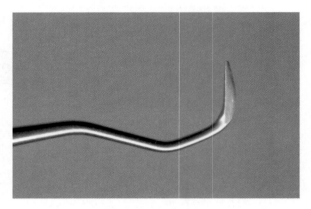

Figure 8-25. Sickle Scaler. A **sickle scaler** is a periodontal instrument used to remove calculus deposits from the crowns of the teeth. The working-end of a sickle scaler has a pointed back, pointed tip, and is triangular in cross section.

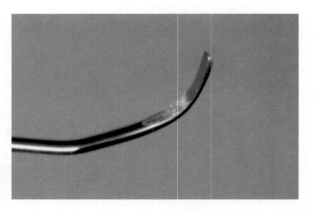

Figure 8-26. Curet. A **curet** is a periodontal instrument used to remove calculus deposits from the crowns and roots of the teeth. The working-end of a curet has a rounded back, rounded toe, and is semicircular in cross section. Two curet subtypes are the universal curet and area-specific curet.

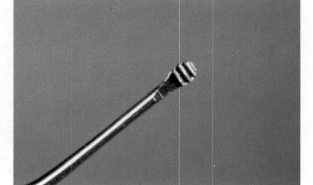

Figure 8-27. A Periodontal File. A **periodontal file** is an instrument used to crush large calculus deposits. Each working-end of a periodontal file has several cutting edges.

References

1. Leigh JP, Miller TR. Occupational illnesses within two national data sets. *Int J Occup Environ Health.* 1998;4(2):99–113.
2. Bernard BP. Musculoskeletal disorders and workplace factors. Cincinnati, OH: NIOSH (National Institute for Occupational Safety); 1997.
3. Kao SY. Carpal tunnel syndrome as an occupational disease. *J Am Board Fam Pract.* 2003;16(6):533–442.
4. Nathan PA, Istvan JA, Meadows KD. A longitudinal study of predictors of research-defined carpal tunnel syndrome in industrial workers: findings at 17 years. *J Hand Surg.* 2005;30(6):593–598.
5. Nathan PA, Meadows KD, Istvan JA. Predictors of carpal tunnel syndrome: an 11-year study of industrial workers. *J Hand Surg.* 2002;27(4):644–651.
6. Roquelaure Y, Mechali S, Dano C, et al. Occupational and personal risk factors for carpal tunnel syndrome in industrial workers. *Scand J Work Environ Health.* 1997;23(5):364–369.
7. Bramson JB, Smith S, Romagnoli G. Evaluating dental office ergonomic. Risk factors and hazards. *J Am Dent Assoc.* 1998;129(2):174–183.
8. Dong H, Barr A, Loomer P, Laroche C, Young E, Rempel D. The effects of periodontal instrument handle design on hand muscle load and pinch force. *J Am Dent Assoc.* 2006;137(8):1123–1130; quiz 70.
9. Dong H, Loomer P, Barr A, Laroche C, Young E, Rempel D. The effect of tool handle shape on hand muscle load and pinch force in a simulated dental scaling task. *Appl Ergon.* 2007;38(5):525–531.
10. Horstman SW, Horstman BC, Horstman FS. Ergonomic risk factors associated with the practice of dental hygiene: a preliminary study. *Prof Safety.* 1997(42):49–53.
11. Liskiewicz ST, Kerschbaum WE. Cumulative trauma disorders: an ergonomic approach for prevention. *J Dent Hyg.* 1997;71(4):162–167.
12. Michalak-Turcotte C. Controlling dental hygiene work-related musculoskeletal disorders: the ergonomic process. *J Dent Hyg.* 2000;74(1):41–48.
13. Simmer-Beck M, Branson BG. An evidence-based review of ergonomic features of dental hygiene instruments. *Work.* 2010;35(4):477–485.
14. van der Beek AJ, Frings-Dresen MH. Assessment of mechanical exposure in ergonomic epidemiology. *Occup Environ Med.* 1998;55(5):291–299.
15. Simmer-Beck M, Bray KK, Branson B, Glaros A, Weeks J. Comparison of muscle activity associated with structural differences in dental hygiene mirrors. *J Dent Hyg.* 2006;80(1):8.
16. Ergonomics and Dental Work. Ontario, Canada: Occupational Health Clinics for Ontario Workers, Inc. (OHCOW); January 12, 2012. Available from: http://www.ohcow.on.ca/uploads/Resource/Workbooks/ERGONOMICS AND DENTAL WORK.pdf.
17. Bobjer O, Johansson SE, Piguet S. Friction between hand and handle. Effects of oil and lard on textured and non-textured surfaces; perception of discomfort. *Appl Ergon.* 1993;24(3):190–202.
18. Fredrick L, Armstrong T. Effect of friction and load on pinch force in hand transfer task. *Ergonomics.* 1995;38(12):2447–2454.
19. Johansson RS, Westling G. Roles of glabrous skin receptors and sensorimotor memory in automatic control of precision grip when lifting rougher or more slippery objects. *Exp Brain Res.* 1984;56(3):550–564.
20. Laroche C, Barr A, Dong H, Rempel D. Effect of dental tool surface texture and material on static friction with a wet gloved fingertip. *J Biomech.* 2007;40(3):697–701.

Section 5
Skill Application

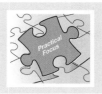

PRACTICAL FOCUS

1. **Working-End Design.** Use nail polish to identify the design elements of several periodontal instruments as illustrated in Figure 8-28 below.
   - Equipment: Ask your instructor to help you assemble the following instruments—a sickle scaler, universal curet, and an area-specific curet.
   - Materials: Four bottles of nail polish in different colors and nail polish remover or orange solvent (to remove nail polish from your instruments at the completion of this activity).
     a. Paint the **lateral surfaces** of each working-end with one color of nail polish.
     b. Use a contrasting color of polish to paint the **face** of each instrument.
     c. Paint the **back** of each instrument.
     d. Paint the **functional shank** on each instrument. Compare the functional shank lengths on the various instruments.
     e. Use a contrasting color of polish of polish to paint the **lower shank** on each instrument.
     f. Ask an instructor to check your work.

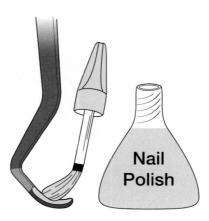

Figure 8-28. Identify Parts of Instrument with Nail Polish. Use different shades of nail polish to mark the following areas of a periodontal instrument: face, back, lateral surfaces, functional shank, and lower shank.

2. **The World of Periodontal Instruments.** The periodontal instruments in your school's kit are only a small sample of the many instrument designs on the market.
   - Select one of the instrument manufacturer's websites listed below.
   - Go to the website and explore at the variety of periodontal instruments available on the site. Select one instrument that is NOT part of the your school's instrument kit.
   - Identify the design characteristics of the instrument.
   - Post the following information in your course instructor's drop box:
     ○ Website
     ○ Instrument selected by item number, product number, or design name and number
     ○ Description of the design characteristics of the working-ends

Some Manufacturer Sites:
- http://www.am-eagle.com
- http://www.dentalez.com/stardental/hygiene

- http://www.jjinstruments.com (click on dental and then select periodontal curettes)
- http://www.hu-friedy.com
- http://www.nordent.com
- http://www.pdtdental.com/products.php
- http://www.premusa.com/dental/instruments.asp
- http://www.smartpractice.com (enter hygiene instruments in the product search box)
3. **Evaluation of Design Characteristics: Instrument Kit.** Assemble a variety of periodontal instruments from your instrument kit, including assessment and calculus removal instruments. For each instrument, determine its classification and intended use by evaluating the design features of the shank and working-end. Enter the information in Table 8-3.

TABLE 8-3. EVALUATION OF INSTRUMENT DESIGN AND CLASSIFICATION

Instrument	Shank Simple or complex? Short or long?	Working-End Pointed tip? Rounded toe?	Classification	Instrument Use Assessment? Calculus removal?
A				
B				
C				
D				
E				
F				
G				
H				
I				
J				
K				
L				
M				
N				

Student Self Evaluation Module 8: Instrument Design and Classification

Student: _____

Date: _____

Instrument 1 = _____

Instrument 2 = _____

Instrument 3 = _____

Instrument 4 = _____

DIRECTIONS: Self-evaluate your skill level as: **S** (satisfactory) or **U** (unsatisfactory).

Criteria				
Instrument	**1**	**2**	**3**	**4**
Identifies each working-end by its design name and number				
Determines if the instrument is balanced				
Working-End	**1**	**2**	**3**	**4**
Identifies the classification of each working-end				
Identifies the parts of the working-end (face, back, lateral surfaces, tip or toe, and cutting edges)				
States the shape of the working-end in cross section				
Shank	**1**	**2**	**3**	**4**
Identifies the functional shank				
Identifies the lower (terminal) shank				
Identifies the shank as simple or complex				

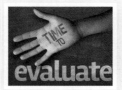

NOTE TO COURSE INSTRUCTORS: To download Module Evaluations for this textbook, go to http://thepoint.lww.com/GehrigFundamentals8e and log on to access the Instructor Resources for *Fundamentals of Periodontal Instrumentation and Advanced Root Instrumentation.*

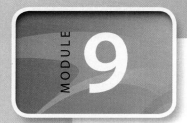

Technique Essentials: Movement and Orientation to Tooth Surface

Module Overview

This module introduces two techniques that are essential to effective periodontal instrumentation: (1) the manner in which the instrument is moved during periodontal instrumentation and (2) the orientation of the instrument to the various tooth surfaces in the dentition during periodontal instrumentation.

- Movement of the instrument involves (a) using the muscles of the hand and arm to move the working-end across the tooth surface, (b) pivoting on the fulcrum finger, and (c) rolling the instrument handle as the working-end moves around the tooth.
- Orientation involves alignment of the instrument to the tooth surface to be instrumented.

Module Outline

Section 1	**Learning Periodontal Instrumentation**	**215**

Section 2	**Moving the Instrument's Working-End**	**219**

The Wrist-Rocking Motion
Skill Building. Wrist-Rock Activation, p. 221
Digital Motion Activation
Skill Building. Digital Motion Activation, p. 222

Section 3	**Rolling the Instrument Handle**	**223**

Skill Building. The Handle Roll, p. 223

Section 4	**Pivoting on the Fulcrum**	**224**

Skill Building. The Hand Pivot, p. 224

Section 5	**Orientation of Instrument to Tooth Surface**	**225**

Angulation of Teeth in Dental Arches
Orientation to Tooth Surface
Skill Building. Alignment to Tooth Surface, p. 229

Section 6	**Skill Application**	**231**

Student Self Evaluation Module 9: Movement and Orientation to
    Tooth Surface

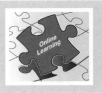

Online resource for this module: Rolling the Instrument Handle for Adaptation
Available at: http://thepoint.lww.com/GehrigFundamentals8e

Key Terms

Psychomotor skills
Brain–body coordination
Skill
Myelination
Automaticity

Motion activation
Wrist-rocking motion
    activation
Digital motion activation
Rolling the instrument handle

Drive finger
Pivot
Tooth surface being
    instrumented

Learning Objectives

- Name and define four stages of psychomotor development described in this module.
- Name and apply five strategies that assist in acquiring psychomotor skills.
- Define motion activation as it relates to periodontal instrumentation.
- Name two types of motion activation commonly used in periodontal instrumentation.
- Define and explain the uses of wrist-rocking motion during periodontal instrumentation.
- Using a pencil or periodontal probe, demonstrate the correct technique for wrist-rocking motion activation.
- When demonstrating a wrist-rocking motion, use correct instrumentation technique such as using the fulcrum finger as a support beam, maintaining correct grasp, and maintaining neutral wrist position.
- Define and explain the uses of digital motion activation during periodontal instrumentation.
- Using a pencil or periodontal probe, demonstrate the correct technique for digital motion activation.
- When demonstrating digital motion activation use correct instrumentation technique such as using the fulcrum finger as a support beam, maintaining correct grasp, and maintaining neutral wrist position.
- Define and explain the use of the handle roll during periodontal instrumentation.
- Using a pen or pencil, demonstrate the handle roll using correct technique including correct modified pen grasp, knuckles-up position, fulcrum finger as a support beam, and neutral wrist position.
- Explain how the teeth are positioned in the dental arches.
- Using a periodontal probe and a typodont or tooth model, correctly orient the working-end of a probe to the various tooth surfaces of the dentition.

Section 1
Learning Periodontal Instrumentation

1. **Exactly what is this skill we call instrumentation?**
   Periodontal instrumentation is a fine motor skill. Fine motor skills—or psychomotor skills—are small movements carried out when the brain, nervous system, and muscles work together. Basically a fine motor skill is about brain–body coordination. The term skill denotes a movement that is complex and the performance of which requires a lot of repeated practice.

   Even as children, we learn fine motor skills, for example, a child who is learning to tie shoelaces. Box 9-1 describes the process a child uses in learning to tie his or her own shoes.

Box 9-1 **Brain–Body Coordination: Learning to Tie Shoelaces**

To learn the skill of shoelace tying, involves a complex sequence of actions that require perceptual information and control of the muscles. The child needs to process the following information:

1. From the brain: What are shoelaces? Why do I need shoelaces? What is my motivation for learning to tie my shoes by myself?

2. From the eyes: Where are the shoelaces on my shoes? What does a correctly tied shoelace look like?

3. From the fingers: What is the shape of a shoelace, how does it feel in my fingers?

4. Next the child needs to combine this information by controlling the muscles of the fingers and hands to move the shoelaces in the correct way.

5. Feedback: An adult or older sibling assists the child by providing feedback on what went wrong and what went right in the child's attempt to tie the shoes.

6. Self-evaluation: The child learns to self-assess how he or she is doing. "What steps did I do correctly?" "What steps did I miss or do incorrectly?" "Does the finished shoelace bow look correct? If not, how does the bow look different from the one that my older sister tied?"

7. In the beginning, shoelace tying will be difficult and require much concentration on the part of the child. Many practice sessions in the art of shoelace tying will be necessary over the coming weeks before the child can successfully tie his shoes without assistance.

---

2. **What information should I know about the development of a psychomotor skill?**
   A. **Psychomotor Skills and the Athlete.** When learning a psychomotor skill, individuals progress through several stages of learning. Athletic coaches know that understanding the stages of psychomotor development help an athlete continue to improve his or her skill.
      1. A good athletic coach sets goals, encourages practice, gives feedback, and provides motivation.
      2. A good coach also helps the athlete understand the different stages of psychomotor development. In a similar manner, knowledge of the stages of psychomotor development makes it easier and less frustrating for a dental hygiene student to learn.
   B. **Stages of Psychomotor Development.** Educational experts—Bloom, Harrow, Simpson, and Thomas—have developed theories for the stages of psychomotor development. Table 9-1 presents a combination of these theories in a simplified form as related to periodontal instrumentation.

TABLE 9-1. STAGES OF PSYCHOMOTOR DEVELOPMENT

Stage	Definition	Example
1. Observing	Mental attention to steps of a psychomotor skill	• The learner studies the steps of a skill. • Examples include reading step-by-step instructions, viewing a video clip, watching a demonstration. • This stage occurs during preclinical instruction in periodontal instrumentation.
2. Imitating	Attempted copying of the psychomotor skill	• The first step in learning a skill. The learner attempts each step in the skill with guidance from step-by-step instructions. • The learner's movements are not smooth or automatic. • The learner receives feedback on performance. • This stage occurs during preclinical instruction in periodontal instrumentation.
3. Practicing	Attempting a psychomotor skill over and over	• The skill is practiced over and over. • The entire sequence is performed repeatedly. • The learner's movements are becoming smoother. • This stage occurs in the preclinical and clinical setting.
4. Adapting	Fine-tuning. Minor adjustments are made to the skill in order to perfect it.	• A mentor is needed to provide an outside perspective on how to improve or adjust in order to perfect the skill. • This stage occurs in the last semester or quarter of clinic.

C. Psychomotor Skills and the Brain
   1. **Muscle Memory.** "Muscle memory" is not a memory stored in your muscles, of course, but rather memories of frequently enacted muscle tasks that are stored in your brain (1).
      a. In order to perform any kind of psychomotor task, we have to activate various portions of our brain.
      b. At first, a new skill feels stiff and awkward. But as we practice, it gets smoother and feels more natural and comfortable.
      c. What practice is doing is helping the brain optimize for this particular psychomotor skill, through a process called myelination. Myelination is the process of forming a myelin sheath around a nerve to allow nerve impulses to move more quickly.

2. Repeated Practice and Myelination
   a. Compelling evidence regarding practice comes from brain scans of expert musicians.
   b. Studies suggest that the estimated amount of practice an expert musician did in childhood and adolescence is correlated with the myelin matter density in the regions of the brain related to finer motor skills.
   c. Most significantly, these studies show a direct correlation between how many hours the musicians practiced and how dense their myelin matter was (2,3).

3. Quality of Practice
   a. Understanding the role of myelin means not only understanding why *quantity* of practice is important to skill improvement—as it takes repetition of the same nerve impulses again and again to work better in unison—but also the *quality* of practice.
   b. Muscle memory doesn't judge whether the learner is performing a skill correctly or incorrectly.
      1. *So if a learner practices poorly for hours on end he or she is going to be really good at making the same mistakes over and over again.*
      2. When the learner repeats mistakes again and again, he or she builds a muscle memory of those mistakes.
   c. Fortunately, experts in the field of learning have discovered a lot about how someone successfully learns a new psychomotor skill.
      1. Some of this research evidence has been known for years, while some evidence comes from very recent studies.
      2. *Table 9-2 summarizes important points on successful learning strategies. Every dental hygiene student should learn and apply these principles.*

4. Automaticity
   a. Automaticity is the ability to perform a psychomotor skill smoothly, easily, and without frustration. Automaticity is important not only in periodontal instrumentation, but in everyday life. Box 9-2 gives an example of everyday automaticity.
   b. The development of automaticity for psychomotor skills depends on high levels of practice. There is no substitute. Ensuring consistent sustained practice is the way to ensure that the learner will become effective at a psychomotor skill (4).
   c. Movements do not become a permanent part of the brain until they are performed many, many, many times. The learner must think about every movement. With repetition, the movements begin to look smoother and the learner feels less awkward (5).

Box 9-2 Automaticity when Driving a Car

- Consider how difficult it would be to navigate an unfamiliar city by car if you had to focus on how hard to press the accelerator and brake, how far to turn the steering wheel, and all the other components of driving that have become automatized.
- Yet, when first learning to drive, the learner does indeed need to visualize and practice each of these component skills for driving.
- Teenagers spend a lot of time practicing the skills of mirror adjustment, accelerating, braking, and steering when learning to drive. Eventually, these skills become automatic.

TABLE 9-2. STRATEGIES THAT MAKE PSYCHOMOTOR LEARNING EASIER

Strategy	Application of Strategy
GUIDANCE	• Follow detailed step-by-step directions for each component skill in periodontal instrumentation (6–10). • Attend to these explicit directions one-by-one in a step-by-step fashion (6–10). • Before beginning practice, recognize what correct skill performance looks like (9). The ***Skill Evaluation Checklists*** at the end of the modules of this book provide one form of guidance.
PRACTICE	• Practice ***frequently*** and get lots of feedback so you practice ***correctly***. • Take it slow at first and expect choppy movements. • Break up the task into parts and concentrate on learning one part really well. Practice that part slowly until you're able to do it well. • Take breaks. Be patient. • Be deliberate and mindful during practice—focus solely on the skill you are practicing (11–16). • Delay gratification; tolerate a short-term discomfort in order to achieve a worthwhile goal.
FEEDBACK	• Obtain specific and timely feedback to assure that your muscle memory is learning the correct technique and not storing an incorrect movement (17,18).
RECOGNITION SELF-ASSESSMENT	• Devote time to develop your ability to recognize and contrast correct vs. incorrect technique; good recognition skills improve performance (9,19–23). The ***Practical Focus*** sections of the modules are designed to develop recognition skills. • Visualize the correct performance of a skill prior to practicing it (19). • Develop accurate self-assessment of your own performance (9,19). Use the ***Skill Evaluation Checklists*** at the end of the modules of this book for self-assessment.
PRACTICE BEYOND "GETTING IT RIGHT"	• Improve performance by frequent, sustained practice. • Practice beyond "getting a skill right" for one module evaluation (4,5). • Make each skilled movement a permanent part of your brain by performing the skill correctly many, many, many times.

Section 2
Moving the Instrument's Working-End

Motion activation is the muscle action used to move the working-end of a periodontal instrument across a tooth surface.

1. **Types of Motion Activation.** Two types of motion activation commonly used in periodontal instrumentation are the wrist-rocking motion and digital motion activation.
    A. **Wrist-Rocking Motion.** Wrist-rocking motion is the most commonly used type of movement used for periodontal instrumentation.
        1. This type of motion activation employs the hand, wrist, and arm—moving as a unit—to produce a rotating motion used to move the working-end across a tooth surface.
            a. As the wrist-rocks to move the instrument, the intraoral finger rest provides hand stability.
            b. Through the use of finger rests dental hygienists can increase stability while also reducing muscular loading (24,25). The closer the finger rest is positioned to the tooth being instrumented, the greater the level of hand control.
        2. A clinician experiences less fatigue using a wrist-rocking motion than if finger movements are used to move the instrument during periodontal instrumentation.
        3. Wrist-rocking motion activation is recommended for calculus removal with hand-activated instruments (24–26).
    B. **Digital Activation.** Digital motion activation—finger activation—is a much less commonly used type of movement for periodontal instrumentation.
        1. This type of activation moves the instrument by making push-pull movements with the thumb, index, and middle fingers. For example, on mandibular teeth, the fingers are used to pull the working-end up the tooth and then a push movement returns the working-end back to its starting position.
        2. Digital motion activation is used whenever physical strength is not required during instrumentation. It is used most commonly with powered instruments such as ultrasonic and sonic instruments. With powered instruments, the machine, rather than the clinician, provides the force necessary for calculus removal.
        3. Digital motion activation also may be used to instrument areas where movement is very restricted, such as when instrumenting furcation areas.
2. **Stroke Length for Periodontal Instrumentation.** It is important to remember that instrumentation strokes are tiny movements. The working-end is moved only a few millimeters with each stroke.

THE WRIST-ROCKING MOTION

Wrist-rocking motion activation is the act of rotating the hand and wrist as a unit to provide the power for an instrumentation stroke (Fig. 9-1). This technique allows the clinician to maintain a neutral upper body posture—shoulders level, upper arm vertical, and forearm horizontal—while keeping the workload on the forearm and wrist rather than on the hand and fingers (25,27).

1. This movement is a rotating motion similar to the action of turning a doorknob.
2. The way the fulcrum finger is used is an important element in the controlled movement of the working-end across a tooth surface.
   a. During motion activation, the fulcrum finger supports the weight of the hand and assists in controlling the movement of the working-end.
   b. Throughout the production of an instrument stroke, the fulcrum finger should remain pressed against the tooth to act as a pivot-point for the motion.
   c. The slight pressure of the finger against the tooth allows the fulcrum to act like a "brake" to stop the movement at the end of each stroke. If the instrument tip flies off of the tooth at the end of a stroke, the clinician did not stop the stroke by pressing down with the fulcrum against the tooth.

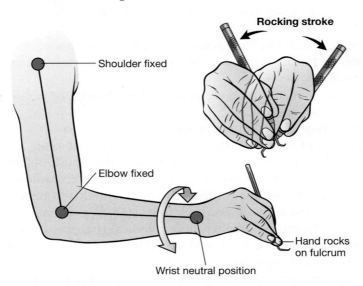

Figure 9-1. The Wrist-Rocking Motion. The arm and hand position for wrist-rocking motion activation. This movement is a rotating motion similar to the action of turning a doorknob.

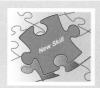

SKILL BUILDING
Wrist-Rock Activation

Directions: This skill building activity is designed to help you experience wrist-rocking motion activation. Keep in mind that the movements in this practice are broad, large movements when compared with the tiny, precise movements used to instrument a tooth.

1. **Get Ready.** Grasp a periodontal probe or pencil with a modified pen grasp in your *dominant hand*. The photographs below show a right-handed clinician.
2. **Get Set: Starting Position**
   - Establish a finger rest with your ring finger on a countertop. Your thumb, middle, and index fingers should be in a neutral position and relaxed. Your ring finger is advanced ahead of the other fingers in the grasp and held straight to act as a support beam for your hand.
   - The photograph in Figure 9-2A shows the starting position, **Position A.**
   - The end of the periodontal probe or pencil should be touching the countertop and the long axis of the periodontal probe or pencil should be perpendicular ($\perp$) to the countertop.
   - Your wrist should be in neutral position—as depicted in Figure 9-1—so that the back of your hand and wrist are in straight alignment and your arm is parallel (=) to the countertop.
3. **Activate Motion**
   - Press your ring finger downward against the counter in preparation for motion.
   - Using a similar motion to turning a doorknob, rotate your hand and wrist as a unit away from your body into Position B shown in Figure 9-2B. As you make this movement, the end of the periodontal probe or pencil lifts off of the countertop.
   - Throughout the motion, your ring finger continues to press down against the countertop and does not lift off the counter.
4. **Reposition for Next Movement.** Return the periodontal probe or pencil to **Position A** by rotating your hand and wrist back toward your body.

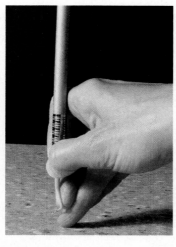

Figure 9-2. A: Wrist Motion Activation. Position A at start of activation.

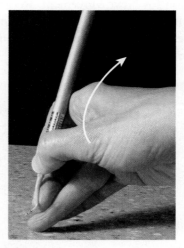

Figure 9-2. B: Wrist Motion Activation. Position B at end of activation.

DIGITAL MOTION ACTIVATION

Digital motion activation is moving the instrument by flexing the thumb, index, and middle fingers.

1. Digital motion activation is used whenever physical strength is not required during instrumentation. It may be used with periodontal probes, explorers, and ultrasonic instruments. With ultrasonic (automated, powered) instruments, the machine, rather than the clinician, provides the force necessary for calculus removal.
2. Digital motion activation also may be used to instrument areas where movement is very restricted, such as when instrumenting the furcation areas of multirooted teeth.

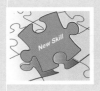

SKILL BUILDING
Digital Motion Activation

Directions: Follow these steps to practice digital motion activation.

1. **Get Ready.** Grasp a periodontal probe or pencil with a modified pen grasp in your *dominant hand*. The photographs below show a right-handed clinician.
2. **Get Set: Starting Position**
   - Establish a finger rest with your ring finger on the edge of a textbook so that the working-end of the probe extends over the side the book. Your thumb, middle, and index fingers should be in a neutral position and relaxed. Your ring finger is advanced ahead of the other fingers in the grasp and held straight to act as a support beam for your hand. Figure 9-3A shows the starting position, **Position A.**
   - Your wrist should be in neutral position so that the back of your hand and wrist are in straight alignment and your arm is parallel (=) to the countertop.
3. **Activate Motion**
   - Press your ring finger downward against the textbook in preparation for motion.
   - Pull the tip of the periodontal probe or pencil upwards by pulling your thumb, index, and middle fingers toward the palm of your hand into **Position B** as shown in Figure 9-3B.
   - Your ring finger should remain motionless pressing down against the textbook.
4. **Reposition for Next Movement.** Return the periodontal probe or pencil to **Position A** by pushing downward with your thumb, index, and middle fingers. Note that you have little strength and your fingers would fatigue quickly when using this type of motion activation.

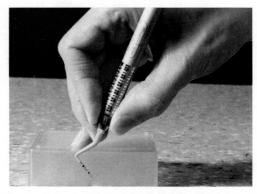

Figure 9-3. A: Digital Activation, Position A.

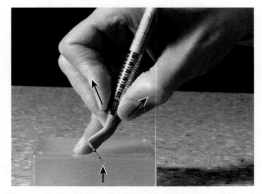

Figure 9-3. B: Digital Activation. Position B.

Section 3
Rolling the Instrument Handle

Rolling the instrument handle is the act of turning the handle between the thumb and index finger. The purpose is to maintain precise contact of the working-end to the tooth surface as it moves around the tooth. Either the index finger *or* the thumb acts as the **drive finger** used to turn the instrument. The finger used to roll the handle determines the direction in which the working-end will turn.

SKILL BUILDING
The Handle Roll

Directions: Figures 9-4 to 9-6 demonstrate how to use the thumb and index finger to roll an instrument. Use a pen with lettering running along its length. The lettering on the pen provides a visual reference point as the pen turns between your fingers.

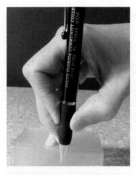

Figure 9-4. Get Ready. Establish a finger rest on a textbook and allow the tip of the pen to extend over the side of the book.
- Grasp the pen so that the lettering is visible between your index finger and thumb.
- *Space your thumb and index finger slightly apart on the pen shaft. Touching or overlapping the fingers makes it more difficult to roll the pen.*

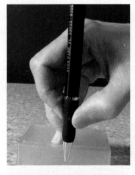

Figure 9-5. Roll in a Clockwise Direction. Roll the pen between your index finger and thumb in a clockwise direction until the lettering is no longer visible. Does your index finger or your thumb act as the drive finger to turn the instrument in a clockwise direction?

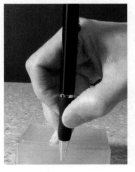

Figure 9-6. Roll in a Counter-Clockwise Direction. Finally, turn the pen in a counter-clockwise direction, back toward the starting position. Continue rolling until the pen has returned to the original starting position. Does your index finger or your thumb act as the drive finger to turn the instrument in a counter-clockwise direction?

Section 4
Pivoting on the Fulcrum

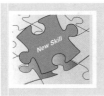

SKILL BUILDING
The Hand Pivot

Directions: This skill building activity will assist you in learning to pivot on your fulcrum finger. As with all movements when working in the oral cavity, the pivot is a tiny movement used to reposition your hand.

A pivot is something, such as a rod, that supports an object as it turns or rotates. For example, spinning around while balancing on one foot like a ballerina. In this example, a foot and leg act as the pivot that supports the rest of the body as it turns. In periodontal instrumentation, the fulcrum finger acts as the **pivot** that supports the hand as it turns.

- Pivoting the hand and arm assists the clinician in keeping the working-end against the tooth as it moves around the tooth.
- Pivoting is used principally when moving around a line angle and onto the proximal surface of a tooth. For example, moving the working-end from the facial surface—around the mesiofacial line angle—and onto the mesial surface of a molar tooth (Figs. 9-7 and 9-8).

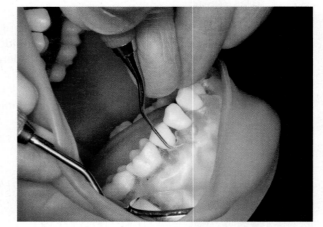

Figure 9-7. Prior to Pivot on Facial Surface.
- The clinician pictured here is moving the working-end across the facial surface of the second premolar.
- Note that while working on the facial surface, only the *underside* of the middle finger is visible on this photo.

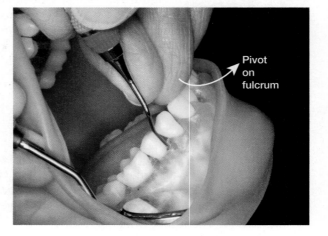

Figure 9-8. After Pivot.
- As the clinician reaches the mesiofacial line angle, he or she pivots on the fulcrum finger to rotate the hand slightly.
- With a slight pivot of the hand, the clinician has moved the working-end from the facial surface onto the mesial surface of the premolar.
- Note that the *side* of the middle finger is visible after the hand pivot.

Section 5
Orientation of Instrument to Tooth Surface

ANGULATION OF TEETH IN DENTAL ARCHES

The placement of the working-end in relation to the tooth surface being instrumented is a critical element in periodontal instrumentation. Much periodontal instrumentation occurs on the root surfaces of the teeth.

1. Correct placement of the working-end to the *root surface being instrumented* is facilitated if the clinician has a clear visual picture of the angulation of the teeth in the dental arches.
   a. As illustrated in Figure 9-9A, a common misconception is that most teeth are positioned vertically in the dental arches. The teeth however, do not sit like fence posts sticking straight down into the soil. This incorrect visual picture of the teeth in the dental arches results in positioning the lower shank incorrectly in relation to the root surface being instrumented.
   b. As illustrated in Figure 9-9B, the teeth usually are tilted in the dental arches. This correct visual picture of the teeth in the dental arches facilitates correct alignment of the lower shank with the root surface being instrumented.
2. Figures 9-10 and 9-11 illustrate the true angulation of the maxillary and mandibular teeth in the dental arches.

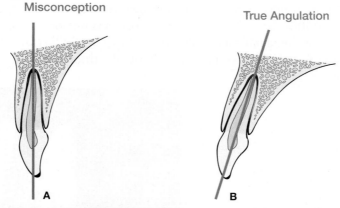

Figure 9-9. Angulation of the Teeth in the Dental Arches. A: Incorrect Visual Picture. A common misconception is that most teeth are positioned vertically in the dental arches. **B: True Angulation.** Most teeth are tilted in the dental arch.

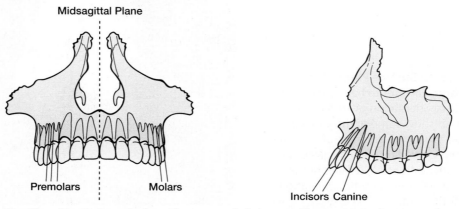

Figure 9-10. Maxillary Teeth Angulation. The roots of all the maxillary teeth incline inward.

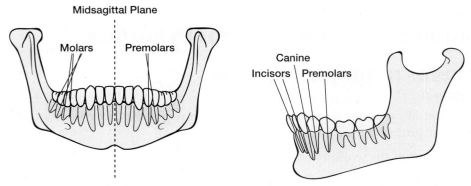

Figure 9-11. Mandibular Teeth Angulation. The roots of the mandibular anterior teeth usually tilt inward. The roots of the mandibular premolars usually are positioned more nearly vertical. The roots of the mandibular molars tilt slightly outward.

ORIENTATION TO TOOTH SURFACE

Initial placement of the working-end against the tooth surface begins by orienting the lower shank with the tooth surface to be instrumented.

1. Orienting the instrument with the tooth surface to be instrumented requires some thought on the part of the clinician.
2. A single tooth has many surfaces, each with its own orientation including the convex, rounded posterior tooth crowns, tapering root surfaces, divergent roots, and root concavities. Figure 9-16 illustrates the many surface orientations of a maxillary first molar when viewed from the facial aspect. Figures 9-12 to 9-18 illustrate incorrect and correct orientation to various tooth surfaces in the dentition.

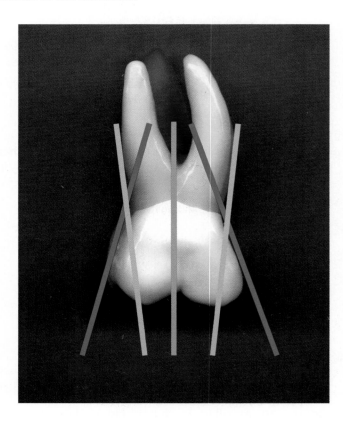

Figure 9-12. Tooth Surface Planes for Instrumentation. Each tooth has many surfaces each with its own orientation or surface plane. The colored lines show some of the surface orientations on the crown and root of a maxillary first molar when viewed from the facial aspect. Note that the orientations of surfaces of the crown differ significantly from the orientations of the surfaces of the root.

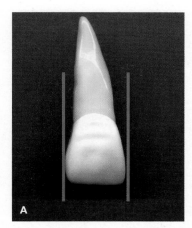
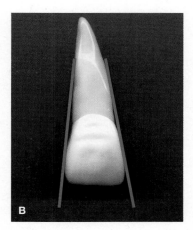

Figure 9-13. Orientation to Proximal Surfaces. A: Incorrect. The red lines indicate incorrect alignment to the distal and mesial surfaces of a maxillary central incisor. **B: Correct.** The green lines indicate correct alignment to the distal and mesial proximal surfaces of a maxillary central incisor.

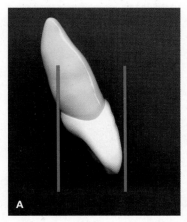
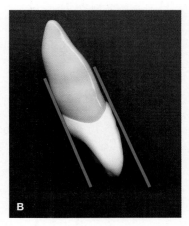

Figure 9-14. Orientation to Facial and Lingual Surfaces. A: Incorrect. The red lines indicate incorrect alignment to the lingual and facial surfaces of a maxillary central incisor. **B: Correct.** The green lines indicate correct alignment to the lingual and facial surfaces of a maxillary central incisor.

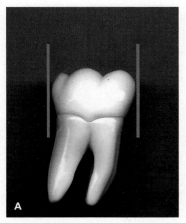
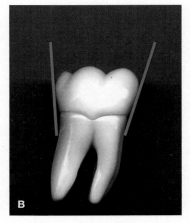

Figure 9-15. Orientation to Proximal Surfaces. A: Incorrect. The red lines indicate incorrect alignment to the distal and mesial surfaces of a mandibular molar. **B: Correct.** The green lines indicate correct alignment to the distal and mesial proximal surfaces of a mandibular molar.

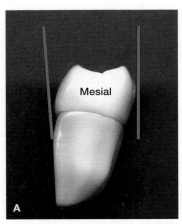
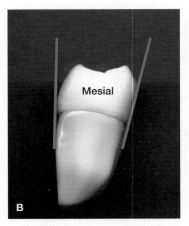

Figure 9-16. Orientation to Facial and Lingual Surfaces. A: Incorrect. The red lines indicate incorrect alignment to the lingual and facial surfaces of a mandibular molar. **B: Correct.** The green lines indicate correct alignment to the lingual and facial surfaces of a mandibular molar.

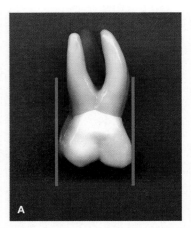
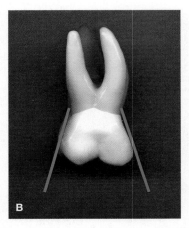

Figure 9-17. Orientation to Proximal Surfaces. A: Incorrect. The red lines indicate incorrect alignment to the distal and mesial surfaces of a maxillary molar. **B: Correct.** The green lines indicate correct alignment to the distal and mesial proximal surfaces of a maxillary molar.

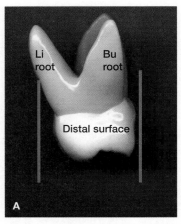
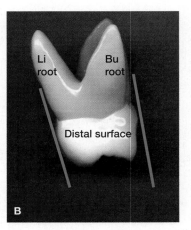

Figure 9-18. Orientation to Facial and Lingual Surfaces. A: Incorrect. The red lines indicate incorrect alignment to the lingual and facial surfaces of a maxillary molar. **B: Correct.** The green lines indicate correct alignment to the lingual and facial surfaces of a maxillary molar.

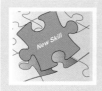

SKILL BUILDING
Alignment to Tooth Surface

Directions: This skill building activity is designed to assist you in learning to align the working-end of a periodontal probe to various tooth surfaces in the dentition. The working-end of a periodontal probe should be positioned parallel to the root surface being instrumented.

- Equipment: A periodontal typodont with flexible or removable gingiva and a periodontal probe
- Practice orienting a periodontal probe to the facial, lingual, mesial, and distal aspects of the first molar in the four posterior sextants and a central incisor tooth in both anterior sextants of the mouth. A few examples are shown below in Figures 9-19 to 9-21.

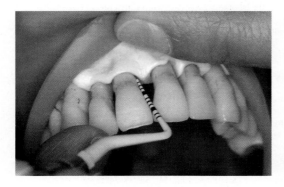

Figure 9-19. Orientation to Mesial Surface of Maxillary Central Incisor.

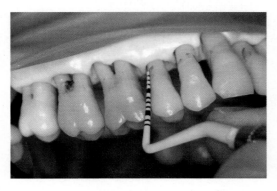

Figure 9-20. Orientation to Distal Surface of Maxillary Second Premolar.

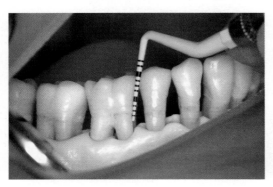

Figure 9-21. Orientation to Mesial Surface of Mandibular Molar.

References

1. Witt JK, Ashe J, Willingham DT. An egocentric frame of reference in implicit motor sequence learning. *Psychol Res.* 2008;72(5):542–552.

2. Bengtsson SL, Nagy Z, Skare S, Forsman L, Forssberg H, Ullen F. Extensive piano practicing has regionally specific effects on white matter development. *Nat Neurosci.* 2005;8(9):1149–1150.

3. Hyde KL, Lerch J, Norton A, et al. The effects of musical training on structural brain development: a longitudinal study. *Ann N Y Acad Sci.* 2009;1169:182–186.

4. Shiffrin RM, Schneider W. Automatic and controlled processing revisited. *Psychol Rev.* 1984;91(2):269–276.

5. Schmidt RA, Lee TD. *Motor learning and Performance: From Principles to Application.* 5th edition. Champaign, IL: Human Kinetics; 2013.

6. Anderson JR. *Rules of the Mind.* Hillsdale, NJ: L. Erlbaum Associates; 1993, ix, 320.

7. Anderson JR. *The Architecture of Cognition.* Mahwah, NJ: Lawrence Erlbaum Associates; 1996, xi, 345.

8. Chambers DW, Glassman P. A primer on competency-based evaluation. *J Dent Educ.* 1997;61(8):651–666.

9. Hauser AM, Bowen DM. Primer on preclinical instruction and evaluation. *J Dent Educ.* 2009;73(3):390–398.

10. Proctor RW, Dutta A. *Skill Acquisition and Human Performance.* Thousand Oaks, CA: Sage; 1995, xvi, 442.

11. Ericsson KA. Deliberate practice and the acquisition and maintenance of expert performance in medicine and related domains. *Acad Med.* 2004;79(10 Suppl):S70–S81.

12. Ericsson KA. An expert-performance perspective of research on medical expertise: the study of clinical performance. *Med Educ.* 2007;41(12):1124–1130.

13. Ericsson KA. Deliberate practice and acquisition of expert performance: a general overview. *Acad Emerg Med.* 2008;15(11):989–994.

14. Ericsson KA, Whyte Jt, Ward P. Expert performance in nursing: reviewing research on expertise in nursing within the framework of the expert-performance approach. *ANS Adv Nurs Sci.* 2007;30(1):E59–E71.

15. Ericsson KA, Williams AM. Capturing naturally occurring superior performance in the laboratory: translational research on expert performance. *J Exp Psychol Appl.* 2007;13(3):115–123.

16. Hashimoto DA, Sirimanna P, Gomez ED, et al. Deliberate practice enhances quality of laparoscopic surgical performance in a randomized controlled trial: from arrested development to expert performance. *Surg Endosc.* 2015;29(11):3154–3162.

17. Ericsson KA, Lehmann AC. Expert and exceptional performance: evidence of maximal adaptation to task constraints. *Ann Rev Psychol.* 1996;47:273–305.

18. van de Ridder JM, Stokking KM, McGaghie WC, ten Cate OT. What is feedback in clinical education? *Med Educ.* 2008;42(2):189–197.

19. Feil PH, Gatti JJ. Validation of a motor skills performance theory with applications for dental education. *J Dent Educ.* 1993;57(8):629–633.

20. Feil PH, Guenzel PJ, Knight GW, Geistfeld R. Designing preclinical instruction for psychomotor skills (I)–theoretical foundations of motor skill performance and their applications to dental education. *J Dent Educ.* 1994;58(11–12):806–812.

21. Knight GW, Guenzel PJ. Discrimination training and formative evaluation for remediation in basic waxing skills. *J Dent Educ.* 1990;54(3):194–198.

22. Knight GW, Guenzel PJ. Design and validation of mirror skills instruction. *J Dent Educ.* 1994;58(10):752–761.

23. Knight GW, Guenzel PJ, Fitzgerald M. Teaching recognition skills to improve products. *J Dent Educ.* 1990;54(12):739–742.

24. Dong H, Barr A, Loomer P, Rempel D. The effects of finger rest positions on hand muscle load and pinch force in simulated dental hygiene work. *J Dent Educ.* 2005;69(4):453–460.

25. *Ergonomics and Dental Work.* Ontario, Canada: Occupational Health Clinics for Ontario Workers, Inc. (OHCOW); 2012 Available from: http://www.ohcow.on.ca/uploads/Resource/Workbooks/ERGONOMICS AND DENTAL WORK.pdf.

26. Sanders MJ, Turcotte CA. Ergonomic strategies for dental professionals. *Work.* 1997;8(1):55–72.

27. Meador HL. The biocentric technique: a guide to avoiding occupational pain. *J Dent Hyg.* 1993;67(1):39–51.

Section 6
Skill Application

Student Self Evaluation Module 9: Movement and Orientation to Tooth Surface

Student: _____

Date: _____

DIRECTIONS: Self-evaluate your skill level as: **S** (satisfactory) or **U** (unsatisfactory).

Criteria	Eval.
Wrist Motion: Uses a pencil to demonstrate wrist motion activation	**Eval.**
Uses modified pen grasp with precise finger placement on the pencil	
Uses ring finger as a support beam	
Maintains neutral wrist position throughout activation	
Digital Motion: Uses a pencil to demonstrate digital motion activation	**Eval.**
Uses modified pen grasp with precise finger placement on the pencil	
Uses ring finger as a support beam	
Maintains neutral wrist position throughout activation	
Pivot: Uses pencil and Figure 9-8A,B to demonstrate pivoting on the fulcrum finger	**Eval.**
Uses modified pen grasp with precise finger placement on the pencil	
Uses ring finger as a support beam	
Maintains neutral wrist position during pivot	
Handle Roll: Demonstrates rolling a pencil in a clockwise and counter-clockwise direction	**Eval.**
Uses modified pen grasp with precise finger placement on the pencil	
Uses ring finger as a support beam	
Maintains neutral wrist position	
Orientation to Tooth Surfaces: Uses a typodont or tooth models and a periodontal probe	**Eval.**
Demonstrates how to correctly orient the probe tip to the anterior teeth in the dentition, including facial lingual, and proximal surfaces	
Demonstrates how to correctly orient the probe tip to the mandibular posterior teeth	
Demonstrates how to correctly orient the probe tip to the maxillary posterior teeth	

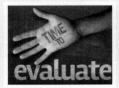

NOTE TO COURSE INSTRUCTORS: To download Module Evaluations for this textbook, go to http://thepoint.lww.com/GehrigFundamentals8e and log on to access the Instructor Resources for *Fundamentals of Periodontal Instrumentation and Advanced Root Instrumentation*.

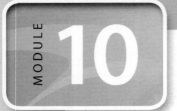

MODULE

10

Technique Essentials: Adaptation

Module Overview

An instrumentation stroke is the act of moving the working-end of a periodontal instrument across a tooth surface. The production of an instrumentation stroke involves several precise techniques. These include (1) motion activation, (2) orientation to the tooth surface, (3) adaptation, and (4) angulation. This module discusses adaptation of the working-end to the tooth surface. Motion activation and orientation to the tooth surface were discussed in Module 9.

Adaptation refers to the positioning of the first 1 or 2 mm of the working-end's lateral surface in contact with the tooth. For successful instrumentation, correct adaptation must be maintained as the working-end is moved over a tooth surface.

Module Outline

Section 1   **Adaptation of the Working-End**   **234**
Adaptation of the Leading-Third of the Working-End
Skill Building. Adaptation to the Tooth Crown, p. 235

Section 2   **Ergonomics of the Handle Roll for Adaptation**   **237**
Skill Building. Maintaining Adaptation to Curved Surfaces, p. 238

Section 3   **Selecting the Correct Working-End**   **240**
Skill Building. Working-End Selection, Posterior Teeth, p. 241

Section 4   **Skill Application**   **243**
Practical Focus: Observation of Clinician Technique
Student Self Evaluation Module 10: Adaptation

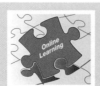

Online videoclips for this module:
- Introduction to Adaptation
- Rolling the Instrument Handle for Adaptation
- Maintaining Adaptation of the Tip/Toe of Working-End
Available at: http://thepoint.lww.com/GehrigFundamentals8e

Key Terms

Adaptation
Leading-third of working-end

Toe-third (curet)
Tip-third (sickle scaler)

Learning Objectives

- Define the term adaptation as it relates to periodontal instrumentation.
- Identify the leading-, middle-, and heel-third of the working-end of a sickle scaler and a curet.
- Using a typodont and an anterior sickle scaler describe and demonstrate correct adaptation of the working-end to the midline and line angle of a mandibular anterior tooth.
- Explain problems associated with incorrect adaptation during periodontal instrumentation.
- Using Figure 10-17 and a pencil demonstrate how to maintain adaptation to curved tooth surfaces while using a correct modified pen grasp and wrist motion activation.
- Given a universal curet and a typodont, explain how to use visual clues to select the correct working-end for use on the distal surface of a mandibular premolar tooth.
- Use precise finger placement on the handle of a periodontal instrument while demonstrating adaptation and selection of the correct working-end for a treatment area:
  - Fingertips of thumb and index finger opposite one another on handle
  - Thumb and index finger do not overlap each other on the handle
  - Pad of middle finger rests lightly on the shank
  - Thumb, index, and middle fingers in a "knuckles-up" position
  - Ring finger is straight and supports weight of the hand

NOTE TO COURSE INSTRUCTOR: PERIODONTAL TYPODONTS FOR TECHNIQUE PRACTICE

One excellent source of periodontal typodonts with flexible gingiva for technique practice is Kilgore International, Inc.: (517) 279-9000 or online at http://www.kilgoreinternational.com. These typodonts are an excellent addition to student instrument kits to be used when learning instrumentation technique and for patient instruction in self-care (home care) techniques in clinic.

- Typodonts allow students to practice techniques such as insertion without danger of injury to the sulcular or junctional epithelium of a partner (1).
- Also, there is the advantage that students can see for themselves the results of improper adaptation on the synthetic gingival tissue.
- In later modules, students can use typodonts to practice instrumentation on root surfaces—the most important and difficult areas of the tooth on which to master instrumentation (2).

Section 1
Adaptation of the Working-End

ADAPTATION OF THE LEADING-THIRD OF THE WORKING-END

Adaptation is the act of placing the first 1 or 2 mm of the working-end's lateral surface in contact with the tooth.

1. The three sections of a working-end are the (1) leading-third, (2) middle-third, and (3) the heel-third. Figure 10-1 presents a bird's eye view—looking down on the face—of a curet and a sickle scaler showing the three sections of each working-end. The leading-third is the anterior portion of the working-end.
2. Correct adaptation of the working-end to the tooth surface requires positioning the working-end so that the *leading-third of the working-end* is in contact with the tooth surface. Figures 10-2 and 10-3 show examples of correct and incorrect adaptation.

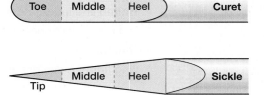

Figure 10-1. Leading Third.
- *On curets,* the leading-third is termed the toe-third of the working-end.
- *On sickle scalers,* the leading-third is termed the tip-third of the working-end.

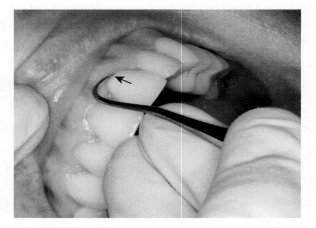

Figure 10-2. Correct Adaptation. The tip-third of this sickle scaler is **correctly** adapted to the facial surface of the incisor tooth.

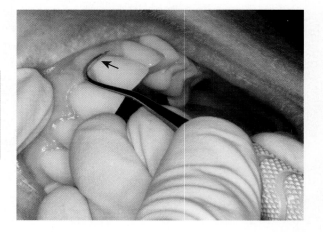

Figure 10-3. Incorrect Adaptation. Here, the middle-third of the working-end is **incorrectly** adapted to the tooth. Note how the instrument tip is sticking out and could injure the soft tissue (ouch!).

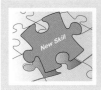

SKILL BUILDING
Adaptation to the Tooth Crown

Directions:

1. Assemble the following equipment: anterior sickle scaler and a dental typodont. Follow the steps illustrated on this and the following page as demonstrated in Figures 10-4 to 10-7.
2. Treatment Area: **RIGHT-handed clinician:** Mandibular anteriors, facial surfaces TOWARD your non-dominant hand; **LEFT-handed clinician:** Mandibular anteriors, facial surfaces AWAY FROM your non-dominant hand

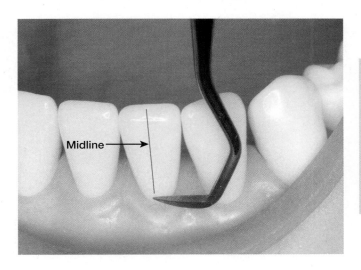

Figure 10-4. Practice correct adaptation on the facial surface.
- Adapt the *tip-third* of the working-end to the midline of the tooth. **This is the correct way to adapt the working-end to the midline.**
- Note that the *middle- and heel-thirds* of the working-end are NOT in contact with the tooth surface.

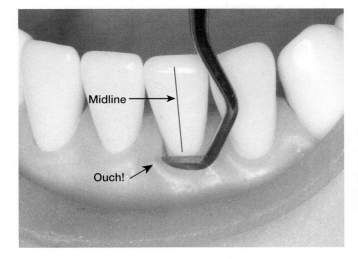

Figure 10-5. Experience the results of incorrect adaptation at the midline.
- Adapt the middle-third of the working-end to the midline of the tooth.
- Look carefully at the instrument. Note that the tip-third of the working-end is NOT adapted to the tooth. **In fact, it is sticking out. This is the incorrect technique.**
- What could happen to the soft tissue if the working-end were incorrectly adapted in this manner?

Figure 10-6. Practice correct adaptation on the line angle.
- Adapt the tip-third of a sickle scaler to the line angle of the tooth. **This is the correct way to adapt the working-end to a line angle.**
- Note that the middle- and heel-thirds of the working-end are not adapted to the tooth.

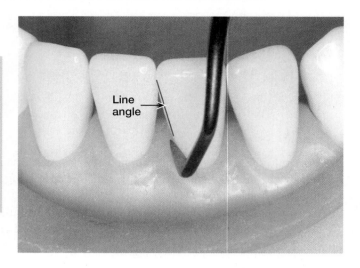

Figure 10-7. Experience the results of incorrect adaptation at the line angle.
- Adapt the middle-third of the working-end to the line angle.
- **This incorrect adaptation is a mistake commonly made by beginning clinicians when moving from the facial surface onto the distal surface.**
- Can you see why this is not the correct technique for adaptation? OUCH!

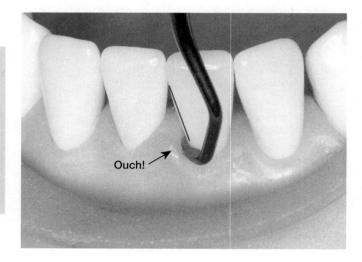

Section 2
Ergonomics of the Handle Roll for Adaptation

The correct grasp allows the clinician to achieve precise control of the working-end during instrumentation and reduce musculoskeletal stress to the hands and fingers (3–8). An important component of the skill of adaptation is rolling the instrument handle to keep the tip- or toe-third adapted to the tooth.

1. Neutral Joint Position Enhances Adaptation. *Precise control when rolling the handle requires the use of the fingertips—not the finger pads—to grasp the instrument handle. Neutral joint position greatly reduces the risk of musculoskeletal injury.*
   - Holding the instrument handle with the *tips* of finger pads enables the clinician to roll the instrument handle between the fingers in a controlled manner.
   - The handle roll is used to position the working-end against the tooth surface in a precise manner. Figure 10-8 shows an ideal pinch grasp using the fingertips to hold the instrument.

2. Hyperextended Joint Position Hinders Adaptation
   - Holding the instrument with joints in a hyperextended position impairs the ability to roll the instrument handle between the thumb and index finger in a precise, controlled manner. Figure 10-9 shows how a hyperextended position causes the fingertips to lift off the instrument handle.
   - An individual with hypermobility must learn to grasp an instrument without having the joint of the thumb or index finger hyperextend with the joint "collapsed inward."

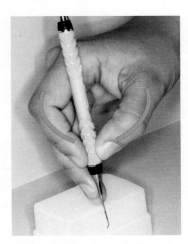

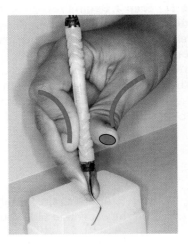

Figure 10-8. Neutral Joint Position. Neutral joint position allows the clinician to hold the instrument handle with the *tips* of the finger pads. This grasp facilitates adaptation and reduces stress to the fingers and hand during instrumentation.

Figure 10-9. Hyperextended Joints. The finger placement shown here hinders control of a periodontal instrument.
- This grasp—with hyperextended joints—makes it extremely difficult to control the position of the working-end with the fingers in this position.
- This collapsed finger position—with hyperextended joints—causes the tips of the finger pads to lift off of the handle, making it very difficult to roll the instrument handle between the fingers.

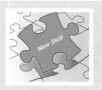

SKILL BUILDING
Maintaining Adaptation to Curved Surfaces

Directions: This activity is designed to simulate rolling an instrument handle between the index finger and thumb for adaptation. This activity uses a pencil and a drawing of the mandibular teeth (Fig. 10-16) to provide practice with adaptation. Follow Figures 10-10 to 10-15.

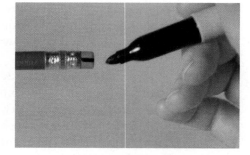

Figure 10-10. Step 1. Prepare a Pencil.
- Use a pen to make a vertical mark on a pencil eraser. The line should extend from the base of the eraser to the top of the eraser.
- In this activity you will try to adapt the **vertical mark** to the drawing in Figure 10-16.

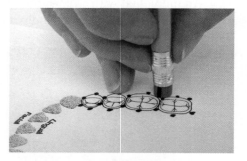

Figure 10-11. Step 2. Begin Practice on the Facial Aspect of the Mandibular First Molar.
- *To understand this exercise, practice first on only the mandibular first molar.*
- Orient the tooth drawing as shown here.
- Establish a fulcrum near the molar tooth.
- Place the black mark so that it "faces" the distofacial line angle of the tooth.

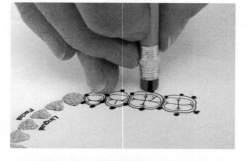

Figure 10-12. Step 3. Adapt to the Facial Aspect.
- Lift the pencil off the paper and slide your fulcrum forward slightly.
- Roll the pencil between your index finger and thumb and return the pencil to the paper so that the black line is "facing" the facial surface.

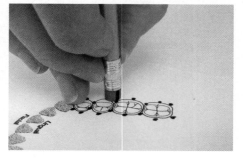

Figure 10-13. Step 4. Adapt to the Mesiofacial Line Angle.
- Lift the pencil off the paper and slide your fulcrum forward slightly.
- Roll the pencil between your index finger and thumb and return the pencil to the paper so that the black line is "facing" the mesiofacial line angle.

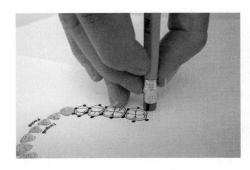

Figure 10-14. **Step 5. Practice Adaptation to the Facial and Lingual Aspects of the Sextant in Figure 10-16.**
- Begin by adapting to the distofacial line angle of the second molar.
- Note that the pictured clinician is fulcruming on the first molar at the beginning of the exercise.
- Continue rolling the handle to adapt to each aspect of all the teeth in the sextant.

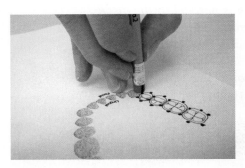

Figure 10-15. **Step 6. Practice Adaptation to the Facial and Lingual Aspects of the Sextant in Figure 10-16.**
- Finish by adapting to the mesiofacial line angle of the first premolar.
- Note that the pictured clinician is fulcruming on an anterior tooth as she finishes off the exercise.

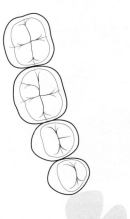

Lingual

Facial

Figure 10-16. **Representation of Mandibular Right Posterior Sextant.** Use this figure to simulate rolling an instrument handle between the index finger and thumb to maintain adaptation to the curved surfaces of the teeth.

Section 3
Selecting the Correct Working-End

Before using a double-ended instrument on a posterior tooth, the clinician first must determine which working-end to use. To select the correct working-end, the clinician observes the relationship of the lower shank to the distal surface of the tooth. The position of the lower shank provides a visual clue to the correct working-end. *It is helpful to use a premolar tooth for working-end selection, as a premolar is more easily viewed than a molar tooth.*

- *Visual Clue for the Correct Working-End: The lower shank is parallel to the distal surface and the functional shank goes "up and over the tooth."* Figure 10-17 shows the correct working-end for the facial aspect of the mandibular right posterior sextant.
- *Visual Clue for the Incorrect Working-End: The lower shank is NOT parallel to the distal surface and the functional shank is "down and around the tooth."* Figure 10-18 shows the incorrect working-end for the facial aspect of the mandibular right posterior sextant.

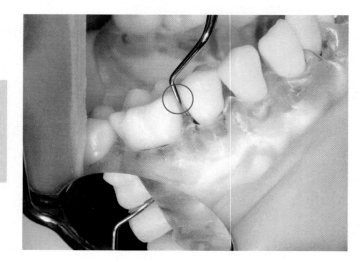

Figure 10-17. Correct Working-End. This photograph shows working-end **A** of the instrument adapted to the distal surface of a mandibular premolar tooth. This is the **CORRECT working-end** because the *lower shank is parallel to the distal surface.*

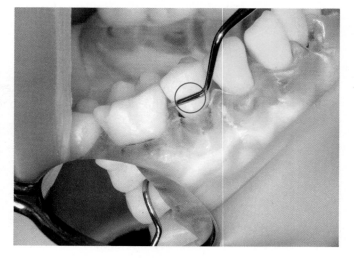

Figure 10-18. Incorrect Working-End. This photograph shows working-end **B** of the instrument adapted to the distal surface of a mandibular premolar tooth. This is the **INCORRECT working-end** because the lower shank is NOT parallel to the distal surface.

Complete the Technique Practice on the following page to gain experience in selecting the correct end of a double-ended instrument.

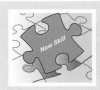

SKILL BUILDING
Working-End Selection, Posterior Teeth

Materials: Ask your instructor to help you pick an instrument for this technique practice. Use a universal curet, such as a Barnhart 1/2 or a Columbia 13/14. If you do not have a universal curet in your instrument kit, you can use a Langer 1/2 or a posterior sickle. Use a typodont to practice working-end selection.

1. **Right-handed clinician:** Mandibular right posterior sextant, facial aspect.
   Left-handed clinician: Mandibular left posterior sextant, facial aspect.
2. Remember: "Me, My patient, My light, My dominant hand, My nondominant hand."
3. Grasp the curet in your dominant hand and establish a finger rest to work on the distal surface of the first premolar.
4. Maintain your finger rest as you randomly select one working-end of the instrument and place it on the distal surface of the first premolar tooth.
5. Assess the visual clues for this working-end.
   - Is the lower shank parallel to the distal surface?
   - Does the functional shank go "up and over the tooth" or "down and around the tooth"?
6. Repeat the process with the other working-end of the instrument.
7. Based on the visual clues, which is the correct working-end?
8. Ask your instructor to check your results.

References

1. Dufour LA, Bissell HS. Periodontal attachment loss induced by mechanical subgingival instrumentation in shallow sulci. *J Dent Hyg.* 2002;76(3):207–212.
2. Ruhling A, Konig J, Rolf H, Kocher T, Schwahn C, Plagmann HC. Learning root debridement with curettes and power-driven instruments. Part II: Clinical results following mechanical, nonsurgical therapy. *J Clin Periodontol.* 2003;30(7):611–615.
3. Baur B, Furholzer W, Jasper I, Marquardt C, Hermsdorfer J. Effects of modified pen grip and handwriting training on writer's cramp. *Arch Phys Med Rehabil.* 2009;90(5):867–875.
4. Canakci V, Orbak R, Tezel A, Canakci CF. Influence of different periodontal curette grips on the outcome of mechanical non-surgical therapy. *Int Dent J.* 2003;53(3):153–158.
5. Chin DH, Jones NF. Repetitive motion hand disorders. *J Calif Dent Assoc.* 2002;30(2):149–160.
6. Gentilucci M, Caselli L, Secchi C. Finger control in the tripod grasp. *Exp Brain Res.* 2003;149(3):351–360.
7. Scaramucci M. Getting a grasp. *Dimens Dent Hyg.* 2008;5(6):24–26.
8. Macdonald G, Wilson SG, Waldman KB. Physical characteristics of the hand and early clinical skills. Their relationship in a group of dental hygiene students. *J Dent Hyg.* 1991;65(8):380–384.

Section 4
Skill Application

PRACTICAL FOCUS
Observation of Clinician Technique

Directions: Analyze the photos for Case 1 (Fig. 10-19A–C) and Case 2 (Fig. 10-20A–C) on this and the following page.

CASE 1. Your friend, Marybeth, has difficulty removing calculus on the mandibular teeth. In addition, she frequently lacerates the papillae when working on the mandibular anteriors. Marybeth simply does not know what she is doing wrong! She asks you to observe her in clinic and give her feedback about the problems she is encountering. The three photos below are typical of your observations as Marybeth worked on the mandibular anteriors, facial, and lingual aspects. What problems, if any, did your observe? How might Marybeth correct these problems?

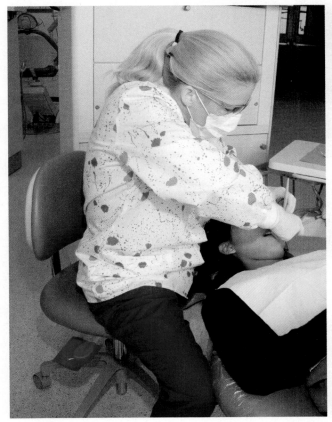
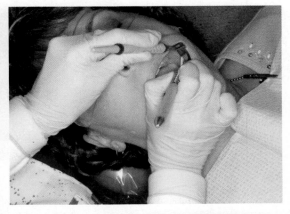
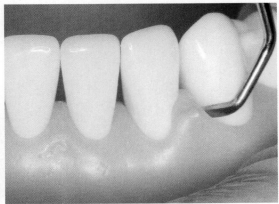

Figure 10-19

CASE 2. Observe a classmate, Marybeth, as she practices determining the correct working-end of an explorer. The three photos below are typical of your observations as Marybeth worked on the mandibular posterior sextant (1). Evaluate each photograph (2). If you find any problems, explain how each problem could be corrected.

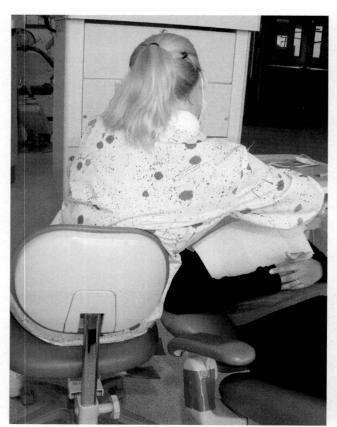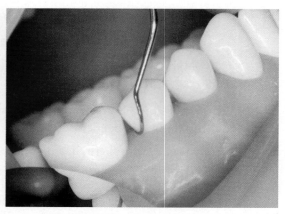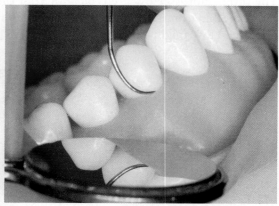

Figure 10-20

Student Self Evaluation Module 10: Adaptation

Student: _____

Date: _____

DIRECTIONS: Self-evaluate your skill level as: **S** (satisfactory) or **U** (unsatisfactory).

Criteria	Eval.
Identifies the (1) tip-third or toe-third, (2) middle-third, and (3) heel-third of the cutting edge on a sickle scaler and a curet	
Using a typodont and an anterior sickle scaler, adapts the tip-third of the cutting edge to the (1) midline and (2) line angle of a canine tooth while maintaining a correct grasp and finger rest	
Given a universal curet, selects the correct working-end for use on the distal surface of a mandibular premolar tooth while maintaining a correct grasp and finger rest	

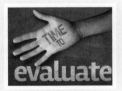

NOTE TO COURSE INSTRUCTORS: To download Module Evaluations for this textbook, go to http://thepoint.lww.com/GehrigFundamentals8e and log on to access the Instructor Resources for *Fundamentals of Periodontal Instrumentation and Advanced Root Instrumentation*.

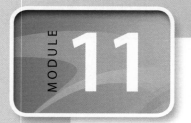

Technique Essentials: Instrumentation Strokes

Module Overview

An instrumentation stroke is the act of moving the working-end of a periodontal instrument over the tooth surface. The three basic directions employed with an instrumentation stroke are vertical, oblique, and horizontal. The three types of instrumentation stroke—assessment, calculus removal, and root debridement—each have unique characteristics and functions during periodontal instrumentation.

Module Outline

Section 1   **The Instrumentation Stroke**   **248**
Characteristics of the Instrument Stroke
Stroke Direction
Types of Instrumentation Strokes

Section 2   **Use of Pressure During Instrumentation**   **253**
Tailoring Pressure to the Task at Hand
The Ergonomics of Stroke Pressure
Skill Building. Assessment Stroke with an Explorer, p. 255

Section 3   **Skill Application**   **258**
Practical Focus: Strategies for Avoiding Injury During Instrumentation
Student Skill Evaluation Module 11: Instrumentation Strokes

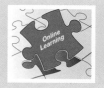

Online resource for this module: Calculus Removal Stroke
Available at: http://thepoint.lww.com/GehrigFundamentals8e

Key Terms

Instrumentation stroke
Junctional epithelium
Vertical strokes
Oblique strokes

Horizontal strokes
Multidirectional strokes
Assessment stroke
Calculus removal stroke

Root surface debridement
  stroke
Residual calculus deposits
"Out of the line of fire"

Learning Objectives

- Using a sickle scaler and a periodontal typodont, demonstrate the three basic stroke directions: vertical, oblique, and horizontal.

- Compare and contrast the functions and characteristics of three types of instrumentation strokes: assessment, calculus removal, and root debridement.

- Demonstrate how to stabilize the hand and instrument to perform an instrumentation stroke by using an appropriate intraoral fulcrum and the ring finger as a "support beam" for the hand.

- Demonstrate the elements of an assessment stroke in a step-by-step manner.

- Use precise finger placement on the handle of a periodontal instrument while demonstrating assessment strokes:

  ○ Finger pads of thumb and index finger opposite one another on handle

  ○ Thumb and index finger do not overlap each other on the handle

  ○ Pad of middle finger rests lightly on the shank

  ○ Thumb, index, and middle fingers in a neutral joint position

  ○ Ring finger is straight and supports weight of the hand

Section 1
The Instrumentation Stroke

CHARACTERISTICS OF THE INSTRUMENT STROKE

The act of moving the working-end of a periodontal instrument against the tooth surface is termed the instrumentation stroke. Instrumentation strokes are used to assess the character of the tooth surface (such as to locate calculus deposits hidden beneath the gingival tissue) and to remove plaque biofilm and calculus deposits from the tooth surfaces.

1. One example of an instrumentation stroke occurs when the working-end of a curet is positioned apical to—beneath—a calculus deposit in preparation for a calculus removal stroke. The instrument stroke occurs as the working-end is moved coronally against the calculus deposit to dislodge it from the tooth surface.
2. The working-end of an explorer is used to make a series of light, flowing instrumentation strokes over the root surface for the purpose of detecting calculus deposits scattered over the root surface of the tooth.
3. An important principle regarding movement of the working-end over a tooth surface relates to the working-end and the junctional epithelium.
   - The junctional epithelium is the soft epithelial tissue that forms the base of a gingival sulcus or periodontal pocket.
   - The cutting edge of a curet or sharp point of an explorer would injure the junctional epithelium and thus, should not come in contact with the soft tissue base of a sulcus or periodontal pocket.

STROKE DIRECTION

An instrumentation stroke may be made in one of three directions. The stroke direction varies depending on the tooth surface being instrumented with the clinician selecting the best stroke direction to access the particular area of the tooth. Figure 11-1 depicts the various stroke directions: vertical, oblique, horizontal, and multidirectional. Figures 11-2 to 11-5 show the three stroke directions in use.

1. Vertical and oblique instrumentation strokes always should be made in a coronal direction away from the soft tissue base of the sulcus or periodontal pocket.
2. Horizontal instrumentation strokes are most useful when working around the line angles of a posterior tooth or at the midline of an anterior tooth. This type of stroke is discussed in more detail in later modules of this book. *It is important to note that the working-end does not come in contact with the junctional epithelium when using a horizontal stroke.*
3. Multidirectional strokes combine the use of all three stroke directions. Multidirectional strokes are very useful when removing plaque biofilm from root surfaces.
   A. The clinician covers the root surface using one stroke direction, followed by a second different stroke direction, and finally uses the third stroke direction.
   B. This technique assures that biofilm is removed from every square millimeter of the root surface.

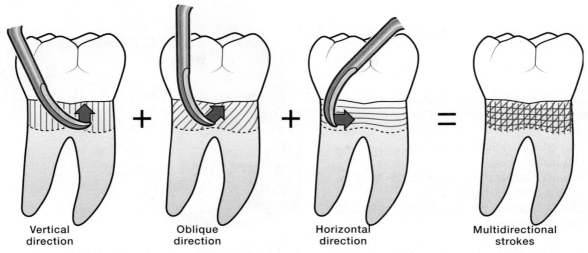

Vertical
direction
+
Oblique
direction
+
Horizontal
direction
=
Multidirectional
strokes

Figure 11-1. Stroke Directions for Instrumentation. Three stroke directions can be used for assessment and calculus removal with a periodontal instrument: vertical, oblique, or horizontal. Multidirectional strokes combine all three stroke directions on the surface of the tooth.

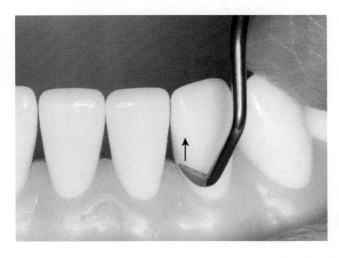

Figure 11-2. Vertical Stroke.
• On *anterior teeth,* vertical strokes are used on the facial, lingual, and proximal surfaces.
• On *posterior teeth,* vertical strokes are used primarily on the mesial and distal surfaces.

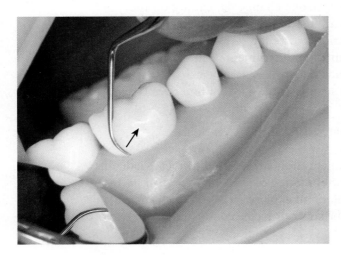

Figure 11-3. Oblique Stroke. Oblique strokes are used most commonly on the *facial and lingual surfaces* of posterior teeth.

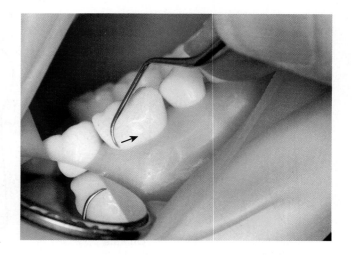

Figure 11-4. Horizontal Stroke on Posterior Tooth. On posterior teeth, horizontal strokes are used:
- Around line angles
- In furcation areas
- In deep pockets that are too narrow to allow vertical or oblique strokes

Figure 11-5 depicts the use of a horizontal stroke on an anterior tooth.

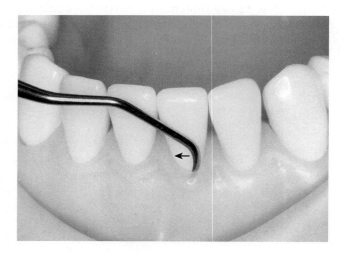

Figure 11-5. Horizontal Stroke on Anterior Tooth.
- The *facial and lingual surfaces* of anterior teeth are difficult to instrument because these teeth have a narrow mesial-distal width. Horizontal strokes are very effective in removing calculus from these narrow root surfaces.
- The working-end is used in a toe-down position. A short, controlled horizontal stroke is made on the tooth surface.

TYPES OF INSTRUMENTATION STROKES

The well-known saying "different strokes for different folks" refers to the fact the different ways of doing something are appropriate for different people. In a similar manner, the characteristics of an instrumentation stroke change depending on the purpose of the stroke. Periodontal instruments are used to assess characteristics of the root surface, remove biofilm and calculus deposits, and refine root surfaces to facilitate soft tissue healing. Each of these functions requires an instrumentation stroke with unique properties. The three types of instrumentation strokes are the assessment stroke, calculus removal stroke, and root debridement stroke. Table 11-1 summarizes the characteristics of these instrumentation strokes.

1. Assessment Stroke: Evaluation of the Characteristics of the Root Surface
   A. Also known as an exploratory stroke.
   B. An Assessment stroke is a type of instrumentation stroke used to locate calculus deposits or other tooth surface irregularities *hidden beneath the gingival margin*.
      1. The fine working-end and flexible shank of an explorer are used to enhance tactile information to the clinician's fingers. The superior tactile conduction of an explorer

makes it the instrument of choice for (1) *initially locating subgingival calculus deposits* and for (2) *re-evaluating tooth surfaces* following calculus removal.

    2. During calculus removal, assessment strokes are used with curets to locate calculus deposits.

        a. When all deposits detectable with a curet have been removed, a definitive evaluation of the root surface should be made using an explorer.

        b. Because the explorer provides superior tactile information, it is common to detect some remaining calculus deposits with an explorer that could not be detected with a curet.

  C. Assessment strokes are characterized by:

    1. Fingers relaxed in the modified pen grasp

    2. Feather-light strokes against the tooth surface; longer strokes in comparison with the short length of calculus removal strokes

2. Calculus Removal Stroke: Remove Supragingival and Subgingival Calculus

  A. A calculus stroke removal is a type of instrumentation stroke used with sickle scalers, universal and area-specific curets to remove calculus deposits from the tooth.

    1. A calculus removal stroke is characterized by a very short, controlled, biting stroke made with firm pressure of the cutting edge against the tooth surface.

    2. The fulcrum finger supports the hand and instrument during a stroke. At the initiation (start) of a stroke, the clinician presses the fulcrum finger down against the tooth.

    3. Each stroke is a tiny movement of the working-end; the working-end only moves a few millimeters. After each calculus removal stroke, the clinician pauses and then uses a feather-light assessment stroke to determine if the deposit has been completely removed.

  B. Calculus removal strokes are not used on tooth surfaces that are free of calculus deposits.

    1. *Instrumentation practice on student partners who have healthy shallow sulci is not recommended since instrumentation practice may result in periodontal attachment loss* (1).

    2. *Periodontal typodonts with flexible "gingiva" are recommended for students learning instrumentation. Periodontal typodonts allow students to practice insertion into periodontal pockets. Instrumentation practice on periodontal typodonts is ideal since skilled instrumentation of root surfaces is vital to successful dental hygiene therapy* (2,3).

3. Root Debridement Stroke: Refine Root Surface to Facilitate Tissue Healing

  A. The root debridement stroke is a type of instrumentation stroke used to remove residual calculus deposits, plaque biofilm, and byproducts from root surfaces exposed due to gingival recession or within deep periodontal pockets. Residual calculus deposits are very tiny deposits remaining on the root surface that can be removed using the lighter pressure of a root debridement stroke.

  B. A root debridement stroke is characterized by:

    1. A shaving stroke made with moderate pressure with the cutting edge against the tooth cementum.

    2. A stroke that is slightly longer than a calculus removal stroke

  C. *Conservation of cementum is an important goal of instrumentation.*

    1. It is currently believed that conservation of cementum enhances healing of the soft tissues after instrumentation. In periodontal health an important function of cementum is to attach the periodontal ligament fibers to the root surface. During the healing process after disease, cementum is thought to contribute to repair of the periodontium (4–8).

2. In addition, research studies indicate that complete removal of cementum from the root surface, exposing the ends of dentinal tubules, may allow bacteria to travel from the periodontal pocket into the pulp in some instances (9).

3. Over the course of many years, overzealous instrumentation can result in removal of all cementum and exposure of the underlying dentin. Within deep periodontal pockets, a plastic "implant" curet or a slim-tipped ultrasonic instrument may be used for plaque removal when no residual calculus deposits are present.

D. *Conservation of cementum should not be confused with a failure to remove calculus deposits.*

1. The goal of periodontal instrumentation is the *complete* removal of calculus deposits and bacterial products contaminating the tooth surfaces.

2. Calculus deposits are always covered with living bacterial biofilms that are associated with continuing inflammation if not removed.

TABLE 11-1. STROKE CHARACTERISTICS WITH HAND-ACTIVATED INSTRUMENTS

	Assessment Stroke	Calculus Removal Stroke	Root Debridement Stroke
Purpose	To assess tooth anatomy; detect calculus and other plaque-retentive factors	To lift calculus deposits off of the tooth surface	To completely remove all residual (remaining) calculus deposits; disrupt plaque biofilm from root surfaces within deep periodontal pockets
Used with	Probes, explorers, curets	Sickle scalers, curets	Area-specific curets
Lateral pressure	Contact with tooth surface, but little pressure	Firm pressure against tooth surface	Moderate pressure against tooth surface
Character	Flowing, feather-light stroke of moderate length	Brief, tiny biting stroke	Shaving stroke of moderate length
Number	Many overlapping strokes to evaluate the entire root surface	Limited to areas with calculus deposits	Many, multidirectional strokes; covering the entire subgingival root surface

Section 2
Use of Pressure During Instrumentation

TAILORING PRESSURE TO THE TASK AT HAND

1. Three Pressure Forces of the Instrumentation Stroke. Three types of force are applied during periodontal instrumentation: (1) pinch pressure of the fingers in the modified pen grasp, (2) pressure of the fulcrum to stabilize the hand, and (3) lateral pressure against the tooth during the instrument stroke. These three forces change according to the task—assessment, calculus removal, or root surface debridement.
   A. Assessment Stroke. Pressure applied during an assessment stroke varies greatly from that used during a calculus removal or root surface debridement stroke.
      1. *Pinch Pressure:* The force of the pinch grasp should be as light as possible during an assessment stroke. Vibrations transmitted from the instrument to the nerves of the fingertips are enhanced by a light grasp.
      2. *Pressure of Fulcrum Against the Stabilizing Tooth:* Apply only light pressure—upward or downward—with the fulcrum finger against a stable tooth surface during an assessment stroke.
      3. *Lateral Pressure Against Surface of Tooth:* As the working-end moves over the tooth surface for assessment, only feather light pressure glides over the tooth surface.
   B. Calculus Removal Stroke
      1. *Pinch Pressure:* The instrument is held with moderate pressure during the execution of a calculus removal stroke.
      2. *Pressure of Fulcrum Against the Stabilizing Tooth:* Apply firm pressure—upward or downward—with the fulcrum finger against a stable tooth surface during the execution of a calculus removal stroke.
      3. *Lateral Pressure Against Surface of Tooth:* As the working-end is adapted to the tooth surface the fingers in the grasp apply a firm pressure so that the cutting edge "bites" into the tooth surface. This lateral—sideways—pressure is applied only briefly just prior to and during the calculus removal stroke (the hand rests between strokes).
   C. Root Surface Debridement Stroke
      1. *Pinch Pressure:* The instrument is held with moderate pressure during the execution of a root surface debridement stroke.
      2. *Pressure of Fulcrum Against the Stabilizing Tooth:* Apply moderate pressure—upward or downward—with the fulcrum finger against a stable tooth surface during the execution of a root surface debridement stroke.
      3. *Lateral Pressure Against Surface of Tooth:* As the working-end is adapted to the tooth surface the fingers in the grasp apply moderate pressure so that the cutting edge will "shave" the root surface. This lateral—sideways—pressure is applied only prior to and during the slightly longer debridement stroke.
2. Balancing the Three Pressure Forces of the Instrumentation Stroke. The three forces used during an instrumentation stroke should be balanced (the force of the pinch grasp, pressure against tooth surface, and that applied with fulcrum finger). If firm lateral pressure is exerted against the tooth surface while the fulcrum finger applies only light pressure, the working-end will fly off the tooth surface during the stroke! Table 11-2 summarizes the balance of forces for instrumentation.

THE ERGONOMICS OF STROKE PRESSURE

1. The Misuse of Constant Pressure
   A. Unfortunately, novice clinicians often apply constant firm pressure—with all three forces—in an attempt to control instrumentation strokes. This use of constant pressure is soon stored in the muscle memory and becomes an ongoing bad habit (10–25).
   B. Researches suggest that use of unnecessary force in a pinch grip is the greatest contributing risk factor in the development of injury among dental hygienists (14,15).
2. When to Apply Pressure. The three most important concepts (Box 11-1) regarding the use of pressure during periodontal instrumentation are:
   A. Gauge the Amount of Pressure. Use as little force as possible to accomplish the task at hand.
   B. Apply only Brief Pressure. *Apply pressure only just prior to and during—NEVER between—instrumentation strokes.*
   C. Relax After Each Stroke. PAUSE and RELAX your fingers between each stroke.

TABLE 11-2. BALANCES OF FORCES WITH INSTRUMENTATION STROKE

	Assessment Stroke	Calculus Removal Stroke	Root Surface Debridement Stroke
Pinch Grasp	Relaxed	Firm (but not "death grip")	Moderate
Fulcrum Pressure	Light	Firm	Moderate
Lateral Pressure	Feather light	Firm	Moderate
Character of Stroke	Long, gliding	Short, biting	Longer, shaving

Box 11-1 Ergonomics of Pressure During Instrumentation

- **Gauge the Amount of Pressure.** Use as little force as possible to accomplish the task at hand.
- **Apply only Brief Pressure.** Apply pressure only just prior to and during—NEVER between—instrumentation strokes.
- **Relax After Each Stroke.** PAUSE and RELAX your fingers between each stroke.

SKILL BUILDING
Assessment Stroke with an Explorer

Directions: Follow the steps in Figures 11-6 to 11-11 to practice an assessment stroke.

- **Right-handed clinicians** work on the mandibular right first molar, facial aspect.
- **Left-handed clinicians** work on the mandibular left first molar, facial aspect.
- Use a periodontal typodont with removable or flexible "gingiva" so that you can practice as if working in a deep periodontal pocket. Use an explorer such as a 11/12-type explorer for this technique practice.
- **Establish a Finger Rest.** Establish an intraoral finger rest near but not directly over the surface to be instrumented. The finger rest should not be positioned in line with the working-end of the instrument to prevent pricking the ring finger with the sharp working-end when making a stroke. Position the finger rest "out of the line of fire" near to the tooth surface to be instrumented.

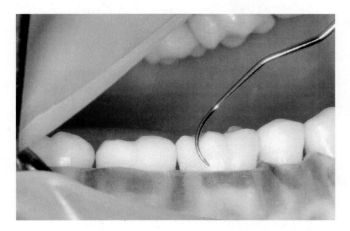

1. **Figure 11-6. Get Ready.** Prepare to assess the facial aspect of the molar. Establish a finger rest and place the working-end of the explorer in the middle-third of the crown. *Place the leading-third of the side of the explorer—**not the point**—against the tooth surface.* The explorer tip should "hug" the tooth surface.

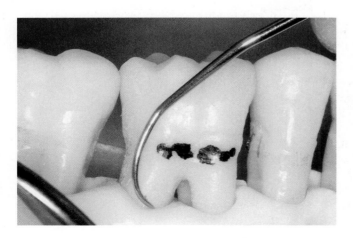

2. **Figure 11-7. Insert.** Gently slide the tip of the explorer beneath the gingival margin keeping the tip against the tooth surface.
   - When working on a periodontal typodont, insert the tip of the explorer well into the "periodontal pocket."
   - *In a real mouth, the explorer is inserted until the back of the working-end touches the junctional epithelium at the base of the pocket.*

3. **Figure 11-8. Make an Assessment Stroke.**
   - Use wrist activation to make an instrumentation stroke, away from the soft tissue at the base of the pocket.
   - As you make the *feather-light* assessment stroke, you will encounter a calculus deposit.
   - As the explorer tip moves over the calculus deposit you will feel tiny vibrations with your fingertips on the shank and handle.

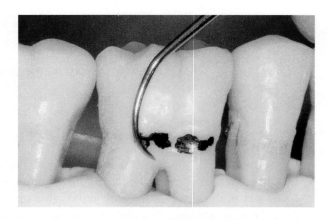

4. **Figure 11-9. Employ Recommended Technique.**
   - *Assessment strokes are overlapping feather-light strokes.*
   - Keep the fingers in your grasp very relaxed when making assessment strokes.
   - A tight grasp will prevent you from feeling calculus deposits. (Tip: If your fingers are blanched, your grasp is too tight.)

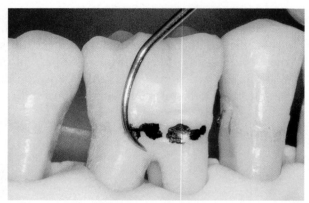

5. **Figure 11-10. Stop the Assessment Stroke.**
   - Stop each stroke just beneath the gingival margin. Tip: your fulcrum finger should NOT lift off of the tooth at the end of a stroke.
   - At the gingival margin, do not remove the explorer tip from the pocket. Removing and reinserting with each stroke will traumatize the gingival tissue.

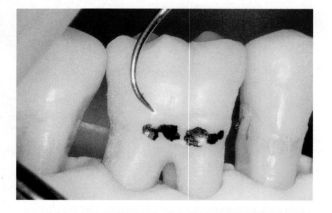

6. **Figure 11-11. Make a Series of Assessment Strokes.**
   - Practice making a series of feather-light strokes across the facial surface.
   - With each stroke, glide to the base of the pocket, make an assessment stroke, stop near gingival margin, and repeat.
   - Remember to *keep your fingers very relaxed in the grasp.*
   - Keep your touch *feather-light against the tooth surface.*

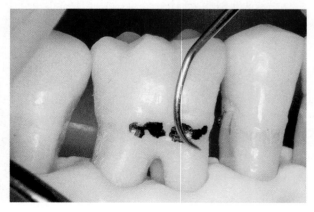

References

1. Dufour LA, Bissell HS. Periodontal attachment loss induced by mechanical subgingival instrumentation in shallow sulci. *J Dent Hyg.* 2002;76(3):207–212.
2. Rucker LM, Gibson G, McGregor C. Getting the "feel" of it: the non-visual component of dimensional accuracy during operative tooth preparation. *J Can Dent Assoc.* 1990;56(10):937–941.
3. Ruhling A, Konig J, Rolf H, Kocher T, Schwahn C, Plagmann HC. Learning root debridement with curettes and power-driven instruments. Part II: Clinical results following mechanical, nonsurgical therapy. *J Clin Periodontol.* 2003;30(7):611–615.
4. Goncalves PF, Gurgel BC, Pimentel SP, et al. Effect of two different approaches for root decontamination on new cementum formation following guided tissue regeneration: a histomorphometric study in dogs. *J Periodontal Res.* 2006;41(6):535–540.
5. Goncalves PF, Gurgel BC, Pimentel SP, et al. Root cementum modulates periodontal regeneration in Class III furcation defects treated by the guided tissue regeneration technique: a histometric study in dogs. *J Periodontol.* 2006;77(6):976–982.
6. Goncalves PF, Lima LL, Sallum EA, Casati MZ, Nociti FH, Jr. Root cementum may modulate gene expression during periodontal regeneration: a preliminary study in humans. *J Periodontol.* 2008;79(2):323–331.
7. Nyman S, Westfelt E, Sarhed G, Karring T. Role of "diseased" root cementum in healing following treatment of periodontal disease. A clinical study. *J Clin Periodontol.* 1988;15(7):464–468.
8. Zaman KU, Sugaya T, Hongo O, Kato H. A study of attached and oriented human periodontal ligament cells to periodontally diseased cementum and dentin after demineralizing with neutral and low pH etching solution. *J Periodontol.* 2000;71(7):1094–1099.
9. Berutti E. Microleakage of human saliva through dentinal tubules exposed at the cervical level in teeth treated endodontically. *J Endod.* 1996;22(11):579–582.
10. Bernard BP. Musculoskeletal disorders and workplace factors. In: U.S. Department of Health and Human Services, ed. Cincinnati, OH: NIOSH (National Institute for Occupational Safety); 1997.
11. Kao SY. Carpal tunnel syndrome as an occupational disease. *J Am Board Fam Pract.* 2003;16(6):533–542.
12. Nathan PA, Istvan JA, Meadows KD. A longitudinal study of predictors of research-defined carpal tunnel syndrome in industrial workers: findings at 17 years. *J Hand Surg.* 2005;30(6):593–598.
13. Nathan PA, Meadows KD, Istvan JA. Predictors of carpal tunnel syndrome: an 11-year study of industrial workers. *J Hand Surg Am.* 2002;27(4):644–651.
14. Sanders MA, Turcotte CM. Strategies to reduce work-related musculoskeletal disorders in dental hygienists: two case studies. *J Hand Ther.* 2002;15(4):363–374.
15. Sanders MJ, Turcotte CA. Ergonomic strategies for dental professionals. *Work.* 1997;8(1):55–72.
16. Graham C. Ergonomics in dentistry, Part 1. *Dent Today.* 2002;21(4):98–103.
17. Hayes M, Cockrell D, Smith DR. A systematic review of musculoskeletal disorders among dental professionals. *Int J Dent Hyg.* 2009;7(3):159–165.
18. Hayes MJ, Smith DR, Cockrell D. Prevalence and correlates of musculoskeletal disorders among Australian dental hygiene students. *Int J Dent Hyg.* 2009;7(3):176–181.
19. Hayes MJ, Smith DR, Cockrell D. An international review of musculoskeletal disorders in the dental hygiene profession. *Int Dent J.* 2010;60(5):343–352.
20. Hayes MJ, Smith DR, Taylor JA. Musculoskeletal disorders and symptom severity among Australian dental hygienists. *BMC Res Notes.* 2013;6:250.
21. Hayes MJ, Smith DR, Taylor JA. Musculoskeletal disorders in a 3 year longitudinal cohort of dental hygiene students. *J Dent Hyg.* 2014;88(1):36–41.
22. Hayes MJ, Taylor JA, Smith DR. Predictors of work-related musculoskeletal disorders among dental hygienists. *Int J Dent Hyg.* 2012;10(4):265–269.
23. Kanteshwari K, Sridhar R, Mishra AK, Shirahatti R, Maru R, Bhusari P. Correlation of awareness and practice of working postures with prevalence of musculoskeletal disorders among dental professionals. *Gen Dent.* 2011;59(6):476–483; quiz 84–85.
24. Khan SA, Chew KY. Effect of working characteristics and taught ergonomics on the prevalence of musculoskeletal disorders amongst dental students. *BMC Musculoskelet Disord.* 2013;14:118.
25. Roquelaure Y, Mechali S, Dano C, et al. Occupational and personal risk factors for carpal tunnel syndrome in industrial workers. *Scand J Work Environ Health.* 1997;23(5):364–369.

Section 3
Skill Application

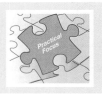

PRACTICAL FOCUS
Strategies for Avoiding Injury During Instrumentation

The very nature of periodontal instrumentation means that the clinician engages in repetitive movements. One of the most damaging aspects of repetitive movements is maintaining the hand, arm, and back muscles in the same positions for extended time periods. Some suggestions for reducing muscle stain are presented in Box 11-2.

Box 11-2 | **Strategies for Avoiding Injury During Instrumentation**

1. **Relax.** Only apply pressure against the tooth surface ***during*** a calculus removal or root debridement stroke. Keep the muscles of the fingers, hand, and wrist relaxed at all other times.

2. **Slow Down.** Calculus removal strokes should **not** be made in a rapid, nonstop manner as if keeping time to a beat.
   - Remember that the faster the pace of the strokes, the more difficult it is to control them.
   - Slow down; take time to precisely make each individual stroke and pause between strokes.
   - Slowing down and pausing between strokes makes each stroke more accurate and lessens stress on the muscles.

3. **Pause**
   - Pause at the end of each calculus removal stroke to relax the muscles. This does not mean taking the hand out of the mouth and laying the instrument down after each stroke. Rather simply relax the muscles to lightly grasp the instrument handle.
   - Relax the hand when repositioning the working-end in preparation for the next stroke. In terms of avoiding musculoskeletal injury, this step is of most importance.

4. **During Instrumentation**
   - Approximately every 20 minutes, stop and return the instrument to the tray setup. Stretch the fingers apart and hold the stretch for a few seconds.
   - Relax the fingers and slowly curl them inward without clenching. Keep the fingers curled for a few seconds before repeating. Repeat several times.
   - Allow a little recovery time between instrumentation-intensive activities to cool and lubricate muscles and tendons. A 10-minute break each hour from instrumentation provides sufficient recovery time. Without short breaks, the need for recovery builds and the threat of injury increases.
   - Rest your eyes periodically by pausing and focusing on distant objects.

Student Self Evaluation Module 11: Instrumentation Strokes

Student: _____

Date: _____

DIRECTIONS: Self-evaluate your skill level as: **S** (satisfactory) or **U** (unsatisfactory).

- **Right-Handed Clinician:** demonstrate on facial surface of the mandibular right first molar
- **Left-Handed Clinician:** demonstrate on facial surface of the mandibular left first molar

Criteria	
Assessment Stroke on Facial Surface of a Mandibular First Molar	**Eval.**
Establishes a correct finger rest and selects the correct working-end of the explorer	
Places explorer working-end in the middle-third of the crown in preparation for insertion	
Pauses to assess finger placement in the modified pen grasp; corrects finger position, if necessary	
Gently inserts the working-end beneath the gingival margin keeping the tip-third against the tooth surface	
Using a relaxed grasp keeps the tip-third in contact with the tooth surface and slides the working-end to the base of the pocket	
Maintaining a relaxed grasp makes a feather-light assessment stroke away from the junctional epithelium	
Stops the assessment stroke just beneath the gingival margin (Fulcrum finger does not lift off of the tooth at the end of a stroke)	
Makes a series of feather-light strokes across the facial surface of the tooth	
Maintains a relaxed grasp with no finger blanching during the entire assessment process of the facial surface	

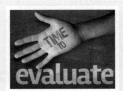

NOTE TO COURSE INSTRUCTORS: To download Module Evaluations for this textbook, go to http://thepoint.lww.com/GehrigFundamentals8e and log on to access the Instructor Resources for *Fundamentals of Periodontal Instrumentation and Advanced Root Instrumentation*.

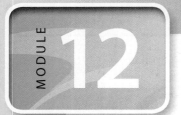

12

Periodontal Probes and Basic Probing Technique

Module Overview

The periodontal probe is a periodontal instrument that is calibrated in millimeter increments and used to evaluate the health of the periodontal tissues. Findings from an examination with a calibrated probe are an important part of a comprehensive periodontal assessment to determine the health of the periodontal tissues. This module presents the design characteristics of calibrated periodontal probes and step-by-step instructions for use of a calibrated periodontal probe.

Module Outline

Section 1   **The Periodontal Probe**   **262**
Design Characteristics and Functions
Probe Designs
Millimeter Markings
Examples of Probe Calibrations

Section 2   **Assessing Tissue Health**   **266**
Review of Periodontal Anatomy in Health
Identification of Periodontal Pockets
Pocket Formation

Section 3   **Reading and Recording Depth Measurements**   **269**
Clinical Probing Depth Measurements
Periodontal Chart
Limitations of Probing Measurements

Section 4   **Probing Technique**   **272**
Alignment and Adaptation
Probing Maxillary Molars
Probing Proximal Root Surfaces
The Walking Stroke
Skill Building. Probing Technique on Posterior Teeth, p. 275
Skill Building. Probing Technique on Anterior Teeth, p. 278

Section 5   **Informed Consent for Periodontal Instrumentation**   **281**

Section 6   **Skill Application**   **284**
Practical Focus: Determining Probing Depths
Student Self Evaluation Module 12: Basic Probing Technique

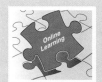

Online resource for this module:
- Periodontal Probe
- Technique with a Periodontal Probe

Available at: http://thepoint.lww.com/GehrigFundamentals8e

Key Terms

Periodontal probe
Junctional epithelium
Attached gingiva
Periodontitis
Periodontal pocket
Gingival pocket

Pseudo-pocket
Apical migration
Probing depth
Periodontal chart
Probing
Walking stroke

Informed consent
Capacity for consent
Written consent
Verbal consent
Informed refusal

Learning Objectives

- Identify the millimeter markings on several calibrated periodontal probes including some probe designs that are not in your school instrument kit.

- Identify factors that can affect the accuracy of periodontal probing.

- Discuss the characteristics of effective probing technique in terms of adaptation and angulation of the tip, amount of pressure needed, instrumentation stroke, and number and location of probe readings for each tooth.

- Using calibrated periodontal probe, demonstrate correct adaptation on facial, lingual, and proximal surfaces and beneath the contact area of two adjacent teeth.

- While using correct positioning, mirror, grasp, and finger rests, demonstrate a walking stroke in all sextants of the dentition.

- Determine a probing depth accurately to within 1 mm of an instructor's reading.

- Differentiate between a normal sulcus and a periodontal pocket and describe the position of the probe in each.

- Define and discuss the terms informed consent, capacity for consent, written consent, and informed refusal as these terms apply to periodontal instrumentation.

NOTE TO COURSE INSTRUCTORS: Please refer to the module on Advanced Probing Techniques for content on advanced assessments with periodontal probes: (1) gingival recession, (2) tooth mobility, (3) oral deviations, (4) width of attached gingiva, (5) clinical attachment level, and (6) furcation involvement.

Section 1
The Periodontal Probe

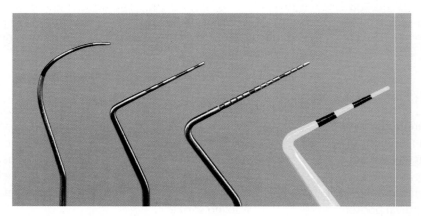

Figure 12-1. Calibrated Periodontal Probes. The **periodontal probe** is a periodontal instrument that is calibrated in millimeter increments and used to evaluate the health of the periodontal tissues.

DESIGN CHARACTERISTICS AND FUNCTIONS

1. Design of Periodontal Probes
   A. A periodontal probe has a blunt, rod-shaped working-end that may be circular or rectangular in cross section and is calibrated with millimeter markings (Fig. 12-1).
   B. The working-end and the shank meet in a defined angle that usually is greater than 90 degrees.
2. Function of Periodontal Probes
   A. Primary Function: Detect Periodontal Pockets to Determine the Health Status of the Periodontium
      1. The most convenient and reliable way of detecting and measuring periodontal pockets is through the use of a periodontal probe. A periodontal probe is used to obtain a physical measurement of the distance between the gingival margin and the base of a periodontal pocket.
      2. In 1958, the eminent periodontist, Orban (1) described the periodontal probe as the "eye of the clinician beneath the gingival margin," an essential part of a complete periodontal examination.
      3. The periodontal probe is the most important clinical tool for obtaining information about the health status of the periodontium. In other words, a determination of whether the tissue is healthy or diseased (2,3).
   B. Other Functions. In addition to measuring periodontal pocket depths, the periodontal probe has numerous other uses in the periodontal assessment (2–4). These other uses of the periodontal probe are explained in the module on advanced probing techniques.
      - Measure clinical attachment loss
      - Measure extent of recession of the gingival margin
      - Measure the width of the attached gingiva
      - Measure the size of intraoral lesions
      - Assess bleeding on probing
      - Determine mucogingival relationships
      - Monitoring the longitudinal response of the periodontium to treatment

PROBE DESIGNS

Different probes, such as Michigan, Williams, Marquis, Goldman-Fox, and Nabers probes, have different dimensions and a different diameter at the tip. The probes pictured in Table 12-1 represent some of the diversity in probe designs. The tip diameters range from 0.28 mm for the Michigan "O" probe to 0.7 mm for the Williams probe (3). Most periodontal probes are made of stainless steel, but some are made of titanium or plastic.

TABLE 12-1. EXAMPLES OF PROBE DESIGNS

Probe	Design Characteristics
Williams Probe 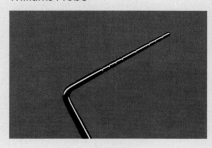	• Prototype for most subsequent probe designs (standard on which later probe designs are based) • Williams was a periodontist who specialized in the study of the relationship between pocket formation and local infection (5) • Thin, round working-end • Millimeter grooves at 1, 2, 3, 5, 7, 8, 9, and 10 mm (markings at 4 and 6 mm are missing to avoid confusion in reading the markings)
University of North Carolina (UNC-12 and UNC-15) Probe 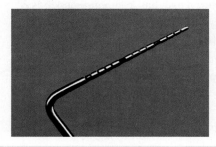	• Preferred probe for use in clinical research • Millimeter markings at each millimeter • UNC-12 color-coded at 4 and 9 mm • UNC-15 color-coded at 4, 9, and 14 mm • Thin, round working-end
World Health Organization (WHO) 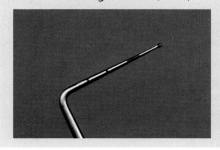	• Has a unique ball-end of 0.5 mm in diameter which is attached to a 16-mm long working-end • Markings at 3.5, 5.5, 8.5, and 11.5 mm • Advocated for use in epidemiology and routine periodontal screening in general dental practice • Thin, round working-end

(continues)

TABLE 12-1. EXAMPLES OF PROBE DESIGNS (*Continued*)

Probe	Design Characteristics
Goldman Fox Probe 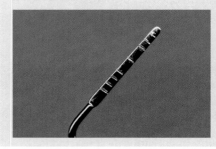	• Millimeter grooves at 1, 2, 3, 5, 7, 8, 9, and 10 mm (markings are 4 and 6 mm are missing) • Flat working-end
Novatech Probe 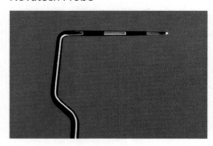	• Unique shank design with upward and right-angled bend to facilitate access to the distal surfaces of molars • Novatech probe pictured has millimeter markings at 3, 6, 9, and 12 mm • Available in a variety of millimeter calibrations
Plastic Probe 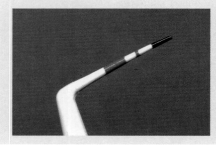	• Color-coded in a variety of millimeter calibrations • PerioWise probe pictured here has millimeter markings at 3, 5, 7, and 10 mm • Round, tapered working-end • Color-coding facilitates reading • Recommended if probing dental implants • Sterilizable for reuse
Electronic Probes 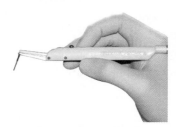 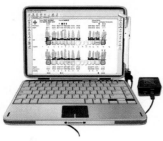	• Computer-assisted probe with digital readouts and computer storage of data • Measurement of the probe depth is made electronically and transferred automatically to the computer (6–10) • Can also record missing teeth, recession, pocket depth, bleeding, suppuration, furcation involvement, mobility, and plaque assessment (Photographs of Florida Probe of courtesy of Florida Probe Corporation)

MILLIMETER MARKINGS

Calibrated probes are marked in millimeter increments and are used like miniature rulers for making intraoral measurements.

1. **Millimeter Markings**
   A. Grooves, colored indentations, or colored bands may be used to indicate the millimeter markings on the working-end of a periodontal probe.
   B. Each millimeter may be indicated on the probe or only certain millimeter increments may be marked (Figs. 12-2 and 12-3).
   C. If uncertain how a probe is calibrated, a millimeter ruler may be used to determine the millimeter markings.
2. **Color-Coding.** Color-coded probes are marked in bands (often black in color) with each band being several millimeters in width.

EXAMPLES OF PROBE CALIBRATIONS

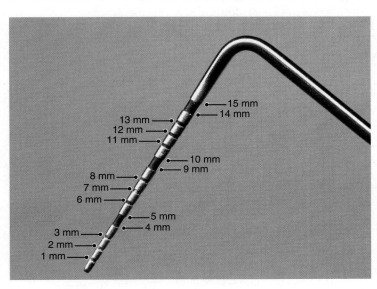

15 mm
14 mm
13 mm
12 mm
11 mm
10 mm
9 mm
8 mm
7 mm
6 mm
5 mm
4 mm
3 mm
2 mm
1 mm

Figure 12-2. Markings at Each Millimeter. The UNC 15 probe has millimeter markings at 1, 2, 3, 4, 5, 6, 7, 8, 9, 10, 11, 12, 13, 14, and 15 millimeters. Colored bands between 4 and 5 mm, 9 and 10 mm, and 14 and 15 mm facilitate reading of the markings.

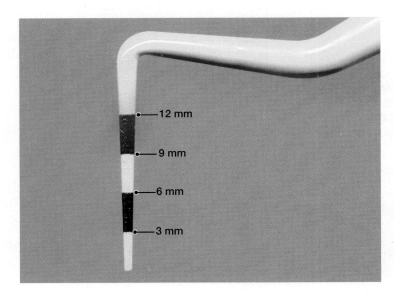

12 mm
9 mm
6 mm
3 mm

Figure 12-3. Color-Coded Probe. This probe is marked in alternating black and yellow bands; each band is 3 mm in length. The millimeter markings are at 3-6-9-12 mm on this particular probe.

Section 2
Assessing Tissue Health

REVIEW OF PERIODONTAL ANATOMY IN HEALTH

The **gingiva** is the tissue that covers the cervical portions of the teeth and the alveolar processes of the jaws (Fig. 12-4).

1. The Free Gingiva. The **free gingiva** is the unattached portion of the gingiva that surrounds the tooth in the region of the cementoenamel junction (CEJ).
   A. The tissue of the free gingiva fits closely around the tooth—in a turtleneck manner—but is not directly attached to it. This tissue, because it is unattached, may be moved gently away from the tooth surface with a periodontal probe.
   B. The free gingiva meets the tooth in a thin rounded edge called the **gingival margin**.
2. The Gingival Sulcus. The **gingival sulcus** is a shallow, V-shaped *space* between the free gingiva and the tooth surface.
3. The Attached Gingiva. The **attached gingiva** is the part of the gingiva that is tightly connected to the cementum on the cervical-third of the root and to the periosteum (connective tissue cover) of the alveolar bone.

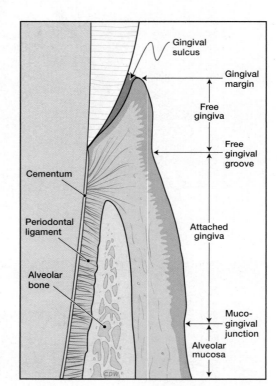

Figure 12-4. The Gingival Tissues in Cross Section. The structures of the healthy periodontium in cross section. The sulcus is a V-shaped, shallow space around the tooth. The base of the sulcus is formed by the junctional epithelium.

IDENTIFICATION OF PERIODONTAL POCKETS

The periodontal probe is the most important clinical tool for obtaining information about the health status of the periodontium.

1. The Healthy Sulcus
   A. In health, the tooth is surrounded by a sulcus. The junctional epithelium (JE) is the tissue that forms the base of the sulcus by attaching to the enamel of the crown near the CEJ.

B. *Anatomically, the gingival sulcus is defined as the distance from the gingival margin to the coronal-most part of the junctional epithelium* (4,11). The true anatomic determination of the bottom of the pocket can be obtained solely through a histologic examination (11).

C. The depth of a clinically normal gingival sulcus is from 1 to 3 mm, as measured using a periodontal probe (Fig. 12-5).

D. Probing depths on the mesial and distal surfaces are slightly deeper than depths on lingual surfaces. Probing depths on facial surfaces exhibit the least depth (2,12).

2. The Periodontal Pocket

A. Periodontitis is a bacterial infection of all parts of the periodontium including the gingiva, periodontal ligament, alveolar bone, and cementum.

1. Clinically periodontitis is identified by the presence of a periodontal pocket—a sulcus that is greater than 3 millimeters (mm) (4).

2. The correct identification of periodontal pockets therefore is fundamental in the recognition of periodontitis.

B. A periodontal pocket is a gingival sulcus that has been deepened by disease. In a periodontal pocket the junctional epithelium forms the base of the pocket by attaching to the root surface somewhere apical to (below) the CEJ. A periodontal pocket results from destruction of alveolar bone and the periodontal ligament fibers that surround the tooth.

C. The depth of a periodontal pocket, as measured by a periodontal probe, will be greater than 3 mm (Fig. 12-6). It is common to have pockets measuring 5 to 6 mm in depth.

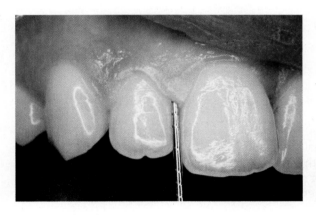

Figure 12-5. Probe in a Healthy Sulcus. This photograph shows a probe inserted into a healthy gingival sulcus, the space between the free gingiva and the tooth. A healthy sulcus is 1 to 3 mm deep, as measured with a periodontal probe.

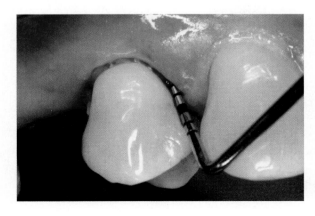

Figure 12-6. Probe in a Periodontal Pocket.
- This photograph shows a probe inserted into a periodontal pocket.
- Bleeding from the pocket's soft tissue wall is a sign of disease. This bleeding was evident upon gentle probing. (Courtesy of Dr. Richard Foster, Guilford Technical Community College, Jamestown, NC)

POCKET FORMATION

1. **Gingival Sulcus.** In health, the junctional epithelial cells attach to the enamel of the tooth crown (Fig. 12-7).
2. **Gingival Pocket.** A gingival pocket is a deepening of the gingival sulcus. The increased probing depth seen in a gingival pocket is due to (1) detachment of the coronal portion of the junctional epithelium from the tooth and (2) increased tissue size due to swelling of the tissue (Fig. 12-8).
3. **Periodontal Pocket.** A periodontal pocket forms as the result of the (1) apical migration of the junctional epithelium and (2) destruction of the periodontal ligament fibers and alveolar bone (Fig. 12-9). Apical migration is the movement of the cells of the junctional epithelium from their normal position—coronal to the CEJ—to a position apical to the CEJ. In periodontitis, the junctional epithelial cells attach to the cementum of the tooth root.

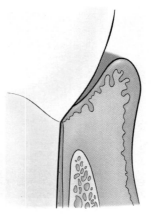

Figure 12-7. Gingival Sulcus.
- In health, the junctional epithelium is located slightly apical to—above—the CEJ.
- The junctional epithelium (JE) attaches along its entire length to the enamel of the crown.

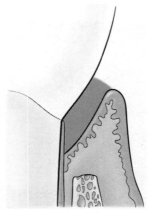

Figure 12-8. Gingival Pocket.
- In gingivitis, the coronal-most portion of the junctional epithelium detaches from the tooth resulting in an increased probing depth.
- Compare the sulcus depth in this illustration with that shown in Figure 12-7.
- In some cases of gingivitis, the gingival tissue swells resulting in an increased probing depth known as a pseudo-pocket.

Figure 12-9. Periodontal Pocket.
- In a periodontal pocket, the junctional epithelium is located on the root somewhere below the CEJ.
- The deeper probing depth of a periodontal pocket is due to the apical migration of the junctional epithelium.

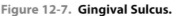

Section 3
Reading and Recording Depth Measurements

CLINICAL PROBING DEPTH MEASUREMENT

A **probing depth** is a measurement of the depth of a sulcus or periodontal pocket (Fig. 12-10). It is determined by measuring the distance from the gingival margin to the base of the sulcus or pocket with a calibrated periodontal probe (4).

1. **Six Zones per Tooth.** Probing depth measurements are recorded for six specific zones on each tooth: (1) distofacial, (2) facial, (3) mesiofacial, (4) distolingual, (5) lingual, and (6) mesiolingual (Box 12-1).
2. **One Reading per Zone.** Only one reading per zone is recorded. If the probing depths vary within a zone, the deepest reading obtained in that zone is recorded. For example, if the probing depths in the facial surface ranged from 3 to 6 mm, only the 6 mm reading would be entered on the chart for the facial area (Fig. 12-11).
3. **Full Millimeter Measurements.** Probing depths are recorded to the nearest full millimeter. Measurements are rounded up to the next higher whole number, for example, a reading of 3.5 mm is recorded as 4 mm or a 5.5 mm reading is recorded as 6 mm.

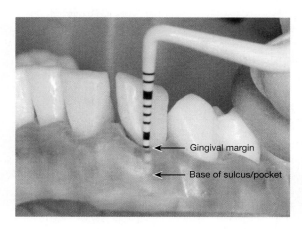

Gingival margin

Base of sulcus/pocket

Figure 12-10. Probing Depth. A probing depth is the distance in millimeters from the *gingival margin* to the base of the sulcus or periodontal pocket as measured with a calibrated probe.

Box 12-1   ## Record Measurements for Six Zones Per Tooth

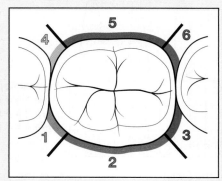

Probing depth measurements are recorded for 6 specific sites on each tooth:

1 - distofacial line angle to the midline of distal surface

2 - facial surface

3 - mesiofacial line angle to the midline of mesial surface

4 - distolingual line angle to the midline of distal surface

5 - lingual surface

6 - mesiolingual line angle to the midline of mesial surface

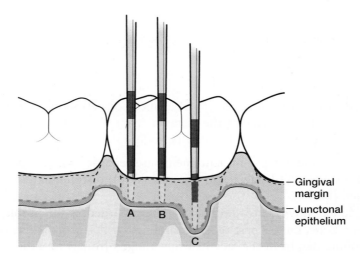

Figure 12-11. Record the Deepest Reading per Zone. In the illustration shown here, the depth of the pocket base varies considerably at points **A**, **B**, and **C** in the facial surface.

• Points **A** and **B** on the facial surface measure 3 mm.
• Point **C** on the facial surface is a 6 mm reading. Since only a single reading can be recorded for the facial surface, the deepest reading at point **C** is recorded for the facial surface.

PERIODONTAL CHART

Probing depth measurements are recorded on a periodontal chart. Most periodontal charts include rows of boxes that are used to record the probing depths on the facial and lingual aspects of the teeth (Fig. 12-12).

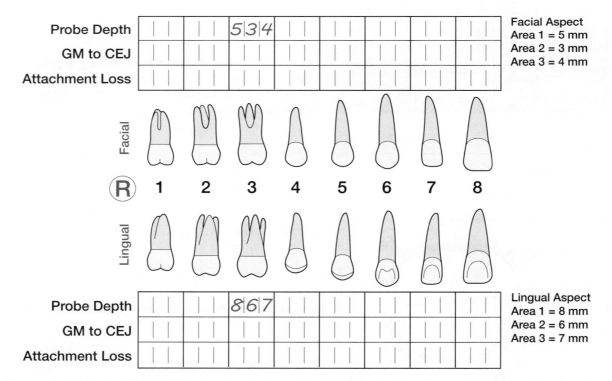

Figure 12-12. Recording Probing Depths. Probing depths for the facial and lingual aspects of the maxillary right first molar are recorded on the periodontal chart shown here.

LIMITATIONS OF PROBING MEASUREMENTS

Probing depth measurements have their limitations. Various factors can affect how accurately probing depths reflect the extent of periodontal destruction (2–4,11,13,14).

1. **Position of the Gingival Margin.** In health, the position of the gingival margin is slightly coronal to (above) the CEJ. *If the gingival margin is not in its normal location, the probing depths will NOT accurately reflect the health of periodontium.*
   A. **Gingival Margin Significantly Coronal to the CEJ.** Frequently the gingival tissue is swollen or overgrown due to gingivitis or drug therapy (15). In such cases, the extent of periodontal destruction is overestimated since the gingival margin is coronal to (above) its normal position.
   B. **Gingival Margin Apical to the CEJ.** In this instance, the gingival margin is apical to (below) its normal location. In situations where recession of the gingival margin is present, probing depth readings can substantially underestimate the true extent of periodontal destruction (16).

2. **Reading Errors Due to Naturally Occurring States**
   A. Reading errors may result from naturally occurring states, such as interference from calculus deposits on the tooth surface, the presence of an overhanging restoration, or the crown's contour (13). Figure 12-13 depicts two states that can interfere with probing.
   B. When a calculus deposit is encountered, the probe is gently teased out and around the deposit or the calculus deposit is removed so that the probe can be inserted to the base of the pocket.

3. **Reading Errors Due to Probing Technique and Equipment**
   A. Technique errors include incorrect angulation and positioning of the probe, incorrect amount of pressure applied to the probe, misreading the probe calibrations, and recording the measurements incorrectly (13).
   B. Other variables that influence measurements include the diameter and shape of the probe, calibration scale of the probe, and the degree of inflammation in the periodontal tissues.
   C. Manufacturing errors can result in the widths of probe markings differing by as much as 0.7 mm between probes (17).
   D. A research study by van Weringh et al. suggests that the diameter of the instrument handle of a probe has an effect on the force exerted with a periodontal probe (18).

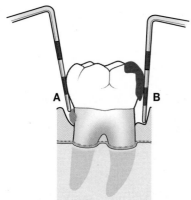

Figure 12-13. Interference with Probe Insertion. Reading errors may result from interference of (**A**) a large calculus deposit or (**B**) overhanging restoration.

Section 4
Probing Technique

ALIGNMENT AND ADAPTATION

1. **Insertion and Adaptation.** Once a probe is inserted into a periodontal pocket, *the working-end is kept parallel to the root surface.* Figures 12-14A and B depict correct and incorrect alignment of a probe to the root surface.
   A. The tip should be kept as flat against the root surface as possible as the working-end is inserted to the base of the pocket.
   B. Even though the probing involves contact of the working-end with the root surface, no pressure should be used with a probing stroke.
2. **Obtaining Alignment on Distal Surfaces Maxillary Molars.** Often it is difficult to align the probe's working-end to the distal surfaces of the maxillary molars because the mandible is in the way. This problem can be overcome by repositioning the instrument handle to the side of the patient's face. This solution is depicted in Figure 12-15.

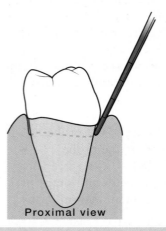
Proximal view

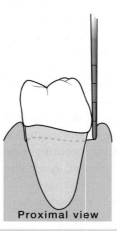
Proximal view

Figure 12-14. A: Correct Adaptation to Proximal Surface. This illustration shows correct adaptation of the probe with the working-end parallel to the root surface.

Figure 12-14. B: Incorrect Adaptation to Proximal Surface. In this example, the probe is not parallel to the root surface resulting in an underestimation of the measurement.

PROBING MAXILLARY MOLARS

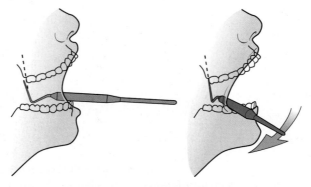

Figure 12-15. Technique for Distal Surfaces of the Maxillary Molars. Often it is difficult to probe the distal surfaces of the maxillary molars because the mandible is in the way. This problem can be overcome by repositioning the instrument handle to the side of the patient's face.

PROBING PROXIMAL ROOT SURFACES

1. Periodontal Pocketing on Proximal Root Surfaces
   A. It is important to assess the proximal surfaces of a tooth since periodontal pockets are common on the mesial and distal surfaces.
   B. *The proximal surfaces should be probed from both the facial and lingual aspects to assure that the entire circumference of the junctional epithelium is assessed* (Fig. 12-16).
2. Technique for Probing Proximal Root Surfaces. *When two adjacent teeth are in contact, a special technique is used to probe the depth of the junctional epithelium directly beneath the contact area.* The two-step technique used on a proximal—mesial or distal—surface is depicted in Figure 12-17.
   A. Step 1: Keeping the working-end of the probe in contact with the proximal root surface, walk the probe across the proximal surface until it touches the contact area (Fig. 12-16A). The area beneath the contact area cannot be probed directly because the probe will not fit between the contact areas of the adjacent teeth.
   B. Step 2: Slant the probe slightly so that the tip reaches under the contact area (Fig. 12-16B). The tip of the probe extends under the contact area while the upper portion touches the contact area. With the probe in this position, *gently press downward to touch the junctional epithelium.*

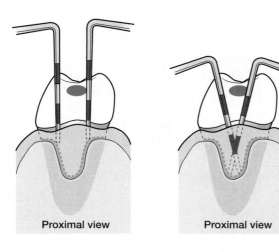

Proximal view   Proximal view

Figure 12-16. Assessing the Proximal Surface. The proximal surface of a tooth is assessed from both the facial and lingual aspects of the dental arch.

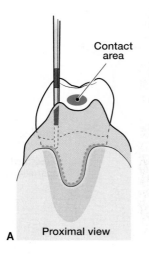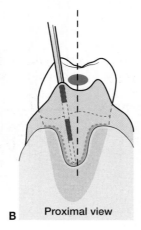

Contact area

A   Proximal view   B   Proximal view

Figure 12-17. Probing the Proximal Surface.
Step 1. Walk the probe across the proximal surface until it touches the contact area of the tooth. In this position, the probe fails to assess the true position of the junctional epithelium beneath the contact area.
Step 2. Slant the working-end of the probe so that the tip extends under the contact area to reach the midline of the proximal surface. With the probe in this position gently press downward to touch the junctional epithelium.

THE WALKING STROKE

Probing is the act of walking the tip of a probe along the junctional epithelium within the sulcus or pocket for the purpose of assessing the health status of the periodontal tissues. Careful probing technique is essential if the information obtained with a periodontal probe is to be accurate.

1. Description of Walking Stroke
   A. The walking stroke is the movement of a calibrated probe around the perimeter of the base of a sulcus or pocket.
   B. Walking strokes are used to cover the entire circumference of the sulcus or pocket base. *It is essential to evaluate the entire circumference of the pocket base— all the way around the entire tooth—because the junctional epithelium is not necessarily at a uniform depth from the gingival margin. In fact, differences in the depths of two neighboring sites along the pocket base are common.*
2. Production of the Walking Stroke
   A. Walking strokes are a series of bobbing strokes made within the sulcus or pocket. The stroke begins when the probe is inserted into the sulcus or periodontal pocket while *keeping the probe tip against and in alignment with the root surface.*
   B. The probe is inserted until the tip encounters the resistance of the junctional epithelium that forms the base of the sulcus or periodontal pocket. The junctional epithelium feels soft and resilient when touched by the probe.
   C. The walking stroke is created by moving the probe up and down ($\updownarrow$) in short bobbing strokes while moving forward in 1 mm increments ($\leftrightarrow$). With each down stroke, the probe returns to touch the junctional epithelium (Fig. 12-18).
   D. The probe is not removed from the sulcus or periodontal pocket with each upward stroke. Removing and reinserting the probe repeatedly can traumatize the tissue at the gingival margin.
   E. The pressure exerted with the probe tip against the junctional epithelium should be between 10 and 20 g. A sensitive scale that measures weight in grams can be used to standardize the probing pressure.
   F. Either wrist or digital (finger) activation may be used with the probe because only light pressure is used when probing.

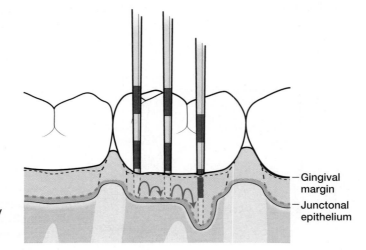

Figure 12-18. The Walking Stroke. The walking stroke is a series of bobbing strokes along the junctional epithelium (JE). Each up-and-down stroke should be approximately 1 to 2 mm in length ($\updownarrow$). The strokes must be very close together, about 1 mm apart ($\leftrightarrow$).

Gingival margin

Junctonal epithelium

SKILL BUILDING
Probing Technique on Posterior Teeth

Directions:

- Follow steps 1 to 11 to practice probing the facial aspect of a mandibular first molar (Figs. 12-19 to 12-29). **Right-handed clinicians:** begin your practice session with the mandibular right posterior sextant, facial aspect. **Left-handed clinicians:** begin your practice session with the mandibular left posterior sextant, facial aspect.
- Remember: "*Me, My patient, My light, My dominant hand, My nondominant hand, My finger rest, My adaptation*"

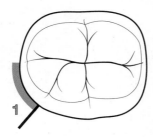

1. **Figure 12-19.** **Locate Zone 1.** Prepare to assess Zone 1 from the distofacial line angle to the midline of the distal surface. Insert the probe near the distofacial line angle of the *first molar*.

   Keep the side of the working-end in contact with the root surface as you gently slide the probe to touch the pocket base.

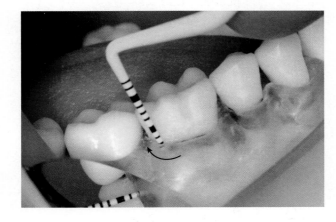

2. **Figure 12-20.** **Begin to probe Zone 1.** Keeping the working-end in contact with the tooth, initiate a series of short, bobbing strokes ***toward the distal surface***. Use a walking stroke, keeping your strokes close together. Gently touch the junctional epithelium with each downward stroke with the probe.

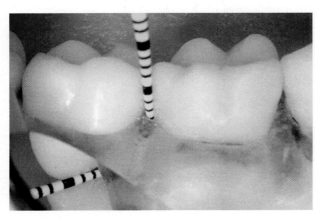

3. **Figure 12-21.** **Walk the probe onto the proximal surface.** Walk the probe across the distal surface until it touches the contact area.

4. **Figure 12-22. Assess beneath the contact area.** Tilt the probe so that the tip reaches beneath the contact area (the upper portion of the probe touches the contact area).

   Gently press downward to touch the junctional epithelium.

   Enter the deepest reading encountered for Area 1 on the periodontal chart.

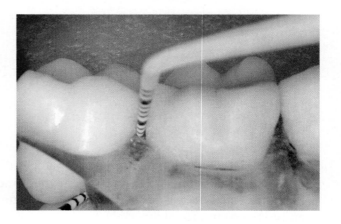

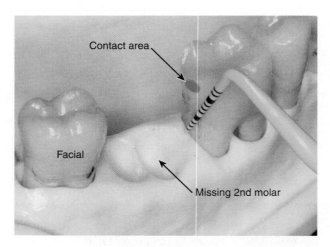

5. **Figure 12-23. Technique check: distal view.** *In this photo, the adjacent tooth has been removed* to provide a view of the correct probe position for assessing the tissue beneath the contact area from the facial aspect. Tilt your probe in a similar manner.

6. **Figure 12-24. Locate Zone 2.** Prepare to assess Zone 2, the facial surface from the distofacial line angle to the mesiofacial line angle.

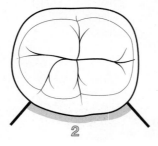

7. **Figure 12-25. Probe Zone 2.** Reposition the probe at the distofacial line angle in preparation for assessing Zone 2, the facial surface.

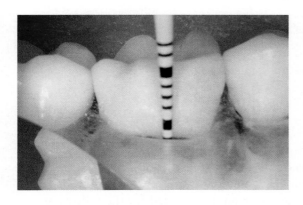

8. **Figure 12-26.** **Continue Across Zone 2.** Starting at the distofacial line angle, make a series of tiny walking strokes across Zone 2—the facial surface—moving in a forward direction toward the mesiofacial line angle.

Record the deepest measurement in Area 2 on the periodontal chart.

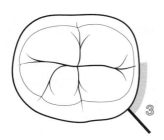

9. **Figure 12-27.** **Locate Zone 3.** Finally, probe Zone 3 from the mesiofacial line angle to the midline of the mesial surface.

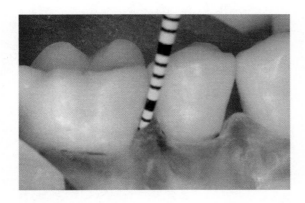

10. **Figure 12-28.** **Probe Zone 3.** Starting at the mesiofacial line angle, walk the probe across the mesial surface until it touches the contact area.

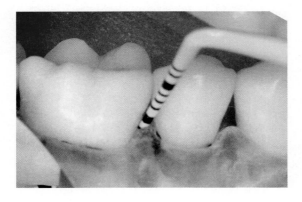

11. **Figure 12-29.** **Area 3. Assess beneath the contact area.** Tilt the probe and extend the tip beneath the contact area. Press down gently to touch the junctional epithelium. *Record the deepest reading for Area 3 on the periodontal chart.*

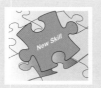

SKILL BUILDING
Probing Technique on Anterior Teeth

Directions:

- Follow steps 1 to 11 below to practice probing a maxillary canine (Figs. 12-30 to 12-40) to practice probing the facial aspect of a maxillary canine. **Divide the facial aspect of each tooth into three zones.** For an anterior tooth, a probing depth measurement is recorded for the following three zones of the facial aspect: (1) distofacial area, (2) facial surface, and (3) mesiofacial area.
  - Begin by probing the distofacial area and record the deepest measurement for this area.
  - Next, probe the facial surface and record the deepest measurement.
  - Finally, probe the mesiofacial area and record the deepest measurement on a periodontal chart.
- *Right-handed clinicians:* begin this practice session with the maxillary right canine, facial aspect. *Left-handed clinicians:* begin this practice session with the maxillary left canine, facial aspect.

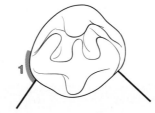

1. **Figure 12-30. Locate Zone 1.** Begin with Zone 1 from the distofacial line angle to the midline of the distal surface of the canine. (This drawing shows the incisal view of a canine.)

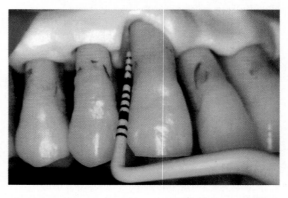

2. **Figure 12-31. Zone 1. Insert at the distofacial line angle.** Begin by inserting the probe at the distofacial line angle of the canine. You are now in position to assess the distal area of the facial aspect.

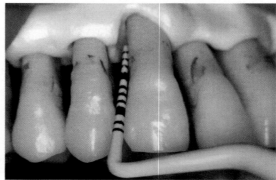

3. **Figure 12-32. Zone 1. Walk toward the distal surface.** Walk the probe across the distal surface until it touches the contact area. Gently touch the junctional epithelium with each downward stroke of the probe.

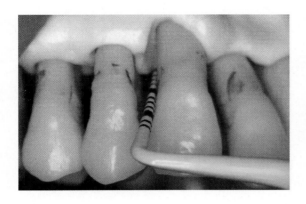

4. **Figure 12-33.** **Zone 1. Assess beneath the contact area.** Tilt the probe and extend the tip beneath the contact area. Press down gently to touch the junctional epithelium. *Record the deepest measurement for Area 1 on the periodontal chart as the distofacial reading.*

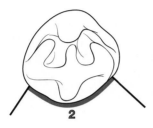

2

5. **Figure 12-34.** **Locate Zone 2.** The second zone is the facial surface, extending from the distofacial line angle to the mesiofacial line angle. (This drawing shows the incisal view of a canine.)

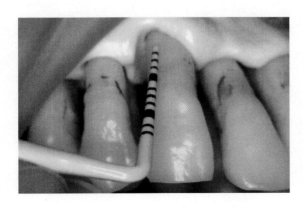

6. **Figure 12-35.** **Zone 2. Reposition the probe at the distofacial line angle.** Remove the probe from the sulcus and reinsert it at the distofacial line angle. You are now in position to probe the facial surface of the canine.

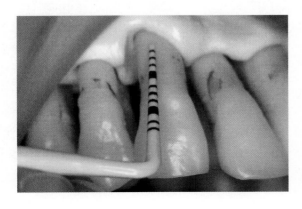

7. **Figure 12-36.** **Zone 2. Assess the facial surface.** Make a series of walking strokes across the facial surface.

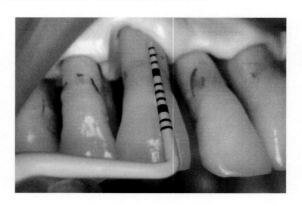

8. **Figure 12-37. Zone 2. Walk toward the mesial surface.** Walk across the facial surface, stopping at the mesiofacial line angle. *Record the deepest reading in Area 2 on the periodontal chart.*

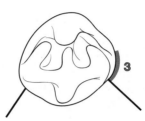

9. **Figure 12-38. Locate Zone 3.** Finally assess Zone 3 from the mesiofacial line angle to the midline of the mesial surface. (This drawing shows the incisal view of a canine.)

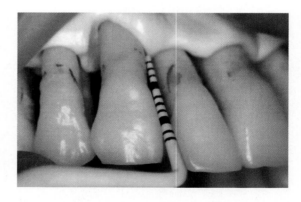

10. **Figure 12-39. Zone 3.** Begin with the probe positioned at the mesiofacial line angle. Walk the probe onto the mesial surface until it touches the contact area.

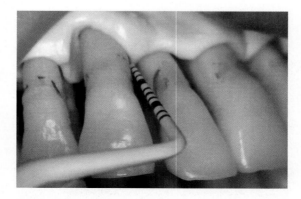

11. **Figure 12-40. Zone 3. Assess beneath the contact area.** On adjacent *anterior teeth,* only a slight tilt is needed to probe the col area. Gently probe the col area. *Record the deepest reading for Zone 3 on the periodontal chart.*

Section 5
Informed Consent for Periodontal Instrumentation

Once the dental hygienist has completed an assessment of the oral status of the patient's periodontium, the next step is to explain the findings to the patient and present treatment recommendations. The core value of "Individual Autonomy and Respect for Human Beings" within the Code of Ethics for the American Dental Hygienists' Association discusses informed consent (19).

1. Informed Consent for Periodontal Instrumentation
   A. It is the responsibility of the dental hygienist to provide complete and comprehensive information about the recommended plan for periodontal instrumentation so that the patient can make a well-informed decision about either accepting or rejecting the proposed treatment.
   B. Informed consent not only involves informing the patient about the expected successful outcomes of periodontal instrumentation, but the possible risks, unanticipated outcomes, and alternative treatments as well. The patient should be made aware of the costs for each of the options involved, which may influence the patient's ultimate decision. Box 12-2 summarizes some of the ethical considerations for informed consent.
2. Capacity for Consent. A patient must also have the capacity to consent.
   A. Capacity for consent—the ability of a patient to fully understand the proposed treatment, possible risks, unanticipated outcomes, and alternative treatments—takes into account the patient's age, mental capacity, and language comprehension.
   B. The patient expects that the proposed periodontal instrumentation will be performed according to the proper standard of care, or that of the "reasonably prudent hygienist."
   C. A dialogue between the patient and the hygienist is the best way to initiate the informed consent process.
3. Documenting Consent
   A. Once the patient is satisfied and agrees to the proposed plan for periodontal instrumentation, it is best if it is written in the patient's chart and signed by the patient and hygienist. This is an example of written consent. Written consent is legally binding and will hold up in a court of law.
   B. Both verbal consent (verbally agreeing to a proposed treatment without any formal written documentation), and implied consent (sitting in a dental chair and opening one's mouth for the hygienist), although acceptable for certain procedures, is not as legally sound as written consent.

Box 12-2 **Ethical Considerations for Informed Consent for the Patient**

- Reasoning/importance of proposed periodontal instrumentation
- Expected outcomes of the proposed periodontal instrumentation
- Risks involved in the proposed periodontal instrumentation
- Possible unexpected results of periodontal instrumentation
- Alternative approaches to periodontal instrumentation
- Possible consequences of refusal of treatment
- Costs of proposed treatment and alternatives
- Patient's capacity to consent (age, mental, language comprehension)
- Written consent by patient

4. **Informed Refusal.** Despite being informed of the proposed treatments, risks, and alternatives, the patient may decide to refuse the treatment plan. This is called "informed refusal."

  A. Autonomy, as defined by the ADHA Code of Ethics guarantees "self-determination" of the patient, and is linked to informed consent (19).

  B. Only after the patient has received informed consent, can a decision be made to either accept or reject the proposed treatment.

  C. Although refusal may not be the optimal choice of the treating hygienist, the patient has a right to make any decision about his/her treatments that only affects him/her personally and does not pose a threat to others. Radiographs, fluoride treatments, and sealants are a few services for which patients have exercised informed refusal.

  D. As a result each dental office should include an informed consent/refusal form as part of the patient treatment record to insure proper documentation.

  E. Figure 12-41 shows an example of an informed consent/informed refusal form.

Informed Consent/Informed Refusal Form

1. I _____ , (name) agree to the proposed dental treatment by _____ , (name) RDH.

2. I fully understand the importance of the proposed treatment. ___Yes ___No

3. I understand that _____ is the expected outcome of the proposed treatment.

4. I understand that the possible risks/and or unanticipated outcomes of the proposed treatment are _____ .

5. The possible treatment alternatives to the proposed treatment are _____ .

6. I have been informed of the costs of the proposed and alternative treatments.   ___Yes ___No

7. I understand the possible consequence(s) of refusal of the proposed treatment is/are_____ .

8. I have the capacity to consent to the proposed treatment. ___Yes ___No

9. I refuse the proposed treatment. ___Yes ___No

10. Please list the treatment you are refusing. _____

_____   _____   _____
Patient Signature   Date   RDH Signature

Figure 12-41. Sample Informed Consent/Informed Refusal Form.

References

1. Orban BJ, Grant DA. *Orban's Periodontics: A Concept-Theory and Practice*. Saint Louis: Mosby, 1972.
2. Hefti AF. Periodontal probing. *Crit Rev Oral Biol Med*. 1997;8(3):336–356.
3. Khan S, Cabanilla LL. Periodontal probing depth measurement: a review. *Compend Contin Educ Dent*. 2009;30(1):12–14, 6, 8–21; quiz 2, 36.
4. Armitage GC. Diagnosis of periodontal diseases. *J Periodontol*. 2003;74(8):1237–1247.
5. Williams CH. Some newer periodontal findings of practical importance to the general practitioner. *J Can Dent Assoc*. 1936;2:333–340.
6. Gibbs CH, Hirschfeld JW, Lee JG, et al. Description and clinical evaluation of a new computerized periodontal probe–the Florida probe. *J Clin Periodontol*. 1988;15(2):137–144.
7. Mullally BH, Linden GJ. Comparative reproducibility of proximal probing depth using electronic pressure-controlled and hand probing. *J Clin Periodontol*. 1994;21(4):284–288.
8. Osborn JB, Stoltenberg JL, Huso BA, Aeppli DM, Pihlstrom BL. Comparison of measurement variability in subjects with moderate periodontitis using a conventional and constant force periodontal probe. *J Periodontol*. 1992;63(4):283–289.
9. Tupta-Veselicky L, Famili P, Ceravolo FJ, Zullo T. A clinical study of an electronic constant force periodontal probe. *J Periodontol*. 1994;65(6):616–622.
10. Wang SF, Leknes KN, Zimmerman GJ, Sigurdsson TJ, Wikesjo UM, Selvig KA. Reproducibility of periodontal probing using a conventional manual and an automated force-controlled electronic probe. *J Periodontol*. 1995;66(1):38–46.
11. Listgarten MA. Periodontal probing: what does it mean? *J Clin Periodontol*. 1980;7(3):165–176.
12. Persson GR. Effects of line-angle versus midproximal periodontal probing measurements on prevalence estimates of periodontal disease. *J Periodontal Res*. 1991;26(6):527–529.
13. Badersten A, Nilveus R, Egelberg J. Reproducibility of probing attachment level measurements. *J Clin Periodontol*. 1984;11(7):475–485.
14. Chamberlain AD, Renvert S, Garrett S, Nilveus R, Egelberg J. Significance of probing force for evaluation of healing following periodontal therapy. *J Clin Periodontol*. 1985;12(4):306–311.
15. Hassell TM, Hefti AF. Drug-induced gingival overgrowth: old problem, new problem. *Crit Rev Oral Biol Med*. 1991;2(1):103–137.
16. Newman MG, Takei HH, Klokkevold PR, Carranza FA. *Carranza's Clinical Periodontology*. 12th ed. St. Louis, MO: Saunders, 2014.
17. van der Zee E, Davies EH, Newman HN. Marking width, calibration from tip and tine diameter of periodontal probes. *J Clin Periodontol*. 1991;18(7):516–552.
18. van Weringh M, Barendregt DS, Rosema NA, Timmerman MF, van der Weijden GA. A thin or thick probe handle: does it make a difference? *Int J Dent Hyg*. 2006;4(3):140–144.
19. *ADHA Bylaws and code of ethics*. Chicago, IL: American Dental Hygienists' Association; 2014.

Section 6
Skill Application

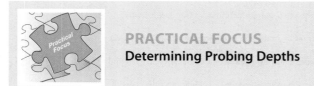

PRACTICAL FOCUS
Determining Probing Depths

1. **Probing Depths.** Using the color-coded probe shown in Figure 12-41, measure and record the probing depths for the three teeth illustrated in Figures 12-42 to 12-45 below.

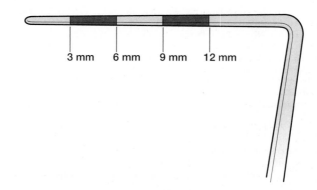

3 mm	6 mm	9 mm	12 mm

Figure 12-42. **Probe Millimeter Markings.**

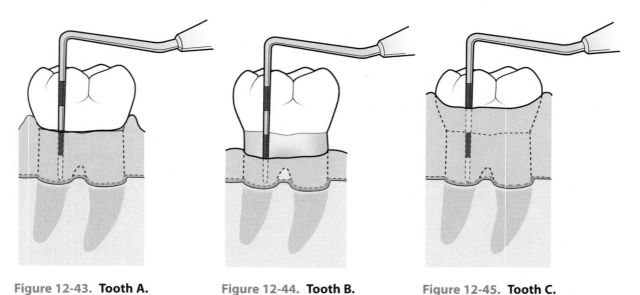

Figure 12-43. **Tooth A.**
Probing Depth = ___ mm

Figure 12-44. **Tooth B.**
Probing Depth = ___ mm

Figure 12-45. **Tooth C.**
Probing Depth = ___ mm

Assess the Probing Depths. Look closely at teeth A, B, and C above.

1. Compare the bone level on these three teeth? Is the level of bone the same or different for these teeth?
2. Compare the probing depths. Do the probing depths provide you with an accurate picture of the amount of bone lost from around each of the teeth?

Student Self Evaluation Module 12: Basic Probing Technique

Student: _____   Anterior Area 1 = _____

Date: _____   Anterior Area 2 = _____

Posterior Area 3 = _____

Posterior Area 4 = _____

DIRECTIONS: Self-evaluate your skill level in each treatment area as: **S** (satisfactory) or **U** (unsatisfactory).

Criteria				
Positioning/Ergonomics	Area 1	Area 2	Area 3	Area 4
Adjusts clinician chair correctly				
Reclines patient chair and assures that patient's head is even with top of headrest				
Positions instrument tray within easy reach for front, side, or rear delivery as appropriate for operatory configuration				
Positions unit light at arm's length or dons dental headlight and adjusts it for use				
Assumes the recommended clock position				
Positions backrest of patient chair for the specified arch and adjusts height of patient chair so that clinician's elbows remain at waist level when accessing the specified treatment area				
Asks patient to assume the head position that facilitates the clinician's view of the specified treatment area.				
Maintains neutral position				
Directs light to illuminate the specified treatment area				
Instrument Grasp: Dominant Hand	Area 1	Area 2	Area 3	Area 4
Grasps handle with tips of finger pads of index finger and thumb so that these fingers are opposite each other on the handle, but do NOT touch or overlap				
Rests pad of middle finger lightly on instrument shank; middle finger makes contact with ring finger				
Positions the thumb, index, and middle fingers in the "knuckles up" convex position; hyper-extended joint position is avoided				
Holds ring finger straight so that it supports the weight of hand and instrument; ring finger position is "advanced ahead of" the other fingers in the grasp				
Keeps index, middle, ring and little fingers in contact; "like fingers inside a mitten"				
Maintains a relaxed grasp; fingers are NOT blanched in grasp				
Finger Rest: Dominant Hand	Area 1	Area 2	Area 3	Area 4
Establishes secure finger rest that is appropriate for tooth to be treated				
Once finger rest is established, pauses to self-evaluate finger placement in the grasp, verbalizes to evaluator his/her self-assessment of grasp, and corrects finger placement if necessary				
Insertion	Area 1	Area 2	Area 3	Area 4
Establishes 0-degree angulation in preparation for insertion				
Gently inserts explorer tip beneath the gingival margin to base of sulcus or pocket				
Probing Technique	Area 1	Area 2	Area 3	Area 4
Orients probe working-end parallel to the root surface being probed				
Keeps tip in contact with the root surface				
Uses small walking strokes within the sulcus or periodontal pocket; maintains the probe beneath the gingival margin with each stroke				
Tilts probe and extends tip beneath contact area to assess interproximal area				
Covers entire circumference of the junctional epithelium with walking strokes				
Maintains neutral wrist position throughout motion activation				
Obtains measurement readings that are within 1 mm of the evaluator's measurements				

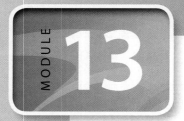

Explorers

Module Overview

Explorers have flexible wire-like working-ends used to detect subgingival calculus deposits and other irregularities for the purpose of assessing the progress and completeness of subgingival periodontal instrumentation. Explorers are also used to assess tooth anomalies, surface irregularities and the integrity of the margins on dental restorations. This module presents the design characteristics of explorers and step-by-step instructions for their use of in the detection of root surface irregularities and calculus deposits.

Module Outline

Section 1   **Explorers**   **288**
Functions and Design Characteristics
The Explorer Tip
Explorer Designs for Root Surface Assessment
The Assessment Stroke: The Feeling Stroke
Subgingival Assessment with an Explorer

Section 2   **Technique Practice—Anterior Teeth**   **293**
Skill Building. Anterior Teeth with Orban-Type Explorer, p. 293
Skill Building. Working-End Selection for Anterior Teeth:
    11/12-Type Explorer, p. 296
Skill Building. Anterior Teeth with 11/12-Type Explorer, p. 298

Section 3   **Technique Practice—Posterior Teeth**   **300**
Skill Building. Working-End Selection for Posterior Teeth:
    11/12-Type Explorer, p. 300
Skill Building. Mandibular Posterior Teeth with 11/12-Type
    Explorer, p. 301
Skill Building. Maxillary Posterior Teeth with 11/12-Type
    Explorer, p. 305

Section 4   **Technique Alerts**   **307**
Horizontal Strokes
Neutral Wrist Position

Section 5   **Detection of Dental Calculus Deposits**   **309**
Types and Characteristics of Calculus Deposits
The Nature of Calculus Formation
Supragingival Calculus Detection
Interpretation of Subgingival Conditions
Reference Table: Undetected Calculus

Section 6	**Detection of Dental Caries** Changing Paradigm for Caries Detection	**314**
Section 7	**Skill Application** Practical Focus Reference Sheet—Explorers Student Self Evaluation Module 13: Explorers	**318**

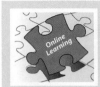

Online resource for this module:
- The ODU 11/12 Explorer
- The 17/23 Orban-Type Explorer

Available at: http://thepoint.lww.com/GehrigFundamentals8e

Key Terms

Assessment instruments

Explorers

Explorer tip

Supragingival
  instrumentation

Subgingival instrumentation

Assessment stroke

Exploratory stroke

Tactile sensitivity

Calculus

Plaque retentive

Supragingival deposits

Subgingival calculus deposits

Residual calculus deposits

Carious lesion

Cavitated lesion

Noncavitated lesion

Learning Objectives

- Given a variety of explorer designs, identify the design characteristics of each explorer and describe the advantages and limitations of the various explorer designs.

- Describe how the clinician can use visual clues to select the correct working-end of a double-ended explorer.

- Demonstrate correct adaptation of the explorer tip.

- Demonstrate an assessment stroke with an explorer while maintaining correct position, correct finger rests, and precise finger placement in the grasp.

- Demonstrate detection of *supra*gingival calculus deposits using compressed air.

- Name and describe several common types of calculus deposit formations.

- Explain why the forceful application of an explorer tip into a carious pit or fissure could be potentially harmful.

Section 1
Explorers

FUNCTIONS AND DESIGN CHARACTERISTICS

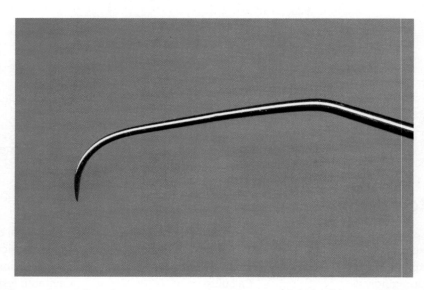

Figure 13-1. Explorer. An explorer is an assessment instrument with a flexible wire-like working-end.

1. Functions of Explorers
   A. Assessment instruments—such as periodontal probes and explorers—are used to determine the health of the periodontal tissues, tooth anatomy, and the texture of tooth surfaces. Figure 13-1 shows one example of an explorer.
   B. Explorers are used to detect, by tactile means, the texture and character of tooth surfaces before, during, and after periodontal instrumentation to assess the progress and completeness of instrumentation.
      1. The explorer's flexible working-end quivers as it is moved over tooth surface irregularities such as dental calculus.
      2. Dental calculus deposits frequently are located subgingivally below the gingival margin where they cannot be detected visually. Since these subgingival calculus deposits cannot be seen, the clinician must rely on his or her sense of touch to find and remove these hidden deposits. The explorer with its highly flexible working-end is the instrument of choice for detection of subgingival calculus deposits.
      3. Explorers also are used to examine tooth surfaces for dental anomalies, and anatomic features such as grooves, curvatures, or root furcations and to assess dental restorations and sealants.
2. Importance of Calculus Detection
   A. Plaque biofilm is the main cause of periodontal disease, however, calculus removal is critical to the successful treatment of periodontal disease. Calculus deposits harboring biofilms are directly related to more than 60% of the disease sites in periodontal disease (1).
   B. The explorer is the best instrument for assessing the texture of the root surface for the detection of biofilm retentive factors such as calculus, defective restorations, surface irregularities, and root caries.

3. Design of Explorers
   A. Explorers are made of flexible metal that conducts vibrations from the working-end to the clinician's fingers resting on the instrument shank and handle.
   B. Explorers are circular in cross section and may have unpaired (dissimilar) or paired working-ends.
   C. The working-end is 1 to 2 mm in length and is referred to as the explorer tip (Fig. 13-2).
   D. *The actual point of the explorer is not used to detect dental calculus; rather the side of explorer tip is applied to the tooth surface.*

THE EXPLORER TIP

For periodontal instrumentation, the explorer tip is defined as 1 to 2 mm of the *side* of the explorer. The tip is adapted to the tooth for detection of dental calculus or root surface irregularities.

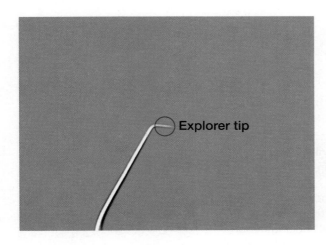

Explorer tip

Figure 13-2. Explorer Tip Design. Explorers are available in a variety of different designs. On this explorer, the tip is bent at a 90-degree angle to the lower shank. Such an explorer design is ideal for subgingival instrumentation. ***The actual point of the explorer is never used for detection of calculus.***

EXPLORER DESIGNS FOR ROOT SURFACE ASSESSMENT

Explorers are available in a variety of design types. Figures 13-3 to 13-5 depict explorer designs commonly used for assessing the texture of the root surface for the detection of biofilm retentive factors such as calculus, defective restoration, surface irregularities, and root caries.

All design types are not well suited to subgingival use; therefore, the clinician should be knowledgeable about the recommended use of each design type.

1. Supragingival instrumentation—use of an instrument coronal to (above) the gingival margin. For example, use of an explorer to examine the margins of restorations or dental sealants.
2. Subgingival instrumentation—use of an instrument apical to (below) the gingival margin. For example, use of an explorer to detect calculus deposits hidden beneath the gingival margin.

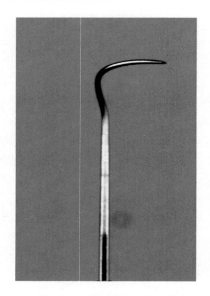

Figure 13-3. Pigtail and Cowhorn Explorers—get their names because they resemble a pig's tail or a bull's horns.
Design Characteristics: Care must be taken not to injure the soft tissue base of the sulcus or pocket with the point of the working-end.
Use:
- Calculus detection in normal sulci or shallow pockets extending no deeper than the cervical-third of the root.
- The curved lower shank causes considerable stretching of the tissue away from the root surface.

Examples: 3ML, 3CH, and 2A.

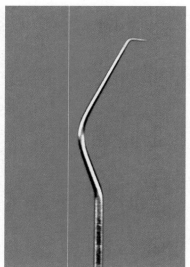

Figure 13-4. Orban-Type Explorer
Design Characteristics:
- The tip is bent at a 90-degree angle to the lower shank; this feature allows the *back of the tip* (instead of the point) to be directed against the soft tissue at the base of the sulcus or pocket.
- The straight lower shank allows insertion in narrow pockets with only slight stretching of the tissue away from the root surface.

Use: Assessment of anterior root surfaces and the facial and lingual surfaces of posterior teeth. Difficult to adapt to the line-angles and proximal surfaces of the posterior teeth.
Examples: 17, 20F, and TU17.

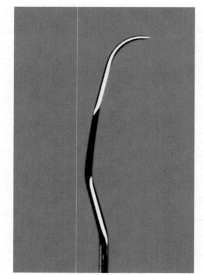

Figure 13-5. 11/12-Type Explorer—an explorer with several advantageous design characteristics:
Design Characteristics:
- Like the Orban-type explorers, the tip is at a 90-degree angle to the lower shank.
- The long complex shank design makes it equally useful when working on anterior and posterior teeth with normal sulci or a deep periodontal pockets.

Use: Assessment of root surfaces on anterior and posterior teeth.
Examples: ODU 11/12 and 11/12AF.

THE ASSESSMENT STROKE: THE FEELING STROKE

An assessment stroke, also called an exploratory stroke, is used to detect calculus deposits or other tooth surface irregularities. Assessment strokes require a high degree of precision. The proper use of an explorer requires feather light, controlled strokes. Table 13-1 summarizes the characteristics of an assessment stroke.

1. During subgingival instrumentation, the clinician relies on his or her sense of touch to locate calculus deposits hidden beneath the gingival margin.
   - *A critical factor of exploring effectively is pressure—the absence of pressure!*
   - The clinician holds the explorer in a very light grasp; light enough so that someone could grasp the instrument handle and slide the explorer from the clinician's grasp.
2. Tactile sensitivity is the ability to detect tooth irregularities by feeling vibrations transferred from the explorer tip to the handle.
   - For example, the explorer tip quivers slightly as it travels over rough calculus deposits on the tooth surface. These vibrations are transmitted from the tip, through the shank, and into the handle.
   - The clinician feels the vibrations with his or her fingertips resting on the handle and instrument shank.
3. The fine working-end and flexible shank of an explorer are used to enhance tactile information to the clinician's fingers.
   - The superior tactile conduction of an explorer makes it the instrument of choice for (1) *initially locating subgingival calculus deposits* and for (2) *re-evaluating tooth surfaces* following calculus removal.
4. *During calculus removal,* the curet may be used for calculus detection.
   - When all deposits detectable with a curet have been removed, a definitive evaluation of the root surface should be made using an explorer.
   - Because the explorer provides superior tactile information, it is common to detect some remaining calculus deposits with an explorer that could not be detected with a curet.

TABLE 13-1. ASSESSMENT STROKE WITH AN EXPLORER	
Grasp	Relaxed grasp; middle finger rests lightly on shank
Adaptation	1 to 2 mm of the side of the tip is adapted
Lateral Pressure	Feather light pressure with working-end against tooth
Activation	Wrist activation is usually recommended, however digital activation is acceptable with an explorer because physical strength is not required for assessment strokes.
Stroke Characteristics	Fluid, sweeping strokes
Stroke Number	Many close, overlapping multidirectional strokes are used to cover every square millimeter of the root surface
Common Errors	AVOID a tight, tense "death grip" on handle
	AVOID applying pressure with the middle finger against the instrument shank as this will reduce tactile information to the finger

SUBGINGIVAL ASSESSMENT WITH AN EXPLORER

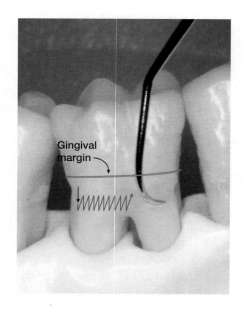

Gingival margin

Figure 13-6. Subgingival Exploring. Subgingival assessment strokes should be short in length and involve many, overlapping strokes covering every square millimeter of the root surface.

Steps for Subgingival Exploration: Feeling What Cannot Be Seen

1. **Get Ready and Insert.** Adapt the explorer tip to the tooth surface above the gingival margin in the middle-third of the crown. Gently slide the tip under the gingival margin.
2. **Insert to Base of Pocket.** Keep the tip constantly in contact with the root surface. Gently slide the explorer in an apical direction until the back of the tip touches the soft tissue base of the sulcus or pocket. The attached tissue will have a soft, elastic feel.
3. **Initiate Assessment Stroke In Coronal Direction.** Move the tip forward slightly and use a vertical or oblique stroke to move the explorer up the surface of the root. Keep the tip in contact with the root surface as you pull the tip up toward the gingival margin. Concentrate, as the tip moves over the tooth surface; be alert for quivers of the tip that indicate a calculus deposit.
4. **Control Stroke Length.** Don't remove the explorer tip from the sulcus or pocket as you make an upward stroke. Removing and reinserting the tip repeatedly can traumatize the tissue at the gingival margin. Bring the explorer tip to a point just beneath the gingival margin and move the tip forward slightly.
5. **Reposition at Base of Pocket.** Maintaining the tip in contact with the tooth surface, return the tip to the base of the sulcus or pocket. As you move the tip, remain alert for tactile information transmitted through the instrument shank.
6. **Divide Root into Apical, Middle, and Cervical Sections.** Keep your assessment strokes short, approximately 2 to 3 mm in length.
   - If you are working within a normal sulcus, your strokes will extend from the base of the sulcus to a point just beneath the gingival margin.
   - Within a pocket, first, explore the portion of the root next to the base of the pocket. Then, move the tip up and explore the mid-section on the root. Finally, assess the section near the gingival margin. The depth of the pocket will determine how many sections—3 mm in height—are needed to cover the entire root surface.
7. **Considerations for Proximal Surfaces.** On the distal and mesial proximal surfaces lead with the point of the explorer tip. Do not "back" into the proximal surface. Your strokes should reach under the contact area, so that half of the proximal surface is explored from the facial aspect and half from the lingual aspect of the tooth.

Section 2
Technique Practice—Anterior Teeth

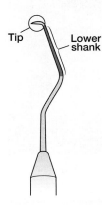

Tip   Lower shank

Figure 13-7. The Orban-Type Explorer. An Orban-type explorer, such as a TU17, is an excellent choice for subgingival assessment of the anterior teeth. The straight lower shank allows insertion in narrow pockets with only slight tissue stretching away from the root surface. The tip design allows the back of the tip—rather than the sharp point—to be directed against the junctional epithelium.

New Skill

SKILL BUILDING
Anterior Teeth with Orban-Type Explorer

Directions:

- Follow the steps depicted in Figures 13-8 to 13-15 to practice exploring the mandibular anterior teeth with an Orban-type explorer.
- Remember: "Me, My patient, My light, My dominant hand, My nondominant hand, My finger rest, My adaptation."

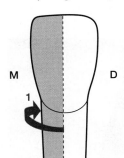

M   D

1

Figure 13-8. Tooth Surface. First practice on the mandibular left central incisor, facial aspect.
- **Right-handed** clinicians—*surface toward.*
- **Left-handed** clinicians—*surface away.*

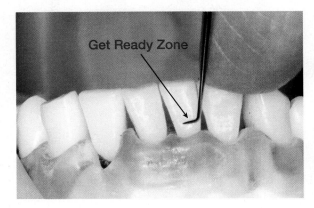

Get Ready Zone

Figure 13-9. Place the Tip in the Get Ready Zone.
- Place the tip on the middle-third of the crown near the midline of the facial surface.
- The point of the explorer should face in the direction of the mesial surface.

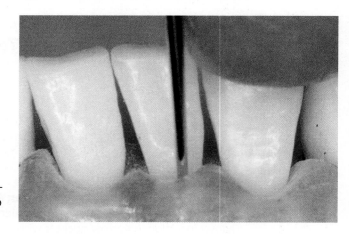

Figure 13-10. Insert. Gently insert the working-end beneath the gingival margin keeping the tip in contact with the tooth surface.

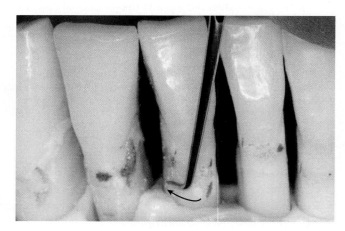
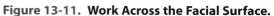

Figure 13-11. Work Across the Facial Surface.
- Make assessment strokes across the facial surface working toward the mesial surface.
- It may be helpful to remove the gingival tissue from the typodont to facilitate practice on the root surfaces.
- As you approach the mesiofacial line angle, roll the instrument handle to maintain adaptation.

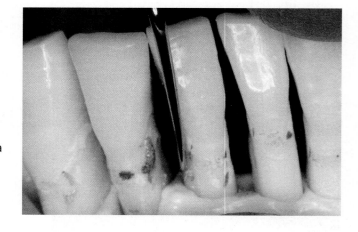

Figure 13-12. Explore the Mesial Surface.
Continue making strokes under the contact area until you have explored at least halfway across the mesial proximal surface. (The other half of the mesial surface is assessed from the lingual aspect of the tooth.)

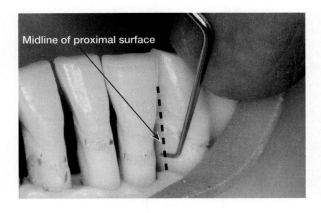

Figure 13-13. Technique Check. This photograph shows a dental typodont with the gingiva removed. Note the position of the explorer tip on the mesial of this canine tooth. Correct technique demands that the explorer reach at least the halfway point of the proximal surface under the contact area.

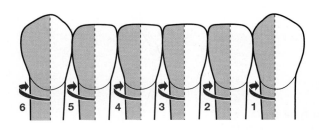

Figure 13-14. Sequence 1. Next, use the sequence shown in this illustration to explore the colored tooth surfaces of the facial aspect. Begin with the left canine and end with the right canine.

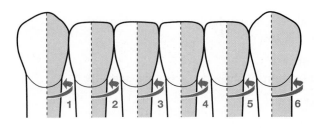

Figure 13-15. Sequence 2. Change your clock position and complete the remaining facial surfaces, beginning with the right canine and ending with the left canine.

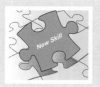

SKILL BUILDING
Working-End Selection for Anterior Teeth: 11/12-Type Explorer

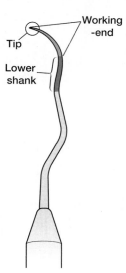

Figure 13-16. An 11/12-Type Explorer. Like the Orban-type explorer, the tip of this explorer is at a 90-degree angle to the lower shank. The ODU 11/12 is a double-ended instrument with mirror image working-ends.

The working-end design of a 11/12-type explorer makes it more challenging to adapt to the anterior teeth than an Orban-type explorer (Fig. 13-16).

- This explorer has a rather long curved working-end.
- It is important to remember that only the terminal 2 mm of the side of tip are actually adapted to the tooth surface.
- Figure 13-17 depicts correct working-end selection. Incorrect working-end selection is shown in Figure 13-18. Box 13-1 summarizes working-end selection.

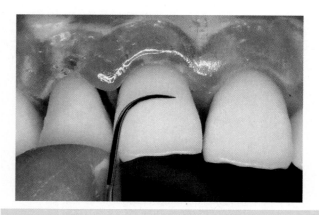

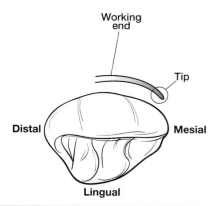

Figure 13-17. Correct Working-End.
- The photo and illustration show the correct working-end for use on the midline of the facial surface to the midline of the mesial surface. (This is the surface away from the right-handed clinician and the surface toward the left-handed clinician.)
- *The correct working-end is 12.* The correct working-end curves inward toward—"wraps around"—the facial surface.

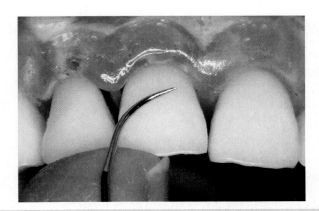
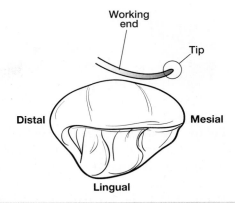

Figure 13-18. Incorrect Working-End.
- The photo and illustration show the incorrect working-end for use on the midline of the facial surface to the midline of the mesial surface. (This is the surface away from the right-handed clinician and the surface toward the left-handed clinician.)
- *The incorrect working-end is 11.* The incorrect working-end curves outward, away from the facial surface.

Box 13-1	Visual Clue Anterior Teeth: "Wrapping" the Working-End

1. A useful visual clue in selecting the correct working-end is to select the working-end that "wraps around" or "curves toward" the tooth surface.
   - ***When using this visual clue, it is vital to understand that the entire working-end does not wrap around the tooth during an assessment stroke. During an assessment stroke, only the tip of the working-end is adapted to the tooth surface.***
   - "Wrapping" the working-end is simply a useful verbal description when explaining working-end selection.

2. Selecting the working-end that curves inward toward the tooth surface facilitates adaptation of the explorer tip to the curved surfaces of the anterior teeth.

3. Using the explorer in this manner is very similar to the way that a universal curet is adapted to the anterior teeth. Thus, this method aids in transfer of the technique from the explorer to the universal curet.

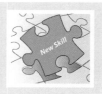

SKILL BUILDING
Anterior Teeth with 11/12-Type Explorer

- Follow the steps depicted in Figures 13-19 to 13-24 to practice exploring the maxillary anterior teeth with a 11/12-type explorer.
- **Right-handed clinicians** begin practice with the surfaces away; **Left-handed clinicians** begin practice with the surfaces toward.
- Remember: "Me, My patient, My light, My dominant hand, My nondominant hand, My finger rest, My adaptation."

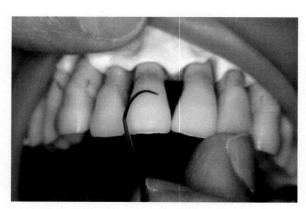

1. **Figure 13-19. Select the Correct Working-End.**
   - Select the correct working-end for use on the midline of the facial surface to the midline of the mesial surface (right-handed clinician: surface away; left-handed clinician: surface toward).
   - The correct working-end is the **12**.

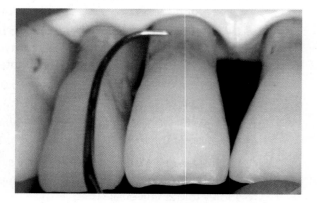

2. **Figure 13-20. Insert and Position for Instrumentation.**
   - Gently insert the #12 working-end to the base of the pocket.
   - Position the tip slightly to the right of the midline with the tip facing toward the mesial surface.
   - Make a series of assessment strokes in the direction of the mesial surface.

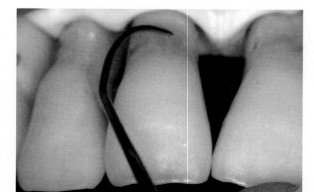

3. **Figure 13-21. Work Across the Facial Surface.**
   - Make assessment strokes across the facial surface.
   - Roll the instrument handle to keep the just the tip of the working-end adapted to the root surface.

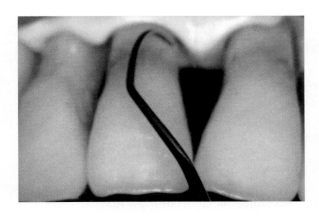

4. **Figure 13-22.** **Move Around the Line Angle.** Roll the instrument handle to move the tip around the mesiofacial line angle.

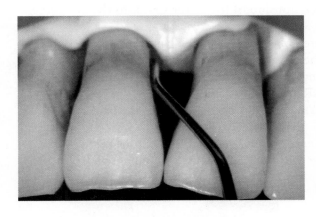

5. **Figure 13-23.** **Assess the Mesial Surface.** Assess at least halfway across the mesial surface from the facial aspect.

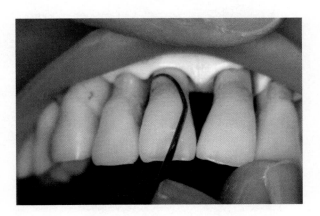

6. **Figure 13-24.** **Assess the Other Half of Tooth.**
   - Select the correct working-end to instrument the surface toward if you are right-handed (or the surface away if you are left-handed).
   - The correct working-end is the **11**.

Section 3
Technique Practice—Posterior Teeth

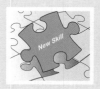

SKILL BUILDING
Working-End Selection for Posterior Teeth: 11/12-Type Explorer

Before using a double-ended explorer on the posterior sextants, the clinician must first determine which working-end to use.

1. To select the correct working-end, observe the relationship of the lower shank to the distal surface of the tooth.
2. Pick a tooth that is easily seen, such as the first premolar tooth. Randomly select one of the explorer working-ends and adapt the tip to the distal surface of the first premolar.
   A. As shown in Figure 13-25, the correct working-end is selected if the lower shank is parallel to the distal surface of the premolar. Refer to Box 13-2.
   B. As shown in Figure 13-26, the incorrect working-end has been selected if the lower shank extends across the facial surface of the premolar.
3. Using the mandibular right posterior sextant as an example, one working-end of the explorer adapts to the facial aspect and the other working-end adapts to the lingual aspect of the sextant.

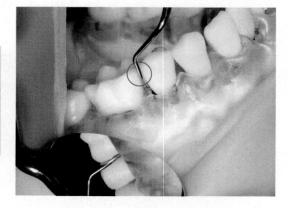

Figure 13-25. Correct Working-End.
Visual Clue to Correct Working-End:
* ***Lower shank*** is parallel to the distal surface of the premolar
* ***Functional shank*** goes "up and over the premolar tooth"

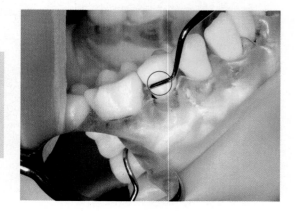

Figure 13-26. Incorrect Working-End.
Visual Clue to Incorrect Working-End:
* ***Lower shank*** is not parallel to distal surface of the premolar
* ***Functional shank*** is "down and around the premolar tooth"

Box 13-2 Working-End Selection on Posterior Teeth

When the working-end is adapted to a distal surface of a posterior tooth, the correct working-end has the following relationship between the shank and the tooth:

- Lower shank is parallel to the distal surface
- Functional shank goes up and over the tooth

Think: "Posterior = Parallel. Functional shank up and over!"

SKILL BUILDING
Mandibular Posterior Teeth with 11/12-Type Explorer

Directions:

- Follow the steps depicted in Figures 13-27 to 13-39 to practice exploring the mandibular right posterior sextant, facial aspect with a 11/12-type explorer.
- Remember: "Me, My patient, My light, My dominant hand, My nondominant hand, My finger rest, My adaptation."

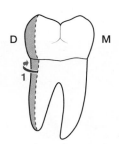

1. **Figure 13-27. Begin with Mandibular First Molar.** As an introduction to exploring the posterior teeth, first practice on the *mandibular right first molar.* The distal surface is completed first, beginning at the distofacial line angle and working onto the distal surface.

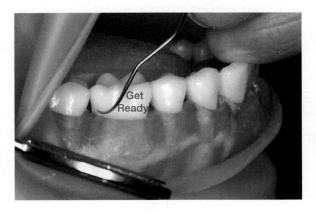

2. **Figure 13-28. Position the Tip Near the Distofacial Line Angle in the Get Ready Zone.**
   - Place the tip in the middle-third of the crown just forward of the distofacial line angle.
   - The tip should aim toward the back of the mouth because this is the direction in which you are working.

3. **Figure 13-29. Insert.**
   - Lower the instrument handle and adapt the "face" of the explorer tip to the tooth surface.
   - Slide the tip beneath the gingival margin.

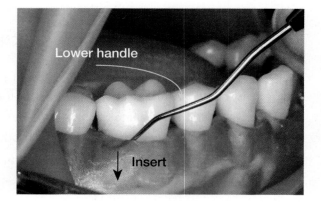

4. **Figure 13-30. Explore Distal Surface.**
   - Return the handle to its normal position.
   - Beginning at the distofacial line angle, make feather-light strokes toward the distal surface.

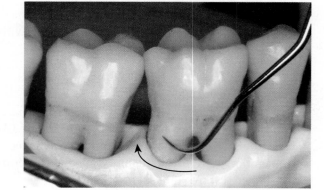

5. **Figure 13-31. Roll the Instrument Handle.**
   - Roll the instrument handle slightly to adapt to the distal surface.
   - Explore at least halfway across the distal surface from the facial aspect. Keep the tip adapted to the tooth surface at all times.

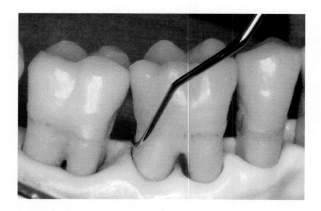

6. **Figure 13-32. Explore the Facial Surface.** You are now ready to explore the facial and mesial surfaces of the tooth, beginning at the distofacial line angle.

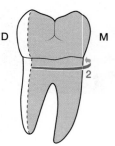

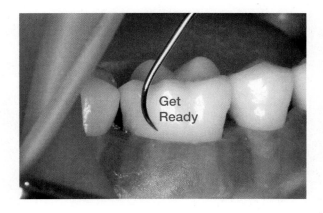

7. **Figure 13-33.** **Reposition the Tip for Facial Surface.**
   - While maintaining your fulcrum, remove the tip from the sulcus and turn it so that it aims toward the front of the mouth.
   - Place the tip in the middle-third of the facial surface with the point facing forward.

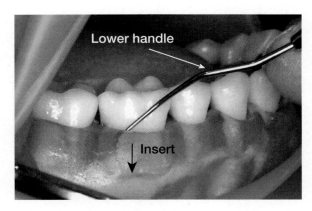

8. **Figure 13-34.** **Insert.**
   - Lower the instrument handle and place the "face" of the explorer against the facial surface in preparation for insertion.
   - Reinsert the tip and reposition it just to the left of the distofacial line angle.

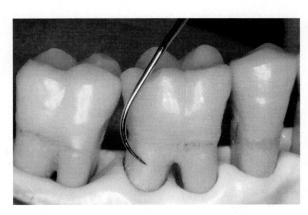

9. **Figure 13-35.** **Explore the Facial Surface.**
   - Return the handle to its normal position.
   - Beginning at the distofacial line angle initiate feather-light strokes.

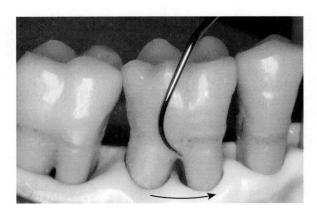

10. **Figure 13-36.** **Roll the Handle.** Continue making feather-light strokes across the facial surface.

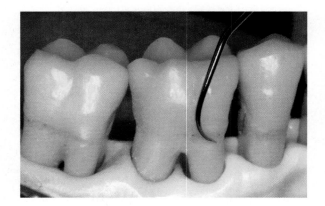

11. **Figure 13-37. Roll the Handle.** As you approach the mesiofacial line angle, roll the handle slightly to maintain adaptation.

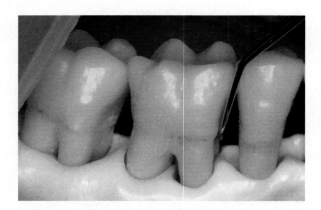

12. **Figure 13-38. Continue Strokes.** Explore at least halfway across the mesial surface from the facial aspect. (The other half of the mesial surface is explored from the lingual aspect.)

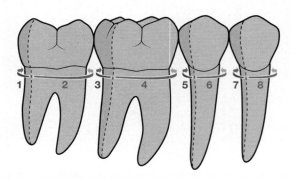

13. **Figure 13-39. Sequence for Sextant.** Next, use the sequence shown in this illustration to explore the facial aspect of the entire sextant, beginning with the posterior-most molar.

SKILL BUILDING
Maxillary Posterior Teeth with 11/12-Type Explorer

Directions:

- Follow the steps depicted in Figures 13-40 to 13-45 to practice exploring the maxillary left posterior sextant, lingual aspect with a 11/12-type explorer.
- Remember: "Me, My patient, My light, My dominant hand, My nondominant hand, My finger rest, My adaptation."

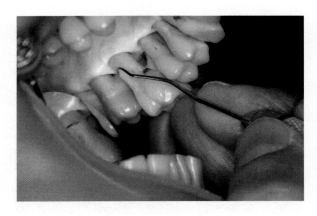

1. **Figure 13-40. Begin at the Distolingual Line Angle.** Position the explorer tip at the distolingual line angle in preparation for assessing the distal surface.

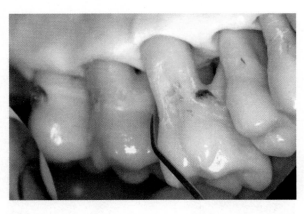

2. **Figure 13-41. Assess the Distal Surface.** Make assessment strokes from the distolingual line angle to the midline of the distal surface.

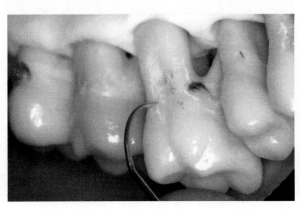

3. **Figure 13-42. Prepare to Assess the Lingual Surface.** Reposition the explorer tip at the distolingual in preparation for assessing the lingual surface.

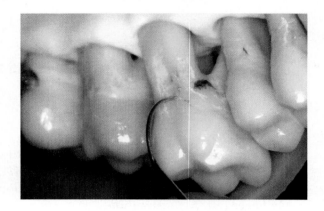

4. **Figure 13-43. Assess the Lingual Surface.** Make assessment strokes across the lingual surface.

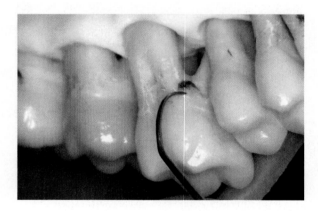

5. **Figure 13-44. Assess the Mesial Surface.** Roll the instrument handle to keep the tip adapted as you work around the mesiolingual line angle. Continue making assessment strokes across the mesial surface.

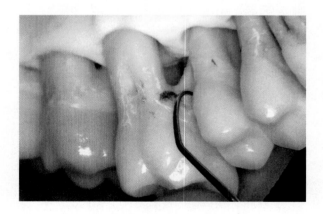

6. **Figure 13-45. Extend Strokes Across Mesial Surface.** Continue assessment strokes at least halfway across the mesial surface.

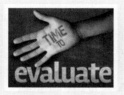

NOTE TO COURSE INSTRUCTOR: Exploration of root concavities and furcation areas is covered in Module 22, Advanced Techniques for Root Surface Debridement.

Section 4
Technique Alerts

HORIZONTAL STROKES

New clinicians often fail to detect calculus deposits that are located (1) near the distofacial or distolingual line angle of posterior teeth and (2) at the midline of the facial or lingual surfaces of anterior teeth. Undetected calculus deposits may result from not overlapping the assessment strokes sufficiently at the line angles and midlines of teeth. Horizontal strokes are extremely useful for calculus detection in these areas. Follow the steps depicted in Figures 13-46 and 13-48 to practice horizontal strokes at the distofacial line angle of a molar tooth and the midline of an anterior tooth.

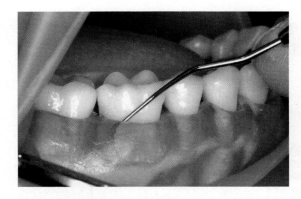

Figure 13-46. Position for Horizontal Strokes. Insert the explorer slightly distal to the distofacial line angle. *Lower the instrument handle until the explorer's point is toward—but not touching—the base of the pocket.* Make several short, controlled horizontal strokes around the line angle.

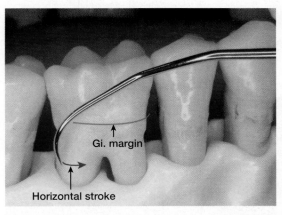

Figure 13-47. Technique Check: Working-End Position. This photograph was taken on a typodont with the gingiva removed so that the explorer working-end is visible. The tip is positioned at the line angle and a short horizontal stroke is made around the line angle. Note that the point of the explorer is toward the base of the pocket and care must be taken not to injure the junctional epithelium with the sharp point.

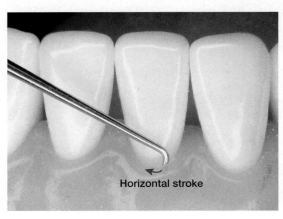

Figure 13-48. Horizontal Strokes: Midline of Anterior Tooth. Insert the explorer tip just distal to the midline.
- Lower the handle until the explorer's point is toward—**but not touching**—the base of the pocket.
- Make several short, controlled horizontal strokes across the midline.

NEUTRAL WRIST POSITION

The most common positioning error when working on the maxillary posterior treatment areas is failing to maintain a neutral wrist position. A failure to maintain neutral wrist position occurs when the clinician bends the wrist rather than (1) assuming the correct clock position (Fig. 13-49) or (2) adjusting the handle position in the grasp. Correct neutral wrist position is shown in Figure 13-50.

Directions: This technique practice allows you to experience the difference in wrist positions that result from using two different handle positions in the grasp.

1. Equipment: an ODU 11/12-type explorer.
2. Right-handed clinicians: maxillary right central incisor, surface away; Left-handed clinicians: maxillary right central incisor, surface toward

Figure 13-49. Incorrect Wrist Position.
Here the clinician is instrumenting the maxillary anterior surfaces away from the clinician.
- Note that the clinician is incorrectly seated in the 8:00 position.
- In this position, the clinician must bend his or her wrist in order to position the lower shank parallel to the distal surface of the tooth.

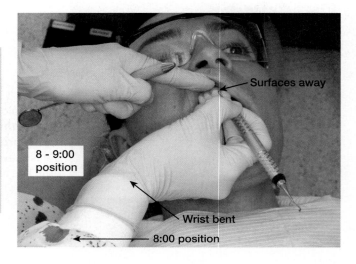

Figure 13-50. Correct Wrist Position.
Here the clinician is seated correctly in the 11 to 12:00 position for the anterior surfaces away.
- Note that the wrist is in neutral position.
- The instrument handle rests securely against the index finger in the "handle-down" orientation.

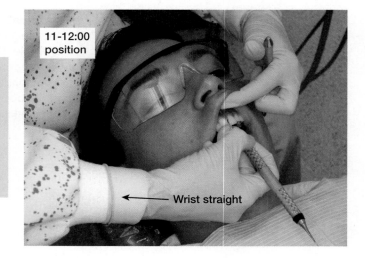

Section 5
Detection of Dental Calculus Deposits

TYPES AND CHARACTERISTICS OF CALCULUS DEPOSITS

Calculus is calcified plaque biofilm that forms as a hard tenacious mass on tooth surfaces and dental prostheses. It is commonly known as tartar. Calculus deposits are plaque retentive, meaning that the outer surface of a calculus deposit is covered with a layer of dental plaque biofilm.

1. *Supra*gingival deposits are calculus deposits located coronal to the gingival margin (above the gingival margin).
   - When dried with a stream of compressed air, supragingival calculus has a rough, chalky appearance that contrasts visually with the smooth enamel surfaces.
   - Wet supragingival calculus is difficult to detect because the wet surface reflects light and blends in with the shiny tooth enamel.
2. *Sub*gingival calculus deposits are hidden beneath the gingival margin within the gingival sulcus or periodontal pocket. (Think "*sub*marines travel beneath the surface of the water".) Subgingival calculus deposits often are flattened in shape due to the pressure of the pocket wall against the tooth.
3. Residual calculus deposits are tiny remnants of a larger calculus deposit remaining on the surface of the root after instrumentation.

THE NATURE OF CALCULUS FORMATION

When attempting to imagine the nature of subgingival deposits, remember that the deposits are built up layer by layer slowly over time.

- Calculus deposits are heavier more often near the CEJ rather than near the junctional epithelium, as deposits near the CEJ have been forming longer than those near the base of the pocket.
- The most common types of calculus formations are spicules, nodules, ledges, rings, veneers, and finger-like formations (2). These formations are described in Box 13-3 and depicted in Figure 13-51.

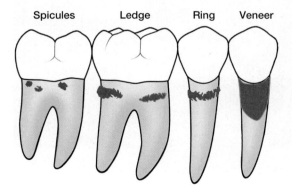

Figure 13-51. Common Calculus Formations. Four common types of calculus formations are spicules, ledges, rings, and veneers.

Box 13-3	Common Calculus Formations

Spicule—an isolated, minute particle or speck of calculus. Commonly found under contact areas, at line angles, and at the midline line of a tooth.

Nodule—larger spicule-type formations with a crusty or spiny surface

Ledge—a long ridge of calculus running parallel to the gingival margin. Common on all tooth surfaces.

Ring—a ridge of calculus running parallel to the gingival margin that encircles the tooth.

Veneer—a thin, smooth coating of calculus with a "shield-like shape" located on a portion of the root surface.

Finger-like formation—a long, narrow deposit running parallel or oblique to the long axis of the root.

SUPRAGINGIVAL CALCULUS DETECTION

Supragingival calculus is detected visually using a good light source, a dental mirror, and compressed air. When wet with saliva, supragingival calculus deposits are difficult to see. To detect these deposits, the clinician should apply a continuous stream of compressed air to the tooth surfaces as they are being visually examined (Fig. 13-52).

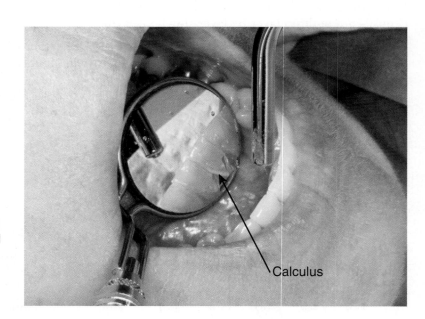

Calculus

Figure 13-52. Use of Compressed Air for Detection of Supragingival Calculus Deposits. Examine the tooth surfaces visually while applying a continuous stream of air with the air syringe.

INTERPRETATION OF SUBGINGIVAL CONDITIONS

The ability to assess the texture of the root surface for the detection of biofilm retentive factors such as calculus, defective restorations, surface irregularities, and root caries is a skill that takes time and concentration to develop. The illustrations and descriptions in Figures 13-53 to 13-58 depict tactile sensations transmitted from the explorer tip to the clinician's fingers.

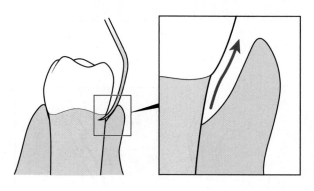

Figure 13-53. Normal Conditions. The fingers do not feel any interruptions in the path of the explorer as it moves from the junctional epithelium to the gingival margin.

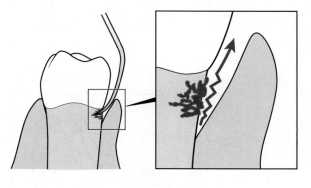

Figure 13-54. Spicules of Subgingival Calculus. The explorer tip transmits a gritty sensation to the clinician's fingers as it passes over fine, granular deposits. This can be compared to the sensation experienced when inline skating over a few pieces of gravel scattered on one area of a paved surface.

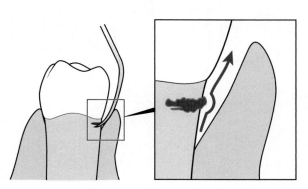

Figure 13-55. Ledge of Subgingival Calculus. As the explorer tip moves along the tooth surface, it moves out and around the raised bump, and returns back to the tooth surface. This is similar to the sensation of skating over speed bumps in a parking lot or over a cobblestone surface.

Figure 13-56. Restoration with Overhanging Margin. The explorer's path is blocked by the overhang and must move away from the tooth surface and over the restoration. This is similar to encountering the edge of a section of pavement that is higher than the surrounding pavement. Your skates must move up and over the higher section of pavement.

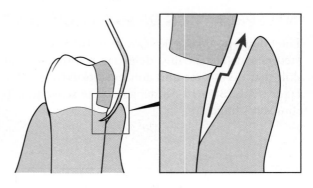

Figure 13-57. Restoration with Deficient Margin. The explorer passes over the surface of the tooth and then dips in to trace the surface of the restoration. This is similar to encountering the edge of a section of pavement that is lower than the surrounding pavement. Your skates must move down onto this section of pavement.

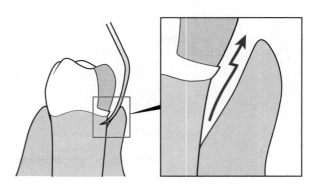

Figure 13-58. Subgingival Carious Lesion (Decay). The explorer dips in and then comes out again as it travels along the root surface. This would be like skating into a pothole, across the pothole, and then back onto the pavement.

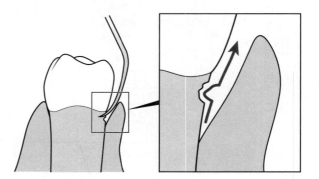

REFERENCE TABLE: UNDETECTED CALCULUS

Errors in exploring technique are the most common cause of a failure to detect subgingival calculus deposits (Table 13-2). As this reference table shows, often a small change in technique makes a big difference in the ability to detect calculus deposits.

TABLE 13–2. CAUSES OF UNDETECTED CALCULUS DEPOSITS	
Location	**Technique Error**
No particular pattern of undetected deposits	• Use of inappropriate explorer for task • "Death-grip" on instrument handle • Middle finger not on shank (fewer vibrations can be felt through handle than through the shank) • Middle finger applying pressure against shank, reducing tactile information • Strokes too far apart (not overlapping)
Undetected deposits at midlines of anteriors, or line angles of posteriors	• Failure to overlap strokes in these areas • Failure to maintain constant adaptation to surface • Not using horizontal strokes in these areas • Failure to roll handle to achieve adaptation when working around the line angle
Undetected deposits on mesial or distal surfaces	• Strokes not extended apical to contact area so that at least one-half of surface is explored from both the facial and lingual aspects
Undetected *supra*gingival deposits	• Failure to use compressed air for a visual inspection of the teeth, esp. facials of maxillary molars and lingual surfaces of mandibular anterior teeth
Undetected deposits at base of sulcus or pocket	• Failure to insert explorer to junctional epithelium before initiating stroke • Incorrect patient head position, especially for anterior treatment areas • Incorrect clinician clock position for the treatment area

Section 6
Detection of Dental Caries

CHANGING PARADIGM FOR CARIES DETECTION

1. Caries Diagnosis
   A. Dental Caries
      1. A carious lesion is a decayed area on the tooth crown or root.
         a. Enamel caries often can be detected visually by changes in the appearance of the enamel. The first visual indication of caries in enamel is generally a small white lesion on smooth surfaces or light to dark brown lesions in pits or fissures (Fig. 13-59) (3).
         b. In more advanced stages caries (Fig. 13-60) can appear as open cavities on enamel, dentin layers, or all the way to the pulp (3).
         c. Root caries are common in older adults and periodontal patients.
   B. Cavitated versus Noncavitated Lesions
      1. A cavitated lesion is a lesion that has lost the outer surface layer of the crown or root of the tooth, leading to a discontinuity in the tooth surface. A dental restoration normally is needed to repair a tooth surface with a cavitated lesion.
      2. A noncavitated lesion is the result of demineralization of an area of tooth surface. This demineralization usually is reversible or can be arrested with proper treatment. Fluorides and the placement of sealants may be used to reverse or arrest the demineralization process.
   C. Caries as a Biofilm Disease. Traditionally, the diagnosis of dental caries entailed detecting only cavitated lesions (4). Over the last decade, however, the caries process became recognized as a biofilm disease.
      1. It is now understood that caries is not one single episode of demineralization that suddenly leads to cavitation, but a continuum of demineralization that ranges from a noncavitated lesion to an obviously cavitated lesion (3).
      2. The primary purpose of caries detection is to identify the disease early in order to halt its progression. Early detection of a lesion at the noncavitated level may allow for remineralization of the lesion without the need for a dental restoration (filling) (3,4). Box 13-4 summarizes prerequisites for early diagnosis of dental caries.

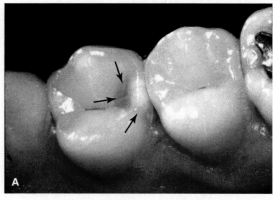
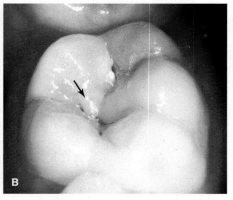

Figure 13-59. Clinical Appearance of Dental Caries. A: The area of the marginal ridge over the contact area of this premolar tooth shows a change in translucency appearing like a brown or gray shadow beneath the surface of the enamel. **B:** This molar tooth shows stained grooves and adjacent demineralization seen as a chalky whiteness surrounding the stained pit.

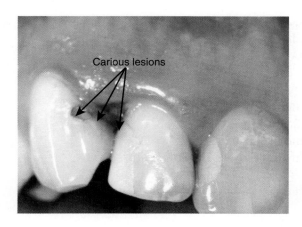

Carious lesions

Figure 13-60. Dental Decay. Smooth surface caries (cavitated lesions) on the canine and lateral incisor. Clinically visible carious lesions should NOT be explored.

Box 13-4 **Prerequisites for Early Caries Diagnosis**

- Good lighting
- Clean tooth surface that is free of biofilm and deposits
- A three-way syringe so that teeth can be viewed both wet and dry
- Sharp eyes
- Blunt explorer or periodontal probe
- Bitewing radiographs

---

2. **Historic Use of a Sharp Dental Explorer for Tactile Detection of Caries.** Historically, the use of the sharp point of an explorer—gently forced into a pit or fissure—was a commonly used caries detection method. The sharp point of the explorer (Fig. 13-61) was placed into the pit or fissure and the presence of a "tug-back" or resistance to removal of the explorer was thought to indicate the presence of decay (5).
   A. **Unreliability of Explorer "Catch" as a Detection Method.**
      1. Research has shown this technique at best to be unreliable for carious lesion detection and at worst potentially damaging (6–15).
      2. *The use of a sharp explorer to diagnose caries in pit and fissure sites is no longer recommended and clinicians instead should rely on "sharp eyes and a blunt explorer or probe"* (Fig. 13-62) (16–18).
         a. Penetration by a sharp explorer can actually cause cavitation in areas that are remineralizing or could be remineralized.
         b. Dental lesions initially develop as a subsurface lesion. Early lesions may be reversed—with meticulous patient self-care and application of fluoride—as long as the thin surface layer over the lesion remains intact (19).
         c. The use of a dental explorer with firm pressure to probe suspicious areas may result in the rupture of the surface layer covering early lesions (19).
   B. **Visual Detection Methods**
      1. Visual signs have proven to be good indicators of the presence of enamel and dentin lesions (20–22).
      2. Detailed visual examination methods record early signs of the carious process such as opacities, brown discolorations, enamel breakdowns, or microcavities without an obvious cavity.

3. The International Caries Detection and Assessment System (ICDAS-II) presents visual guidelines for the diagnosis of carious lesions on all tooth surfaces at all stages of severity (14,15,19,23,24). The ICDAS-II may be accessed online at http://www.icdas.org.

3. New Detection Aids
   A. To date, no one form of diagnosis is reliable in detecting all carious lesions or determining if a lesion is active or arrested (21,25).
   B. Noninvasive detection aids currently available include visual detection, radiographs, laser fluorescence, quantitative light-induced fluorescence, subtraction radiography, and electrical caries measurements (26). The ideal caries detection method has yet to be identified but it is likely that dental hygienists will see new developments in the future.

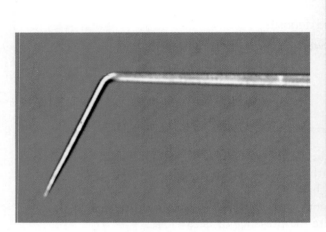

Figure 13-61. Sharp Explorer. The use of an explorer with a sharp pointed tip is no longer recommended for caries detection.

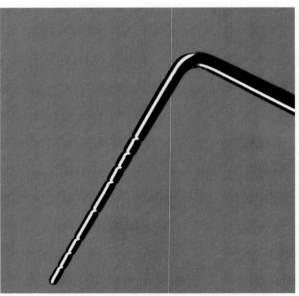

Figure 13-62. Blunt Probe. A blunt probe or explorer is the recommended instrument for caries detection.

4. The Dental Hygienist and the Changing Paradigm for Caries Detection
   A. Dental hygienists are quite skilled in the detection of calculus, and the use of an explorer is a critical part of this calculus detection skill set.
   B. It is important for the dental hygienist to realize that the use of an explorer to detect calculus in no way compares to the older use of a sharp explorer tip to detect dental caries since most calculus detection requires the gentle use of the side of the tip of the explorer rather than forceful use of the sharp explorer tip.
   C. Thus in spite of the changing paradigm for caries detection, dental hygienists should continue to locate calculus deposits with an explorer, in the traditional manner, to help prevent and control periodontal diseases.

References

1. Wilson TG, Harrel SK, Nunn ME, Francis B, Webb K. The relationship between the presence of tooth-borne subgingival deposits and inflammation found with a dental endoscope. *J Periodontol*. 2008;79(11):2029–2035.
2. Gurgan CA, Bilgin E. Distribution of different morphologic types of subgingival calculus on proximal root surfaces. *Quintessence Int*. 2005;36(3):202–208.
3. Fejerskov O. Concepts of dental caries and their consequences for understanding the disease. *Community Dent Oral Epidemiol*. 1997;25(1):5–12.
4. Ismail AI. Clinical diagnosis of precavitated carious lesions. *Community Dent Oral Epidemiol*. 1997;25(1):13–23.
5. Baum L, Phillips RW, Lund MR, Phillips RW. *Textbook of Operative Dentistry*. 2nd ed. Philadelphia, PA: Saunders; 1985. viii, 603.
6. Aleksejuniene J, Gorovenko M. Caries detection techniques and clinical practice. *Pract Proced Aesthet Dent*. 2009;21(1): 26–28.
7. Berg JH, Swift EJ, Jr. Critical appraisal: current caries detection devices. *J Esthet Restor Dent*. 2010;22(5):464–470.
8. Braga MM, Mendes FM, Ekstrand KR. Detection activity assessment and diagnosis of dental caries lesions. *Dent Clin North Am*. 2010;54(3):479–493.
9. Ekstrand K, Qvist V, Thylstrup A. Light microscope study of the effect of probing in occlusal surfaces. *Caries Res*. 1987;21(4):368–374.
10. Neuhaus KW, Ellwood R, Lussi A, Pitts NB. Traditional lesion detection aids. *Monogr Oral Sci*. 2009;21:42–51.
11. Pitts NB. Implementation. Improving caries detection, assessment, diagnosis and monitoring. *Monogr Oral Sci*. 2009;21: 199–208.
12. Pitts NB. How the detection, assessment, diagnosis and monitoring of caries integrate with personalized caries management. *Monogr Oral Sci*. 2009;21:1–14.
13. Selwitz RH, Ismail AI, Pitts NB. Dental caries. *Lancet*. 2007;369(9555):51–59.
14. Shivakumar K, Prasad S, Chandu G. International Caries Detection and Assessment System: A new paradigm in detection of dental caries. *J Conserv Dent*. 2009;12(1):10–16.
15. Topping GV, Pitts NB. Clinical visual caries detection. *Monogr Oral Sci*. 2009;21:15–41.
16. Kuhnisch J, Goddon I, Berger S, et al. Development, methodology and potential of the new Universal Visual Scoring System (UniViSS) for caries detection and diagnosis. *Int J Environ Res Public Health*. 2009;6(9):2500–259.
17. Pitts NB. Are we ready to move from operative to non-operative/preventive treatment of dental caries in clinical practice? *Caries Res*. 2004;38(3):294–304.
18. World Health Organization. *Oral Health Surveys: Basic Methods*. 5th edition. ed. Geneva: World Health Organization; 2013. vii, 125.
19. Zero DT, Fontana M, Martinez-Mier EA, et al. The biology, prevention, diagnosis and treatment of dental caries: scientific advances in the United States. *J Am Dent Assoc*. 2009;140(Suppl 1):25S–34S.
20. Ekstrand KR, Ricketts DN, Kidd EA. Occlusal caries: pathology, diagnosis and logical management. *Dent Update*. 2001;28(8):380–387.
21. Ekstrand KR, Zero DT, Martignon S, Pitts NB. Lesion activity assessment. *Monogr Oral Sci*. 2009;21:63–90.
22. Nyvad B, Machiulskiene V, Baelum V. Reliability of a new caries diagnostic system differentiating between active and inactive caries lesions. *Caries Res*. 1999;33(4):252–260.
23. Pitts N. "ICDAS"–an international system for caries detection and assessment being developed to facilitate caries epidemiology, research and appropriate clinical management. *Community Dent Health*. 2004;21(3):193–198.
24. Committee IC. Rational and evidence for the International Detection and Assessment System (ICDAS II)2005 December 31, 2015. Available from http://www.icads.org.
25. NIH Consensus Development Conference on Diagnosis and Management of Dental Caries Throughout Life. Bethesda, MD, March 26–28, 2001. Conference Papers. *J Dent Educ*. 2001;65(10):935–1179.
26. Neuhaus KW, Longbottom C, Ellwood R, Lussi A. Novel lesion detection aids. *Monogr Oral Sci*. 2009;21:52–62.

Section 7
Skill Application

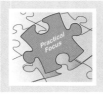

PRACTICAL FOCUS

Diagramming Calculus Deposits. This activity will help you to develop tactile detection skills and the ability to form a mental picture of the deposits you detect.

Directions:

1. Begin by creating some objects that will represent tooth roots with calculus deposits.
   * If possible, locate some discarded pieces of old copper or PVC plumbing pipes. The maintenance department at your college or university might be able to supply some.
   * Use synthetic calculus to create "ledges and spicules of calculus" on the surface of the copper tubes.
   * The "calculus deposits" should have a random pattern and each copper tube should have a unique pattern of "deposits."
   * Allow the "calculus" to dry overnight. Obtain a small *opaque* trash bag.
2. Put an explorer, a copper tube, and both of your hands inside the trash bag.
   * Use your mirror hand to hold the copper tube. Grasp the explorer in your other hand and establish a finger rest on the side of the copper tube.
   * Initiate assessment strokes along the surface of the tube.
   * As you form a mental picture of the "calculus deposits" diagram them on a piece of paper on which you have drawn a rectangle representing the copper tube.
   * Indicate the location and relative size of the "calculus deposits" on the tube.
3. Finally, remove the copper tube from the bag.
   * Compare the actual "calculus deposits" to your drawing (Fig. 13-63). How did you do? Repeat this activity with different copper tubes to improve your detection and visualization skills.

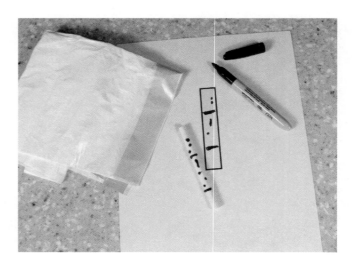

Figure 13-63. Check your diagram. Compare the actual deposits on the copper tube with your diagram.

REFERENCE SHEET—EXPLORERS

Explorers are used to detect, by tactile means, the texture and character of tooth surfaces before, during, and after periodontal instrumentation to assess the progress and completeness of instrumentation. Box 13-5 provides a summary of explorer use.

Box 13-5 | Reference Sheet for Explorers

General Technique for Calculus Detection:

- Use a relaxed grasp, resting your middle finger lightly on the shank.
- Use the side of the explorer tip, not the actual point.
- Cover every millimeter of the root surface with light, flowing strokes.

Anterior Teeth:

- **Working-End Selection:** Working-end "wraps" around the tooth curving toward the tooth surface
- **Sequence:** Begin with the surfaces toward you. Start on the canine on the opposite side of the mouth and work toward yourself. (Right-handed: left canine, mesial surface; Left-handed: right canine, mesial surface)

Posterior Teeth:

1. **Working-End Selection:** Lower shank is parallel to tooth surface ("posterior parallel")
2. **Sequence:** Begin with the posterior-most tooth in the sextant. On each tooth, do the distal surface first, followed by facial and mesial (or lingual and mesial) surfaces.

Student Self Evaluation Module 13: Explorers

Student: _____   Date = _____

DIRECTIONS: Self-evaluate your skill level in each treatment area as: **S** (satisfactory) or **U** (unsatisfactory).

Criteria				
Positioning/Ergonomics	**Area 1**	**Area 2**	**Area 3**	**Area 4**
Adjusts clinician chair correctly				
Reclines patient chair and assures that patient's head is even with top of headrest				
Positions instrument tray within easy reach				
Assumes the recommended clock position				
Positions backrest of patient chair for the specified arch and adjusts height of patient chair so that clinician's elbows remain at waist level when accessing the specified treatment area				
Asks patient to assume the head position that facilitates the clinician's view of the specified treatment area.				
Directs light to illuminate the specified treatment area				
Instrument Grasp: Dominant Hand	**Area 1**	**Area 2**	**Area 3**	**Area 4**
Grasps handle with tips of finger pads of index finger and thumb				
Rests pad of middle finger lightly on instrument shank				
Positions the thumb, index, and middle fingers in the "knuckles up" convex position; hyper-extended joint position is avoided				
Holds ring finger straight so that it supports the weight of hand and instrument; ring finger position is "advanced ahead of" the other fingers in the grasp				
Keeps index, middle, ring, and little fingers in contact; "like fingers inside a mitten"				
Maintains a relaxed grasp; fingers are NOT blanched in grasp				
Finger Rest: Dominant Hand				
Establishes secure finger rest that is appropriate for tooth to be treated				
Once finger rest is established, pauses to self-evaluate finger placement in the grasp, verbalizes to evaluator his/her self-assessment of grasp, and corrects finger placement if necessary				
Prepare for Instrumentation ("Get Ready")				
Selects correct working-end for tooth surface to be instrumented				
Places the working-end in the "Get Ready Zone" while using a correct finger rest for the treatment area				
Exploring Technique	**Area 1**	**Area 2**	**Area 3**	**Area 4**
Maintains a relaxed grasp to make feather light, overlapping strokes of an appropriate length				
Stops each assessment stroke beneath the gingival margin(to avoid trauma to the gingival margin); does NOT remove tip from sulcus/pocket with each stroke				
Maintains adaptation of tip; pivots and rolls handle as needed to maintain adaptation				
Covers entire root surface with assessment strokes				
Uses appropriate sequence in the sextant				
Uses overlapping strokes at midlines of anterior teeth, under the contact area, and at line angles of posterior teeth				
Maintains neutral wrist position throughout motion activation				
Ethics and Professionalism				
Punctuality, appearance, demeanor, attitude, composure, honesty				

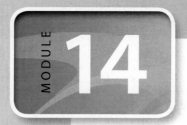
Technique Essentials: Supragingival Calculus Removal

Module Overview

Moving the instrument working-end over the tooth surface to remove a supragingival calculus deposit involves several small motor skills. For successful instrumentation, correct adaptation and angulation of the working-end and application of force must be maintained throughout the instrumentation stroke. The module discusses the elements of an instrumentation stroke for *supragingival* calculus removal including angulation, force, and stabilization.

Module Outline

Section 1   **Supragingival Calculus Deposits**   **323**

Section 2   **Relationship of the Instrument Face to the Tooth Surface**   **324**

Picturing the Tooth and Working-End in Cross Section
Correct Angulation for Calculus Removal
Angulation Errors that Result in Tissue Injury or Incomplete Calculus Removal

Section 3   **Application of Force for Calculus Removal**   **327**

Pinch Force, Stabilization, and Lateral Pressure
Relaxation of Force Between Strokes

Section 4   **Stroke Pattern for Supragingival Calculus Removal**   **329**

A Large Supragingival Calculus Deposit: Dividing Up the Work
Step-by-Step Sequence for Supragingival Calculus Removal

Section 5   **Skill Application**   **332**

Practical Focus: Practice in Establishing Angulation and Maintaining Adaptation

Online resource for this module:
- Calculus removal stroke
- Calculus removal strokes: sheet calculus

Available at: http://thepoint.lww.com/GehrigFundamentals8e

Key Terms

Supragingival calculus
  deposits
Periodontium

Angulation
Pinch pressure
Stabilization

Lateral pressure
Burnished calculus deposit

Learning Objectives

- Given a drawing of the healthy periodontium in cross section (similar to that shown in Fig. 14-1) correctly label all the structures depicted in the illustration.

- Define the term angulation as it relates to the use of a sickle scaler for supragingival periodontal instrumentation.

- Explain the problems associated with using an angulation greater than 90 degrees for calculus removal.

- Explain the problems associated with using an angulation less than 45 degrees for calculus removal.

- Describe the correct approach for removing a large supragingival calculus deposit and differentiate this technique from a different approach that leads to burnishing of the deposit.

- List from memory the sequence of steps used for supragingival calculus removal as outlined in Figure 14-9.

Section 1
Supragingival Calculus Deposits

Supragingival calculus deposits are those deposits located coronal to the gingival margin, usually on the crowns of the teeth.

- Supragingival deposits (Figs. 14-1 to 14-3) range from light deposits to heavy accumulations of calculus.
- Sickle scalers and curets are recommended for removal of light deposits. Sickle scalers, periodontal files, and powered ultrasonic and sonic instruments are used for removal of heavy accumulations of supragingival calculus.

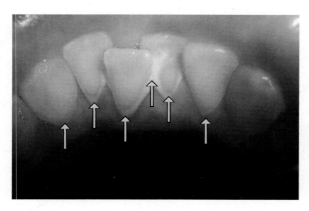

Figure 14-1. Light Supragingival Calculus Deposits. A very common site of supragingival calculus deposits is on lingual surfaces of the mandibular anterior teeth. Thoroughly drying the teeth with compressed air assists the clinician in locating these deposits.

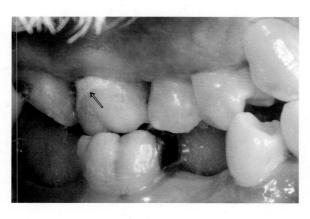

Figure 14-2. Thin Layer of Supragingival Calculus Deposits. Another common site of supragingival deposit formation is on the facial surface of the maxillary first molar. The deposit pictured here is a thin layer of white calculus. Use of indirect vision with a mirror is very helpful in detecting these deposits.

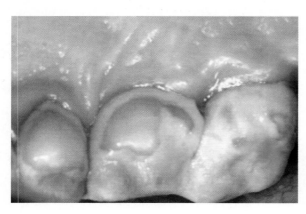

Figure 14-3. Heavy Supragingival Calculus Deposits. This photograph shows heavy accumulations of supragingival calculus on the lingual aspect of these maxillary posterior teeth.

Section 2
Relationship of the Instrument Face to the Tooth Surface

PICTURING THE TOOTH AND WORKING-END IN CROSS SECTION

- The tissues that surround and support a tooth in the dental arch are known as the periodontium. The components of the periodontium are the gingiva, periodontal ligament, cementum, and the alveolar bone.
- To picture the placement of the working-end against the tooth, the hygienist must mentally picture the cross section of the tooth, periodontium, and the instrument working-end (1).
- Figure 14-4 depicts a tooth and healthy periodontium in cross section. Figure 14-5 shows the working-end of a sickle scaler in cross section.

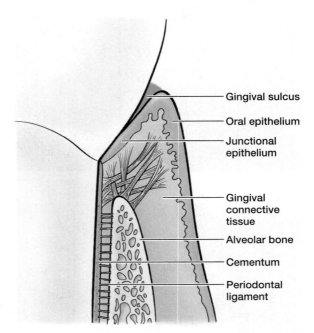

Figure 14-4. Healthy Periodontium in Cross Section. Illustrated here are the structures of a healthy periodontium.

- Gingival sulcus
- Oral epithelium
- Junctional epithelium
- Gingival connective tissue
- Alveolar bone
- Cementum
- Periodontal ligament

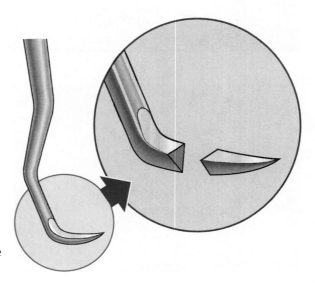

Figure 14-5. Cross Section of a Sickle Scaler. A sickle scaler is triangular in cross section.

CORRECT ANGULATION FOR CALCULUS REMOVAL

Angulation refers to the relationship between the face of a calculus removal instrument and the tooth surface to which it is applied.

- *For calculus removal, the face-to-tooth surface angulation is an angle between 45 and 90 degrees.*
- The ideal angulation for calculus removal is between 60 and 80 degrees. Figure 14-6 depicts the correct angulation for calculus removal.

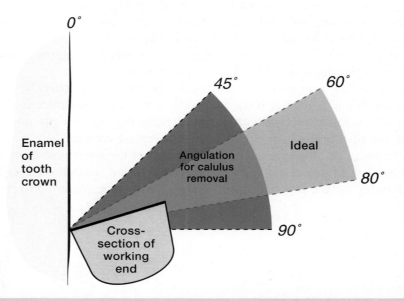

Figure 14-6. Angulation of the Working-End for Calculus Removal.
- The **correct** *face-to-tooth surface angulation* is greater than 45 degrees and less than 90 degrees.
- Correct angulation allows the cutting edge to bite into the calculus deposit and fracture it from the tooth surface.

ANGULATION ERRORS THAT RESULT IN TISSUE INJURY OR INCOMPLETE CALCULUS REMOVAL

Incorrect angulation of the working-end to the tooth surface is a technique error that results in negative consequences during patient treatment.

1. **Angulation Greater than 90 Degrees.** If the face-to-tooth surface angulation is greater than 90 degrees, one cutting edge will be in contact with the soft tissue lining of the periodontal pocket, injuring the tissue. Figure 14-7 illustrates this technique error.
2. **Angulation Less than 45 Degrees.** If the face-to-tooth surface angulation is less than 45 degrees, the cutting edge will slide over the surface of a calculus deposit, rather than biting into it. This technique error is shown in Figure 14-8.
   A. Incorrect angulation of less than 45 degrees removes only the outermost layer of a calculus deposit, leaving behind the bulk of the deposit.
      1. Calculus deposits form over time in irregular layers, so ordinarily the outermost layer is rough and jagged. It is the rough characteristic of the calculus deposit that enables it to be detected with an explorer. As the explorer tip moves over a deposit, the tip vibrates as it passes across the jagged surface.
      2. When incorrect technique results in the removal of the outermost layer of a calculus deposit, the remaining calculus is left with a smooth surface. The smooth outer surface is very difficult to detect with an explorer or to remove.

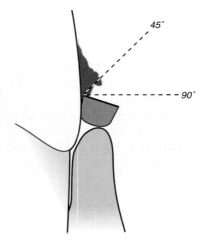

Figure 14-7. Incorrect Angulation for Calculus Removal—Angle Greater than 90 Degrees. The **incorrect** *face-to-tooth surface angulation* shown in this illustration is greater than 90 degrees. The face is tilted away from the root surface. In this position, calculus removal will be difficult and tissue trauma is likely.

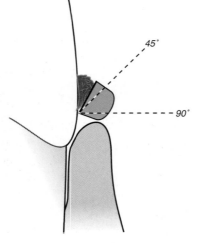

Figure 14-8. Incorrect Angulation for Calculus Removal— Angle Less than 45 Degrees. The **incorrect** *face-to-tooth surface angulation* shown here is less than 45 degrees. The face is tilted too close to the root surface. In this position, the cutting edge cannot bite into the deposit; instead, the face slips over the calculus deposit.

Section 3
Application of Force for Calculus Removal

PINCH FORCE, STABLIZATION, AND LATERAL PRESSURE

Three types of force are applied during periodontal instrumentation: (1) pinch pressure of the fingers in the modified pen grasp, (2) pressure of the fulcrum to stabilize the hand, and (3) lateral pressure against the tooth during the instrument stroke. Figure 14-9 summarizes the use of force during an instrumentation stroke for calculus removal.

1. **Three Forces of Instrumentation**
   A. Pinch pressure is the pressure exerted by the fingers in the modified grasp when holding the instrument handle (2).
   B. Stabilization is the act of preparing for an instrumentation stroke by (1) locking the joints of the ring finger and (2) pressing the fingertip against a tooth surface to provide control for the instrumentation stroke.
      1. **Stabilizing the Fulcrum Finger.** This is accomplished by locking the joints of the fulcrum finger so that the finger can function as a "support beam" for the hand during the instrumentation stroke.
      2. **Stabilizing the Hand and Instrument**
         a. This is accomplished by pressing the tip of the fulcrum finger against the tooth surface.
         b. The extent of the pressure against the tooth ranges from light to firm depending upon the type of stroke used.
         c. If the fulcrum finger lifts of the tooth at the end of a stroke, the clinician is not pressing down against the tooth with the fulcrum finger as the stroke is completed.
      3. **Lateral Pressure Against the Tooth Surface**
         a. Lateral pressure against the tooth surface is created by applying pressure with the *index finger and thumb* inward against the instrument handle prior to and throughout the instrumentation stroke.
         b. Both fingers must apply pressure equally against the handle or the instrument will be difficult to control.
   C. Lateral pressure is the act of applying equal pressure with the index finger and thumb inward against the instrument handle to press the *tip-third of the cutting edge* against the tooth surface prior to and throughout an instrumentation stroke.
      1. **The Task Determines the Amount of Lateral Pressure**
         a. The instrument classification and instrumentation task determine the amount of lateral pressure needed during instrumentation.
            a. Assessment—requires a feather light touch against the tooth surface.
            b. Calculus removal—requires firm lateral pressure against the tooth surface.
            c. Root debridement—requires less lateral pressure than a calculus removal stroke.
         b. More pressure applied against the handle and by the fulcrum finger against the tooth results in more pressure against the tooth surface or calculus deposit. Lateral pressure against the tooth surface will range from light to firm; however, heavy pressure is never recommended.

2. Lateral Pressure and Adaptation During Calculus Removal
   A. Effective calculus removal depends on a combination of (1) correct adaptation of the tip-third of the cutting edge, (2) firm lateral pressure, and (3) correct angulation. With ideal lateral pressure and angulation, a calculus deposit is fractured from the tooth surface.
   B. As the tip-third of the cutting edge is adapted to the tooth surface, the fingers in the grasp apply a firm pressure so that the cutting edge "bites" into the tooth surface. This lateral—sideways—pressure is applied only briefly just prior to and during the calculus removal stroke.
   C. The short, biting stroke of a calculus removal stroke is balanced with a firm grasp and firm downward or upward pressure against the stabilizing tooth.
   D. Inadequate lateral pressure and/or incorrect angulation result in incomplete calculus removal.

RELAXATION OF FORCE BETWEEN STROKES

The techniques of stabilization and lateral pressure are used only (1) immediately prior to beginning a calculus removal stroke and (2) during the production of a calculus removal stroke.

1. *The finger muscles should be relaxed between strokes and when returning the working-end to the base of the sulcus after completing a stroke.*
2. Maintaining constant pressure with the fulcrum finger or when grasping the handle is very stressful to the muscles of the hand and wrist.
3. PAUSE and RELAX your fingers between each stroke.
   A. Unfortunately, novice clinicians often apply constant firm pressure—with all three forces—in an attempt to control instrumentation strokes. This use of constant pressure is soon stored in the muscle memory and becomes an ongoing bad habit (3–18).
   B. Researches suggest that use of unnecessary force in a pinch grip is the greatest contributing risk factor in the development of injury among dental hygienists (17,18).

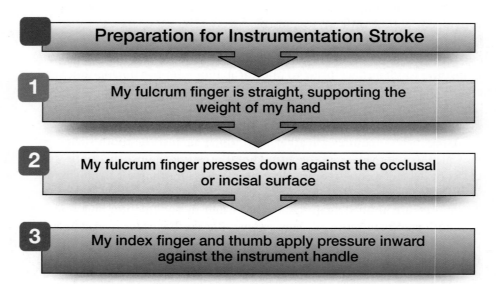

Figure 14-9. Application of Force in Preparation for an Instrumentation Stroke. Three forces are applied during an instrumentation stroke. These three forces must be balanced for an effective stroke.

Section 4
Stroke Pattern for Supragingival Calculus Removal

A LARGE SUPRAGINGIVAL CALCULUS DEPOSIT: DIVIDING UP THE WORK

Often a calculus deposit will be too large to be removed as a single piece.

1. Incorrect Approach: Removing the Large Deposit Layer-by-Layer
   A. Attempting to remove a large calculus deposit by removing the outer layers of the deposit is the *incorrect* approach to calculus removal.
   B. A calculus deposit that has had the outermost layer removed is termed a burnished calculus deposit. Figure 14-10 shows a burnished calculus deposit.
      1. *All calculus deposits, including burnished deposits, are highly porous formations that retain living plaque biofilms that are associated with continuing inflammation (periodontal disease). All calculus deposits must be removed in order for the tissues of the periodontium to heal.*
      2. A burnished deposit, with its smooth outer layer, is much more difficult to remove than a nonburnished calculus deposit. It is best, therefore, to avoid burnishing a deposit by using correct angulation with the working-end during instrumentation.
2. Correct Approach: Removing the Large Deposit in Sections
   1. *Large calculus deposits should be removed in sections using a series of short, firm instrumentation strokes* (Fig. 14-11).
   2. The calculus in one section should be completely removed before moving on to the next section.

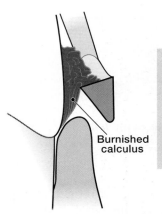

Figure 14-10. Incorrect Technique: Remove Outer Layer.
- The deposit *should not be removed in layers* since removing the outermost layer will leave the deposit with a smooth surface.
- A calculus deposit that has had the outermost layer removed is referred to as a burnished deposit.
- Burnished calculus is difficult to remove since the cutting edge tends to slip over the smooth surface of the deposit.

Burnished calculus

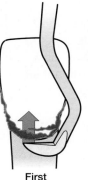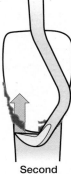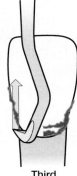

First section   Second section   Third section

Figure 14-11. Correct Technique: Remove Large Deposit in Sections.
- Large calculus deposits should be removed in sections.
- Use a series of calculus removal strokes to remove the deposit one section at a time.

STEP-BY-STEP SEQUENCE FOR SUPRAGINGIVAL CALCULUS REMOVAL

Step-by-Step Sequence for Supragingival Calculus Removal. Figure 14-12 summarizes the concepts for supragingival calculus removal in a step-by-step manner.

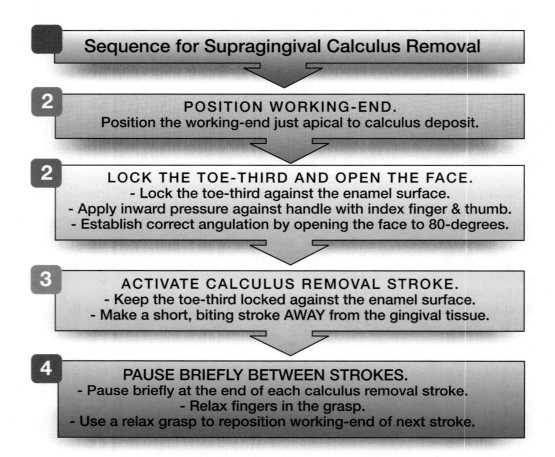

Sequence for Supragingival Calculus Removal

2   POSITION WORKING-END.
Position the working-end just apical to calculus deposit.

2   LOCK THE TOE-THIRD AND OPEN THE FACE.
- Lock the toe-third against the enamel surface.
- Apply inward pressure against handle with index finger & thumb.
- Establish correct angulation by opening the face to 80-degrees.

3   ACTIVATE CALCULUS REMOVAL STROKE.
- Keep the toe-third locked against the enamel surface.
- Make a short, biting stroke AWAY from the gingival tissue.

4   PAUSE BRIEFLY BETWEEN STROKES.
- Pause briefly at the end of each calculus removal stroke.
- Relax fingers in the grasp.
- Use a relax grasp to reposition working-end of next stroke.

Figure 14-12.   Step-By-Step Sequence for Supragingival Calculus Removal.

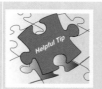

NOTE TO COURSE INSTRUCTORS: This textbook has separate modules devoted to each instrument design classification (sickle scalers, universal curets, area-specific curets, periodontal files, and instruments for advanced root instrumentation). Each of these modules provides step-by-step instructions for instrument use and does not rely on the content from any previous instrument module. ***This module structure means that the instrument modules can be covered in any order that you prefer.*** In addition, it is not necessary to include all modules. For example, if periodontal files are not part of your school's instrument kit, this module does not need to be included in the course.

References

1. Rucker LM, Gibson G, McGregor C. Getting the "feel" of it: the non-visual component of dimensional accuracy during operative tooth preparation. *J Can Dent Assoc.* 1990;56(10):937–941.
2. Dong H, Barr A, Loomer P, Rempel D. The effects of finger rest positions on hand muscle load and pinch force in simulated dental hygiene work. *J Dent Educ.* 2005;69(4):453–460.
3. Bernard BP. Musculoskeletal disorders and workplace factors. A critical review of epidemiologic evidence for work-related musculoskeletal disorders of the neck, upper extremity, and lower back. Cincinnati, OH: NIOSH (National Institute for Occupational Safety); 1997.
4. Graham C. Ergonomics in dentistry, Part 1. *Dent Today.* 2002;21(4):98–103.
5. Hayes M, Cockrell D, Smith DR. A systematic review of musculoskeletal disorders among dental professionals. *Int J Dent Hyg.* 2009;7(3):159–165.
6. Hayes MJ, Smith DR, Cockrell D. Prevalence and correlates of musculoskeletal disorders among Australian dental hygiene students. *Int J Dent Hyg.* 2009;7(3):176–181.
7. Hayes MJ, Smith DR, Cockrell D. An international review of musculoskeletal disorders in the dental hygiene profession. *Int Dent J.* 2010;60(5):343–352.
8. Hayes MJ, Smith DR, Taylor JA. Musculoskeletal disorders and symptom severity among Australian dental hygienists. *BMC Res Notes.* 2013;6:250.
9. Hayes MJ, Smith DR, Taylor JA. Musculoskeletal disorders in a 3 year longitudinal cohort of dental hygiene students. *J Dent Hyg.* 2014;88(1):36–41.
10. Hayes MJ, Taylor JA, Smith DR. Predictors of work-related musculoskeletal disorders among dental hygienists. *Int J Dent Hyg.* 2012;10(4):265–269.
11. Kanteshwari K, Sridhar R, Mishra AK, Shirahatti R, Maru R, Bhusari P. Correlation of awareness and practice of working postures with prevalence of musculoskeletal disorders among dental professionals. *Gen Dent.* 2011;59(6):476–483; quiz 84–85.
12. Kao SY. Carpal tunnel syndrome as an occupational disease. *J Am Board Fam Pract.* 2003;16(6):533–542.
13. Khan SA, Chew KY. Effect of working characteristics and taught ergonomics on the prevalence of musculoskeletal disorders amongst dental students. *BMC Musculoskelet Disord.* 2013;14:118.
14. Nathan PA, Istvan JA, Meadows KD. A longitudinal study of predictors of research-defined carpal tunnel syndrome in industrial workers: findings at 17 years. *J Hand Surg.* 2005;30(6):593–598.
15. Nathan PA, Meadows KD, Istvan JA. Predictors of carpal tunnel syndrome: an 11-year study of industrial workers. *J Hand Surg.* 2002;27(4):644–651.
16. Roquelaure Y, Mechali S, Dano C, et al. Occupational and personal risk factors for carpal tunnel syndrome in industrial workers. *Scand J Work Environ Health.* 1997;23(5):364–369.
17. Sanders MA, Turcotte CM. Strategies to reduce work-related musculoskeletal disorders in dental hygienists: two case studies. *J Hand Ther.* 2002;15(4):363–374.
18. Sanders MJ, Turcotte CA. Ergonomic strategies for dental professionals. *Work.* 1997;8(1):55–72.

Section 5
Skill Application

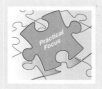

PRACTICAL FOCUS
Practice in Establishing Angulation and Maintaining Adaptation

This activity is designed to help you develop the ability to establish angulation and maintain adaptation to a curved object similar in size to a posterior molar tooth.

Equipment:

- An inexpensive marker (such as a Sharpie marker), an anterior instrument, a pad of paper
- Draw a line around the marker about 1½ in (12 mm) from the top of the pen (see photographs below). Imagine that the line is the CEJ of a mandibular molar tooth.

Instructions: Follow Steps 1 to 6 for this technique practice.

1. Sit in a comfortable seated position with the paper tablet on your lap. Hold the pen with your *nondominant* hand and stabilize the opposite end of the marker on the paper.
2. **Grasp** an anterior instrument and establish a finger rest on the top of the marker (Fig. 14-13).
3. **Adapt the tip-third of the cutting edge** just above the line on the marker.
4. **Establish correct angulation.** Look down at the pen top and tilt the instrument face toward the marker until the face meets the side of the marker at a 70- to 80-degree angle.
5. Use wrist motion to activate a short (3 mm) instrumentation stroke along the surface of the marker in an upward direction away from the line representing the CEJ.
6. Make a series of strokes around the circumference of the marker, beginning each stroke near the line on pen (Fig. 14-14).
   - Imagine that you are working across the facial surface of a molar toward the proximal surface.
   - Roll the instrument handle in order to keep the tip-third of the cutting edge adapted to the marker.

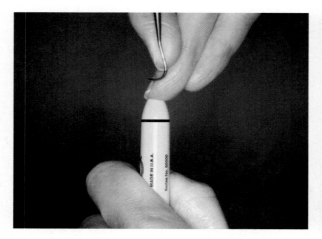

Figure 14-13. Establish a Fulcrum.

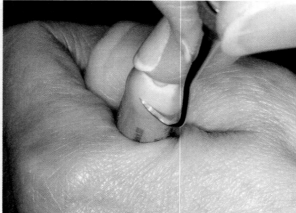

Figure 14-14. Activate a Series of Strokes.

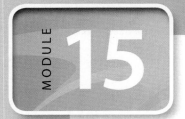

MODULE

15

Sickle Scalers

Module Overview

This module presents the design characteristics of anterior and posterior sickle scalers and step-by-step instructions for using sickle scalers to remove deposits from the enamel surfaces of the anterior and posterior teeth. Module 14—Technique Essentials: Supragingival Calculus Removal—should be completed prior to beginning this module.

Module Outline

Section 1 **Sickle Scalers**   335
General Design Characteristics
Working-End Design
Innovations in Sickle Scaler Design

Section 2 **Calculus Removal Concepts**   338
Revisiting the Instrument Grasp
Characteristics of the Calculus Removal Stroke

Section 3 **Technique Practice—Anterior Teeth**   341
Skill Building. Establishing a 70- to 80-Degree Angulation to an
    Anterior Tooth, p. 339
Skill Building. Technique on Anterior Tooth Surfaces, p. 340
Recipe for Artificial Dental Calculus, p. 342

Section 4 **Maintaining Adaptation to Proximal Surfaces**   345
Skill #1. Adapting the Tip-Third to the Midline of a Tooth
Skill #2. Rolling the Handle to Maintain Adaptation to Proximal
    Surface
Skill #3. Positioning the Tip-Third Beneath the Margin of the Papillary
    Gingiva

Section 5 **Technique Practice—Posterior Teeth**   349
Skill Building. Choosing the Correct Working-End of a Posterior
    Sickle Scaler, p. 347
Skill Building. Establishing 70- to 80-Degree Angulation to a
    Posterior Tooth, p. 349
Skill Building. Application of the Cutting Edges to the Posterior
    Teeth, p. 350
Skill Building. Technique for Posterior Teeth, p. 351

Section 6 **Technique Practice—Primary Teeth**   356
Skill Building. Technique for Primary Teeth, p. 354

Practical Focus: Working-End Selection and Angulation
Reference Sheet—Sickle Scalers
Student Self Evaluation Module 15: Sickle Scalers

Online resources for this module:

- Sickle Scalers
- Anterior Sickle Scaler
- Posterior Sickle Scaler
- Calculus Removal Stroke
- Calculus Removal Strokes: Sheet Calculus
- "Laying Down" vs. "Standing up" on Your Fulcrum

Available at: http://thepoint.lww.com/GehrigFundamentals8e

Key Terms

Sickle scaler   Posterior sickle scaler   Inner cutting edge
Anterior sickle scaler   Outer cutting edge

Learning Objectives

- Given a variety of sickle scaler instruments, identify the design characteristics.
- List the uses and limitations of sickle scalers.
- List characteristics of a calculus removal stroke.
- List from memory the sequence of steps used for calculus removal as outlined in Figure 15-4.
- Given a posterior sickle scaler, demonstrate how to use visual clues to identify the correct working-end.
- Demonstrate correct adaptation and angulation of a sickle scaler.
- Explain why the lower shank of a sickle scaler should be tilted slightly toward the tooth surface being instrumented to obtain correct angulation.
- Demonstrate correct use of a sickle scaler in the anterior sextants while maintaining correct position, correct finger rests, and precise finger placement in the grasp.
- Demonstrate the three skills used to maintain adaptation to the proximal surfaces.
- Demonstrate correct use of a sickle scaler in the posterior sextants while maintaining correct position, correct finger rests, and precise finger placement in the grasp.

NOTE TO COURSE INSTRUCTOR: There is a separate module devoted to each design classification (sickle scalers, universal curets, area-specific curets, periodontal files) and modules covering advanced probing techniques and advanced root instrumentation. Each module provides step-by-step instructions for instrument use and does not rely on the content from any previous instrument module. ***This module structure means that the instrument modules can be covered in any order that you prefer.**** In addition, if an instrument classification is not part of your school's instrument kit, this module may be omitted from the course.

Section 1
Sickle Scalers

GENERAL DESIGN CHARACTERISTICS

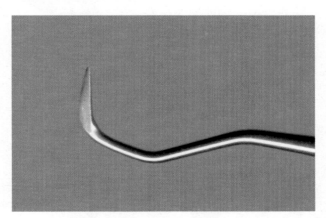

Figure 15-1. Sickle Scaler. The working-end of a sickle scaler.

1. Functions of Sickle Scalers
   A. A sickle scaler is a periodontal instrument used to remove calculus deposits from the crowns of the teeth (Figs. 15-1 and 15-2).
   B. Sickle scalers are restricted to use on enamel surfaces and should NOT be used on root surfaces.
2. Design Characteristics of Sickle Scalers
   A. **Working-End Design.** The working-end of a sickle scaler has several unique design characteristics (Table 15-1).
      1. A pointed back; some newer sickle scaler designs have working-ends with rounded backs
      2. A pointed tip
      3. A triangular cross section
      4. Two cutting edges per working-end
      5. The face is perpendicular to the lower shank
   B. Anterior and Posterior Instrument Designs
      1. Anterior sickle scalers are designed for use on anterior treatment sextants.
         a. Often they are single-ended instruments since only one working-end is needed to instrument the crowns of the anterior teeth.
         b. It is common, however, to combine two different anterior sickles on a double-ended instrument.
      2. Posterior sickle scalers are designed for use on posterior sextants, but they also may be used on anterior teeth.
         c. Usually two posterior sickles are paired on a double-ended instrument (the working-ends are mirror images of one another).
         d. For example, the Jacquette 34 is paired with the Jacquette 35 (the working-end of the Jacquette 34 is a mirror image of the working-end of the Jacquette 35).
3. Examples of Sickle Scaler Instruments
   A. Anterior sickle scalers—OD-1, Jacquette-30, Jacquette-33, Nevi 1, Whiteside-2, USC-128, Towner-U15, Goldman-H6, and Goldman-H7
   B. Posterior sickle scalers—Jacquette 34/35, Jacquette 14/15, Jacquette 31/32, Nevi 2, Ball 2/3, Mecca 11/12, and the Catatonia 107/108

WORKING-END DESIGN

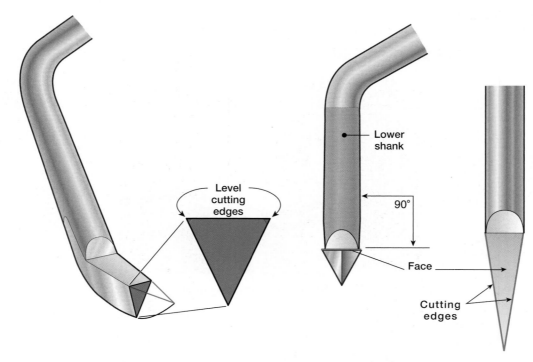

Figure 15-2. **Design Characteristics of Sickle Scalers.**

TABLE 15-1. DESIGN CHARACTERISTICS OF THE SICKLE SCALER	
Cross Section	Triangular cross section; this design limits use to above the gingival margin since the pointed tip and back could cause tissue trauma
Working-End	Pointed back and tip
	Two cutting edges per working-end
Face	Face is perpendicular to the lower shank so that cutting edges are level with one another; *level cutting edges mean that the lower shank must be tilted slightly toward the tooth surface to establish correct angulation*
Application	Anterior teeth—only one single-ended instrument is needed
	Posterior teeth—one double-ended instrument is needed
Primary Functions	Removal of medium- to large-sized calculus deposits
	Excellent for calculus removal on the (1) proximal surfaces of anterior crowns and (2) enamel surfaces apical to the contact areas of posterior teeth
	Debridement of enamel surfaces; NOT recommended for use on root surfaces

INNOVATIONS IN SICKLE SCALER DESIGN

Instrument manufacturers are continuously striving to introduce instruments that are more ergonomic in design and efficient at calculus removal. One of the most recent innovations in sickle scaler design is the Nevi series of instruments (Table 15-2).

TABLE 15-2. NEVI SERIES OF SICKLE SCALERS

Instrument	Characteristics
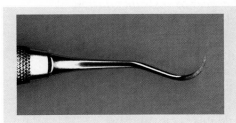	**Nevi 1: Sickle End** • Sickle-end of the Nevi 1 instrument • Rigid shank • Small, thin sickle • Use on coronal surfaces of anterior teeth
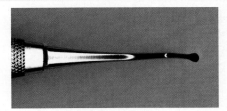	**Nevi 1: Disc End** • Disk-end of the Nevi 1 instrument • All surfaces are sharp on the disk-end • *Supra*gingival use on lingual surfaces of anterior teeth
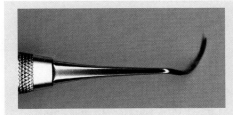	**Nevi 2** • Paired, mirror-image working-ends • Thin, curved sickles for use on posterior teeth • Long cutting edge facilitates access to proximal tooth surfaces • Use on coronal surfaces of posterior teeth
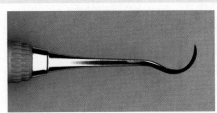	**Nevi 3** • Paired, mirror-image working-ends • Thin, curved sickles for use on posterior teeth • Long cutting edge facilitates access to proximal tooth surfaces • Use on coronal surfaces of posterior teeth • Excellent for use on pediatric patients
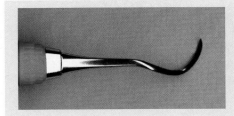	**Nevi 4** • Paired, mirror-image working-ends • Strong, curved sickles for use on posterior teeth • Rigid working-end and shank • Removal of medium- or large-size deposits

Section 2
Calculus Removal Concepts

REVISITING THE INSTRUMENT GRASP

1. Why is this chapter reviewing the grasp again—it is easy—isn't it?
   A. By this time in their preclinical instruction most students think of the instrument grasp as an easy skill learned at the beginning of the course that deserves little thought.
   B. The modified pen grasp, however, *is most often the first aspect of instrumentation to be found in error* during an observation of novice and experienced clinicians (1).
2. What is so important about the grasp anyway?
   A. *The modified pen grasp, however, has a crucial impact on a clinician's effectiveness in removing calculus deposits* (2). Effective instrumentation relies on precise finger position in the grasp (3–7). Precise finger placement is demonstrated in the photograph and illustration shown in Figure 15-3.
   B. Imprecise finger position in the grasp hinders effective calculus removal thus resulting to overworking of the fingers and musculoskeletal injury.
   C. *Prior to initiating an instrumentation stroke, all clinicians should pause for a minute to self-assess their modified pen grasp.*

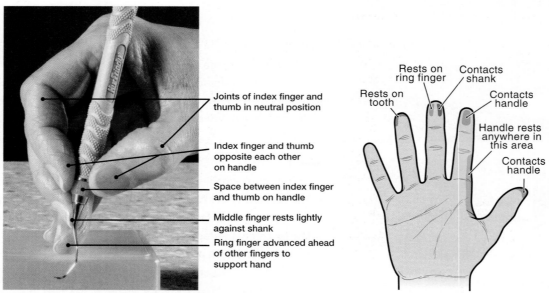

Figure 15-3. Precise Grasp Points for Modified Pen Grasp. Precise finger placement in the modified pen grasp is critical to successful periodontal instrumentation and prevention of injury to the clinician.

CHARACTERISTICS OF THE CALCULUS REMOVAL STROKE

Before beginning the step-by-step technique practice with sickle scalers, review the
(1) characteristics of the calculus removal stroke and (2) steps for calculus removal. These
concepts are the same for use of sickle scalers and universal curets (Table 15-3 and Fig. 15-4).

TABLE 15-3. THE CALCULUS REMOVAL STROKE WITH SICKLE SCALER

Stabilization	Apply pressure with the index finger and thumb inward against the instrument handle and press the tip of the fulcrum finger against the tooth surface
Adaptation	Tip-third of cutting edge is adapted
Angulation	70 to 80 degrees; for sickle scalers the lower shank must be tilted slightly toward the tooth surface to achieve correct angulation
Lateral Pressure for Calculus Removal	Moderate to firm pressure against the tooth surface is maintained during the short, controlled calculus removal stroke made away from the soft tissue
	When making a stroke the instrument handle moves slightly away from the tooth surface being instrumented; for example when working on a facial surface the instrument handle moves slightly toward the cheek or lip and not toward the facial surface
Characteristics	Controlled strokes, short in length
Stroke Direction	Vertical strokes are most commonly used on anterior teeth and on the mesial and distal surfaces of posterior teeth; stroke direction is *away from the soft tissue (in a coronal direction)*
	Oblique strokes are most commonly used on the facial and lingual surfaces of posterior teeth; *away from the soft tissue (in a coronal direction)*
	Horizontal strokes are used at the line angles of posterior teeth and the midlines of the facial or lingual surfaces of anterior teeth, stroke direction is *parallel to the gingival margin but never touching the soft tissue base of the sulcus or pocket*
Stroke Number	Strokes should be limited to areas where calculus is present; use the minimum number of strokes needed to remove calculus deposits

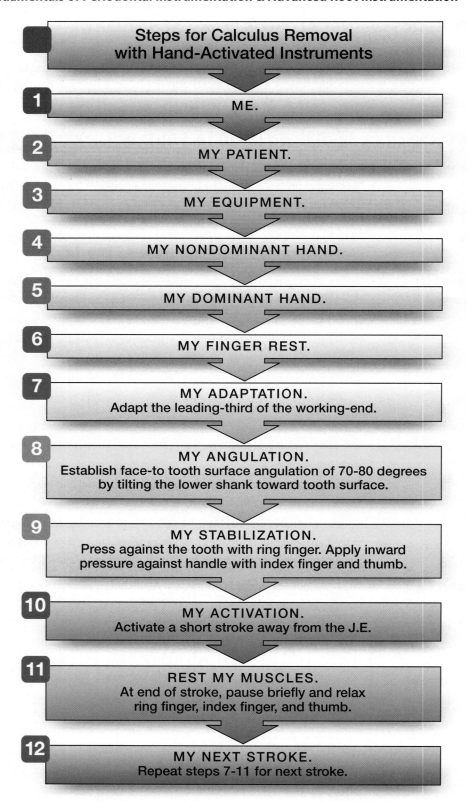

Steps for Calculus Removal with Hand-Activated Instruments

1. ME.

2. MY PATIENT.

3. MY EQUIPMENT.

4. MY NONDOMINANT HAND.

5. MY DOMINANT HAND.

6. MY FINGER REST.

7. MY ADAPTATION.
Adapt the leading-third of the working-end.

8. MY ANGULATION.
Establish face-to tooth surface angulation of 70-80 degrees by tilting the lower shank toward tooth surface.

9. MY STABILIZATION.
Press against the tooth with ring finger. Apply inward pressure against handle with index finger and thumb.

10. MY ACTIVATION.
Activate a short stroke away from the J.E.

11. REST MY MUSCLES.
At end of stroke, pause briefly and relax ring finger, index finger, and thumb.

12. MY NEXT STROKE.
Repeat steps 7-11 for next stroke.

Figure 15-4. Flow Chart for Calculus Removal with Sickles and Universal Curets.

Section 3
Technique Practice—Anterior Teeth

SKILL BUILDING
Establishing a 70- to 80-Degree Angulation to an Anterior Tooth

The relationship of a sickle scaler's face to the lower shank should be kept in mind when establishing angulation of the working-end to the tooth surface (Figs. 15-5 to 15-7).

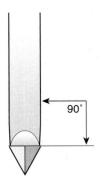

90°

Figure 15-5. Working-End Design. In establishing correct angulation, it is important to remember that *on a sickle scaler the face of the working-end is at a 90-degree angle to the lower shank*.

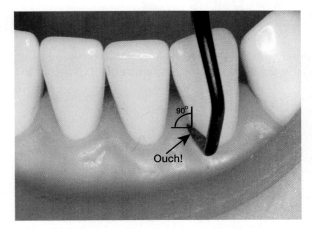

90°

Ouch!

Figure 15-6. Incorrect Angulation.
- Positioning the lower shank parallel to the mesial tooth surface results in a face-to-tooth surface angulation of 90 degrees.
- This angulation means that the other cutting edge could traumatize the soft tissue and calculus removal will be less efficient.

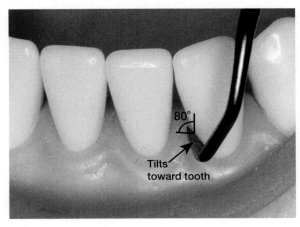

80°

Tilts toward tooth

Figure 15-7. Correct Angulation.
- *Correct angulation is achieved by tilting the lower shank slightly toward the mesial surface.* In this position the face-to-tooth surface angulation is between 70 and 80 degrees.
- With this angulation, the other cutting edge tilts toward the mesial surface and away from the soft tissue.

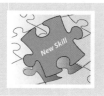

SKILL BUILDING
Technique on Anterior Tooth Surfaces

Directions:

- Figure 15-8 depicts working-end application to anterior surfaces.
- Follow Figures 15-9 to 15-17 to practice use of an anterior sickle scaler on the mandibular anterior teeth. Box 15-1 shows a recipe for artificial calculus.
- Remember: "Me, My patient, My light, My dominant hand, My nondominant hand, My finger rest, My adaptation."

APPLICATION OF THE CUTTING EDGES

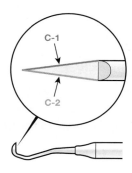

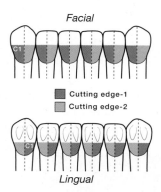

Figure 15-8. Application to Anterior Surfaces. The working-end of an anterior sickle has two cutting edges (C1 and C2). The illustration on the right indicates how the two cutting edges are applied to the tooth surfaces of the anterior teeth.

1. **Figure 15-9. Tooth.** As an introduction to using a sickle scaler on the anterior teeth, first practice on the *mandibular left canine, facial aspect*. **Right-handed clinicians**—*surface toward*. **Left-handed clinicians**—*surface away*.

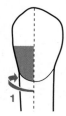

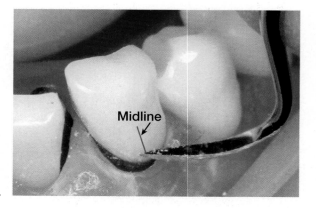

2. **FIGURE 15-10. Position Working-End Near the Midline of the Incisor.**
   - Establish a 70- to 80-degree instrument face-to-tooth surface angulation.
   - Aim the tip toward the mesial surface of the tooth.

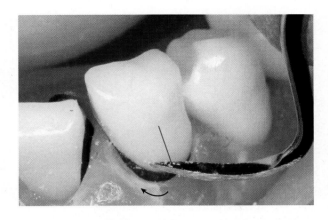

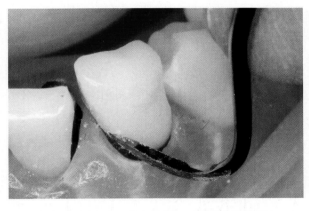

3. **Figure 15-11. Continue Across the Facial Surface.**
   - Use overlapping strokes as you work across the facial surface in the direction of the mesial surface.
   - Roll the instrument handle slightly between strokes to maintain adaptation.

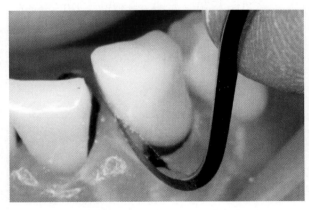

4. **Figure 15-12. Roll the Instrument Handle.** As you approach the mesiofacial line angle, roll the instrument handle to maintain adaptation of the tip-third of the working-end.

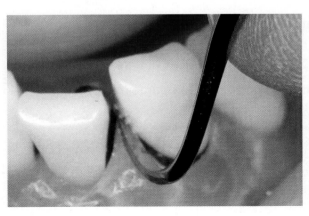

5. **Figure 15-13. Instrument the Mesial Surface.**
   - Check to make sure that you have maintained an angulation of 70 to 80 degrees.
   - Technique check: Keep the tip-third of the cutting edge adapted to the mesial surface. Using the middle-third of the cutting edge might result in trauma to the tissue of the interdental papilla.

6. **Figure 15-14. Instrument Under the Contact Area.** Continue strokes until you work at least halfway across the mesial surface. (The other half of the mesial surface will be instrumented from the lingual aspect of the tooth.)

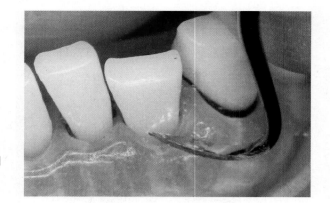

7. **Figure 15-15. Continue with Lateral Incisor.** Move the working-end to the midline of the lateral incisor and proceed in a similar manner with this tooth.

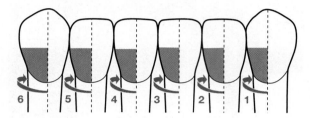

8. **Figure 15-16. Sequence.** Next, use the sequence shown in this illustration to instrument the colored tooth surfaces of the facial aspect. Begin with the left canine and end with the right canine.

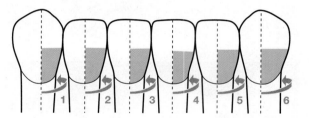

9. **Figure 15-17. Sequence.** Change your clock position and complete the remaining facial surfaces, beginning with the right canine and ending with the left canine.

Box 15-1 **Recipe for Artificial Dental Calculus**

Create realistic artificial dental calculus for use on typodonts using the following ingredients:

- Plaster of Paris
- Oil-based paint (to give the artificial calculus material color)
- Texture additive for paint
- Shellac

Combine 1 teaspoon of each ingredient to create enough artificial calculus for one typodont. Apply immediately and allow artificial calculus to dry overnight.

Section 4
Maintaining Adaptation to Proximal Surfaces

SKILL #1
Adapting the Tip-Third to the Midline of a Tooth

When using a sickle scaler it is important to remember that the tooth surface is curved. *This curvature means that in most cases only the tip-third of the cutting edge can be adapted to the tooth surface.* This is especially true with anterior teeth since these teeth are narrow in width (mesial to distal measurement). Figures 15-18A,B depict incorrect versus correct adaptation.

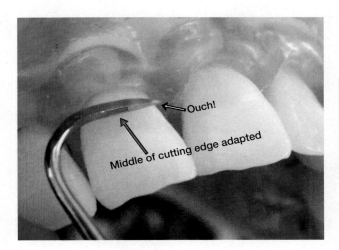

Figure 15-18. A: Incorrect Adaptation. In this photo the middle-third of the cutting edge is adapted to the facial surface. This incorrect technique may result in tissue trauma since the tip-third is not adapted and can "catch and tear" the soft tissue.

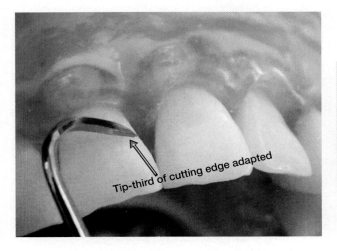

Figure 15-18. B: Correct Adaptation. In this photo the tip-third of the cutting edge is adapted to the facial surface. *Note that when the tip-third of the cutting edge is adapted the middle-third is NOT adapted.* Correct adaptation greatly lessens any occurrence of tissue trauma.

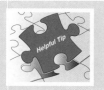

SKILL #2
Rolling the Handle to Maintain Adaptation to Proximal Surfaces

A second common technique error is failure to maintain adaptation of the tip-third (or toe-third) of the cutting edge to a proximal—mesial or distal—surface of a tooth. This technique error occurs when the clinician fails to roll the instrument handle when making strokes around the line angle of the tooth (Figs. 15-19A,B). Correct technique involves rolling the instrument handle in a series of tiny movements to maintain adaptation as strokes are made around the line angle and onto the proximal surface (Fig. 15-19C).

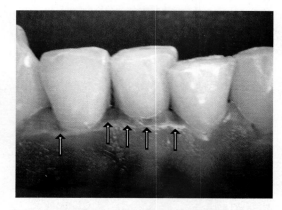

Figure 15-19. A: Tissue Trauma. The tissue trauma seen in this photograph results from failure to maintain adaptation of the tip-third of the cutting edge to the tooth surface.

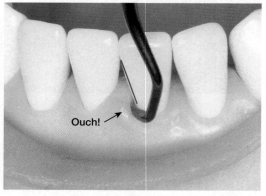

Figure 15-19. B: Incorrect Adaptation
- A common error is failure to roll the instrument handle when working around a line angle and onto the proximal tooth surface.
- *This technique error results in the middle-third of the cutting edge being adapted to the tooth, while the tip-third is NOT adapted.*
- This technique error results in injury to the soft tissue. OUCH!

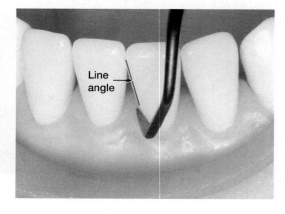

Figure 15-19. C: Correct Adaptation
- Correct technique involves rolling the instrument handle in a series of tiny movements to continuously adjust adaptation of the tip-third to the tooth surface.
- Note when the tip-third is correctly adapted the *middle- and heel-thirds of the working-end are NOT adapted* to the tooth surface.

SKILL #3
Positioning the Tip-Third Beneath the Margin of the Papillary Gingiva

A clinician must consider the anatomy of the gingival tissues during instrumentation (Fig. 15-20). Novice clinicians often fail to consider that the papillae are part of the free gingiva and thus, are unattached to the tooth surface (Figs. 15-21 and 15-22).

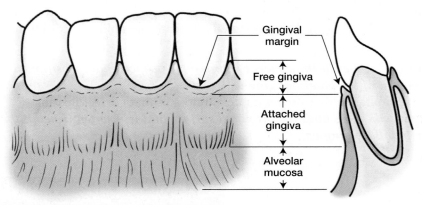

Figure 15-20. Anatomy of the Gingiva. The papillae are part of the free gingiva with a sulcus separating the soft tissue and the tooth surface.

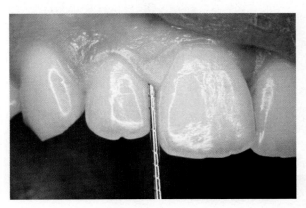

Figure 15-21. Healthy Papillae. In health the papillae have a scalloped (wavy) contour.
- The pointed papillae "hide" the mesial and distal surfaces from view.
- This photo shows a periodontal probe inserted in the sulcus. The probe tip is adapted to the mesial surface of the lateral incisor. In this position, the probe tip is beneath the margin of the pointed papilla.

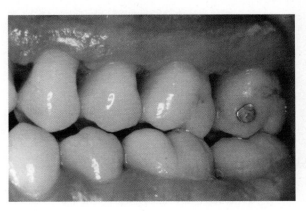

Figure 15-22. Blunted Papillae. In this photo, the papillae are blunted (missing).
- In this case, the working-end can be adapted easily to a mesial or distal surface with no papillae "hiding" these proximal surfaces from view.
- When a pointed papilla is present the clinician inserts the sickle's working-end beneath the margin of the pointed papilla.

The third common technique error is failure to position the working-end beneath the margin of the papillary gingiva. Instrumentation of proximal tooth surfaces (mesial or distal surfaces) adjacent to the papillary gingiva may be challenging to new clinicians.

Incorrect Technique: There is a tendency for a new clinician to "trace the pointed contours of the papilla" with the working-end as shown in the photo in Figure 15-23.

- Note that the working-end is not beneath the margin of the papillary gingiva in Figure 15-23.
- In a similar manner, some patients employ incorrect flossing technique by not wrapping the floss and not inserting it beneath the margin of the papillary gingiva.

Correct technique—as depicted in Figure 15-24—involves positioning the cutting edge against the proximal surface with the working-end beneath the pointed projection of the papillary gingiva.

- Note in Figure 15-24, *the tip-third hugs the proximal surface and is positioned beneath the margin of the papillary gingiva.*
- The technique is similar to that used with dental floss in that correct flossing technique, in that, *the floss hugs the proximal surface and is inserted beneath the margin of the papillary gingiva.*

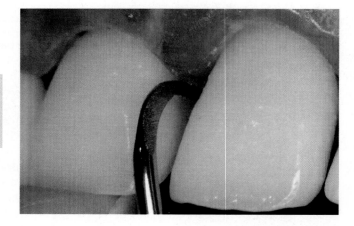

Figure 15-23. Incorrect Technique. Incorrect technique on the proximal surface with *the tip-third tracing the margin of the papilla*.

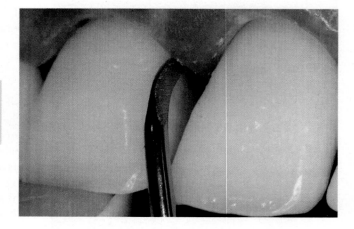

Figure 15-24. Correct Technique. Correct technique on the proximal surface with *the tip-third beneath the margin of the papilla*.

Section 5
Technique Practice—Posterior Teeth

SKILL BUILDING
Choosing the Correct Working-End of a Posterior Sickle Scaler

Method 1: The Lower Shank as a Visual Clue
When a working-end of a posterior sickle scaler is adapted to a distal surface, the correct working-end has the following relationship between the shank and the tooth:

- Lower shank is parallel to the distal surface
- Functional shank goes up and over the tooth
- *Think: Posterior = Parallel. Functional shank up and over!*

Correct working-end selection of a posterior sickle scaler is shown in Figure 15-25. Figure 15-26 shows the incorrect working-end for the distal surface of the mandibular right second premolar, facial aspect.

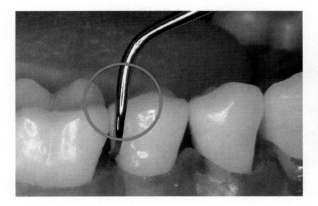

Figure 15-25. Visual Clue for the Correct Working-End.
- The correct working-end is selected when the **lower shank is parallel** to the distal surface.
- The **functional shank goes "up and over the tooth."**

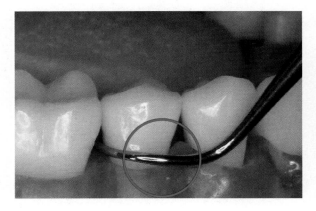

Figure 15-26. Visual Clue for the Incorrect Working-End.
- The incorrect working-end is selected if the **lower shank is not parallel** to the distal surface.
- The **functional shank is "down and around the tooth."**

Method 2: The Inner and Outer Cutting Edges as a Visual Clue
There is a second method for choosing the correct working-end of a posterior sickle scaler. For this method, the cutting edges provide the visual clue (Box 15-2). It is not important whether a clinician uses Method 1 or Method 2 to select the working-end. Each clinician should use the method that is easiest for him or her.

The bends in the functional shank of a posterior sickle scaler cause one of the cutting edges to be nearer to the handle than the other. Each working-end has two cutting edges, an inner and outer cutting edge (Fig. 15-27).

1. The outer cutting edge is the one that is *farther* from the instrument handle.
2. The inner cutting edge is the one that is *closer* to the instrument handle.

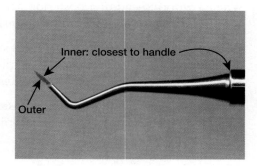

Inner: closest to handle

Outer

Figure 15-27. Inner and Outer Cutting Edges. To identify the cutting edges, **hold the instrument so that you are looking down on the face of the working-end**. One of the cutting edges will be nearer to the instrument handle than the other.

Box 15-2 **The Inner and Outer Cutting Edges as a Visual Clue**

The ***inner cutting edge*** is used to instrument the ***distal surfaces***.

The ***outer cutting edge*** is used to instrument the ***facial, lingual, and mesial surfaces***.

SKILL BUILDING
Establishing 70- to 80-Degree Angulation to a Posterior Tooth

The relationship of a posterior sickle scaler's face to the lower shank should be kept in mind when establishing angulation of the working-end to the tooth surface (Figs. 15-28 to 15-30). Ideally, the cutting edge-to-tooth angulation is between 70 and 80 degrees.

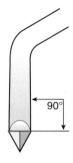

Figure 15-28. Working-End Design of a Posterior Sickle Scaler. In establishing correct angulation, it is important to remember that on a posterior sickle scaler *the face of the working-end is at a 90-degree angle to the lower shank.*

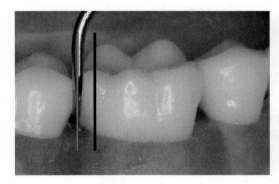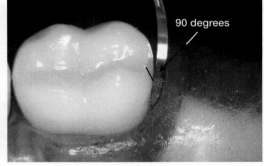

Figure 15-29. Incorrect Angulation. Because the lower shank of a posterior sickle scaler is at a 90-degree angle to face, positioning the lower shank parallel to the tooth surface results in an incorrect angulation of 90 degrees.

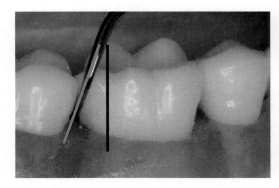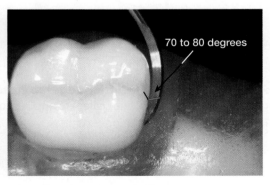

Figure 15-30. Correct Angulation. Correct angulation is achieved by tilting the lower shank slightly toward the tooth surface to be instrumented. In this position the face-to-tooth surface angulation is correct, between 70 and 80 degrees.

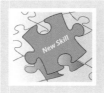

APPLICATION OF THE CUTTING EDGES

All four cutting edges of a posterior sickle scaler are used for calculus removal on the posterior sextants. Figures 15-31 and 15-32 depict application of the cutting edges to the mandibular right posterior sextant. Note that both cutting edges of one working-end—Working-end A—are used on the facial aspect of a tooth while the cutting edges of the other working-end—Working B—are used on the lingual aspect of the same tooth.

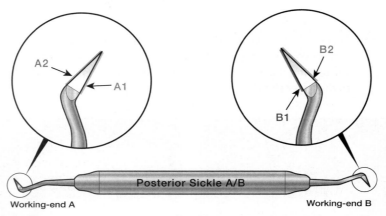

Figure 15-31. Four Cutting Edges of a Posterior Sickle Scaler. A posterior sickle scaler has two working-ends. Working-end A has two cutting edges (A1 and A2). Working-end B has two cutting edges (B1 and B2).

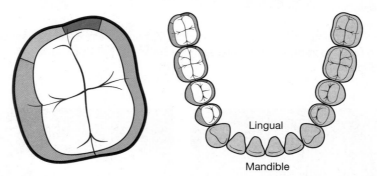

Figure 15-32. Application of Cutting Edges to Posterior Surfaces. These illustrations indicate how the cutting edges of a posterior sickle scaler are applied to the tooth surfaces of the mandibular right first molar and the mandibular right posterior sextant.

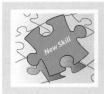

SKILL BUILDING
Technique for Posterior Teeth

Directions:

• Follow steps 1 to 11 to practice use of a posterior sickle scaler on the mandibular right posterior sextant (Figs. 15-33 to 15-43).
• Remember: "Me, My patient, My light, My dominant hand, My nondominant hand, My finger rest, My adaptation."

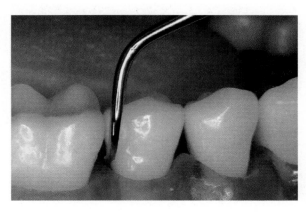

1. **Figure 15-33. Select the Correct Working-End.** When using the lower shank as a visual clue, use a tooth that is easily seen, such as the distal surface of the second premolar to select the correct working-end.

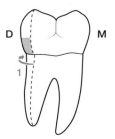

2. **Figure 15-34. Begin with Mandibular First Molar.** As an introduction to the posterior sickle, first practice on the *mandibular right first molar*. The distal surface is completed first, beginning at the distofacial line angle and working onto the distal surface.

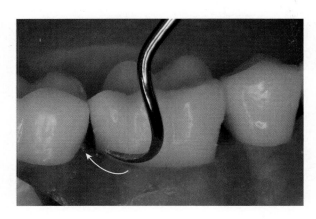

3. **Figure 15-35. Position the Working-End Near the Distofacial Line Angle.**
   • Establish a face-to-tooth surface angulation of between 70 and 80 degrees.
   • The tip should aim toward the back of the mouth because this is the direction in which you are working.

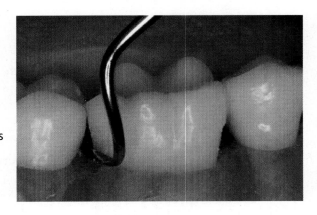

4. **Figure 15-36.** **Continue Strokes.**
   - Continue making a series of short, precise calculus removal strokes.
   - Remember to roll the instrument handle when working around the distofacial line angle and onto the distal surface.

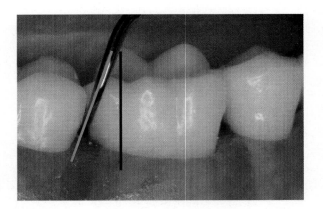

5. **Figure 15-37.** **Technique Check: Distal Surface.**
   - The sickles' face should be at a 70- to 80-degree angulation to the distal surface.
   - *To obtain this angulation, the lower shank will be tilted toward the distal surface.*

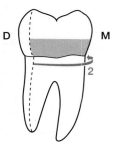

6. **Figure 15-38.** **Instrumentation of the Facial Surface.** Next instrument the facial and mesial surfaces of the tooth, beginning at the distofacial line angle.

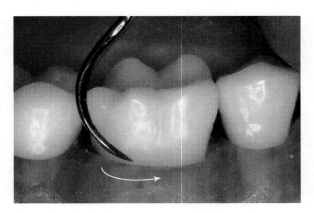

7. **Figure 15-39.** **Reposition the Working-End at the Line Angle.**
   - While maintaining your fulcrum, lift the working-end away from the tooth and turn it so that it aims toward the front of the mouth.
   - Reposition the working-end at the distofacial line angle.

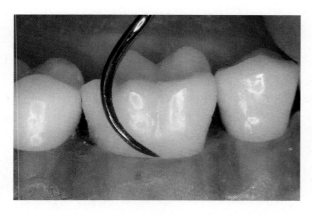

8. **Figure 15-40.** **Work Across Facial Surface.**
   - Continue working across the facial surface. Remember to maintain adaptation at all times.
   - As you approach the mesiofacial line angle, roll the handle slightly to maintain adaptation.

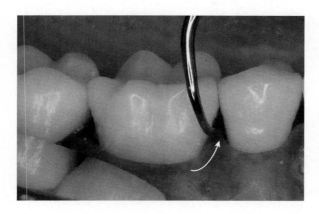

9. **Figure 15-41.** **Instrument the Mesial Surface.**
   - Tilt the lower shank slightly toward the mesial surface to maintain correct angulation.
   - Check the shank position to assure that you have maintained a 70- to 80-degree face-to-tooth surface angulation.

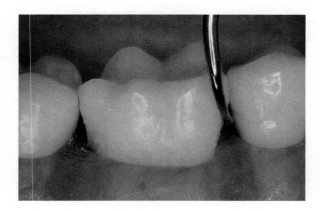

10. **Figure 15-42.** **Continue Strokes.** Work at least halfway across the mesial surface from the facial aspect. (The other half will be instrumented from the lingual aspect.)

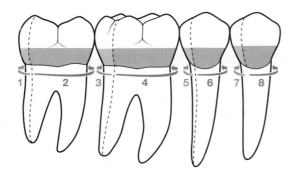

11. **Figure 15-43.** **Sequence for Sextant.** Next, use the sequence shown in this illustration to instrument the facial aspect of the entire sextant, beginning with the posterior-most molar. This sequence allows you to instrument the sextant in an efficient manner.

Section 6
Technique Practice—Primary Teeth

Instrumentation of primary teeth presents some unique challenges. These include the smaller size of the primary crowns as well as the rougher enamel surfaces and cementoenamel junctions on primary teeth (Figs. 15-44 and 15-45).

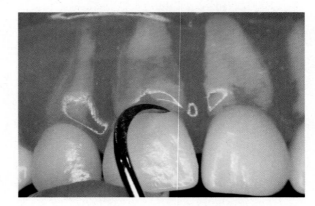

Figure 15-44. Primary Anteriors. The Nevi 1 is a small, thin anterior sickle scaler that works well for the tiny crowns of primary anterior teeth.

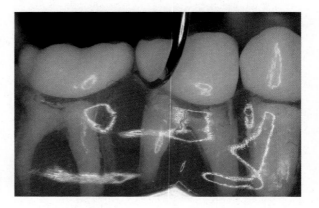

Figure 15-45. Primary Molars. The Nevi 3 posterior sickle scaler has a thin curved working-end that adapts well to primary molars.

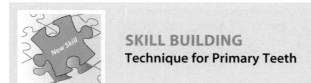

SKILL BUILDING
Technique for Primary Teeth

Equipment: Typodont with primary or mixed dentition and anterior and posterior sickle scalers.

Directions: Practice the use a posterior sickle scaler on primary molar teeth as shown in Figures 15-46 to 15-49.

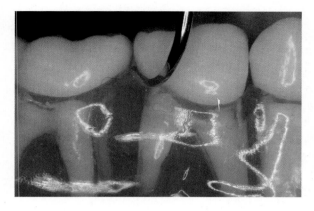

1. Figure 15-46. **Get Ready.**
   - Select the correct working-end and begin instrumentation at the distofacial line angle.
   - Work from the distofacial line angle to halfway across the distal surface.

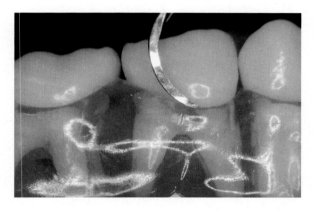

2. Figure 15-47. **Instrument the Facial Surface.**
   - After completing the distal surface, reposition the working-end at the distofacial line angle.
   - Make short, precise strokes across the facial surface.

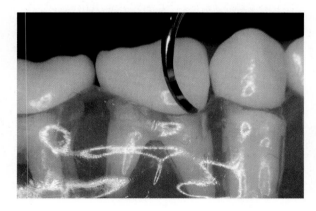

3. Figure 15-48. **Roll Instrument Handle at the Mesiofacial Line Angle.** At the mesiofacial line angle, roll the instrument handle to maintain adaptation as the working-end moves on to the mesial surface.

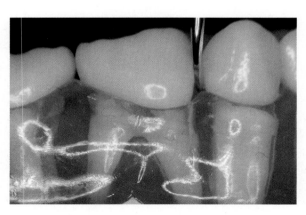

4. Figure 15-49. **Instrument the Mesial Surface.** Make short strokes at least halfway across the mesial surface from the facial aspect.

References

1. Leiseca C. How not to overwork your hands. Use a little leverage during periodontal instrumentation. *RDH*. 2014;5(43):2–6.
2. Dong H, Barr A, Loomer P, Rempel D. The effects of finger rest positions on hand muscle load and pinch force in simulated dental hygiene work. *J Dent Educ*. 2005;69(4):453–460.
3. Baur B, Furholzer W, Jasper I, Marquardt C, Hermsdorfer J. Effects of modified pen grip and handwriting training on writer's cramp. *Arch Phys Med Rehabil*. 2009;90(5):867–875.
4. Canakci V, Orbak R, Tezel A, Canakci CF. Influence of different periodontal curette grips on the outcome of mechanical non-surgical therapy. *Int Dent J*. 2003;53(3):153–158.
5. Dong H, Loomer P, Villanueva A, Rempel D. Pinch forces and instrument tip forces during periodontal scaling. *J Periodontol*. 2007;78(1):97–103.
6. Gentilucci M, Caselli L, Secchi C. Finger control in the tripod grasp. *Exp Brain Res*. 2003;149(3):351–360.
7. Karwowski W, Marras WS. *The Occupational Ergonomics Handbook*. Boca Raton, FL: CRC Press; 1999. xxii, 2065.

Section 7
Skill Application

PRACTICAL FOCUS
Working-End Adaptation and Angulation

- **Task 1:** Assess the adaptation shown in Figures 15-50 and 15-51. Is the adaptation of the cutting edge correct or incorrect?
- **Task 2:** What is the tooth-to-face angulation of the sickle scalers shown in Figures 15-52 and 15-53?

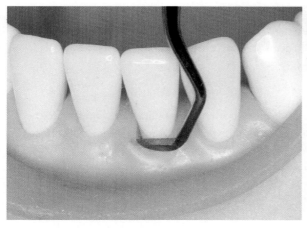

Figure 15-50. Is the Working-End Correct or Incorrect?

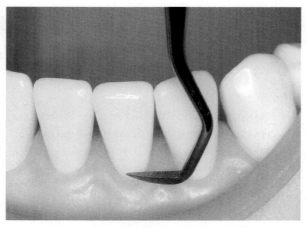

Figure 15-51. Is the Working-End Correct or Incorrect?

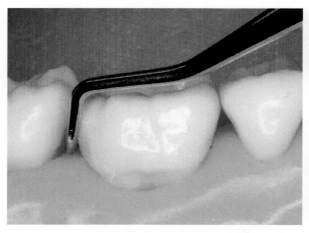

Figure 15-52. Is the Tooth-To-Face Angulation of the Cutting Edge to the Distal Surface of the First Molar Correct or Incorrect?

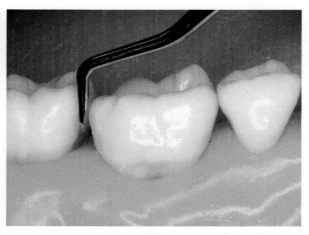

Figure 15-53. Is the Tooth-To-Face Angulation of the Cutting Edge to the Distal Surface of the First Molar Correct or Incorrect?

REFERENCE SHEET—SICKLE SCALERS

Use of Sickle Scalers:
- Sickle scalers are used to remove medium- and large-size calculus deposits from the crowns of posterior teeth.
- The pointed tip provides good access to mesial and distal surfaces apical to the contact areas.
- Sickle scalers are NOT recommended for use on root surfaces.

Basic Concepts:
- Tilt the lower shank slightly toward the tooth surface to establish correct face-to-tooth surface angulation.
- Maintain adaptation of the tip-third of the cutting edge to the tooth surface.
- Before initiating a calculus removal stroke, press down with your fulcrum finger and apply pressure against the instrument handle with the index finger and thumb to create lateral pressure against the tooth surface.
- Activate the calculus removal stroke using wrist motion activation.
- Relax your fingers between each calculus removal stroke.

Anterior Teeth:
- Sequence: Begin with the surfaces toward your nondominant hand. Start on the canine on opposite side of the mouth and work toward yourself. (Right-handed clinicians start with the left canine, mesial surface; Left-handed clinicians start with the right canine, mesial surface)

Posterior Teeth:
- Sequence: Begin at the distofacial line angle of the posterior-most tooth in the sextant and work toward the distal surface. Reposition at the distofacial line angle and complete the facial (or lingual) and mesial surfaces of the tooth, working toward the front of the mouth.

NOTE TO COURSE INSTRUCTOR: Refer to Module 22, Calculus Removal: Concepts, Planning, and Patient Cases, for patient cases relating to calculus removal.

Student Self Evaluation Module 15: Sickle Scalers

Student: _____   Date = _____

DIRECTIONS: Self-evaluate your skill level in each treatment area as: **S** (satisfactory) or **U** (unsatisfactory).

Criteria				
Positioning/Ergonomics	**Area 1**	**Area 2**	**Area 3**	**Area 4**
Adjusts clinician chair correctly				
Assumes the recommended clock position				
Positions backrest of patient chair for the specified arch and adjusts height of patient chair so that clinician's elbows remain at waist level when accessing the specified treatment area				
Asks patient to assume the head position that facilitates the clinician's view of the specified treatment area.				
Directs light to illuminate the specified treatment area				
Instrument Grasp: Dominant Hand	**Area 1**	**Area 2**	**Area 3**	**Area 4**
Grasps handle with tips of finger pads of index finger and thumb				
Rests pad of middle finger lightly on instrument shank				
Positions the thumb, index, and middle fingers in the "knuckles up" convex position; hyper-extended joint position is avoided				
Holds ring finger straight so that it supports the weight of hand and instrument; ring finger position is "advanced ahead of" the other fingers in the grasp				
Maintains a relaxed grasp; fingers are NOT blanched in grasp				
Finger Rest: Dominant Hand				
Establishes secure finger rest that is appropriate for tooth to be treated				
Once finger rest is established, pauses to self-evaluate finger placement in the grasp, verbalizes to evaluator his/her self-assessment of grasp, and corrects finger placement if necessary				
Prepare for Instrumentation ("Get Ready")				
Selects correct working-end for tooth surface to be instrumented				
Places the working-end in the "Get Ready Zone" while using a correct finger rest for the treatment area				
Adaptation, Angulation, and Instrument Stroke	**Area 1**	**Area 2**	**Area 3**	**Area 4**
Correctly orients the lower shank to the tooth surface to be instrumented				
Initiates a stroke in a coronal direction by positioning the working-end beneath a calculus deposit, "locking the tip" against tooth surface and using an angulation between 45 and 80 degrees				
Uses rotating motion to make a short, biting stroke in a coronal direction to snap a deposit from the tooth; does NOT close face toward tooth surface during activation; uses whole hand as a unit, does NOT pull with thumb and index finger				
Maintains appropriate lateral pressure against the tooth throughout the stroke while maintaining control of the working-end				
Precisely stops each individual stroke and pauses briefly (at least 3 seconds) to relax grasp before repositioning working-end beneath calculus deposit; strokes should be short				
Maintains neutral wrist position throughout motion activation				
Maintains correct adaptation as instrument strokes progress around tooth surface; pivots and rolls instrument handle as needed				
Thoroughly instruments proximal surface under each contact area				
Uses appropriate sequence for the specified sextant				
Keeps hands steady and controlled during instrumentation so that working-end moves with precision, regardless of nervousness				
Ethics and Professionalism				
Punctuality, appearance, demeanor, attitude, composure, honesty				

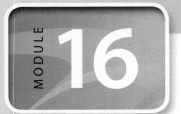

MODULE

16

Technique Essentials: Subgingival Calculus Removal

Module Overview

Periodontal instrumentation for the removal of subgingival plaque biofilm and dental calculus is an important component of nonsurgical periodontal therapy. Subgingival instrumentation requires much greater skill on the part of the clinician than that needed to remove supragingival calculus deposits. This module presents the following significant concepts for subgingival instrumentation: (1) importance of the sense of touch, (2) insertion beneath the gingival margin, (3) theoretical concepts of subgingival instrumentation, (4) a systematic stroke pattern, and (5) production of a calculus removal stroke.

Module Outline

Section 1 | **The Sense of Touch for Subgingival Instrumentation** | **364**
Subgingival Calculus: "The Hidden Enemy"
Visualizing the Unseen

Section 2 | **Inserting a Curet Beneath the Gingival Margin** | **366**
Angulation for Insertion
Preparation for Insertion: The Get Ready Zone
Flow Chart. Insertion in Preparation for Instrumentation
Skill Building. Insertion of a Curet Beneath the Gingival Margin, p. 369

Section 3 | **The Theory Behind Subgingival Instrumentation** | **372**
Why is Subgingival Instrumentation So Important?
How Do I Know When Subgingival Instrumentation is Complete?
Healing After Periodontal Instrumentation

Section 4 | **Systematic Pattern for Subgingival Calculus Removal** | **375**
Width of an Instrumentation Stroke
Instrumentation Zones and Multidirectional Strokes

Section 5 | **Production of a Calculus Removal Stroke** | **378**
Angulation for Calculus Removal
Preparation for a Calculus Removal Stroke
A Calculus Removal Stroke: The Sequence of Events
Skill Building. Initiating a Calculus Removal Stroke, p. 381
Flow Chart: Sequence for Calculus Removal Stroke

Online resources for this module:
- Calculus removal stroke
- Calculus removal strokes: sheet calculus
- Calculus removal strokes: subgingival calculus deposits
- Laying down versus "standing up" on your fulcrum

Available at: http://thepoint.lww.com/GehrigFundamentals8e

Key Terms

Periodontium
Insertion
Get Ready Zone
Out of the line of fire
Periodontal instrumentation

Appointment for
   re-evaluation
Nonresponsive disease sites
Residual calculus deposits
Instrumentation zones

Multidirectional strokes
Crosshatch pattern
Stabilization
Lateral pressure

Learning Objectives

- Explain the importance of learning to rely on the sense of touch for successful performance of sub-gingival instrumentation.

- Define the terms insertion and Get Ready Zone as they apply to periodontal instrumentation.

- On a periodontal typodont, demonstrate the steps used for insertion beneath the gingival margin as outlined in Figure 16-5.

- Define and state the objectives of periodontal instrumentation. Explain why complete removal of all subgingival biofilms and calculus deposits is so important to successful periodontal instrumentation.

- Explain why "tissue response" rather than "root smoothness" is the standard for successful subgingival instrumentation.

- Discuss the importance of a re-evaluation appointment in the treatment of patients with subgingival calculus deposits.

- Define the term nonresponsive disease sites and name signs that indicate that nonresponsive sites are present at a re-evaluation appointment.

- Describe the types of healing that may result following successful instrumentation of root surfaces.

- Explain the importance of instrumenting the root surface in the series of narrow strips, known as instrumentation zones.

- Define and explain the significance of multidirectional strokes in subgingival stroke removal.

- On a periodontal typodont, correctly demonstrate the following skills for subgingival instrumentation while maintaining precise finger placement in the grasp and correct fulcruming technique:
(1) insertion beneath the gingival margin (2) placement of the working-end in the Get Ready Zone, (3) calculus removal technique including locking the toe-third against the root surface, opening the face for a correct cutting edge-to tooth surface angulation, and engaging a short, biting stroke, (4) use of instrumentation zones, (5) and use of multidirectional strokes.

- Discuss the ways in which a clinician's choice of words can facilitate or hinder communication with patients regarding dental hygiene care. Give several examples of word choices that help or hinder the patient's understanding of the procedure of periodontal instrumentation.

Section 1
The Sense of Touch for Subgingival Instrumentation

SUBGINGIVAL CALCULUS: "THE HIDDEN ENEMY"

1. Subgingival deposits are calculus deposits located apical to (below) the gingival margin. Other terms that have been used for deposits apical to the gingival margin are submarginal calculus or serumal calculus.
   A. Distribution and Location
      1. The distribution of subgingival deposits may be localized in certain areas or generalized throughout the mouth.
      2. Subgingival calculus deposits are hidden beneath the gingival margin, thus, hiding them from the clinician's view and making deposit removal much more challenging.
      3. Although subgingival deposits may be found anywhere on the root surface, deposits commonly are located: (1) just apical to the cementoenamel junction (CEJ), (2) on line angles, and (3) within furcation areas and root concavities (Fig. 16-1).
   B. Shape. The shape of subgingival deposits is most often flattened. It is thought that the shape of the deposit may be guided by pressure of the pocket wall against the deposit.
2. Effects of Calculus on the Periodontium
   A. *The surface of a calculus deposit at the microscopic level is quite irregular in contour and is always covered with disease-causing bacteria.*
   B. As dental calculus deposits build up, they create more and more areas of plaque biofilm retention that are difficult or impossible for a patient to clean.
3. Pathologic Potential. Since a layer of living bacterial plaque biofilm always covers a calculus deposit, dental calculus plays a significant role as a local contributing factor in periodontal disease. It is difficult to bring either gingivitis or periodontitis under control in the presence of dental calculus and the importance of removing these deposits in patients with gingivitis and periodontitis cannot be overemphasized.

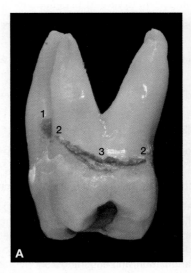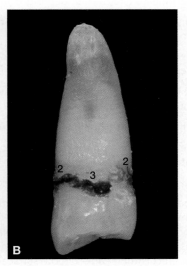

Figure 16-1. Subgingival Calculus Deposits. Surfaces where subgingival calculus commonly is located include those labeled on the maxillary molar (photo A) and premolar (photo B): **1.** coronal to furcation areas, **2.** at line angles, and **3.** apical to the CEJ. (Reprinted with permission from Scheid, RC, Weiss G. *Woelfel's Dental Anatomy.* 8th ed. Philadelphia, PA: Lippincott Williams & Wilkins, 2012.)

VISUALIZING THE UNSEEN

Subgingival calculus removal requires much greater skill on the part of the clinician than supragingival removal. When thinking about performing subgingival instrumentation there is a difficult truth that all clinicians "must come to grips with." *This important concept is that—unless working with a dental endoscope—the clinician cannot SEE the working-end of the instrument beneath the gingival margin.*

1. Relying on the Sense of Touch
   A. For many individuals, the visual "seeing" sense is their dominant sense (the sense that they reply on more than any other).
   B. *For successful subgingival instrumentation, the clinician must learn to rely on his or her sense of touch and make this sense dominant.*
   C. With the working-end hidden beneath the gingival tissue, the dental hygienist needs to be able to visualize the position of the working-end in his or her mind's eye (1).

2. Visualizing in Cross Section
   A. To picture the placement of the working-end against the root surface, the hygienist must mentally picture the cross section of the tooth, periodontium, and the instrument working-end (1). The tissues that surround and support a tooth in the dental arch (Fig. 16-2) are known as the periodontium. The components of the periodontium are the gingiva, periodontal ligament, cementum, and the alveolar bone.
   B. Much subgingival instrumentation is performed within periodontal pockets in an oral cavity that has diseased periodontal tissues. Figure 16-2 depicts periodontitis (diseased tissue with periodontal pockets) and this unhealthy periodontium in cross section.

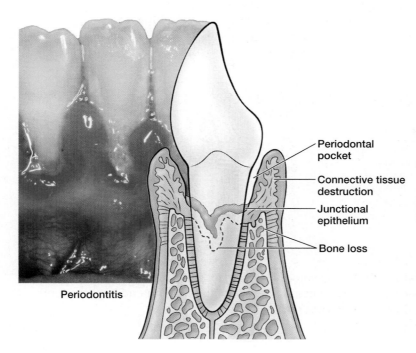

Periodontitis

Periodontal pocket

Connective tissue destruction

Junctional epithelium

Bone loss

Figure 16-2. An Unhealthy Periodontium in Cross Section. Much subgingival instrumentation is performed on an unhealthy periodontium such as the one pictured here. The clinician must visualize the tooth in cross section to successfully work beneath the gingival margin within the periodontal pocket.

Section 2
Inserting a Curet Beneath the Gingival Margin

ANGULATION FOR INSERTION

1. **Insertion** is the act of gently sliding the working-end of an explorer or curet beneath the gingival margin into the gingival sulcus or periodontal pocket.
   A. Care must be used during insertion to prevent injury to the soft tissue. The working-end should be kept in contact with the tooth surface during insertion.
   B. Curets are the primary calculus removal instruments for *sub*gingival instrumentation.
2. *During insertion, the face-to-tooth surface angulation is an angle between 0 and 40 degrees.* Figure 16-3 illustrates the proper angulation for insertion.
   A. During insertion, the face of a curet is held against the tooth surface as closely as possible. It should hug the tooth surface throughout the entire process of insertion.
   B. The 0- to 40-degree angle used for insertion also is referred to as a **closed angle** since the face is closed against the tooth surface.
3. There are several important steps in preparing for insertion beneath the gingival margin. Figure 16-5 summarizes the steps involved in inserting the working-end beneath the gingival margin.
   A. Establishing a secure finger rest near the tooth to be instrumented.
   B. Selecting the correct working-end of a double-ended instrument.
   C. Preparing for insertion by placing the working-end on the crown of the tooth in the "*Get Ready Zone.*"

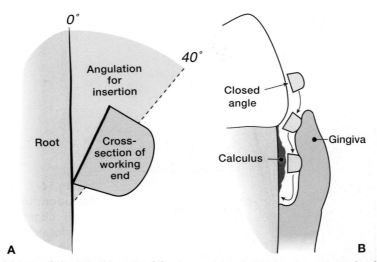

Figure 16-3. Angulation of the Working-End for Insertion. A, During insertion, the face-to-tooth surface angulation should be an angle between 0- and 40-degrees. **B**, The face of the working-end hugs the tooth surface as it slides gently to the base of a periodontal pocket.

PREPARATION FOR INSERTION: THE GET READY ZONE

The Get Ready Zone is an area of the crown where the working-end is positioned *prior* to insertion. *The Get Ready Zone is located in the middle-third of the crown of the tooth.* Figures 16-4A–B show the Get Ready Zones for three teeth on the facial and proximal surfaces.

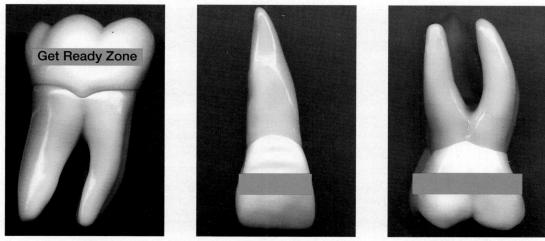

Figure 16-4. A: Insertion Get Ready Zones on Facial Surfaces. Shown here—shaded in *green*—are the Get Ready Zones prior to insertion for the facial surfaces of a mandibular first molar, maxillary central incisor, and maxillary first molar.

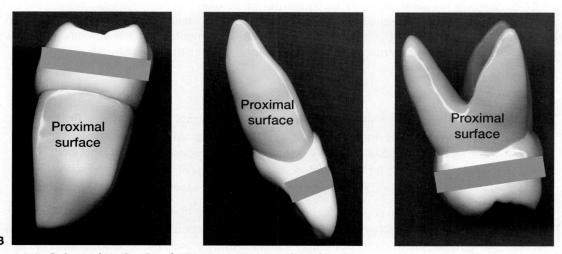

Figure 16-4. B: Insertion Get Ready Zones on Proximal Surfaces. Shown here—shaded in *green*—are the Get Ready Zones prior to insertion for proximal surfaces of a mandibular first molar, maxillary central incisor, and maxillary first molar.

FLOW CHART. INSERTION IN PREPARATION FOR INSTRUMENTATION

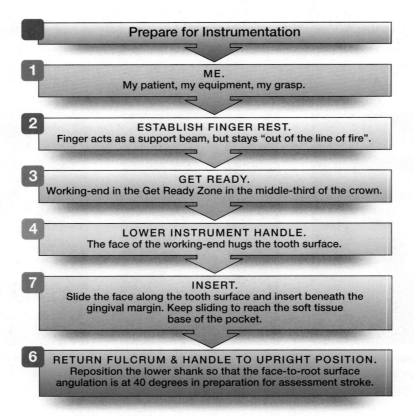

Prepare for Instrumentation

1
ME.
My patient, my equipment, my grasp.

2
ESTABLISH FINGER REST.
Finger acts as a support beam, but stays "out of the line of fire".

3
GET READY.
Working-end in the Get Ready Zone in the middle-third of the crown.

4
LOWER INSTRUMENT HANDLE.
The face of the working-end hugs the tooth surface.

7
INSERT.
Slide the face along the tooth surface and insert beneath the gingival margin. Keep sliding to reach the soft tissue base of the pocket.

6
RETURN FULCRUM & HANDLE TO UPRIGHT POSITION.
Reposition the lower shank so that the face-to-root surface angulation is at 40 degrees in preparation for assessment stroke.

Figure 16-5. Steps in Preparation for an Instrumentation Stroke. This flow chart summarizes the steps involved in inserting the working-end beneath the gingival margin. Small, explicit steps that clearly define the instrumentation technique facilitate learning periodontal instrumentation (2). Envisioning the steps prior to attempting a skill assists the learner in accurately performing the instrumentation skill.

NOTE TO COURSE INSTRUCTOR: Periodontal Typodonts for Technique Practice
One excellent source of periodontal typodonts with flexible gingiva for technique practice is Kilgore International, Inc.: 800-892-9999 or online at http://www.kilgoreinternational.com. These typodonts are an excellent addition to student instrument kits to be used when learning instrumentation technique and for patient instruction in self-care (home care) techniques.

Typodonts allow students to practice techniques such as insertion without danger of injury to the sulcular or junctional epithelium of a partner (3). Also, there is the advantage that students can see for themselves the results of improper adaptation. Periodontal typodonts with flexible or removable gingiva, allow students to practice instrumentation on root surfaces—the most important and difficult areas of the tooth on which to master instrumentation (4).

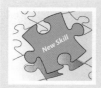

SKILL BUILDING
Insertion of a Curet Beneath the Gingival Margin

Equipment: Periodontal typodont and a universal curet (4). *If the typodont has removable gingiva, first, practice insertion and then, remove the gingiva so that you can see the working-end of the instrument on the root.*

- Follow steps depicted in Figures 16-6 to 16-13 to practice insertion on the distal and facial tooth surfaces of a mandibular first molar. **Right-handed clinician:** Mandibular right posterior sextant, facial aspect; **Left-handed clinician:** Mandibular left posterior sextant, facial aspect.
- Remember: "Me. My patient. My light. My dominant hand. My nondominant hand."
- The finger rest should not be positioned directly in line with the working-end to prevent injury to the ring finger (a finger stick) when making a stroke. *Position the finger rest "out of the line of fire" near to the tooth surface to be instrumented.*

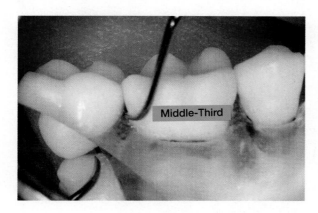

Middle-Third

1. **Figure 16-6. Get Ready for Insertion on Distal Surface.**
   - Turn the toe of working-end toward the distal surface.
   - In preparation for insertion, the working-end is placed in the *Get Ready Zone* in the middle-third of the crown.
   - In this case, the Get Ready Zone is at the distofacial line angle in the middle-third of the crown.

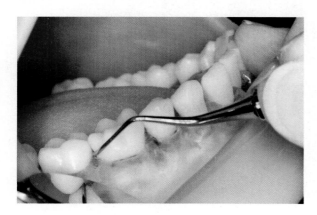

2. **Figure 16-7. Prepare for Insertion on Distal Surface.**
   - Lower your hand and the instrument handle *until the face-to-tooth surface angulation is near to 0 degrees.* (For insertion, it may be necessary to fulcrum briefly on the facial surface.)
   - The face of the instrument should hug the distal surface.

3. **Figure 16-8. Insert on Distal Surface.**
   - Maintaining your hand position gently slide the working-end beneath the gingival margin and onto the distal surface of the root.
   - *Imagine the face of the working-end sliding along the distal surface, all the way to the base of the pocket.*

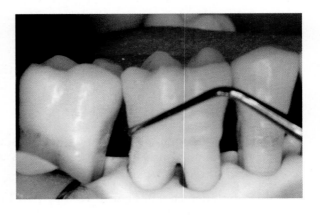

4. **Figure 16-9. Return Fulcrum Finger and Handle to Upright Position.**
   - Return your fulcrum to the occlusofacial line angle of a nearby tooth as you reposition the handle to an upright position (5).
   - Reposition the lower shank so that the face-to-root surface angulation is about 40 degrees in preparation for an assessment stroke.

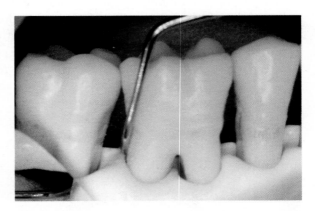

5. **Figure 16-10. Get Ready for Insertion on Facial Surface.**
   - Turn the working-end so that the toe of the curet is "pointing toward" the front of the mouth.
   - Place the working-end in the **Get Ready Zone** on the middle-third of the facial surface.

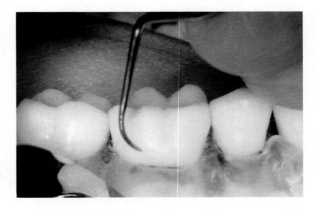

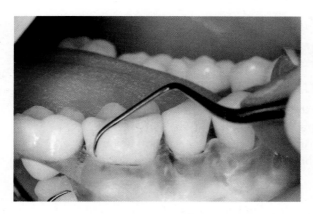

6. **Figure 16-11. Prepare for Insertion on Facial Surface.**
   - Lower your hand and the instrument handle until the curet toe is pointing toward the gingival margin. (For insertion, it may be necessary to fulcrum briefly on the facial surface.)
   - Insert at a 0-degree angulation with the lower shank close to the tooth.
   - *The face of the instrument should hug the facial surface.*

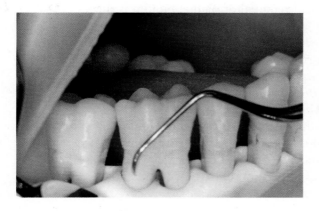

7. **Figure 16-12. Insert on Facial Surface.**
   - Maintaining your hand position gently slide the working-end beneath the gingival margin and onto the facial surface of the root.
   - *Imagine the face of the working-end sliding along the facial surface, all the way to the base of the pocket.*

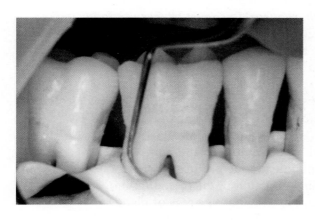

8. **Figure 16-13. Return Fulcrum Finger and Handle to Upright Position.**
   - Return your fulcrum to the occlusofacial line angle of a nearby tooth as you reposition the handle to an upright position.
   - Reposition the lower shank so that the face-to-root surface angulation is about 40 degrees in preparation for an assessment stroke.

Section 3
The Theory Behind Subgingival Instrumentation

WHY IS SUBGINGIVAL INSTRUMENTATION SO IMPORTANT?

1. Objective of Periodontal Instrumentation. Periodontal instrumentation (periodontal debridement) is defined as the removal or disruption of plaque biofilm, its byproducts, and biofilm retentive calculus deposits from coronal tooth surfaces and root surfaces to re-establish periodontal health and restore a balance between the bacterial flora and the host's immune responses.
   A. Mechanical Removal of Plaque Biofilms. The objective of subgingival periodontal instrumentation is the physical removal of calculus deposits, microorganisms, and their products to prevent and treat periodontal infections.
      1. Because of the structure of biofilms, physical removal of plaque biofilm is the most effective mechanism of control.
      2. Most subgingival plaque biofilm located within periodontal pockets cannot be reached by toothbrushes, floss, or mouth rinses.
         a. *For this reason, frequent periodontal instrumentation of subgingival root surfaces to remove or disrupt plaque biofilms mechanically is an essential component of the treatment of most patients with periodontitis.*
         b. In fact, periodontal instrumentation is likely to remain the most important component of nonsurgical periodontal therapy for the foreseeable future.
   B. Mechanical Removal of All Calculus Deposits. The removal of all calculus deposits from tooth surfaces is a critical component of periodontal instrumentation and must be part of any plan for dental hygiene care.
      1. Calculus deposits harbor living bacterial biofilms; thus, if the calculus remains, so do the pathogenic bacteria, making it impossible to re-establish periodontal health (6–8).
      2. *In order to re-establish periodontal health, root surfaces must be free of plaque biofilm and all calculus deposits.* Subgingival periodontal instrumentation must cover every square millimeter of the root surface.
      3. Calculus removal is always a fundamental part of periodontal therapy.
2. Rationale for Subgingival Instrumentation. The scientific basis for performing periodontal instrumentation includes all points listed below.
   A. To arrest the progress of periodontal disease by removing plaque biofilms and plaque biofilm retentive calculus deposits.
   B. To induce positive changes in the subgingival bacterial flora (count and content).
   C. To create an environment that assists in maintaining tissue health and/or permits the gingival tissue to heal, thus, eliminating inflammation in the periodontium.
   D. To increase the effectiveness of patient self-care by eliminating areas of plaque biofilm retention that are difficult or impossible for the patient to clean.
   E. To prevent recurrence of disease during periodontal maintenance. Periodontal maintenance refers to continuing patient care provided by the dental team to help the patient with periodontitis maintain periodontal health.
3. Re-evaluation of Subgingival Periodontal Instrumentation
   A. Response to periodontal instrumentation is normally delayed, since it takes some time for the body's defense mechanisms to respond to the treatment.
   B. Because of this delay time in healing, the dental hygienist is obligated to re-evaluate the results of subgingival instrumentation after a period of healing to ensure that all calculus deposits and biofilm retentive features (such as faulty restorations) have been removed and to identify any other measures that might be needed.

HOW DO I KNOW WHEN SUBGINGIVAL INSTRUMENTATION IS COMPLETE?

1. Assessment with an Explorer
   A. Smoothness of the Root Surface
      1. During subgingival instrumentation, many clinicians use an explorer to feel for the presence of remaining calculus deposits.
      2. Exploration of the entire root surface is one means for locating remaining deposits of calculus beneath the gingival margin. The clinician uses his or her sense of touch to detect roughness on the root surface.
      3. It is important to understand the difference between an assessment technique—use of an explorer to detect roughness—versus determining that subgingival instrumentation has reestablished an environment for health of the periodontium.
         a. *The true measure of successful subgingival instrumentation is the response of the tissue to that instrumentation procedure.*
         b. Root smoothness is a measure clinicians use during subgingival instrumentation to locate calculus deposits and gauge the effectiveness of calculus removal.
            1. But "smoothness" does not in itself indicate if instrumentation has been successful. It is a misconception that a feeling of "smoothness" is an indication of complete calculus removal (9). Rather, tissue response is the only true indicator of the effectiveness of subgingival instrumentation.
            2. Clinicians must remember that we are dealing with the control of plaque biofilms. For organisms the microscopic size of bacteria—that have multiple mechanisms for attachment to the root surface—no root surface is ever truly "smooth."
2. Tissue Response: The True Check for Effective Subgingival Instrumentation
   A. *The successful end point of subgingival instrumentation is to return the tissues of the periodontium to a state of health. In this context, health means periodontal tissues that are healed and free of inflammation.*
      1. Patients who had tissue inflammation and periodontal pockets—prior to subgingival instrumentation—require an appointment for re-evaluation 4 to 6 weeks after periodontal instrumentation
      2. Periodontal tissue healing does not occur overnight, and in most cases it is not possible to determine the true tissue response for at least 1 month after the completion of periodontal instrumentation.
   B. Managing Nonresponsive Disease Sites. During the re-evaluation, members of the dental team may identify nonresponsive disease sites.
      1. Nonresponsive disease sites are areas in the periodontium that show deeper probing depths, continuing loss of attachment, or continuing clinical signs of inflammation in spite of the subgingival instrumentation performed 1 month earlier.
         a. Despite the best efforts of the dental hygienist, root surfaces may still harbor residual (remaining) calculus deposits. Hopefully when the patient returns for re-evaluation, he or she has been doing a good job of daily biofilm control and the health of the tissues is greatly improved.
         b. In the presence of improved tissue health—with little or greatly reduced bleeding—the detection of any residual calculus deposits is much easier.
         c. At each re-evaluation or maintenance appointment, the goal is to remove all calculus deposits and biofilms from the root surfaces (Box 16-1).

2. *Signs of tissue inflammation—redness, bleeding—can be indications that some calculus deposits remain on the root surface* (6,8).
3. Nonresponsive sites should be carefully rechecked for thoroughness of self-care and rechecked for the presence of residual calculus deposits. Healing of the periodontium will not occur when calculus remains on a root surface (6,8).
4. *If calculus is found at a nonresponsive site, additional periodontal instrumentation should be performed to locate and remove the deposit(s).*

Box 16-1   ## Complete Calculus Removal is the Goal

- The objective of periodontal instrumentation is the complete removal of calculus deposits and plaque biofilms for the prevention and treatment of periodontal diseases.
- The tissues of the periodontium cannot heal in the presence of calculus or biofilms—complete calculus removal is always the goal of periodontal instrumentation.
- Tissue healing does not happen over night.
- Re-evaluation and maintenance appointments are required to monitor for new or nonresponsive disease sites.

HEALING AFTER PERIODONTAL INSTRUMENTATION

1. After thorough periodontal instrumentation, some healing of the periodontal tissues normally occurs.
2. Clinically, periodontal instrumentation can result in reduced probing depths. Figure 16-14 shows examples of various soft tissue responses to subgingival instrumentation.
3. *It is important to realize that following periodontal instrumentation, normally there is NO new formation of alveolar bone, cementum, or periodontal ligament.*

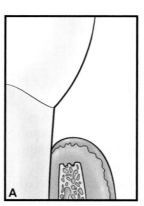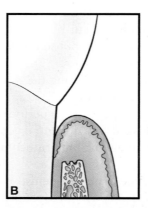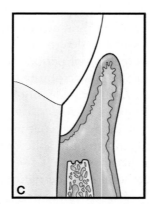

Figure 16-14. Soft Tissue Responses to Thorough Periodontal Debridement. This figure shows some of the possible tissue changes that can occur following thorough periodontal debridement. **A:** There can be complete resolution of the inflammation resulting in shrinkage of the tissue and a shallow probing depth. **B:** There can be readaptation of the tissues to the root surface by epithelium tissue. **C:** There can be very little change in the level of the soft tissues resulting in a residual periodontal pocket. (Used with permission from Nield-Gehrig JS. *Foundations of Periodontics for the Dental Hygienist.* 4th ed. Philadelphia, PA: Lippincott Williams & Wilkins; 2016.)

Section 4
Systematic Pattern for Subgingival Calculus Removal

Locating and removing subgingival calculus deposits is a challenging task since the clinician is working beneath the gingival margin and cannot see the calculus deposits or root surface. For this reason, the clinician must adopt a very systematic pattern of instrumentation strokes. A haphazard stroke pattern will result in missed calculus deposits and unsuccessful treatment of the root surface.

WIDTH OF AN INSTRUMENTATION STROKE

1. Misconception: "Roots are tiny, so I only need to make a few strokes, don't I?"
   A. Contact Area with Root Surface
      1. Many hygienists *incorrectly* assume that they can instrument a 3- to 4-mm wide strip of the root surface with each instrumentation stroke.
      2. In reality, the working-end of a periodontal instrument contacts the tooth in a very narrow 1- to 2-mm strip during the production of a stroke.
         a. *The root surface curves outward in certain places and inward in others. These convexities and concavities only permit adaptation of the toe-third of a cutting edge to the root surface. Figure 16-15 depicts a root surface, note that only the narrow strip—shaded in purple—is in contact with the cutting edge of the curet.*
         b. Regardless of whether the stroke direction is vertical, oblique, or horizontal, the cutting edge only contacts the same 1- to 2-mm strip with each instrumentation stroke.
   B. So, if the area of contact is so tiny how do I make sure to cover the entire root surface with instrumentation strokes?
      1. For successful root instrumentation the clinician visualizes the root surface covered in a series of narrow strips.
      2. Depending on the direction of the stroke, the narrow strips may be vertical, horizontal, or oblique in length (Fig. 16-16).

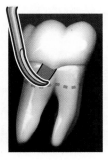

Figure 16-15. Contact Area of the Working-End. It is only possible to adapt the toe-third of a cutting edge to the curved surface of the root. Thus, the working-end of a periodontal instrument contacts the tooth in a very narrow 1- to 2-mm strip during the production of a stroke.

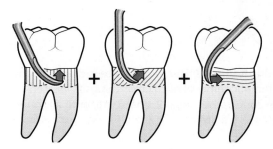

Figure 16-16. Imagine the Root Surface Divided into a Series of Narrow Strips. For complete biofilm and calculus removal the working-end should contact the root surface in a series of narrow strips 1 to 2 mm in width.

INSTRUMENTATION ZONES AND MULTIDIRECTIONAL STROKES

1. Use of Instrumentation Zones for Subgingival Instrumentation
   A. Use Systematic Approach
      1. It is helpful to think of the root surface as being divided into a series of long narrow strips known as instrumentation zones.
      2. *Each instrumentation zone is only as wide as the toe-third of the instrument's cutting edge.*
   B. Use of Instrumentation Zones for Calculus Removal. The surface of the root is divided into a pattern of instrumentation zones for the systematic removal of calculus deposits. The steps in employing calculus removal strokes in a series of narrow strips is as follows:
      1. Begin in "instrumentation zone 1."
         a. Use an assessment stroke with a curet to locate the calculus deposit closest to the soft tissue base of the periodontal pocket.
         b. Calculus deposits adjacent to the junctional epithelium are removed first; those near the gingival margin are removed last.
      2. Place the curet working-end beneath a deposit in zone 1.
         a. Use a tiny calculus removal stroke to snap the entire deposit or a section of a deposit from the root surface.
         b. Reassess the area with the curet using a relaxed assessment stroke.
      3. Continue working in a coronal direction until all deposits in zone 1 have been removed. Figure 16-17 depicts the technique of using instrumentation zones for subgingival calculus removal.
      4. Once you have completed zone 1, repeat the process in zone 2. Continue instrumenting each narrow zone in a similar manner until all zones on this aspect of the tooth have been completed.

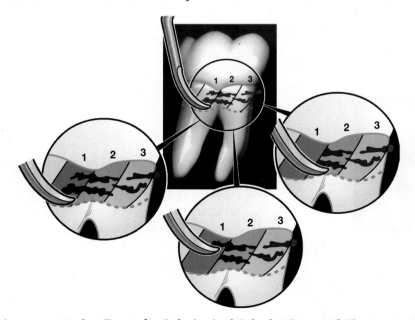

Figure 16-17. Instrumentation Zones for Subgingival Calculus Removal. The root surface is divided into a pattern of instrumentation zones—narrow strips—for the systematic removal of calculus deposits located beneath the gingival tissues. First, all deposits are removed from zone 1, then zone 2, and so on, until all zones are completed.

2. **Use of Multidirectional Strokes**
   A. **Multidirectional strokes** are a series of overlapping strokes produced by a sequence of vertical, oblique, and horizontal strokes.
      1. The three strokes are used, one by one in succession when assessing and instrumenting subgingival root surfaces. For example, the clinician might begin by using vertical strokes, then oblique strokes, followed by horizontal strokes.
         a. Figure 16-18 depicts the use of these strokes in succession to create the multidirectional stroke pattern.
         b. The pattern created by the series of overlapping strokes is sometimes referred to as a **crosshatch pattern**.
      2. The purpose of multidirectional strokes is to assure that every millimeter of the root surface is covered for complete calculus and biofilm removal.
3. **Planning a Calculus Removal Appointment**
   In planning a calculus removal appointment, the clinician should plan to treat only those tooth surfaces from which the calculus deposits can be completely removed. *All calculus deposits should be definitely removed from one tooth before starting instrumentation on a second tooth.* As many calculus removal appointments as needed should be scheduled to treat the entire dentition.

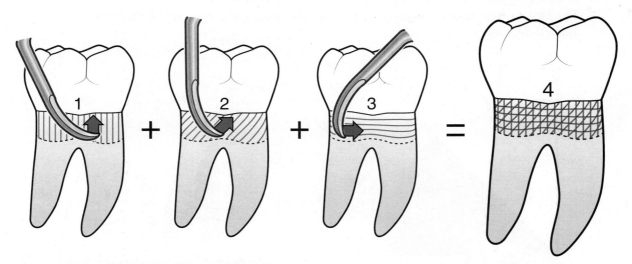

Figure 16-18. Multidirectional Stroke Pattern. The sequential use of three stroke directions results in an overlapping pattern of strokes to assure that every millimeter of the root surface is instrumented.

Section 5
Production of a Calculus Removal Stroke

ANGULATION FOR CALCULUS REMOVAL

1. Angulation During Assessment of the Tooth Surface
   A. Once a curet is inserted to the base of a periodontal pocket, it is used with an assessment stroke to detect calculus deposits on the root surface. Assessment strokes are made in a direction that is away from the junctional epithelium.
   B. For assessment strokes, the face-to-tooth surface angulation is approximately 40 degrees.
2. Angulation for Calculus Removal
   A. *For calculus removal, the face-to-tooth surface angulation is an angle between 45 and 90 degrees.*
   B. The ideal angulation for calculus removal is between 60 and 80 degrees. Figure 16-19 depicts the correct angulation for calculus removal.
3. Angulation for Root Debridement
   A. Root debridement strokes are used to remove subgingival plaque biofilm, residual calculus deposits, or surface irregularities from the root surface.
   B. *The face-to-root surface angulation for root debridement is an angle between 60 and 70 degrees.*

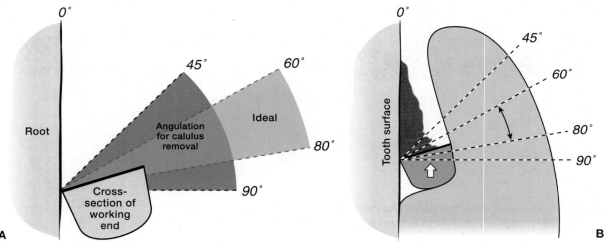

Figure 16-19. Angulation of the Working-End for Calculus Removal. For calculus removal, the face-to-tooth surface angulation should be an angle between 45 and 90 degrees.
- The correct *face-to-tooth surface angulation* is greater than 45 degrees and less than 90 degrees.
- Correct angulation allows the cutting edge to bite into the calculus deposit and fracture it from the tooth surface without injuring the soft tissue lining of the periodontal pocket.
- Note that the working-end is positioned apical to (beneath) the calculus deposit.

PREPARATION FOR A CALCULUS REMOVAL STROKE

1. **Preparation for a Calculus Removal Stroke.** Two elements used during the production of an instrumentation stroke are stabilization and lateral pressure. Figure 16-20 summarizes use of these elements.
   A. Stabilization is the act of preparing for an instrumentation stroke by locking the joints of the ring finger and pressing the fingertip against a tooth surface to provide control for the instrumentation stroke.
      1. Stabilization allows the hand and instrument to function as a unit.
      2. Stabilization provides the control necessary for an effective instrumentation stroke.
   B. Lateral pressure is the act of applying equal pressure with the index finger and thumb inward against the instrument handle to press the working-end against a calculus deposit or tooth surface prior to and throughout an instrumentation stroke.
2. **Skills Involved in the Calculus Removal Stroke.** Many fine psychomotor skills are involved in the production of a calculus removal stroke. Box 16-2 summarizes the series of steps in a calculus removal stroke.

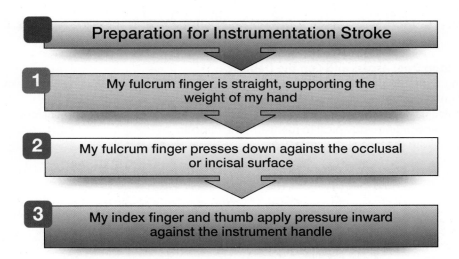

Figure 16-20. Flow Chart: Preparation for Instrumentation Stroke.

Box 16-2   ## Steps in a Calculus Removal Stroke

A calculus removal stroke involves these steps:

1. **Assess.** Employ an assessment stroke ("feeling stroke") away form the junctional epithelium until a calculus deposit is encountered.
2. **Cup.** Cup the calculus deposit with the face of the curet.
3. **Stroke.** Create a calculus removal stroke by (a) locking the toe-third against the tooth surface, (b) opening the face to the correct 70- to 80-degree angulation while (c) making a short, biting stroke away from the base of the pocket.

A CALCULUS REMOVAL STROKE: THE SEQUENCE OF EVENTS

Figures 16-21 and 16-22 detail the process of initiating, making, and finishing a calculus removal stroke. Figure 16-25 summarizes the entire sequence of events that comprise a calculus removal stroke.

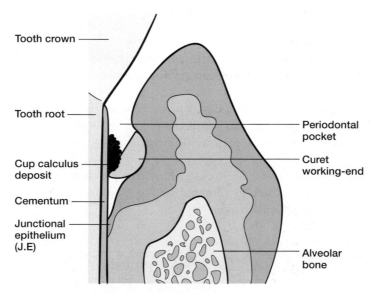

Figure 16-21. Step One: Assess and Cup the Deposit.
- After inserting a curet to the base of the pocket, employ a light assessment ("feeling") stroke over the root surface until encountering a calculus deposit.
- Size up the calculus deposit with an assessment stroke to determine its size and dimensions.
- Position the curet working-end apical to (beneath) the deposit.
- Cup the deposit with the face of the curet.

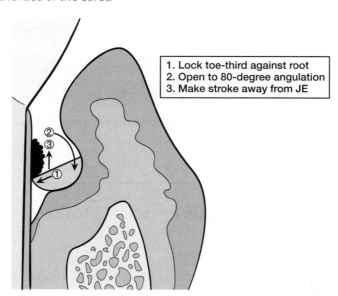

Figure 16-22. Step Two: Stroke. Reassess your grasp to assure that your fingers are precisely positioned in the grasp and that the fulcrum is straight, supporting your hand.
- Prepare for a calculus removal stroke by locking the toe-third against the tooth surface (step 1).
- Activate a stroke by opening the face to a 70- to 80-degree angulation (step 2) while making a short, biting stroke away from the base of the pocket (step 3).

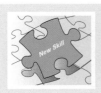

SKILL BUILDING
Initiating a Calculus Removal Stroke

Directions: Follow the steps depicted in Figure 16-23 and 16-24 to practice a calculus removal stroke. *A series of colored dots represent the calculus deposits in the photos.*

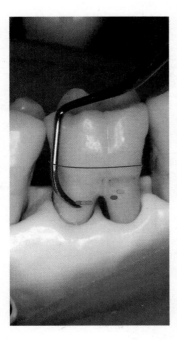

Figure 16-23. **Remove a Calculus Deposit.**
Step 1: Position. Position the toe-third of working-end beneath the distal-most portion of the calculus deposit.
- Only a portion of the deposit is removed with each stroke.
- In this case, the *magenta dot* will be removed with the first stroke. Cup the deposit with the working-end.
Step 2: Lock On and Activate.
- "Lock" the toe-third of the working-end against the facial surface of the root.
- ***Activate a stroke by opening the face to a 70- to 80-degree angulation while making a short, biting stroke away from the base of the pocket.***
- Keep the toe-third locked against the facial surface throughout the short, biting stroke.
Step 3: Make a Single Calculus Removal Stroke. Each calculus removal stroke should be a short, biting stroke to lift the deposit from the tooth.

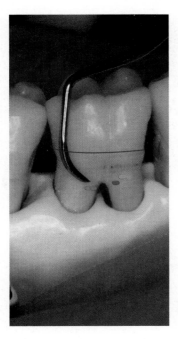

Figure 16-24. **End Stroke and Relax.**
- End each stroke with precision, by pressing down with your fulcrum finger against the occlusolingual line angle of the crown.
- ***Each stroke is distinct; make only one short upward stroke and then pause. Do NOT make a series of continuous back and forth strokes.***
- ***Make a single calculus removal stroke, stop the stroke, and immediately relax your fingers in the grasp.***
- Pause for at least 3 seconds after each stroke to prevent strain to the muscles of your hand. To assure that you take time to relax between strokes, stop and silently think: "1-one thousand, 2-one thousand, 3-one thousand."
The next step is to position the toe-third of the working-end beneath the *green dot.* Remove the green "deposit" and continue with the *orange dot.*

FLOW CHART: SEQUENCE FOR CALCULUS REMOVAL STROKE

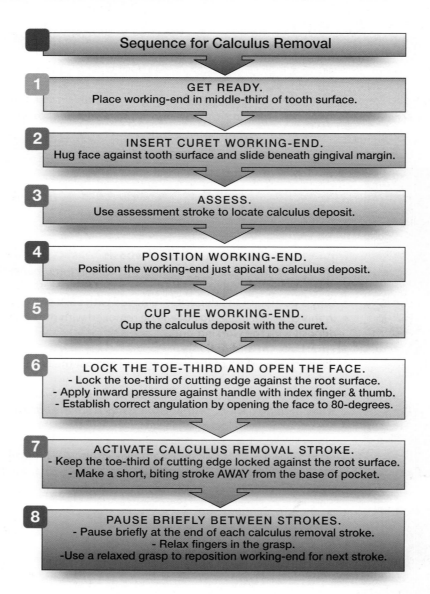

Sequence for Calculus Removal

1 GET READY.
Place working-end in middle-third of tooth surface.

2 INSERT CURET WORKING-END.
Hug face against tooth surface and slide beneath gingival margin.

3 ASSESS.
Use assessment stroke to locate calculus deposit.

4 POSITION WORKING-END.
Position the working-end just apical to calculus deposit.

5 CUP THE WORKING-END.
Cup the calculus deposit with the curet.

6 LOCK THE TOE-THIRD AND OPEN THE FACE.
- Lock the toe-third of cutting edge against the root surface.
- Apply inward pressure against handle with index finger & thumb.
- Establish correct angulation by opening the face to 80-degrees.

7 ACTIVATE CALCULUS REMOVAL STROKE.
- Keep the toe-third of cutting edge locked against the root surface.
- Make a short, biting stroke AWAY from the base of pocket.

8 PAUSE BRIEFLY BETWEEN STROKES.
- Pause briefly at the end of each calculus removal stroke.
- Relax fingers in the grasp.
- Use a relaxed grasp to reposition working-end for next stroke.

Figure 16-25. Flow Chart Showing Sequence of Skills Involved in Calculus Removal.

References

1. Rucker LM, Gibson G, McGregor C. Getting the "feel" of it: the non-visual component of dimensional accuracy during operative tooth preparation. *J Can Dent Assoc.* 1990;56(10):937–941.
2. Hauser AM, Bowen DM. Primer on preclinical instruction and evaluation. *J Dent Educ.* 2009;73(3):390–398.
3. Dufour LA, Bissell HS. Periodontal attachment loss induced by mechanical subgingival instrumentation in shallow sulci. *J Dent Hyg.* 2002;76(3):207–212.
4. Ruhling A, Konig J, Rolf H, Kocher T, Schwahn C, Plagmann HC. Learning root debridement with curettes and power-driven instruments. Part II: Clinical results following mechanical, nonsurgical therapy. *J Clin Periodontol.* 2003;30(7):611–615.
5. Dong H, Barr A, Loomer P, Rempel D. The effects of finger rest positions on hand muscle load and pinch force in simulated dental hygiene work. *J Dent Educ.* 2005;69(4):453–460.
6. Checchi L, Montevecchi M, Checchi V, Zappulla F. The relationship between bleeding on probing and subgingival deposits. An endoscopical evaluation. *Open Dent J.* 2009;3:154–160.
7. Fujikawa K, O'Leary TJ, Kafrawy AH. The effect of retained subgingival calculus on healing after flap surgery. *J Periodontol.* 1988;59(3):170–175.
8. Wilson TG, Harrel SK, Nunn ME, Francis B, Webb K. The relationship between the presence of tooth-borne subgingival deposits and inflammation found with a dental endoscope. *J Periodontol.* 2008;79(11):2029–2035.
9. Sherman PR, Hutchens LH Jr, Jewson LG. The effectiveness of subgingival scaling and root planing. II. Clinical responses related to residual calculus. *J Periodontol.* 1990;61(1):9–15.

Section 6
Skill Application

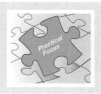

PRACTICAL FOCUS
Word Choice for Explaining Periodontal Instrumentation to Patients

There are several aspects relating to word choice—or terminology—to consider when talking with patients about dental hygiene care and periodontal instrumentation.

1. **Word Choice Pertaining to Dental Hygiene Care.** Dental hygienists hope that patients will value the care that they provide. The value a patient perceives may be influenced by the way that the hygienist refers to those services.
   a. Using words such as "dental cleaning" or "prophy" minimizes the perceived value of hygiene care. Hygienists do not simply "shine the teeth" as the phrase "clean the teeth" implies.
   b. Word choices such as "dental hygiene services" or "dental hygiene therapies" better convey the complex, therapeutic nature of dental hygiene care.
   c. Instead of saying, "Can we set up your next cleaning appointment?" consider a statement such as "Let's set up your next dental hygiene appointment to care for the health of your mouth and prevent disease."
2. **Word Choice Pertaining to Periodontal Instrumentation.** A second consideration is the mental images that the hygienist's words create in the patient's mind.
   a. Words such as "scale" and "root plane" do not clarify the treatment procedure for the patient, but they may conjure up very negative mental pictures. For example, hearing that his teeth are going to be "root planed" might cause a patient to picture layers of his teeth being shaved away the way a wood plane shaves off layers of wood. The terms "scale and root plane your teeth" might cause the patient to envision the planned treatment as something very aggressive and uncomfortable.
   b. Even the phase "periodontal instrumentation of the teeth" does nothing to explain the procedure to the patient. On the positive side, "instrument" may not produce the negative mental images that the forceful sounding terms "scale and root planning" can elicit.
   c. The ideal solution to "word use" when explaining periodontal instrumentation is simply to EXPLAIN in everyday words how the patient will benefit from the procedure. For example, showing the patient the tissue inflammation in his or her own mouth and explaining how biofilms cause disease. An explanation that treatment for periodontal disease involves using dental instruments to remove biofilm and calculus deposits from beneath the gum line can help clarify these procedures.

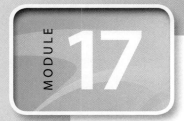

Universal Curets

Module Overview

This module presents the design characteristics of universal curets and step-by-step instructions for using universal curets to remove small- or medium-sized calculus deposits from the anterior and posterior teeth. Module 16: Technique Essentials: Subgingival Calculus Removal should be completed prior to beginning this module.

Module Outline

Section 1   **Universal Curets**   **387**
General Design Characteristics
Working-End Design
Selecting a Universal Curet for a Particular Task

Section 2   **Calculus Removal Concepts**   **390**
Characteristics of the Calculus Removal Stroke

Section 3   **Technique Practice—Posterior Teeth**   **392**
Skill Building. Selecting the Correct Working-End for a Posterior
     Tooth, p. 392
Establishing 70- to 80-Degree Angulation
Application of the Cutting Edges to the Posterior Teeth
Skill Building. Step-By-Step Technique on Mandibular First
     Molar, p. 396
Skill Building. Step-By-Step Technique on Maxillary First
     Molar, p. 401

Section 4   **Technique Alert—Lower Shank Position**   **403**
Incorrect Technique
Correct Technique

Section 5   **Technique Practice—Anterior Teeth**   **405**
Skill Building. Selecting the Correct Working-End for an Anterior
     Tooth, p. 405
Application of the Cutting Edges to the Anterior Teeth
Skill Building. Step-By-Step Technique on a Maxillary Central
     Incisor, p. 408

Section 6   **Technique Alert—Horizontal Strokes**   **410**
Skill Building. Horizontal Strokes Below the Gingival Margin, p. 410

Skill Application

Practical Focus
Reference Sheet—Universal Curets
Student Self Evaluation Module 17: Universal Curets

Online resources for this module:
* Selecting the Working-End
* Universal Curets
* The Columbia 13/14 Universal Curet
Available at: http://thepoint.lww.com/GehrigFundamentals8e

Key Terms

Universal curet
Outer cutting edge
Inner cutting edge

Learning Objectives

* Given a variety of universal curets, identify the design characteristics of each instrument.

* Discuss the advantages and limitations of the design characteristics of universal curets.

* Name the uses of universal curets.

* Describe how the clinician can use visual clues to select the correct working-end of a universal curet on anterior and posterior teeth.

* Given a variety of universal curets to choose from and a task (location, depth, and size of calculus deposits), select the best instrument for the specified task.

* Explain why the lower shank of a universal curet should be tilted slightly toward the tooth surface being instrumented to obtain correct angulation.

* Using a universal curet, demonstrate correct adaptation and use of calculus removal strokes on the anterior teeth while maintaining correct position, correct finger rests, and precise finger placement in the grasp.

* Using a universal curet, demonstrate correct adaptation and use of calculus removal strokes on the posterior teeth while maintaining correct position, correct finger rests, and precise finger placement in the grasp.

* Using a universal curet, demonstrate horizontal calculus removal strokes at the distofacial line angles of posterior teeth and at the midlines on the facial and lingual surfaces of anterior teeth.

Section 1
Universal Curets

GENERAL DESIGN CHARACTERISTICS

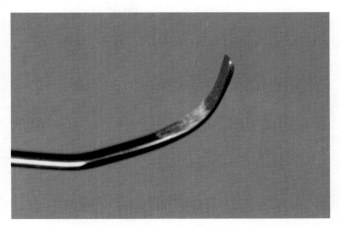

Figure 17-1. The working-end of a universal curet.

1. Functions of Universal Curets
   A. A universal curet is a periodontal instrument used to remove small and medium-sized calculus deposits (Figs. 17-1 and 17-2).
      1. Universal curets can be used both supragingivally and subgingivally—on crown and root surfaces.
      2. A universal curet usually is a double-ended instrument with paired, mirror image, working-ends.
   B. Universal curets are one of the most frequently used and versatile of all the calculus removal instruments. This type of curet is called "universal" because it can be applied to both anterior and posterior teeth. In other words, this type of curet is used universally throughout the entire mouth.
2. Design Characteristics. The working-end of a universal curet has several unique design characteristics. The design characteristics are summarized in Table 17-1.
   A. A rounded back
   B. A rounded toe
   C. A semicircular cross section
   D. Two cutting edges per working-end
   E. The face is at a 90-degree angle to the lower shank and as a result, the two cutting edges are level with one another.
3. Examples of Universal Curet Instruments. Some examples of universal curet instruments are the Columbia 4R/4 L; Columbia 13/14; Rule 3/4; Barnhart 1/2; Barnhart 5/6; Younger-Good 7/8; Indiana University 13/14; McCalls 13/14; Bunting 5/6; Mallery 1/2; Langer 1/2; Langer 3/4; Langer 5/6, and Langer 17/18.

WORKING-END DESIGN

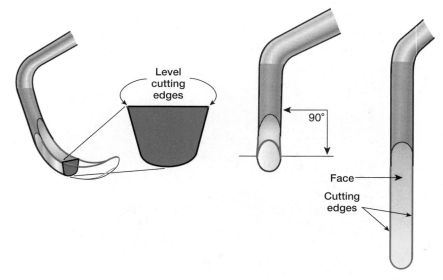

Figure 17-2. Design Characteristics of a Universal Curet.

TABLE 17-1. REFERENCE SHEET: UNIVERSAL CURET	
Cross Section	Semicircular cross section; this design allows the working-end to be used both supragingivally and subgingivally
Working-End	Rounded back and toe Two working cutting edges per working-end
Face	Face is at a 90-degree angle to the lower shank and as a result, the two cutting edges on a working-end are level with one another Since the face is perpendicular to the lower shank, **the lower shank must be tilted slightly toward the tooth surface to establish correct angulation**
Cutting Edges	Two **parallel cutting edges** meet in a rounded toe
Application	One double-ended instrument is used on both anterior and posterior teeth
Primary Functions	**Instrumentation of crown and root surfaces** Removal of small- to medium-sized calculus deposits

SELECTING A UNIVERSAL CURET FOR A PARTICULAR TASK

In selecting a universal curet for a particular calculus removal task, consider its design characteristics such as the curve of the working-end, length of the lower shank, and degree of bend in the shank. The photographs in Figures 17-3 to 17-5 compare two universal curets, demonstrating how the design characteristics of the lower shank impact instrument selection for a particular task.

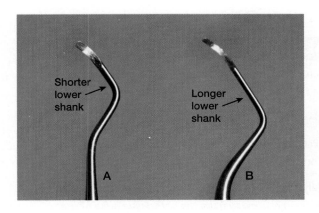

Figure 17-3. Two Universal Curet Designs.
- **Instrument A:** has a short lower shank and working-end
- **Instrument B:** has a long lower shank and working-end

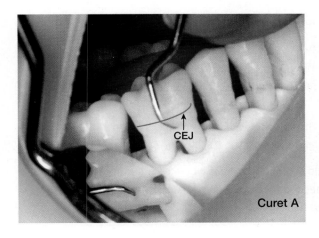

Figure 17-4. Shorter Lower Shank Length.
Instrument A is an excellent choice for removal of supragingival calculus removal and removal of deposits in normal sulci and shallow pockets. CEJ, cementoenamel junction.

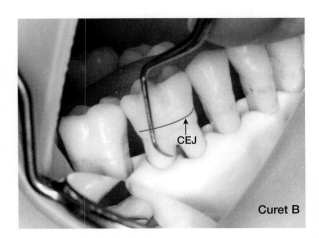

Figure 17-5. Longer Lower Shank Length.
Instrument B, with its longer lower shank, is an excellent choice of removal of deposits in deep pockets.

Section 2
Calculus Removal Concepts

CHARACTERISTICS OF THE CALCULUS REMOVAL STROKE

Before beginning the step-by-step technique practice with a universal curet, review the (1) characteristics of the calculus removal stroke and (2) steps for calculus removal. These concepts are summarized in Table 17-2 and in a flow chart format in Figure 17-6.

TABLE 17-2. THE CALCULUS REMOVAL STROKE WITH A UNIVERSAL CURET	
Stabilization	Apply pressure with the index finger and thumb inward against the instrument handle and press the tip of the fulcrum finger against the tooth surface
Adaptation	Toe-third of cutting edge is adapted to crown or root surface
Angulation	70 to 80 degrees; for universal curets the lower shank must be tilted slightly toward the tooth surface to achieve correct angulation
Lateral Pressure for Calculus Removal	Moderate to firm pressure against the tooth surface is maintained during the short, controlled calculus removal stroke made *away from the soft tissue base of the junctional epithelium*
Characteristics	Powerful controlled strokes, short in length
Stroke Direction	Vertical strokes are most commonly used on anterior teeth and on the mesial and distal surfaces of posterior teeth
	Oblique strokes are most commonly used on the facial and lingual surfaces of posterior teeth
	Horizontal strokes are used at the line angles of posterior teeth and the midlines of the facial or lingual surfaces of anterior teeth
Stroke Number	Calculus removal strokes should be limited to areas where calculus is present; use the minimum number of strokes needed to remove calculus deposits (fewer strokes = less stress to the muscles of the hand)

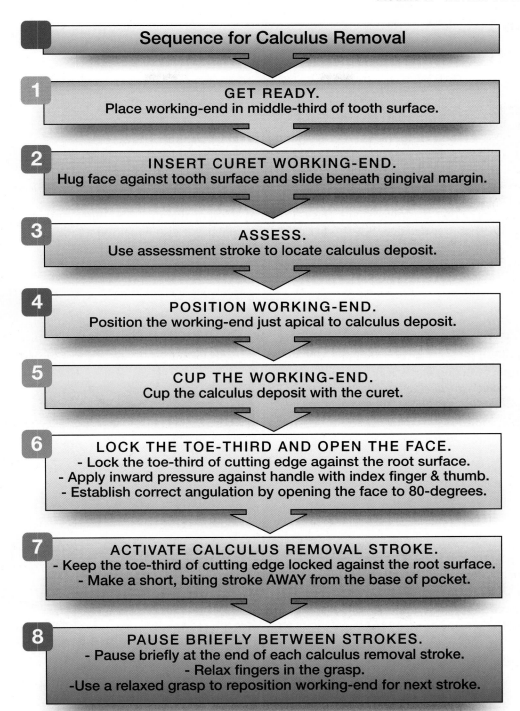

Sequence for Calculus Removal

1 GET READY.
Place working-end in middle-third of tooth surface.

2 INSERT CURET WORKING-END.
Hug face against tooth surface and slide beneath gingival margin.

3 ASSESS.
Use assessment stroke to locate calculus deposit.

4 POSITION WORKING-END.
Position the working-end just apical to calculus deposit.

5 CUP THE WORKING-END.
Cup the calculus deposit with the curet.

6 LOCK THE TOE-THIRD AND OPEN THE FACE.
- Lock the toe-third of cutting edge against the root surface.
- Apply inward pressure against handle with index finger & thumb.
- Establish correct angulation by opening the face to 80-degrees.

7 ACTIVATE CALCULUS REMOVAL STROKE.
- Keep the toe-third of cutting edge locked against the root surface.
- Make a short, biting stroke AWAY from the base of pocket.

8 PAUSE BRIEFLY BETWEEN STROKES.
- Pause briefly at the end of each calculus removal stroke.
- Relax fingers in the grasp.
-Use a relaxed grasp to reposition working-end for next stroke.

Figure 17-6. Flow Chart for Calculus Removal with a Universal Curet. This flow chart reviews the skills involved in the production of a subgingival calculus removal stroke. JE, junctional epithelium.

Section 3
Technique Practice—Posterior Teeth

SKILL BUILDING
Selecting the Correct Working-End for a Posterior Tooth

There are two methods for recognizing the correct working-end of a universal curet. The clinician may use either the lower shank (Figs. 17-7 and 17-8) or the inner and outer cutting edges (Fig. 17-9) as a visual clue. Box 17-1 provides a summary of visual method #1.

Method 1: The Lower Shank as a Visual Clue

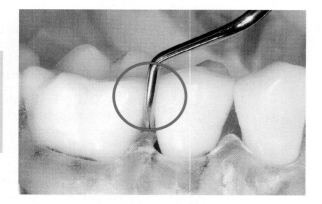

Figure 17-7. Visual Clue for the Correct Working-End.
- The correct working-end is selected when the *lower shank is parallel* to the distal surface
- The *functional shank goes "up and over the tooth."*

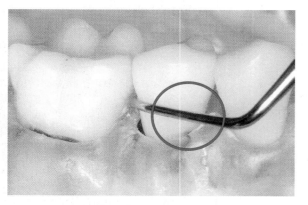

Figure 17-8. Visual Clue for the Incorrect Working-End.
- The incorrect working-end is selected if the *lower shank is not parallel*
- The *functional shank is "down and around the tooth."*

Box 17-1   The Lower Shank as a Visual Clue

When the working-end is adapted to a distal surface:
- Lower shank is parallel to the distal surface
- Functional shank goes up and over the tooth

Think: Posterior = Parallel. Functional shank up and over!

Method 2: The Inner and Outer Cutting Edges as a Visual Clue

There is a second method for recognizing the correct working-end of a universal curet. For this method, the cutting edges provide the visual clue. Box 17-2 provides a summary of visual method #2. It is not important whether a clinician uses Method 1 or Method 2 to select the working-end. Each clinician should use the method that is easiest for him or her.

The bends in the functional shank of a universal curet cause one of the cutting edges to be nearer to the handle than the other. Each working-end has two cutting edges, an inner and outer cutting edge (Fig. 17-9).

1. The outer cutting edge is the one that is *farther* from the instrument handle.
2. The inner cutting edge is the one that is *closer* to the instrument handle.

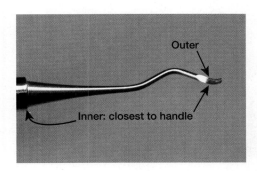

Figure 17-9. **Inner and Outer Cutting Edges.** To identify the cutting edges, hold the instrument *so that you are looking down on the face of the working-end*. One of the cutting edges will be nearer to the instrument handle than the other.

Box 17-2	The Inner and Outer Cutting Edges as a Visual Clue

- The ***inner cutting edges*** are used to instrument the ***distal surfaces***.
- The ***outer cutting edges*** are used to instrument the ***facial, lingual, and mesial surfaces***.

ESTABLISHING 70- TO 80-DEGREE ANGULATION

The relationship of a universal curet's face to the lower shank should be kept in mind when establishing correct angulation of the working-end to the tooth surface (Figs. 17-10 to 17-12).

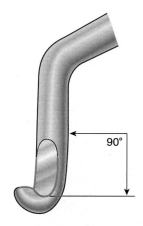

Figure 17-10. Relationship of the Face to the Lower Shank. In establishing correct angulation, it is important to remember that *on a universal curet the face of the working-end is at a 90-degree angle to the lower shank*.

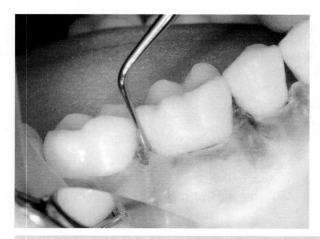
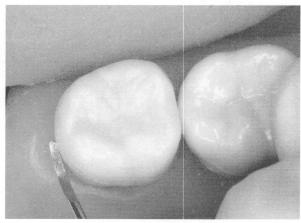

Figure 17-11. Incorrect angulation. Because the lower shank is at a 90-degree angle to face, *positioning the lower shank parallel to the tooth surface results in an angulation of 90-degrees.*

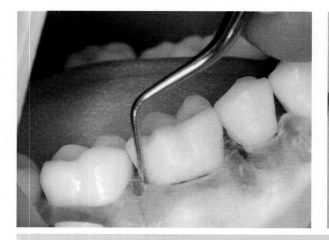
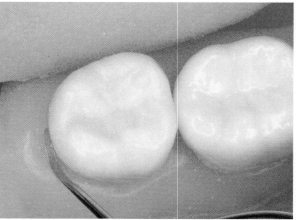

Figure 17-12. Correct angulation. Correct angulation is *achieved by tilting the lower shank slightly toward the tooth surface* to be instrumented. In this position the face-to-tooth surface angulation is between 70 and 80 degrees.

APPLICATION OF THE CUTTING EDGES TO THE POSTERIOR TEETH

All four cutting edges of a universal curet are used for calculus removal on the posterior sextants. Figures 17-13 and 17-14 depict application of the cutting edges to the mandibular right posterior sextant.

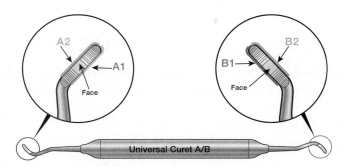

Figure 17-13. **Four Cutting Edges of a Universal Curet.** A universal curet has two working-ends. Working-end A has two cutting edges (A1 and A2). Working-end B has two cutting edges (B1 and B2).

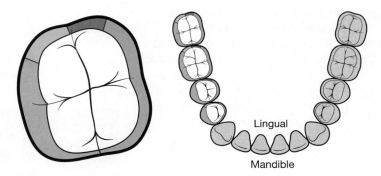

Figure 17-14. **Application of Cutting Edges to Posterior Surfaces.** These illustrations indicate how the cutting edges of a universal curet are applied to the tooth surfaces of the mandibular first molar and the mandibular right posterior sextant.

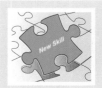

SKILL BUILDING
Step-By-Step Technique on Mandibular First Molar

- Follow steps 1 to 19—shown in Figures 17-15 to 17-33—to practice use of a universal curet on the mandibular right posterior sextant.
- *Use a periodontal typodont (1,2). Practice insertion with the gingiva in place, then remove the gingiva to practice making calculus removal strokes on the cervical thirds of the roots.*
- Remember: "Me, My patient, My light, My dominant hand, My nondominant hand, My finger rest, My adaptation."

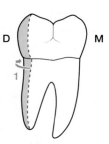

1. **Figure 17-15. Begin with Mandibular First Molar.** As an introduction to the universal curet, first practice on the *mandibular right first molar.* The distal surface is completed first, beginning at the distofacial line angle and working onto the distal surface.

2. **Figure 17-16. Get Ready.**
   - Turn the toe of the working-end toward the distal surface.
   - Place the working-end in the **Get Ready Zone** in the middle-third of the crown. In this case, the Get Ready Zone is at the distofacial line angle in the middle-third of the crown.

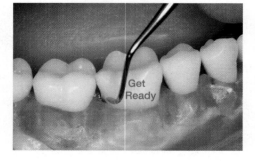

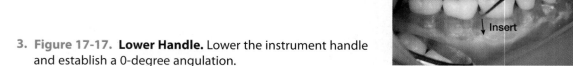

3. **Figure 17-17. Lower Handle.** Lower the instrument handle and establish a 0-degree angulation.

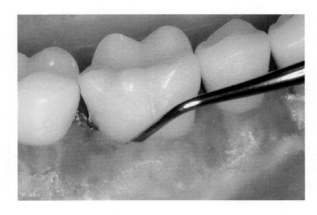

4. **Figure 17-18. Insert.** Gently slide the working-end beneath the gingival margin and onto the distal surface of the root.

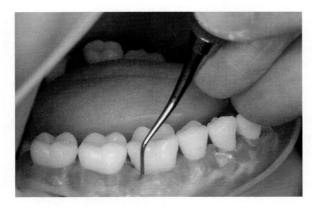

5. **Figure 17-19. Re-establish Handle Position.** Return handle to its normal upright position in preparation for initiation of calculus removal strokes.

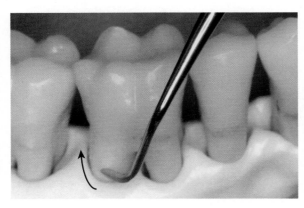

6. **Figure 17-20. Establish Angulation and Lock Toe-Third.**
   - Establish an 80-degree face-to-root surface angulation by tilting the lower shank slightly toward the distal surface.
   - Adapt the toe-third of the working-end to the distofacial line angle. Imagine "locking" the toe-third against the tooth surface.

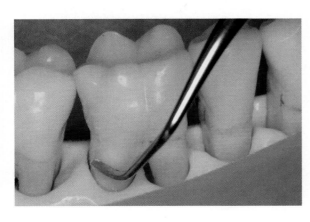

7. **Figure 17-21. Roll Handle.** Roll the instrument handle to maintain adaptation as strokes are made around the distofacial line angle.

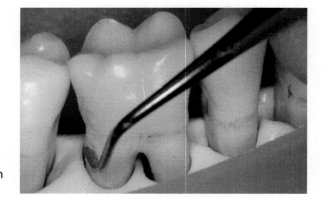

8. **Figure 17-22. Continue Strokes Across Distal Surface.** Continue making short, precise strokes on the distal surface.

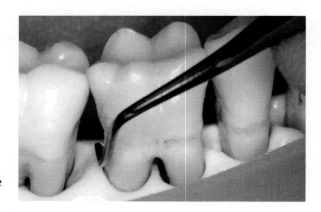

9. **Figure 17-23. Work Across the Distal Surface.** Work at least halfway across the distal surface from the facial aspect. The other half of the distal surface is instrumented from the lingual aspect.

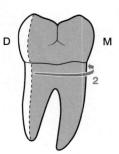

10. **Figure 17-24. Instrumentation of the Facial Surface.** Next, instrument the facial and mesial surfaces of the first molar, beginning at the distofacial line angle.

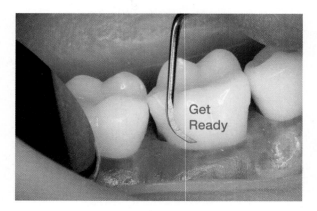

11. **Figure 17-25. Get Ready for Facial Surface.**
    - Turn the working-end so that the toe of the curet aims toward the front of the mouth.
    - Place the working-end in the Get Ready Zone on the middle-third of the facial surface near the line angle.

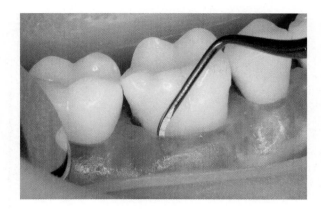

12. **Figure 17-26.** **Insert.**
    - Gently slide the working-end beneath the gingival margin.
    - Imagine the face sliding along the facial surface all the way to the base of the pocket.

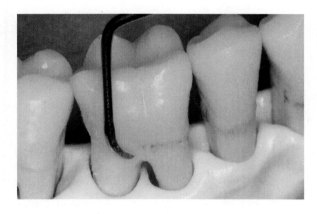

13. **Figure 17-27.** **Establish Angulation and Lock Toe-Third.**
    - Establish an 80-degree face-to-root surface angulation *by tilting the lower shank slightly toward the facial surface*.
    - Adapt the toe-third of the working-end to the distofacial line angle. *Imagine "locking" the toe-third against the tooth surface*.

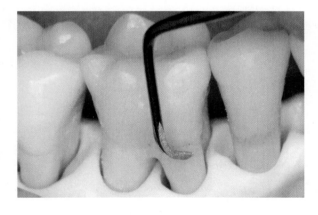

14. **Figure 17-28.** **Make Strokes Across the Facial Surface.** Initiate a series of short, precise strokes across the facial surface.

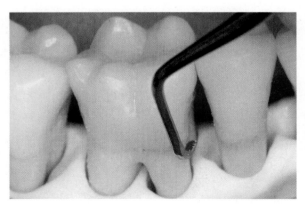

15. **Figure 17-29.** **Instrument the Facial surface.** Roll handle at line angle.
    - As you approach the mesiofacial line angle, roll the handle slightly to maintain adaptation.
    - Keep the toe-third "locked" against the tooth surface.

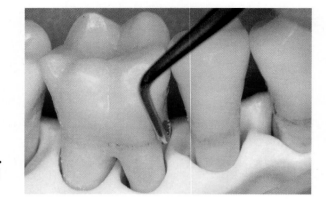

16. **Figure 17-30. Work Across the Mesial Surface.** Make a series of precise strokes across the mesial surface.

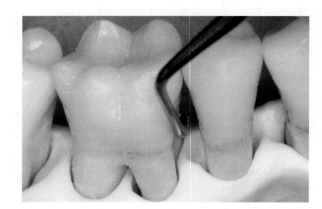

17. **Figure 17-31. Work to Midline of Mesial Surface.** Work at least halfway across the mesial surface from the facial aspect.

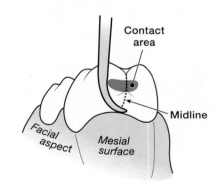

18. **Figure 17-32. Technique Check.** Make sure that your strokes extend past the midline of the mesial proximal surface.
    - Work at least halfway across the mesial surface from the facial aspect while maintaining proper angulation.
    - The other half of the mesial surface will be instrumented from the lingual aspect.

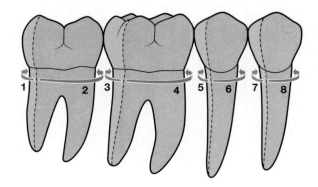

19. **Figure 17-33. Sequence for Sextant.** Next, use the sequence shown in this illustration to instrument the facial aspect of the entire sextant, beginning with the posterior-most molar. This sequence allows you to instrument the sextant in an efficient manner.

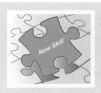

SKILL BUILDING
Step-By-Step Technique on Maxillary First Molar

- Follow steps 1 to 6—shown in Figures 17-34 to 17-39—to practice use of a universal curet on the maxillary right posterior sextant.
- Use a periodontal typodont (1,2). Practice insertion with the gingiva in place, then remove the gingiva to practice making calculus removal strokes on the cervical thirds of the roots.
- Remember: "Me, My patient, My light, My dominant hand, My nondominant hand, My finger rest, My adaptation."

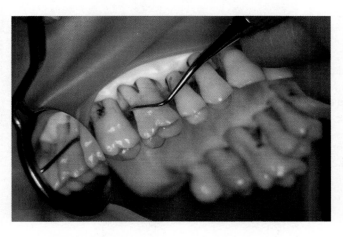

1. **Figure 17-34. Get Ready and Insert.**
   - Turn the toe toward the distal surface. Position the working-end in the Get Ready Zone.
   - Raise the instrument handle and establish a 0-degree angulation.
   - Gently slide the working-end beneath the gingival margin.

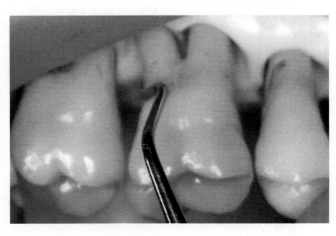

2. **Figure 17-35. Establish Angulation and Lock-Toe Third.**
   - Establish an 80-degree angulation.
   - Adapt the toe-third of the working-end to the distofacial line angle. Imagine "locking" the toe-third against the tooth surface.

3. Figure 17-36. **Instrument the Distal Surface.**
Instrument from the distofacial line angle to the midline of the distal surface.

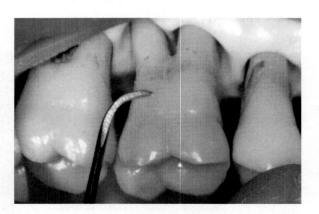

4. Figure 17-37. **Get Ready for Facial Surface.**
   - Turn the working-end so the toe aims toward the front of the mouth.
   - Place the working-end in the Get Ready Zone on the middle-third of the facial surface near the distofacial line angle.
   - Gently slide the working-end beneath the gingival margin all the way to the base of the pocket.

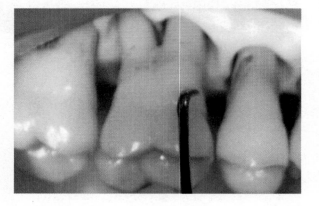

5. Figure 17-38. **Instrument the Facial Surface.**
   - Work across the facial surface.
   - As you approach the mesiofacial line angle, roll the handle slightly to maintain adaptation.

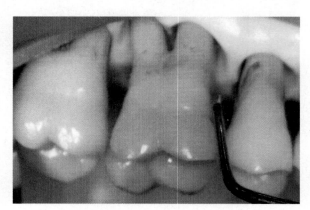

6. Figure 17-39. **Instrument the Distal Surface.**
Work from the mesiofacial line angle to the midline of the mesial surface.

Section 4
Technique Alert—Lower Shank Position

Adapting the working-end to the facial and lingual root surfaces of the mandibular posterior teeth is challenging for two reasons: (1) the clinician's hand position may block the view of the mandibular lingual surfaces and (2) the rounded posterior crowns (Fig. 17-40) make it difficult to instrument the root surfaces of these teeth. Figures 17-41 and 17-42 depict incorrect technique. Figures 17-43 and 14-44 depict correct shank alignment to root surface.

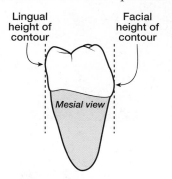

Lingual height of contour   Facial height of contour

Mesial view

Figure 17-40. Height of Contour on Molars. *This illustration shows a side view of a molar, looking at the mesial surface.* Note that the crown protrudes over—overhangs—the root surface.

INCORRECT TECHNIQUE

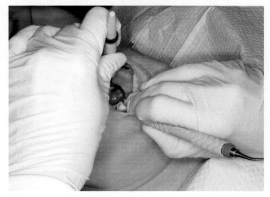

Figure 17-41. Incorrect Handle Position. Inexperienced clinicians often will tilt the instrument handle down in an attempt to obtain a better view of the mandibular lingual surfaces. Note that the clinician's ring finger is "collapsed" and not acting as a support beam for the hand.

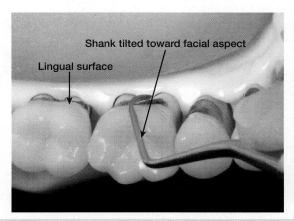

Shank tilted toward facial aspect

Lingual surface

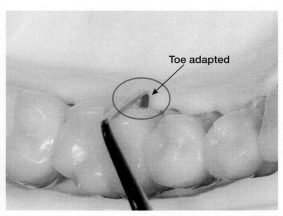

Toe adapted

Figure 17-42. Incorrect Technique: Handle Tilted Toward Clinician. Tilting the instrument handle toward the clinician causes the lower shank to hit the crown of the tooth. In this position it is not possible to adapt the working-end to the root surface since the root is smaller in diameter than the crown. The lower shank simply rocks against the occlusal surface of the crown causing the working-end to lift off of the root surface without engaging the calculus deposit.

CORRECT TECHNIQUE

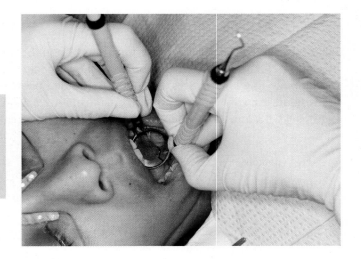

Figure 17-43. Correct Handle Position. When working on the lingual surfaces, keep the handle in the normal position and use the mirror for indirect vision. Note that the clinician's ring finger is upright and supporting the hand in the grasp.

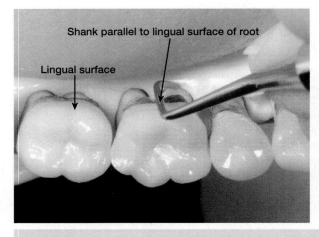

Shank parallel to lingual surface of root

Lingual surface

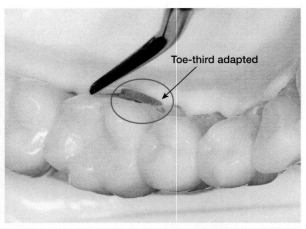

Toe-third adapted

Figure 17-44. Correct Technique Produces an Unimpeded Stroke.
- With the handle in the correct position, the lower shank is not in contact with either the lingual or occlusal surfaces of the tooth crown.
- In this position is it easy to make oblique or vertical instrumentation strokes upward along the root surface without rocking against the occlusal surface of the crown.

Section 5
Technique Practice—Anterior Teeth

Adapting a universal curet to the anterior teeth requires a technique that is different from that used with other instruments. For this reason, some clinicians prefer not to use universal curets on the anterior sextants. The complex shank design of the universal curet, however, sometimes facilitates access to the lingual root surfaces of the mandibular anterior teeth. Additionally, it is efficient to use a single instrument for both the anterior and posterior teeth.

SKILL BUILDING
Selecting the Correct Working-End for an Anterior Tooth

Method 1: Lower Shank as a Visual Clue
The first method uses the lower shank as a visual clue. The visual clue for the correct working-end is shown in the drawing and photo in Figure 17-45. The visual clue for the incorrect working-end is shown in the drawing and photo in Figure 17-46.

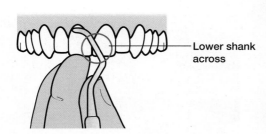

Lower shank across

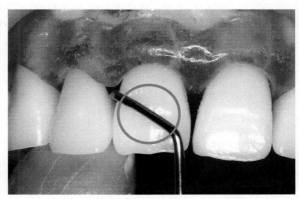

Figure 17-45. Lower Shank as Visual Clue: Correct Working-End.
- When using a universal curet on anterior teeth, the correct working-end is selected if the **lower shank is across the tooth surface**.
- *Think: "Universal curet = anterior across."*

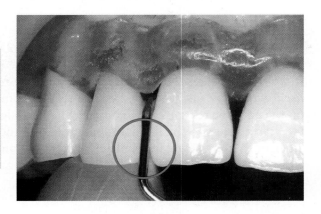

Figure 17-46. Lower Shank as a Visual Clue: Incorrect Working-End.
- This photo shows the **incorrect** working-end of a universal curet adapted to the distal surface of the central incisor.
- In this position, the cutting edge is not correctly adapted to the tooth surface.

Method 2: The Inner and Outer Cutting Edges as a Visual Clue

There is a second method for selecting the correct working-end of a universal curet. For this method, the cutting edges provide the visual clue (Fig. 17-47). Box 17-3 provides a summary of visual method #2. It is not important whether a clinician uses Method 1 or Method 2 to select the working-end. Each clinician should use the method that is easiest for him or her.

The bends in the functional shank of a universal curet cause one of the cutting edges to be nearer the handle than the other. Each working-end has two cutting edges, an inner and an outer cutting edge.

- The **outer cutting edge** is the one that is *farther from the instrument handle.*
- *Only the outer cutting edges—the edges farthest from the handle—are used to instrument the anterior teeth.*

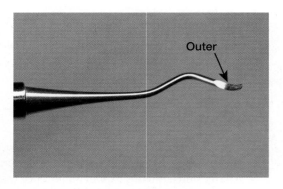

Outer

Figure 17-47. Outer Cutting Edge.
- To identify the outer cutting edge, hold the instrument so that you are looking down at the face of the working-end.
- *Only the outer cutting edges are used to instrument the anterior teeth.*

Box 17-3 **Outer Cutting Edge as Visual Clue**

When using a universal curet on anterior teeth, only the ***outer cutting edges*** are used.

APPLICATION OF THE CUTTING EDGES TO THE ANTERIOR TEETH

Only one cutting edge per working-end (Fig. 17-48) is used on the anterior sextants when working with a universal curet. The visual clues for the correct working-end are (1) the lower shank goes across the tooth surface and (2) only the outer cutting edge is used (Fig. 17-49).

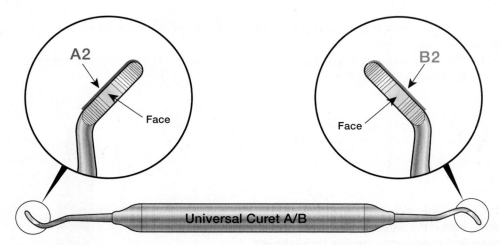

Figure 17-48. Cutting Edges. On a universal curet, *only one cutting edge per working-end is used on anterior tooth surfaces*.

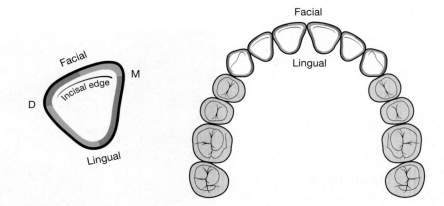

Figure 17-49. Application to Anterior Surfaces. The illustration indicates how the working-ends of a universal curet are applied to the anterior tooth surfaces. *For each aspect, one working-end is used on the surfaces toward the clinician and the opposite working-end is used on the surfaces away from the clinician.*

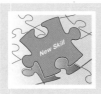

SKILL BUILDING
Step-By-Step Technique on a Maxillary Central Incisor

- Follow steps 1 to 8—shown in Figures 17-50 to 17-57—to practice use of a universal curet on the maxillary anterior teeth.
- Remember: "Me, My patient, My light, My dominant hand, My nondominant hand, My finger rest, My adaptation."

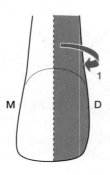

1. **Figure 17-50. Tooth.** As an introduction to using a universal curet on the anterior teeth, first practice on the *maxillary right central incisor, facial aspect*. **Right-handed clinicians**—*surface away*. **Left-handed clinicians**—*surface toward*.

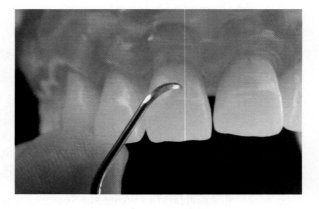

2. **Figure 17-51. Get Ready and Insert.** Select the correct working-end and place it in the Get Ready Zone.

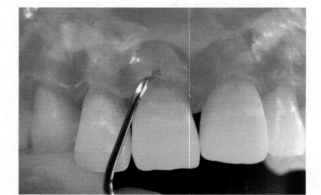

3. **Figure 17-52. Insert.** Insert the working-end to the base of the pocket.

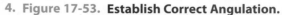

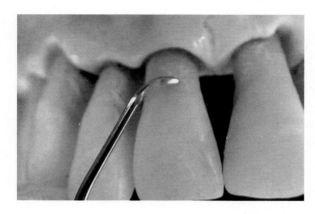

4. **Figure 17-53. Establish Correct Angulation.**
   - Adapt the toe-third to the root surface. Imagine "locking" the toe-third against the root surface.
   - Instrument from the midline of the facial surface toward the mesial surface.

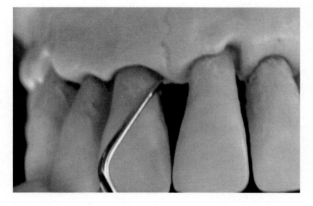

5. **Figure 17-54. Roll Handle at Line Angle.** Roll the handle slightly to maintain adaptation of the toe-third to the line angle.

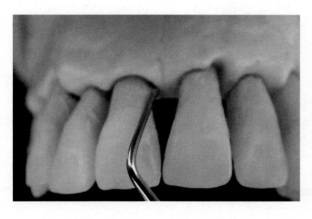

6. **Figure 17-55. Mesial Surface.** Work at least halfway across the mesial surface. The other half of the mesial surface will be instrumented from the lingual aspect of the tooth.

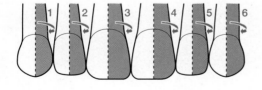

7. **Figure 17-56. Sequence.** Use the sequence shown in this illustration to instrument the colored tooth surfaces of the facial aspect. Begin with the left canine and end with the right canine.

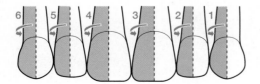

8. **Figure 17-57. Sequence.** Complete the remaining facial surfaces, beginning with the right canine and ending with the left canine.

Section 6
Technique Alert—Horizontal Strokes

- Novice clinicians often fail to remove calculus deposits that are located:
  - Near the distofacial or distolingual line angles of posterior root surfaces
  - At the midlines of the facial and lingual surfaces of anterior root surfaces
- Horizontal calculus removal strokes are extremely useful for calculus removal in these areas.

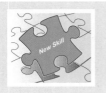

SKILL BUILDING
Horizontal Strokes Below the Gingival Margin

Directions: Follow the directions below to practice making horizontal calculus removal strokes at the distofacial line angle of the mandibular first molar (Figs. 17-58 and 17-59).

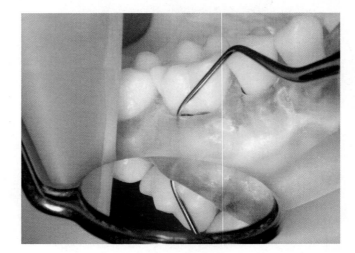

Figure 17-58. Establish Handle Position.
Insert the curet slightly distal to the distofacial line angle. Lower the instrument handle until the curet working-end is oriented with the toe toward—but not touching—the base of the sulcus or pocket.

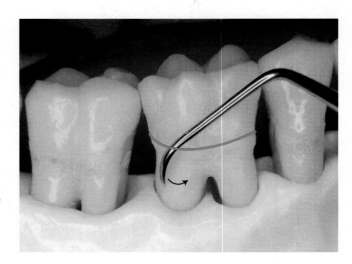

Figure 17-59. Make Several Horizontal Strokes. Begin a calculus removal stroke slightly distal to the distofacial line angle. Make several short, controlled strokes around the distofacial line angle.

Directions: Follow the directions below to practice making horizontal strokes at the midline of the facial surface of a central incisor (Figs. 17-60 and 17-61).

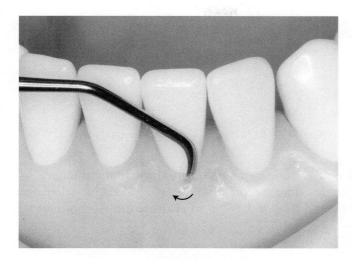

Figure 17-60. **Horizontal Strokes on Facial Surface.** Insert the working-end just distal to the midline. Lower the handle until the curet toe is toward—but not touching—the base of the sulcus. Make several short, controlled horizontal strokes across the midline of the facial surface.

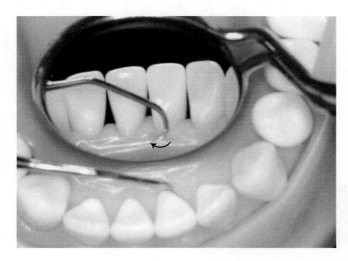

Figure 17-61. **Horizontal Strokes on Lingual Surface.** Lower the handle until the curet toe is toward—but not touching—the base of the sulcus. Make several short, controlled horizontal strokes across the midline of the lingual surface.

Section 7
Skill Application

PRACTICAL FOCUS

Imagine that you have been assigned to observe a second year student, Ling, as she performs periodontal debridement on a patient.

- The photographs in Figures 17-62 to 17-66 are characteristic of Ling's instrumentation technique. What feedback could you give to Ling about her instrumentation technique and instrument selection?
- Hint: use the probing depths indicated in Figures 17-62 and 17-63 to evaluate Ling's choice of instruments for the task.

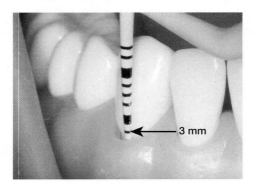

Figure 17-62. Color Coded Probe.

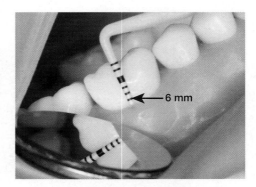

Figure 17-63. Color Coded Probe.

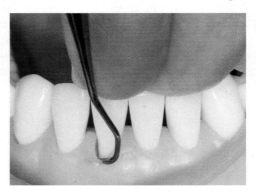

Figure 17-64. Sickle Scaler.

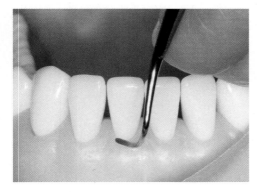

Figure 17-65. Universal Curet.

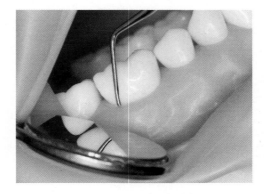

Figure 17-66. Universal Curet.

REFERENCE SHEET—UNIVERSAL CURETS

Use of Universal Curets:

A universal curet is a periodontal instrument used to remove light and medium calculus deposits from the crowns and roots of the teeth.

Basic Concepts:

1. Tilt the lower shank slightly toward the tooth surface to establish correct face-to-tooth surface angulation.
2. Insert the working-end beneath the gingival margin at a 0-to-40-degree angulation.
3. Maintain adaptation of the toe-third of the cutting edge to the tooth surface.
4. Activate the calculus removal stroke away from the junctional epithelium using wrist motion activation.
5. Relax your fingers between each calculus removal stroke.

Anterior Teeth:

1. Select the correct working-end:
   - Method 1: When adapted on a proximal surface, the lower shank goes across the tooth *(Anterior = Across)*.
   - Method 2: Only the outer cutting edges are used to instrument the anterior teeth.
2. Sequence: Begin with the surfaces toward your nondominant hand. Start on the canine on opposite side of the mouth and work toward yourself. (Right-handed clinicians start with the left canine, mesial surface; Left-handed clinicians start with the right canine, mesial surface).

Posterior Teeth:

1. Select the correct working-end:
   - Method 1: The lower shank is parallel to the tooth surface *(Posterior = Parallel. Functional shank up and over!)*
   - Method 2: The inner cutting edges are used on the distal surfaces. The outer cutting edges are used on the facial, lingual, and mesial surfaces.
2. Sequence: Begin at the distofacial line angle of the posterior-most tooth in the sextant and work toward the distal surface. Reposition at the distofacial line angle and complete the facial (or lingual) and mesial surfaces of the tooth, working toward the front of the mouth.

References

1. Dufour LA, Bissell HS. Periodontal attachment loss induced by mechanical subgingival instrumentation in shallow sulci. *J Dent Hyg.* 2002;76(3):207–212. PubMed PMID: 12271866.
2. Ruhling A, Konig J, Rolf H, Kocher T, Schwahn C, Plagmann HC. Learning root debridement with curettes and power-driven instruments. Part II: Clinical results following mechanical, nonsurgical therapy. *J Clin Periodontol.* 2003;30(7):611–615. PubMed PMID: 12834498.

Student Self Evaluation Module 17: Universal Curets

Student: _____   Date: _____

DIRECTIONS: Self-evaluate your skill level in each treatment area as: **S** (satisfactory) or **U** (unsatisfactory).

Criteria				
Positioning/Ergonomics	**Area 1**	**Area 2**	**Area 3**	**Area 4**
Adjusts clinician and patient chairs and equipment correctly				
Assumes the recommended clock position				
Instrument Grasp: Dominant Hand	**Area 1**	**Area 2**	**Area 3**	**Area 4**
Grasps handle with tips of finger pads of index finger and thumb				
Rests pad of middle finger lightly on instrument shank				
Positions the thumb, index, and middle fingers in the "knuckles up" convex position; hyper-extended joint position is avoided				
Finger Rest: Dominant Hand				
Establishes secure finger rest that is appropriate for tooth to be treated				
Once finger rest is established, pauses to self-evaluate finger placement in the grasp, verbalizes to evaluator his/her self-assessment of grasp, and corrects finger placement if necessary				
Prepare for Instrumentation ("Get Ready")				
Selects correct working-end for tooth surface to be instrumented				
Places the working-end in the "Get Ready Zone" while using a correct finger rest for the treatment area				
Insertion	**Area 1**	**Area 2**	**Area 3**	**Area 4**
Establishes 0-degree angulation (face hugs tooth surface) in preparation for insertion				
Gently inserts curet toe beneath the gingival margin to base of sulcus or pocket				
Adaptation, Angulation, and Instrument Stroke	**Area 1**	**Area 2**	**Area 3**	**Area 4**
Assesses the root surface with curet using light, sweeping assessment strokes away from the junctional epithelium				
Initiates a stroke in a coronal direction by positioning the working-end beneath a calculus deposit, "locking the toe" against tooth surface and using an angulation between 45 and 80 degrees				
Uses rotating motion to make a short, biting stroke in a coronal direction to snap a deposit from the tooth; does NOT close face toward tooth surface during activation; uses whole hand as a unit, does NOT pull with thumb and index finger				
Maintains appropriate lateral pressure against the tooth throughout the stroke while maintaining control of the working-end				
Precisely stops each individual stroke and pauses briefly (at least 3 seconds) to relax grasp before repositioning working-end beneath calculus deposit; strokes should be short and working-end remains beneath the gingival margin (to avoid trauma to gingival margin): does NOT remove working-end from the pocket with each stroke				
Maintains neutral wrist position throughout motion activation				
Maintains correct adaptation as instrument strokes progress around tooth surface; pivots and rolls instrument handle as needed				
Thoroughly instruments proximal surface under each contact area				
Uses appropriate sequence for the specified sextant				
Keeps hands steady and controlled during instrumentation so that working-end moves with precision, regardless of nervousness				
Demonstrates horizontal strokes at the midlines of anterior teeth and the line angles of posterior teeth				
Ethics and Professionalism				
Punctuality, appearance, demeanor, attitude, composure, honesty				

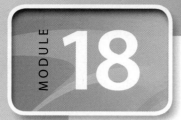

MODULE

18

Advanced Probing Techniques

Module Overview

The comprehensive periodontal assessment is one of the most important functions performed by dental hygienists. This module begins with a review of the periodontal attachment system in health and attachment loss in disease. Other module sections describe techniques for advanced assessments with periodontal probes including: (1) bleeding on gentle probing, (2) level of the free gingival margin, (3) oral deviations, (4) tooth mobility, (5) furcation involvement, (6) clinical attachment levels, and (7) width of the attached gingiva.

Module Outline

Section 1   **The Periodontal Attachment System**   **417**
Attachment in Health
Loss of Attachment in Disease
Alveolar Bone Support in Health and Disease

Section 2   **Assessments with Calibrated Probes**   **420**
Comprehensive Periodontal Assessment
Measuring Oral Deviations
Assessing Tooth Mobility
Assessing Bleeding on Probing
Determining the Level of the Free Gingival Margin

Section 3   **Assessments that Require Calculations**   **427**
Clinical Attachment Levels
Calculating Clinical Attachment Levels
Documenting Clinical Attachment Levels
Calculating the Width of the Attached Gingiva

Section 4   **Assessments with Furcation Probes**   **432**
Furcation Involvement
Review of Root Furcation Morphology
Radiographic Evidence of Furcation Involvement
Design Characteristics of Furcation Probes
Working-End Selection: Nabers Probes
Skill Building. Technique Practice with Furcation Probes, p. 438
Four Classifications of Furcation Involvement
Documentation of Furcation Involvement

Practical Focus: Calculation of Clinical Loss of Attachment
Practical Focus: Fictitious Patient Case Mr. Temple
Practical Focus: Fictitious Patient Case Mrs. Blanchard
Skill Evaluation Module 18: Advanced Probing Techniques

Key Terms

Periodontal attachment system
Junctional epithelium
Fibers of the gingiva
Periodontal ligament fibers
Alveolar bone
Loss of attachment
Comprehensive periodontal assessment

Mobility
Horizontal tooth mobility
Vertical tooth mobility
Mobility-rating scales
Clinical attachment level
Clinical attachment loss
Attached gingiva
Bifurcation

Trifurcation
Furcation area
Furcation involvement
Furcation arrows
Furcation probe

Learning Objectives

- Discuss the uses of calibrated and furcation probes in performing a periodontal assessment.

- Describe the rationale for assessing tooth mobility.

- Demonstrate the technique for assessing tooth mobility and use a mobility rating scale to classify the extent of mobility.

- Describe the rationale and technique for determining the level of the gingival margin.

- Describe the consequences of loss of attachment to the tooth.

- Given the probing depth measurements and gingival margin levels for a tooth, compute the clinical attachment loss.

- Describe the rationale for furcation detection.

- Demonstrate correct technique for use of a furcation probe on a periodontal typodont and classify furcation involvement according to severity.

- Use advanced probing techniques to accurately assess a student partner's periodontium.

- For simulated patient cases, use periodontal measurements to differentiate a healthy periodontium from periodontitis and record these findings on a periodontal chart.

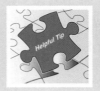

The Skill Application section of this module includes two fictitious patient cases for analysis and practice in calculation of clinical attachment levels. Additional fictitious patient cases and practice opportunities in calculating clinical attachment levels are found in Module 22, Fictitious Patient Cases.

Section 1
The Periodontal Attachment System

ATTACHMENT IN HEALTH

The periodontal attachment system is a group of structures that work together to attach the teeth to the maxilla and mandible (Fig. 18-1). To remain in the oral cavity, each tooth must be attached by:

1. Junctional epithelium—the epithelium that attaches the gingiva to the tooth.
2. Fibers of the gingiva—a network of fibers that brace the free gingiva against the tooth and unite the free gingiva with the tooth root and alveolar bone.
3. Periodontal ligament fibers—the fibers that surround the root of the tooth. These fibers attach to the bone of the socket on one side and to the cementum of the root on the other side.
4. Alveolar bone—the bone that surrounds the roots of the teeth. It forms the bony sockets that support and protect the roots of the teeth.

LOSS OF ATTACHMENT IN DISEASE

Loss of attachment is damage to the structures that support the tooth. Loss of attachment occurs in periodontitis and is characterized by (1) relocation of the junctional epithelium to the tooth root, (2) destruction of the fibers of the gingiva, (3) destruction of the periodontal ligament fibers, and (4) loss of alveolar bone support from around the tooth. The changes that occur in the alveolar bone in periodontal disease are significant because loss of bone height eventually can result in tooth loss. Table 18-1 summarizes the status of the attachment structures in health versus that of disease. Figures 18-2 to 18-5 depict the changes in the level of the alveolar bone and gingival margin in health and disease.

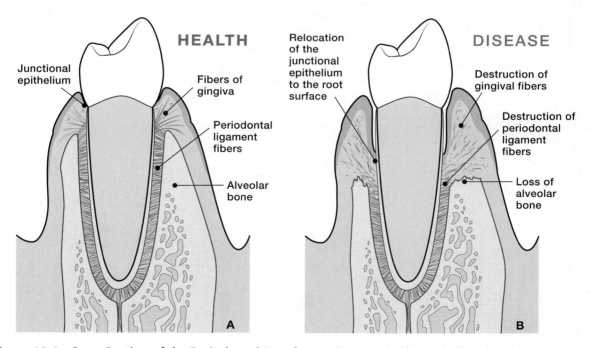

Figure 18-1. Cross Section of the Periodontal Attachment System. A: The periodontal attachment system in health. **B:** Destruction of the periodontal attachment system in disease.

TABLE 18-1. ATTACHMENT STRUCTURES IN HEALTH AND DISEASE

Attachment in Health	Attachment in Disease
Junctional epithelium attaches to enamel at base of sulcus	Junctional epithelium attaches to cementum at base of periodontal pocket
Fibers brace the tissue against the crown	Fiber destruction, tissue lacks firmness
Many fibers attach root to bone of socket	Fewer fibers remain to hold tooth in socket
Most of the root is surrounded by bone; the tooth is firmly held in its socket.	Part of the root is surrounded by bone; the tooth may be movable in its socket

ALVEOLAR BONE SUPPORT IN HEALTH AND DISEASE

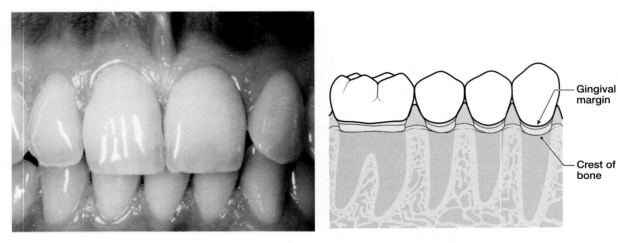

Figure 18-2. Bone Support in Health. In health, most of root is surrounded by bone. The crest of the alveolar bone is located very close to the crowns, only 1 to 2 mm apical to (below) the CEJs of the teeth.

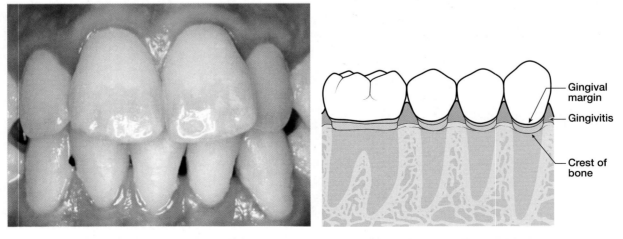

Figure 18-3. Bone Support in Gingivitis. In gingival disease, there is no loss of alveolar bone and the crest of the alveolar bone remains only 1 to 2 mm apical to (below) the CEJs of the teeth.

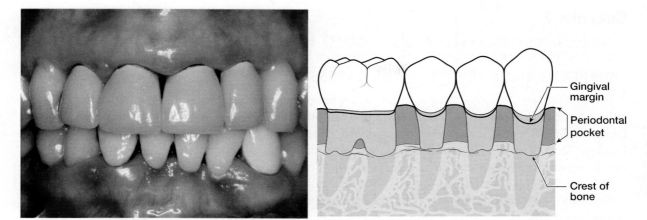

Figure 18-4. Bone Loss and Pocket Formation in Periodontitis. In periodontitis, bone is destroyed and the teeth are not well supported in the arch. In this example of bone loss, the gingival margin has remained near the CEJ creating deep periodontal pockets. Note that the tissues in the photograph are very swollen (edema) due to inflammation.

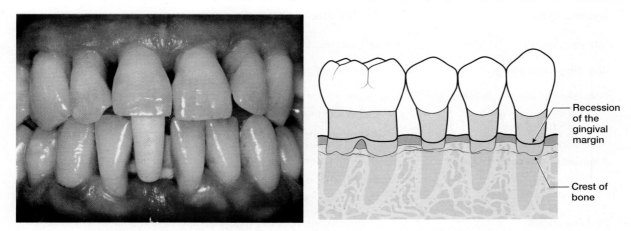

Figure 18-5. Loss of Bone and Recession of the Gingival Margin in Periodontitis. In this example of periodontitis, the gingival margin has receded and the tooth roots are visible in the mouth. Note that the probing depth is less in this example, however, the alveolar bone is at the same level. Only the level of the gingival margin differs between Figures 18-4 and 18-5. The tissues in this photograph are fibrotic, an indication of chronic inflammation of the tissues.

Section 2
Assessments with Calibrated Probes

COMPREHENSIVE PERIODONTAL ASSESSMENT

A comprehensive periodontal assessment is an intensive clinical periodontal evaluation used to gather information about the periodontium. The comprehensive periodontal assessment normally includes clinical features such as probing depth measurements, bleeding on probing, presence of exudate, level of the free gingival margin and the mucogingival junction, tooth mobility, furcation involvement, presence of calculus, and plaque biofilm, gingival inflammation, radiographic evidence of alveolar bone loss, and presence of local contributing factors (1,2). *Much of the information collected during the comprehensive periodontal assessment involves the use of periodontal probes.* Table 18-2 summarizes the role of periodontal probes in the comprehensive periodontal assessment.

TABLE 18-2. USES OF PERIODONTAL PROBES IN THE COMPREHENSIVE PERIODONTAL ASSESSMENT

Assessment	Technique
Intraoral lesions	Measurement of the size of pathologic lesions
Bleeding on probing	Bleeding on gentle probing indicates gingival inflammation
Recession of the gingival margin	Measurement from the free gingival margin to the cementoenamel junction A clinical indicator of loss of attachment
Amount of attached gingiva	Determination of the width of the attached gingiva (the part of the gingiva that is tightly connected to the cementum on the cervical-third of the root and to the periosteum of the alveolar bone).
Probing depth	Measurement from free marginal gingiva to the base of the sulcus or periodontal pocket; deepest reading is recorded for each of six zones per tooth (distofacial, facial, mesiofacial, distolingual, lingual, mesiolingual)
Clinical attachment level	Measurement from the cementoenamel junction to the base of the sulcus or periodontal pocket Measuring from a fixed point—the CEJ—more accurately reflects the true extent of the bone support, especially when recession of the free gingival margin is present
Distance between teeth	Measurement of distances between teeth or migration of teeth with severe periodontal disease
Furcation involvement	Detection of bone loss between the roots of multirooted teeth A specialized curved furcation probe—the Nabers probe—is used to detect furcation involvement

MEASURING ORAL DEVIATIONS

A calibrated probe is used to determine the size of an intraoral lesion or deviation. Figures 18-6 to 18-8 depict the use of a periodontal probe to determine the size of pathologic intraoral lesions.

- When an oral lesion is observed in a patient's mouth, this finding should be recorded in the patient's chart. Information recorded should include the (1) date, (2) size, (3) location, (4) color, and (5) character of the lesion, as well as, (6) any information provided by the patient (e.g., duration, sensation, or oral habits).
- For example: "*January 12, 2015: a soft, red, papillary lesion located on the buccal mucosa opposite the maxillary left first premolar, measuring 5 mm in an anterior–posterior direction and 6 mm in a superior–inferior direction. Patient states that she was unaware of the lesion.*"
- It is best to use anatomic references, rather than "length" or "width," to document your measurements on the chart (e.g., as the anterior–posterior measurement and the superior–inferior measurement).

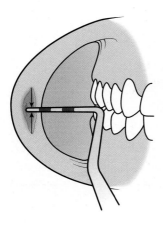

Figure 18-6. Determining Dimensions of a Lesion. Use a periodontal probe to determine the dimensions of the lesion (e.g., the anterior–posterior measurement and the superior–inferior measurement).

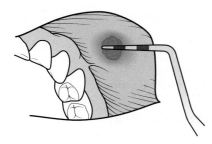

Figure 18-7. Determining the Height of a Raised Lesion. Place the probe tip on normal tissue alongside of the deviation. Imagine a line at the highest part of the deviation, and record this measurement as the height.

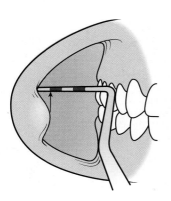

Figure 18-8. Determining the Depth of a Sunken Lesion. Carefully place the probe tip in the deepest part. Imagine a line running from edge to edge of the deviation. The depth is the distance from this imaginary line to the base of the deviation.

ASSESSING TOOTH MOBILITY

Mobility is the loosening of a tooth in its socket. Mobility may result from loss of bone support around the tooth. Most periodontal charts include boxes for documenting tooth mobility.

1. Horizontal tooth mobility is the ability to move the tooth in a facial to lingual direction in its socket.
   A. Horizontal tooth mobility is assessed by putting the handles of two dental instruments on either side of the tooth and applying alternating moderate pressure in the facial–lingual direction against the tooth, first with one, than the other instrument handle (Figs. 18-9 and 18-10). Clinicians often pair the blunt handles of a probe and a mirror to test for mobility.
   B. Mobility can be observed by using an adjacent tooth as a stationary point of reference during attempts to move the tooth being examined.
2. Vertical tooth mobility—the ability to depress the tooth in its socket—is assessed using the end of an instrument handle to exert pressure against the occlusal or incisal surface of the tooth (Fig. 18-11).
3. Even though the periodontal ligament allows some slight movement of the tooth in its socket, the amount of this natural tooth movement is so slight that it cannot be seen with the naked eye. Thus, when visually assessing mobility, the clinician should expect to find no visible movement in a periodontally healthy tooth. Note that all teeth have a normal physiological tooth movement of 0.5 mm due to the periodontal ligament. This normal movement is not recorded on the chart.
4. There are many mobility-rating scales for recording clinical visible tooth mobility on a periodontal chart. One useful rating scale is indicated in Table 18-3.

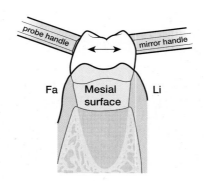

Figure 18-9. Assessing Horizontal Tooth Mobility. Horizontal tooth mobility is assessed by putting the handles of two dental instruments on either side of the tooth and applying alternating moderate pressure in the facial–lingual direction against the tooth, first with one, than the other instrument handle.

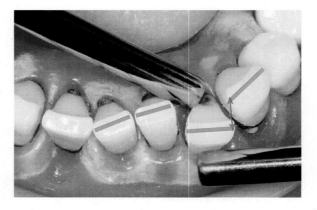

Figure 18-10. Observing Horizontal Tooth Mobility. Mobility can be observed by using an adjacent tooth as a stationary point of reference during attempts to move the tooth being examined.

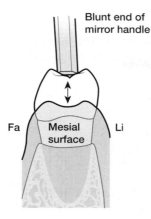

Blunt end of
mirror handle

Fa   Mesial
surface   Li

Figure 18-11. Assessing Vertical Tooth Mobility.
Use the end of an instrument handle to exert pressure against the occlusal surface or incisal edge of the tooth.

TABLE 18-3. A SCALE FOR RATING VISIBLE TOOTH MOBILITY	
Classification	**Description**
Class I	Slight mobility, up to 1 mm of horizontal displacement in a facial–lingual direction (Due to the periodontal ligament, all teeth have a slight physiological movement of less than 1 mm)
Class 2	Moderate mobility, greater than 1 mm but less than 2 mm of horizontal displacement in a facial–lingual direction
Class 3	Severe mobility, greater than 2 mm of displacement in a facial–lingual direction or vertical displacement (tooth depressible in the socket)

ASSESSING BLEEDING ON PROBING

- Bleeding on gentle probing represents bleeding from the soft tissue wall of a periodontal pocket where the wall of the pocket is ulcerated (i.e., where portions of the epithelium have been destroyed). Bleeding on gentle probing is a clinical sign of gingival inflammation (Fig. 18-12).
- Bleeding can occur immediately after the site is probed or can be slightly delayed in occurrence. An alert clinician will observe each site for a few seconds before moving on to the next site.

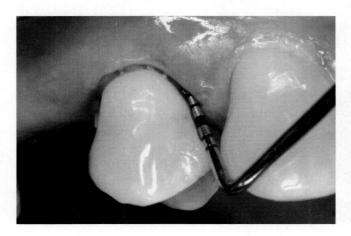

Figure 18-12. Bleeding on Gentle Probing.
Bleeding may be visible immediately when a site is probed or might not be evident for about 10 seconds after a site is probed. Bleeding may appear as a tiny spot or profuse bleeding. Most periodontal charts have a row of boxes that are used to document sites that bleed; bleeding may be indicated with a red dot. (Courtesy of Dr. Richard Foster, Guilford Technical Community College, Jamestown, NC.)

DETERMINGING THE LEVEL OF THE FREE GINGIVAL MARGIN

1. **Gingival Margin Level in Relation to the CEJ.** The level of the free gingival margin in relationship to the cementoenamel junction (CEJ) should be recorded on the dental chart.

2. **Changes in the Gingival Margin Level.** The level of the free gingival margin can change over time in response to trauma, medications, or disease. Three possible relationships exist between the gingival margin and the CEJ of the tooth.

    A. **Gingival margin is slightly coronal to the CEJ.** This is the natural position of the gingival margin and represents the expected position of the gingival margin in the absence of disease or trauma (Fig. 18-13).

    B. **Gingival margin significantly covers the CEJ.** The position of the gingival margin may be significantly coronal to the CEJ due to: (1) swelling (edema), (2) an overgrowth of the gingival tissues caused by certain medications that a patient takes to treat a medical condition, and/or (3) an increase in the fibrous connective tissue of the gingiva due to a long-standing inflammation of the tissue (Fig. 18-14).

    C. **Gingival margin is significantly apical to the CEJ.** When the gingival margin is significantly apical to the CEJ, a portion of the root surface is exposed in the mouth. This relationship is known as **recession of the gingival margin** (Fig. 18-15).

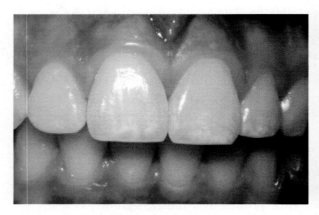

Figure 18-13. Natural Position. The gingival margin is at its normal position, slightly coronal to the CEJ.

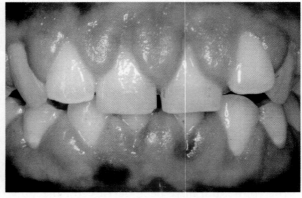

Figure 18-14. Gingival Enlargement. The gingival margin is significantly coronal to the CEJ.

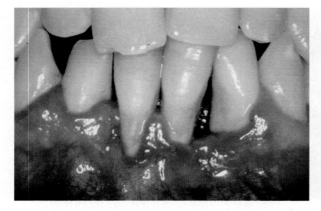

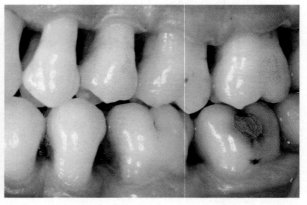

Figure 18-15. Recession of the Gingival Margin. These photos show two examples of recession of the gingival margin leading to exposure of root surfaces to the oral environment.

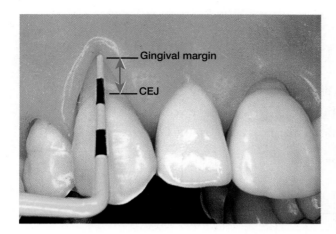

Gingival margin

CEJ

Figure 18-16. Measuring Recession of the Gingival Margin. The extent of recession of the gingival margin is measured in millimeters from the gingival margin to the CEJ. Note in the photograph the gingival margin has receded away from the CEJ, so that the root of the tooth is exposed in the mouth. The probe is *not* pushing the tissue away from the CEJ, rather it is simply used to measure the amount that the tissue has receded.

3. **Determining the Level of the Free Gingival Margin.** The technique for determining the level of the free gingival margin is depicted in Figure 18-16 and outlined in Box 18-1.
4. **Recording the Gingival Margin on a Periodontal Chart**
   A. Customarily, the notations 0, −, or + are used to indicate the position of the gingival margin on a periodontal chart (Box 18-2).
   B. Most periodontal charts include rows of boxes that are used to record the level of the free gingival margin on the facial and lingual aspects. In addition, the level may be indicated on the facial and lingual aspects of the teeth by a line (Fig. 18-17).

Box 18-1 Technique for Determining the Level of the Gingival Margin

When tissue swelling or recession is present, a periodontal probe is used to measure the distance the gingival margin is apical or coronal to the CEJ. Keep in mind that the natural or expected level of the gingival margin in the absence of disease or trauma is slightly coronal to the CEJ.

1. **For gingival recession.** If gingival recession is present, the distance between the CEJ and the gingival margin is measured using a calibrated periodontal probe. This distance is recorded as the gingival margin level.

2. **For gingival enlargement.** If gingival enlargement is present, the distance between the CEJ and the gingival margin is also measured using a calibrated periodontal probe. This distance is estimated using the following technique:
   A. Position the tip of the probe at a 45-degree angle to the tooth surface.
   B. Slowly move the probe tip beneath the gingival margin until the junction between the enamel and cementum is detected as a slight discrepancy in the smoothness of the tooth surface.
   C. Measure the distance between the gingival margin and the CEJ. This distance is recorded as the gingival margin level.

| Box 18-2 | Notations that Indicate the Position of the Free Gingival Margin |

- A zero (**0**) indicates the free gingival margin is slightly coronal to the CEJ
- A negative number (**–**) indicates the free gingival margin significantly covers the CEJ
- A positive number (**+**) indicates the free gingival margin is apical to the CEJ (recession)

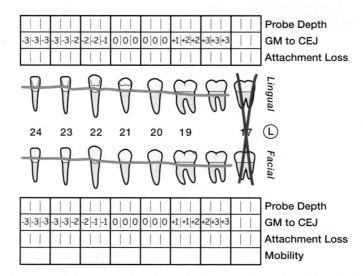

Figure 18-17. Sample Periodontal Chart Indicating the Level of the Gingival Margin. Shown above is an example of how the level of the free gingival margin might be indicated on a periodontal chart for the mandibular left quadrant. There are six total chart entries per tooth, three entries for the facial aspect and three entries for the lingual aspect of each tooth. GM to CEJ = measurement from the gingival margin to the cementoenamel junction.

- The gingival margin levels are indicated in the row of boxes labeled ***"GM to CEJ"—gingival margin to cementoenamel junction***. In addition, a red line on the chart indicates the level of the gingival margin.
- In this example, the level of the gingival margin is significantly coronal to the CEJ on teeth 22, 23, and 24. The gingival margin level is normal for teeth 20 and 21. Recession of the gingival margin is present on teeth 18 and 19.

Section 3
Assessments that Require Calculations

Information collected during the comprehensive periodontal assessment is used to make certain calculations that provide valuable information about the health of the periodontal tissues. The most common findings that require some calculations are the clinical attachment level (CAL) and width of the attached gingiva.

CLINICAL ATTACHMENT LEVELS

1. **Definition.** The clinical attachment level is a clinical measurement of the true periodontal support around the tooth as measured with a periodontal probe.
   A. The CAL provides an estimate of a tooth's stability and the loss of bone support.
   B. Two terms are commonly used in conjunction with the periodontal support system—clinical attachment level and clinical attachment loss. Both of these terms may be abbreviated as CAL and can be used synonymously.
      1. Clinical attachment loss is the extent of periodontal support that has been destroyed around a tooth.
      2. As an example of the use of these two terms, a clinician might report that the "*clinical attachment levels* were calculated for the facial surface of tooth 32 and there is 6 mm of *clinical attachment loss*."
2. **Significance of Clinical Attachment Levels**
   A. *An attachment level measurement is a more accurate indicator of the periodontal support around a tooth than is a probing depth measurement.* Box 18-3 outlines a comparison of probing depths and clinical attachment levels.
      1. Probing depths are measured from the free gingival margin to the base of the sulcus or pocket.
         a. The position of the gingival margin may change with tissue swelling, overgrowth of tissue, or recession of tissue.
         b. Since the position of the gingival margin can change (move coronally or apically), probing depths do not provide an accurate means to monitor changes in periodontal support over time in a patient.
      2. Clinical attachment levels provide an accurate means to monitor changes in periodontal support over time. The CAL is calculated from measurements made from a fixed point on the tooth that does not change (i.e., the CEJ of the tooth).
   B. The presence of loss of attachment is a critical factor in distinguishing between gingivitis and periodontitis.
      1. Inflammation with no attachment loss is characteristic of gingivitis.
      2. Inflammation with attachment loss is characteristic of periodontitis.

> ### Box 18-3 Comparison of Probing Depths and Clinical Attachment Levels
>
> Monitoring the periodontal support of teeth over time is a vital component of long-term care of patients with periodontal disease. There are two measurements used to describe the amount of periodontal support for teeth: (1) probing depths and (2) clinical attachment levels. Clinicians should be aware that the use of probing depths alone may not be in some patients' best interests.
>
> - **Probing depths** alone are not reliable indicators of the amount of periodontal support for a tooth. Probing depths are measured from the gingival margin; the position of the gingival margin often changes over time. Changes in the level of the gingival margin occur with gingival swelling, overgrowth of gingiva, or gingival recession. So, a change in probing depth over time may indicate a change in the amount of periodontal support for a tooth, but it may also only indicate that there has been some change in the level of the gingival margin (which may well be unrelated to the actual periodontal support of the tooth).
> - **Clinical attachment levels** are the preferred and more accurate indicator of the actual amount of periodontal support for a tooth. CAL measurements are made from a fixed point that does not change (i.e., the CEJ of the tooth). Therefore, when there is a change in the CAL over time, this change reflects an accurate measurement of a true change in the periodontal support of a tooth.

CALCULATING CLINICAL ATTACHMENT LEVELS

1. A competent clinician must understand the procedure for determining the clinical attachment level for the three possible relationships of the gingival margin to the CEJ. Figures 18-18 to 18-20 depict the three relationships.
   - A. The gingival margin may be (1) at its normal level slightly coronal to (above) the CEJ, (2) apical to (below) the CEJ, or (3) significantly cover the CEJ.
   - B. Two measurements are used to calculate the clinical attachment level:
     - a. the probing depth and
     - b. the level of the gingival margin (distance from CEJ to gingival margin).
   - C. Note that both of these measurements are routinely taken and documented on a periodontal chart.
2. Customarily, the notations 0, −, or + are used to indicate the position of the gingival margin on a periodontal chart (Box 18-4).

> ### Box 18-4 Notations that Indicate the Position of the Free Gingival Margin
>
> - A zero (0) indicates the free gingival margin is slightly coronal to the CEJ
> - A negative number (−) indicates the free gingival margin significantly covers the CEJ
> - A positive number (+) indicates the free gingival margin is apical to the CEJ (recession)

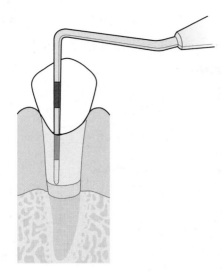

Figure 18-18. Calculating CAL When the Gingival Margin is at the Normal Level. When the gingival margin at its natural location—slightly coronal to the CEJ—no calculations are needed since the probing depth and the clinical attachment level are equal.

For example:
Probing depth measurement: 6 mm
Gingival margin level: 0 mm*
Clinical attachment loss: 6 mm

*gingival margin is at the normal level, therefore no gingival tissue needs to added or taken away (0).

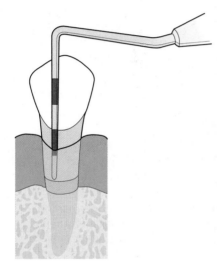

Figure 18-19. Calculating CAL in the Presence of Recession of the Gingival Margin. When recession of the gingival margin is present, the CAL is calculated by ADDING the probing depth to the gingival margin level.

For example:
Probing depth measurement: 4 mm
Gingival margin level: +2 mm*
Clinical attachment loss: 6 mm

*2 mm of tissue needs *to be added* for the gingival margin to be at its normal level.

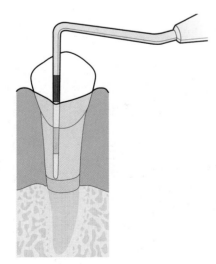

Figure 18-20. Calculating CAL When the Gingival Margin Covers the CEJ. When the gingival margin is significantly coronal to the CEJ, the CAL is calculated by SUBTRACTING the gingival margin level from the probing depth.

For example:
Probing depth measurement: 9 mm
Gingival margin level: −3 mm*
Clinical attachment loss: 6 mm

*3 mm of tissue needs *to be taken away* for the gingival margin to be at its normal level.

DOCUMENTING CLINICAL ATTACHMENT LEVELS

On the sample periodontal chart shown in Figure 18-21, all three possible relationships of the gingival margin to the CEJ are demonstrated.

- On tooth 28—the gingival margin is at the level of the CEJ on the facial and lingual aspects of tooth 28. (Thus a zero is noted on the chart for the facial and lingual aspects of this tooth.)
- On teeth 25 to 27—the gingival margin covers the CEJ. (Thus a negative sign (–) on the chart is used to indicate that the gingival margin is coronal to the CEJ.)
- On teeth 29 and 31—the gingival margin is apical to (below) the CEJ. (Thus a plus sign (+) on the chart is used to indicate that the gingival margin is apical to the CEJ.)

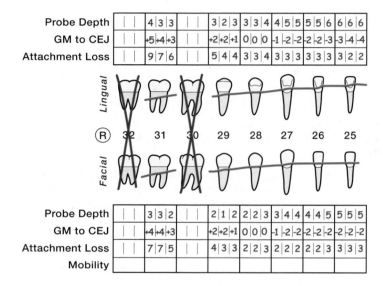

Probe Depth			4	3	3				3	2	3	3	3	4	4	5	5	5	5	6	6	6	6
GM to CEJ			+5	+4	+3				+2	+2	+1	0	0	0	-1	-2	-2	-2	-2	-3	-3	-4	-4
Attachment Loss			9	7	6				5	4	4	3	3	4	3	3	3	3	3	3	3	2	2

Lingual

Ⓡ 32 31 30 29 28 27 26 25

Facial

Probe Depth			3	3	2				2	1	2	2	2	3	3	4	4	4	4	5	5	5	5
GM to CEJ			+4	+4	+3				+2	+2	+1	0	0	0	-1	-2	-2	-2	-2	-2	-2	-2	-2
Attachment Loss			7	7	5				4	3	3	2	2	3	2	2	2	2	2	3	3	3	3
Mobility																							

Figure 18-21. Sample Periodontal Chart. The chart shown above depicts how the following information might be indicated on a periodontal charting of the mandibular right sextant: (1) probing depth measurements, (2) measurement of the level of the free gingival margin to the cementoenamel junction (GM to CEJ), and (3) calculated clinical attachment levels. The clinical attachment levels are calculated based on the measurements for the probing depths and level of the free gingival margin.

CALCULATING THE WIDTH OF THE ATTACHED GINGIVA

1. Description. The attached gingiva is the part of the gingiva that is tightly connected to the cementum on the cervical-third of the root or to the periosteum (connective tissue cover) of the alveolar bone. The attached gingiva lies between the free gingiva and the alveolar mucosa, extending from the base of the sulcus (or pocket) to the mucogingival junction. The alveolar mucosa can be detected visually by its deep red color and shiny appearance.
   A. The functions of the attached gingiva are to keep the free gingiva from being pulled away from the tooth and to protect the gingiva from trauma.
   B. The width of the attached gingiva is not measured on the palate since it is not possible to determine where the attached gingiva ends and the palatal mucosa begins.
   C. *The attached gingiva does not include any portion of the gingiva that is separated from the tooth by a crevice, sulcus, or periodontal pocket.*
2. Significance. The width of the attached gingiva on a tooth surface is an important clinical feature for the dentist to keep in mind when planning many types of restorative procedures. If there is no attached gingiva on a tooth surface, the dentist is limited in the types of restorations that can be placed. Therefore, it is important to use the information collected during the comprehensive periodontal assessment to calculate this clinical feature.
3. Method of Calculation. The method for calculation is shown in Box 18-5. Note that the information needed to calculate the width of the attached gingiva already would have been recorded during the periodontal assessment (Figs. 18-22A and B).

Box 18-5 **Width of the Attached Gingiva**

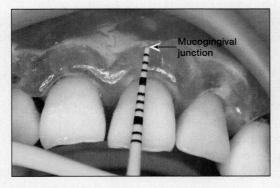

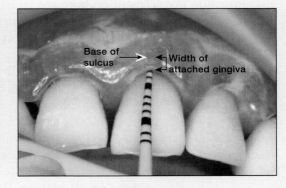

Figure 18-22. A: Total Width of Gingiva.   **Figure 18-22. B: Probing Depth**

Method: Calculate the width of the attached gingiva by subtracting the probing depth from the total width of the gingiva.

Step 1: Measure the total width of the gingiva from the gingival margin to the mucogingival junction. *In the example shown in Figure 18-22A, this measurement is 4 mm.*

Step 2: Measure the probing depth (from the gingival margin to the base of the pocket). *In the example shown in Figure 18-22B, this measurement is 2 mm.*

Step 3: Calculate the width of the attached gingiva by subtracting the probing depth from the total width of the gingiva. *In the example pictured above, the width of the attached gingiva is 4 mm minus 2 mm equaling 2 mm of attached gingiva.*

Section 4
Assessments with Furcation Probes

FURCATION INVOLVEMENT

A furcation is the place on a multirooted tooth where the root trunk divides into separate roots. Most molar teeth are multirooted, but some maxillary premolar teeth also develop with two roots creating the potential for a furcation involvement on some premolars also. The furcation is termed a bifurcation on a two-rooted tooth and a trifurcation on a three-rooted tooth.

1. The furcation area is the space—apical to the root trunk—between two or more roots.
    A. Teeth typically have one, two, or three roots. Anterior teeth usually have one root. Mandibular molars have two roots. Typically, maxillary molars have three roots.
    B. The area of a multirooted tooth that extends from the CEJ to the entrance of the furcation is termed the **root trunk** (Fig. 18-23).
    C. The entrance to a furcation may be as little as 3 to 4 mm apical to (below) the CEJ.
2. In health, the furcation area cannot be probed because it is filled with alveolar bone and periodontal ligament fibers.
3. Furcation involvement is a loss of alveolar bone and periodontal ligament fibers in the space between the roots of a multirooted tooth. Bone loss in the furcation area may be hidden beneath the gingival tissue or—when recession of the gingival margin is present—the furcation area may be clinically visible in the mouth (Fig. 18-24).
    A. Furcation involvement occurs on a multirooted tooth when periodontal infection invades the area between and around the roots, resulting in loss of attachment and loss of alveolar bone between the roots of the tooth.
        1. Mandibular molars are usually bifurcated (mesial and distal roots), with potential furcation involvement on both the facial and lingual aspects of the tooth (Fig. 18-25).
        2. Maxillary molar teeth are usually trifurcated (mesiobuccal, distobuccal, and palatal roots) with potential furcation involvement on the facial, mesial, and distal aspects of the tooth (Fig. 18-26).
        3. Maxillary first premolars can have bifurcated roots (buccal and palatal roots) with the potential for furcation involvement on the mesial and distal aspects of the tooth. Approximately 60% of maxillary first premolars have a buccal and lingual root (3).
    B. Furcation involvement frequently signals a need for periodontal surgery after completion of nonsurgical therapy, so detection and documentation of furcation involvement is a critical component of the comprehensive periodontal assessment.
4. The ability to mentally visualize root furcation morphology is important for effective assessment and instrumentation of periodontal patients. The location of root furcations (Box 18-6) has been the subject of several studies (3–7).

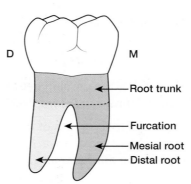

Figure 18-23. Anatomy of a Mandibular First Molar.
The root trunk extends from the CEJ to the entrance of the bifurcation. Mandibular molars have distal and mesial roots.

REVIEW OF ROOT FURCATION MORPHOLOGY

Box 18-6 **Root Furcation Morphology**

Mandibular Molars

Mandibular molars have two roots with furcation areas on the facial and lingual surfaces between the mesial and distal roots.

Maxillary First Premolars

Maxillary first premolars that are bifurcated have a buccal and palatal root. When bifurcated, the roots of a maxillary first premolar separate many millimeters apical to the cementoenamel junction.

Maxillary Molars (Buccal View)

Maxillary molar teeth usually are trifurcated with **mesiobuccal, distobuccal, and palatal** (lingual) **roots**.

Maxillary Molars (Proximal View)

On the mesial surface of a maxillary molar, the furcation is located more toward the lingual surface.

On the distal surface of a maxillary molar, the furcation is located near the center of the tooth.

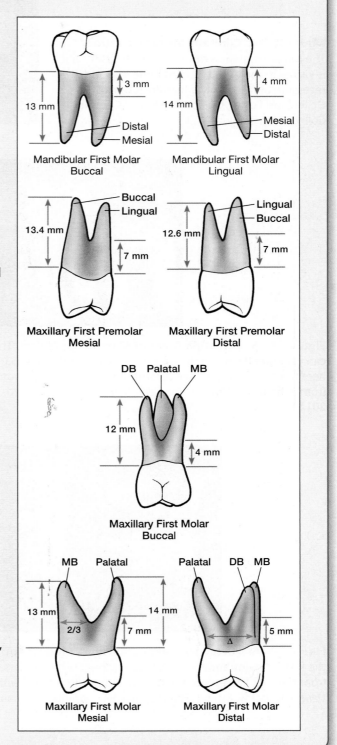

Mandibular First Molar
Buccal

Mandibular First Molar
Lingual

Maxillary First Premolar
Mesial

Maxillary First Premolar
Distal

Maxillary First Molar
Buccal

Maxillary First Molar
Mesial

Maxillary First Molar
Distal

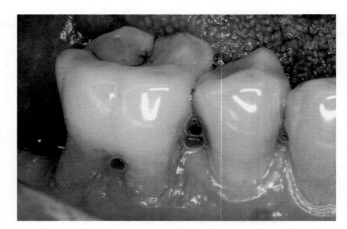

Figure 18-24. Clinically Visible Furcation. The furcation area of this mandibular first molar is visible in the mouth due to bone loss and recession of the gingival margin. (Courtesy of Dr. Richard Foster, Guilford Technical Community College, Jamestown, NC.)

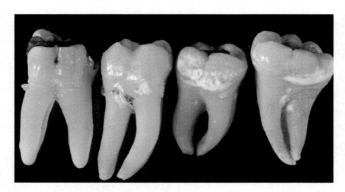

Figure 18-25. Furcation Areas of Mandibular Molars. The entrance to the furcation area of molar tooth can vary greatly in size due to the varying degrees of separation of the roots. The mandibular molars shown here from left to right have divergent roots, straighter roots, and fused roots. (Reprinted with permission from Scheid, RC, Weiss G. *Woelfel's Dental Anatomy*. 8th ed. Philadelphia, PA: Lippincott Williams & Wilkins; 2012.)

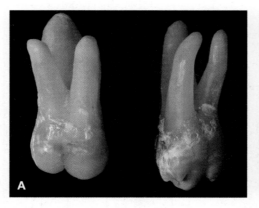
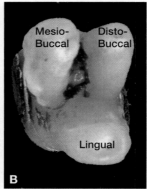

Figure 18-26. Furcation Areas of Maxillary Molars. A: The furcation areas of two maxillary molars showing the furcation entrance from the facial aspect of the molars. **B:** Aerial view of a maxillary molar looking down from the root apices into the furcation area. (Reprinted with permission from Scheid, RC, Weiss G. *Woelfel's Dental Anatomy*. 8th ed. Philadelphia, PA: Lippincott Williams & Wilkins; 2012.)

RADIOGRAPHIC EVIDENCE OF FURCATION INVOLVEMENT

1. A classic study by Ross and Thompson (8) showed that furcation involvement occurs three times more frequently among maxillary molars than among mandibular molars.
   A. Many molars with furcation involvement functioned well from 5 to 24 years (8).
   B. In the Ross/Thompson study furcation involvement was detected more frequently in maxillary molars by radiographic examination than by clinical examination. On the other hand, furcation involvement was detected more frequently in mandibular molars by clinical examination than by radiographic examination.
2. In health, the furcation area cannot be probed because it is filled with alveolar bone and periodontal ligament fibers (Fig. 18-27).
3. When radiographs of maxillary molars are observed, *a small, triangular radiographic shadow pointing toward the furcation* is sometimes noted over either the mesial or distal roots in the proximal furcation area. These small triangular radiographic shadows are called furcation arrows.
   A. Because the furcation arrow seldom appears over uninvolved furcations, the appearance of a furcation arrow indicates that there is proximal bony furcation involvement (9).
   B. However, absence of the furcation arrow image does not necessarily mean an absence of a bony furcation involvement because the arrow was not seen in a large number of furcations with involvement (9).
4. On a radiograph, a triangular radiolucency in the furcation of a molar indicates furcation involvement. Figures 18-28 to 18-32 show examples of radiographic evidence of furcation involvement.
5. Occasionally, a radiograph may show evidence of a molar with fused roots (Fig. 18-33).

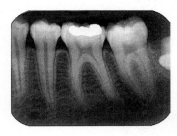

Figure 18-27. Periodontium in Health. In health, the alveolar bone and periodontal ligament fill the furcation area between the roots.

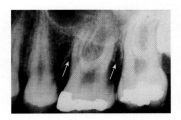

Figure 18-28. Furcation Involvement: Radiolucent Arrows on Proximal Surfaces. The *yellow arrows* on this radiograph indicate the furcation arrows on the proximal surfaces of a maxillary first molar.

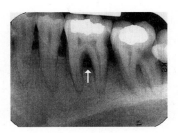

Figure 18-29. Furcation Involvement: Triangular Radiolucency. A triangular radiolucency in the bifurcation of a mandibular first molar indicates furcation involvement.

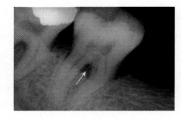

Figure 18-30. Furcation Involvement: Triangular Radiolucency. A triangular radiolucency in the bifurcation of a mandibular molar indicates furcation involvement.

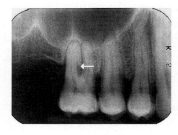

Figure 18-31. Furcation Involvement: Triangular Radiolucency. This radiograph shows furcation involvement on a maxillary first molar. (Courtesy of Dr. Robert P. Langlais.)

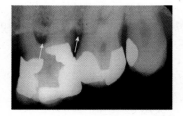

Figure 18-32. Furcation Involvement. The maxillary second molar on this radiograph shows a radiolucent arrow on the mesial proximal surface and a triangular radiolucency in the furcation.

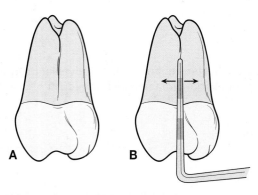

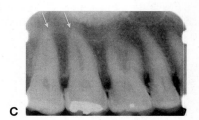

Figure 18-33. Fused Maxillary Roots. A: The concavity formed by fused roots on the distal proximal surface of a maxillary molar. **B:** Probe tip in the concavity. **C:** Radiograph showing fused roots on maxillary molars.

DESIGN CHARACTERISTICS OF FURCATION PROBES

A furcation probe is a type of periodontal probe used to evaluate the bone support in the furcation areas of bifurcated and trifurcated teeth.

1. Furcation probes have curved, blunt-tipped working-ends that allow easy access to the furcation areas.
2. The Nabers N1 and N2 furcation probes are the traditional instruments used for measuring the horizontal depth of bone loss in a furcation area (Figs. 18-34 to 18-36).

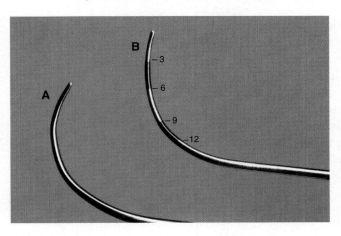

Figure 18-34. Nabers N2 Furcation Probes. Probe **B** has black bands from 3 to 6 mm and 9 to 12 mm. Furcation probes with millimeter markings often are used in research studies.

Other furcation probes, like Probe **A,** do not have millimeter markings.

WORKING-END SELECTION: NABERS PROBES

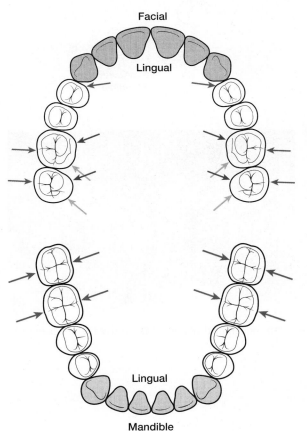

Figure 18-35. Nabers Probe Selection for the Maxillary Teeth. For maxillary first premolar and molars:
- The N2 is used for assessment of facial and lingual furcation areas.
- The N1 is used for assessment of mesial and distal furcation areas.

Figure 18-36. Nabers Probe Selection for the Mandibular Teeth. For mandibular molars, the N2 is used for assessment of facial and lingual furcation areas.

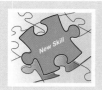

SKILL BUILDING
Technique Practice With Furcation Probes

Directions:

1. Practice with a periodontal typodont or mount an acrylic mandibular molar, maxillary first premolar, and maxillary first molar in modeling clay or plaster. Mount the teeth so that the furcation areas are exposed.
2. Position the probe at the gingival line at a location near where the furcation is suspected.
3. Direct the probe beneath the gingival margin. At the base of the pocket, rotate the probe tip toward the tooth to turn the tip into the entrance of the furcation.
4. Refer to the diagrams and photographs shown in Figures 18-37 to 18-41 for guidance in accessing the furcation areas of mandibular and maxillary molars and the maxillary first premolars.

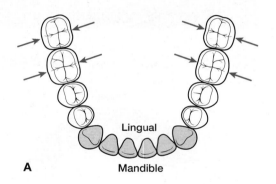

Figure 18-37. A–C: Access to the Furcation on the Buccal and Lingual Aspects of a Mandibular Molar. The furcation area of a mandibular molar is located between the mesial and distal roots. The furcation area can be entered from both the buccal and lingual aspects of the molar tooth as indicated by the *purple arrows* on illustration 18-37A.

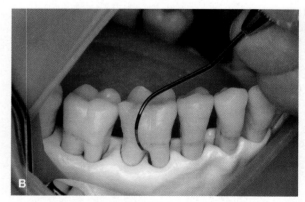

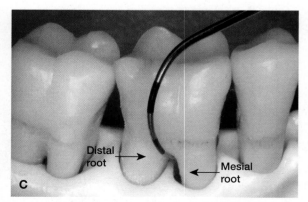

Figure 18-37. B and C: A furcation probe placed between the mesial and distal roots on the facial aspect of the mandibular first molar.

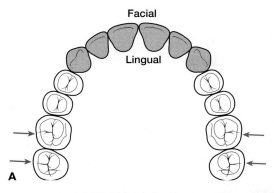

Figure 18-38. A–C: Access to the Furcation on the Buccal Aspect of a Maxillary Molar. Maxillary molars have three roots: a distobuccal, mesiobuccal, and a palatal (lingual) root. Enter the furcation between the distobuccal and mesiobuccal roots from the facial aspect as indicated by the *purple arrows* in Figure 18-38A.

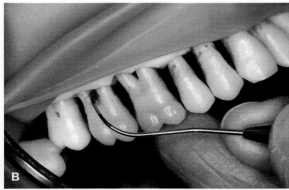

Figure 18-38. B and C. Furcation probe placed between the mesial and distal roots on the facial aspect of a maxillary first molar.

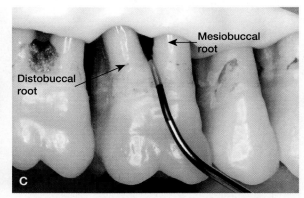

Figure 18-39. A–C: Access to the Furcation on the Distal Aspect of a Maxillary Molar. The distal proximal furcation of a maxillary molar is accessed from the lingual aspect. The N1 furcation probe wraps around the palatal root to enter the furcation between the distobuccal and palatal roots as indicated by the *orange arrows* in Figure 18-39A.

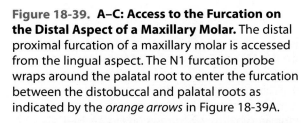

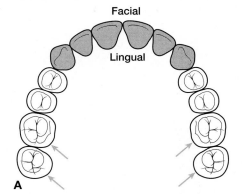

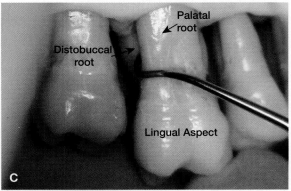

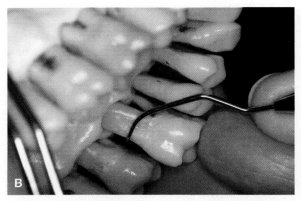

Figure 18-39. B and C. Furcation probe placed between the distofacial and the palatal roots on the lingual aspect of a maxillary first molar, note how the probe tip wraps around the palatal root.

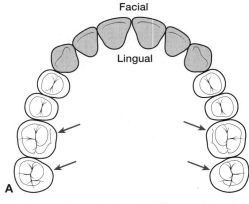

Figure 18-40. A–C: Access to the Furcation on the Mesial Aspect of a Maxillary Molar. The mesial proximal furcation of a maxillary molar is accessed from the lingual aspect. The N1 furcation probe is inserted between the mesiobuccal and palatal roots as indicated by the *red arrows* in Figure 18-40A.

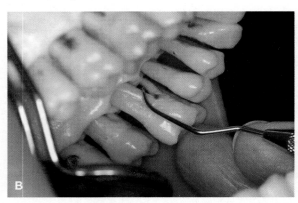

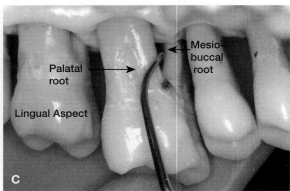

Figure 18-40. B and C: A furcation probe placed between the palatal and mesiobuccal roots on the lingual surface of a maxillary first molar.

Figure 18-41. A–C: Access to the Furcation on the Mesial Aspect of the Maxillary First Premolar. A maxillary first premolar may have a buccal and a palatal root. The proximal furcation is entered from the lingual aspect of the tooth as indicated by the *teal arrows* on Figure 18-41A.

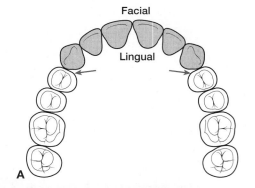

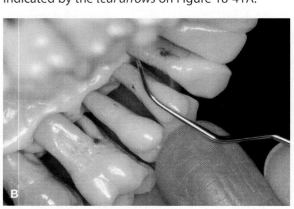

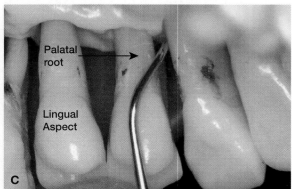

Figure 18-41. B and C: A furcation probe placed between the palatal and facial roots of a maxillary first premolar (note: many maxillary first premolars have only one root).

FOUR CLASSIFICATIONS OF FURCATION INVOLVEMENT

Furcation involvement should be recorded on a periodontal chart using a scale that quantifies the *severity (or extent) of the furcation invasion.* Furcation involvement rating scales are based on the horizontal measurement of attachment loss in the furcation (10,11). Table 18-4 shows a common furcation-rating scale based on four grades and charting symbols that may be used to indicate the grade on a periodontal chart (12).

TABLE 18-4. SCALE AND CHARTING SYMBOLS FOR RATING FURCATION INVOLVEMENT

Grade		Description	Symbol
I		The curvature of the concavity—just above the furcation entrance—on the root trunk can be felt with the probe tip; however, the probe penetrates the furcation no more than 1 mm. (Key: JE, junctional epithelium)	∧
II		The probe penetrates into the furcation greater than 1 mm—extending approximately 1/3 of the width of the tooth—but is not able to pass completely through the furcation.	△
III		In *mandibular molars,* the probe passes completely through the furcation between the mesial and distal roots. In *maxillary molars,* the probe passes between the mesiobuccal and distobuccal roots and touches the palatal root.	▲
IV		Same as a Class III furcation except that the entrance to the furcation area is visible clinically due to recession of the gingival margin.	◆

DOCUMENTATION OF FURCATION INVOLVEMENT

On the sample periodontal chart shown in Figure 18-42, all four classes of furcation involvement are represented.

- Tooth 2 has a Class IV furcation involvement on the facial aspect.
- Tooth 3 has a Class I furcation involvement on the facial aspect between the mesiobuccal and distobuccal roots.
- On the lingual aspect, tooth 2 has a Class III furcation involvement between the distobuccal and palatal roots and a Class II furcation involvement between the mesiobuccal and palatal roots.

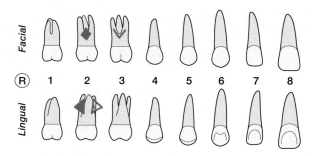

Figure 18-42. Periodontal Chart Indicating Furcation Involvement.

References

1. Armitage GC. Diagnosis of periodontal diseases. *J Periodontol.* 2003;74(8):1237–1247.
2. ADHA (or American Dental Hygienists' Association). *Standards for Clinical Dental Hygiene Practice.* Chicago, IL; ADHA, 2008.
3. Scheid R, Weiss G. *Woelfel's Dental Anatomy Its Relevance to Dentistry.* 8th ed. Philadelphia, PA: Lippincott Williams & Wilkins; 2011:520 p.
4. Dunlap RM, Gher ME. Root surface measurements of the mandibular first molar. *J Periodontol.* 1985;56(4):234–238.
5. Gher MW, Jr., Dunlap RW. Linear variation of the root surface area of the maxillary first molar. *J Periodontol.* 1985;56(1):39–43.
6. Plagmann HC, Holtorf S, Kocher T. A study on the imaging of complex furcation forms in upper and lower molars. *J Clin Periodontol.* 2000;27(12):926–931.
7. Santana RB, Uzel MI, Gusman H, Gunaydin Y, Jones JA, Leone CW. Morphometric analysis of the furcation anatomy of mandibular molars. *J Periodontol.* 2004;75(6):824–829.
8. Ross IF, Thompson RH, Jr. Furcation involvement in maxillary and mandibular molars. *J Periodontol.* 1980;51(8):450–454.
9. Hardekopf JD, Dunlap RM, Ahl DR, Pelleu GB, Jr. The "furcation arrow". A reliable radiographic image? *J Periodontol.* 1987;58(4):258–261.
10. Glickman I. Clinical periodontology; the periodontium in health and disease, recognition, diagnosis and treatment of periodontal disease in the practice of general dentistry. Philadelphia, PA: Saunders; 1953:1019 p.
11. Hamp SE, Nyman S, Lindhe J. Periodontal treatment of multirooted teeth. Results after 5 years. *J Clin Periodontol.* 1975;2(3):126–135.
12. Newman MG, Takei HH, Klokkevold PR, Carranza FA. *Carranza's Clinical Periodontology.* 11th ed. St. Louis, MO: Saunders Elsevier; 2012.

Section 5
Skill Application

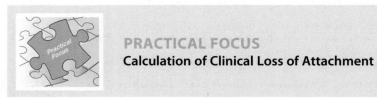

PRACTICAL FOCUS
Calculation of Clinical Loss of Attachment

Using the probe shown in Figure 18-43, calculate the clinical loss of attachment (CAL) for the teeth depicted in Figures 18-44A–C.

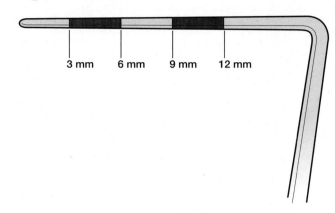

3 mm   6 mm   9 mm   12 mm

Figure 18-43. Probe Calibrations.

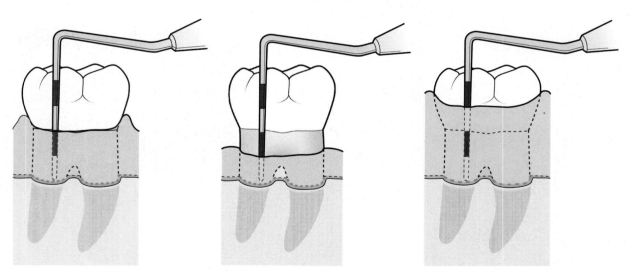

Figure 18-44. A: Tooth A.

Figure 18-44. B: Tooth B.

Figure 18-44. C: Tooth C.

Tooth A		Tooth B		Tooth C	
Probing Depth	=	Probing Depth	=	Probing Depth	=
GM to CEJ	=	GM to CEJ	=	GM to CEJ	=
Attachment Loss	=	Attachment Loss	=	Attachment Loss	=

PRACTICAL FOCUS
Fictitious Patient Case Mr. Temple

Directions: Use Figures 18-45A to D to answer the case questions for fictitious patient, Mr. Temple.

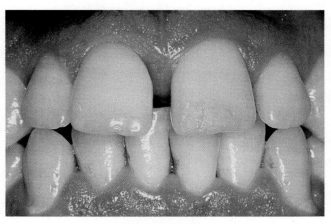

Figure 18-45A

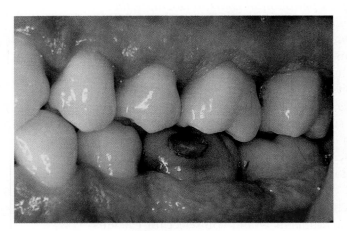

Figure 18-45B

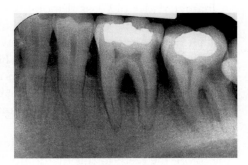

Figure 18-45C

Mr. Temple: Assessment Data

1. Generalized bleeding upon probing.
2. Deposits
   A. Moderate supragingival plaque on all teeth. Light subgingival plaque on all surfaces with moderate subgingival plaque on the proximal surfaces on all teeth.
   B. Supragingival calculus deposits—light calculus on lingual surfaces of mandibular anteriors.
   C. Subgingival calculus deposits—small-sized deposits on all teeth; medium-sized deposits on all proximal surfaces.

Mr. Temple: Periodontal Chart

4	3	5	5	4	6	6	6	6	6	5	6	6	6	6	8	9	8	8	7	7			Probe Depth
0	0	0	0	0	0	0	0	0	0	0	0	0	0	0	0	0	0	0	0	0			GM to CEJ
																							Attachment Loss

| | 24 | 23 | 22 | 21 | 20 | 19 | 18 | 17 | (L) |

4	3	4	4	4	5	4	2	4	5	4	5	5	5	6	7	8	7	7	6	7			Probe Depth
0	0	0	0	0	0	+1	+3	+1	0	0	0	0	0	0	0	0	0	0	0	0			GM to CEJ
																							Attachment Loss
															2		1						Mobility

Figure 18-45D. Mr. Temple's Periodontal Chart. Mr. Temple's periodontal chart for the mandibular left quadrant.

Mr. Temple: Case Questions

1. *Use the information recorded on Mr. Temple's periodontal chart to calculate the clinical attachment loss on the facial and lingual aspects for teeth 18 to 24 and enter this information on Mr. Temple's periodontal chart in Figure 18-45D.*
2. Describe the characteristics of the Class I mobility on tooth 18. Describe the characteristics of Class II mobility on tooth 19.
3. Describe the characteristics of the furcation involvement on teeth 18 and 19 (i.e., what does this level of furcation involvement look like in the mouth?)
4. Does the assessment data indicate healthy sulci or periodontal pockets in this quadrant? Explain which data you used to determine the presence of sulci or pockets?
5. If the gingival margin level information had NOT been documented on this chart, would the probing depth measurements, alone, be an accurate indicator of the level of bone support present? Why?
6. Based on the assessment information, which type of explorer would you select to explore the teeth in this quadrant? Which instruments would you select for calculus removal in this quadrant: sickle scalers, universal curets, and/or area-specific curets? Explain your rationale for instrument selection.

PRACTICAL FOCUS
Fictitious Patient Case Mrs. Blanchard

Directions: Use Figures 18-46A-C to answer the case questions for fictitious patient, Mrs. Blanchard.

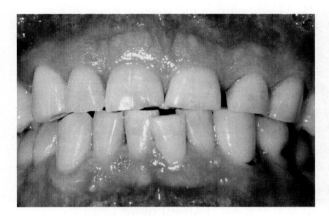

| **Figure 18-46A** | **Figure 18-46B** |

Mrs. Blanchard: Assessment Data

1. Generalized bleeding upon probing.
2. Deposits
   A. Light supragingival plaque on all teeth. Light subgingival plaque on all surfaces.
   B. Supragingival calculus deposits—light calculus on lingual surfaces of mandibular anteriors and facial surfaces of maxillary molar.
   C. Subgingival calculus deposits—small-sized deposits on all teeth

Note to Course Instructor: Additional patient cases and opportunities for practice in calculating clinical attachment levels are found in Module 22, Fictitious Patient Cases.

Mrs. Blanchard: Periodontal Chart

																							Mobility
3	2	3	2	1	3	3	2	4	5	5	3	4	3	5	4	5	6						**Probe Depth**
+4	+5	+4	+5	+6	+5	+4	+5	+4	+3	+4	+3	+2	+2	+1	+1	+1	+1						**GM to CEJ**
																							Attachment Loss

Facial

9 10 11 12 13 14 15 16 (L)

Lingual

4	3	4	3	3	4	4	3	5	6	5	4	5	4	5	5	6	7						**Probe Depth**
+4	+5	+4	+5	+6	+5	+4	+5	+4	+3	+4	+3	+2	+2	+1	+1	+1	+1						**GM to CEJ**
																							Attachment Loss

Figure 18-46. C: Mrs. Blanchard's Periodontal Chart. Mrs. Blanchard's periodontal chart for the mandibular left quadrant.

Mrs. Blanchard: Case Questions

1. *Use the information recorded on Mrs. Blanchard's chart to calculate the clinical attachment loss on the facial and lingual aspects for teeth 9 to 14 and enter this information on Mrs. Blanchard's periodontal chart in Figure 18-46C.*
2. When assessing tooth 14 for mobility, up to 1 mm of horizontal movement in a facial–lingual direction was evident. Determine the classification of mobility for tooth 14 and enter it on the chart.
3. What class furcation involvement is present on the facial aspect of tooth 14? No furcation involvement is present between the mesiobuccal root and the palatal root. In addition, there is no furcation involvement between the distobuccal root and the palatal root. How would you explain this finding?
4. Does the assessment data indicate healthy sulci or periodontal pockets in this quadrant? Explain which data you used to determine the presence of sulci or pockets?
5. If the gingival margin level information had NOT been documented on this chart, would the probing depth measurements, alone, be an accurate indicator of the level of bone support present? Why?
6. Based on the assessment information, which type of explorer would you select to explore the teeth in this quadrant? Which instruments would you select for calculus removal in this quadrant: sickle scalers, universal curets, and/or area-specific curets? Explain your rationale for instrument selection.

Skill Evaluation Module 18: Advanced Probing Techniques

Student: _____   Date = _____

Evaluator: _____

PART 1—PROBING DEPTH MEASUREMENTS ON STUDENT PARTNER

Evaluator assigns a tooth number in each quadrant to be probed on student partner (six reading per tooth).

S = student probing depth reading is within 1 mm of the evaluator's finding for the tooth.
U = student probing depth reading is not within 1 mm of the evaluator's finding for the tooth

QUADRANT	ASPECT	TOOTH #	STUDENT READINGS			EVALUATOR READINGS		
1	Facial	#						
	Lingual							
2	Facial	#						
	Lingual							
3	Facial	#						
	Lingual							
4	Facial	#						
	Lingual							

OPTIONAL GRADE PERCENTAGE CALCULATION—PART 1

Total number of readings within 1 mm of evaluator's measurement _____. (Possible 24 pts.)

PART 2A—FURCATIONS ASSESSMENT ON PERIODONTAL TYPODONT

On a periodontal typodont, use furcation probe to assess a mandibular first molar (2 possible points) and a maxillary first molar (3 possible points). S = correct technique. U = incorrect technique.

PART 2B—CALCULATING ATTACHMENT LOSS

Calculate the clinical attachment loss for teeth A, B, and C below. S = correct calculation. U = incorrect calculation.

	Tooth A		**Tooth B**		**Tooth C**
Probing Depth	= 2 mm	Probing Depth	= 3 mm	Probing Depth	= 6 mm
GM to CEJ	= +5 mm	GM to CEJ	= +4 mm	GM to CEJ	= −3 mm
Attachment Loss	=	Attachment Loss	=	Attachment Loss	=

OPTIONAL GRADE PERCENTAGE CALCULATION—PART 2

Total number of S evaluations for technique with furcation probe _____. (Possible 5 points.)

Total number of correct CAL calculations _____. (Possible 3 points.)

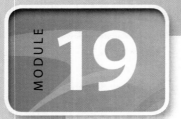

Area-Specific Curets

Module Overview

This module presents the design characteristics of area-specific curets and step-by-step instructions for using area-specific curets to remove subgingival calculus deposits from the anterior and posterior teeth. Module 16, "Technique Essentials: Subgingival Calculus Removal" should be completed before beginning this module.

Module Outline

Section 1 **Area-Specific Curets**   452

General Design Characteristics
Working-End Design
Relationship of Face to Lower Shank
Skill Building. Identifying the Lower Cutting Edge, p. 455
The Gracey Curet Series
Application and Comparison of Gracey Curet Designs

Section 2 **Technique Practice—Anterior Teeth**   459

**Skill Building. Selecting the Correct Working-End for an
     Anterior Tooth, p. 459**
Application of the Cutting Edges to Anterior Teeth
**Skill Building. Step-By-Step Technique on Maxillary Central
     Incisor, p. 461**

Section 3 **Technique Practice—Posterior Teeth**   463

Application of the Cutting Edges to Posterior Teeth
**Skill Building. Selecting the Correct Working-End for a Posterior
     Tooth, p. 464**
**Skill Building. Step-By-Step Technique on Mandibular First
     Molar, p. 465**
**Skill Building. Use of Horizontal Strokes Below the Gingival
     Margin, p. 470**
**Skill Building. Step-By-Step Technique on Maxillary First
     Molar, p. 471**

Section 4 **Instrumentation Techniques on Root Surfaces**   474

Three Types of Instrumentation Strokes for Root Instrumentation
Tailoring Stroke Pressure to the Task at Hand

Section 5 **Production of a Root Debridement Stroke**   477

Use of Multidirectional Strokes on Root Surfaces
Skill Building. Root Debridement Strokes, p. 478

| **Section 6** | **Design Overview: Scalers and Curets** | **479** |

| **Section 7** | **Skill Application** | **481** |

Practical Focus. Fictitious Patient Case
Reference Sheet—Area-Specific Curets
Student Self Evaluation Module 19: Area-Specific Curets

Online resources for this module:
- Calculus removal strokes: subgingival calculus deposits
- Laying down versus "standing up" on your fulcrum
- Area-Specific Curets
- Use of Gracey 11/12 Curet
- The Gracey 13/14 Area-Specific Curet

Available at: http://thepoint.lww.com/GehrigFundamentals8e

Key Terms

Area-specific curet

Working cutting edge

Nonworking cutting edge

Lower cutting edge

Learning Objectives

- Given a variety of area-specific curets, identify the design characteristics of each instrument.
- Discuss the advantages and limitations of the design characteristics of area-specific curets.
- Name the uses of area-specific curets.
- Explain why a set of area-specific curets is needed to instrument the entire dentition.
- Describe how the clinician can use visual clues to select the correct working-end of an area-specific curet on anterior and posterior teeth.
- Using area-specific curets, demonstrate correct adaptation and use of calculus removal strokes on the anterior teeth while maintaining correct position, correct finger rests, and precise finger placement in the grasp.
- Using area-specific curets, demonstrate correct adaptation and use of calculus removal strokes on the posterior teeth while maintaining correct position, correct finger rests, and precise finger placement in the grasp.
- Using area-specific curets, demonstrate horizontal calculus removal strokes at the distofacial line angles of posterior teeth and at the midlines on the facial and lingual surfaces of anterior teeth.
- Given any sickle scaler, universal curet, or area-specific curet identify its function and where it should be used on the dentition.

- Please refer to Module 20, for content on the design and use of periodontal files.
- Refer to Module 20, for content on Langer curets, Gracey designs with extended shanks and miniature working-ends, Curvettes, and debridement curets.
- Refer to Module 21 for content on the anatomy of root surfaces/ root concavities and instrumentation of bi- and trifurcated roots.
- Refer to Module 22 for fictitious patient cases relating to calculus removal.

Section 1
Area-Specific Curets

GENERAL DESIGN CHARACTERISTICS

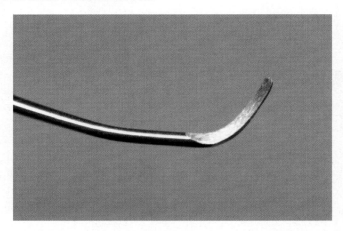

Figure 19-1. The Working-end of an Area-specific Curet.

1. Functions of Area Specific Curets
   A. An area-specific curet is a periodontal instrument used to remove light to moderate calculus deposits from the crowns and roots of the teeth (Fig. 19-1).
   B. *The name "area-specific" signifies that each instrument is designed for use only on certain teeth and certain tooth surfaces. For this reason several area-specific curets are required to instrument the entire mouth.*
2. Design Characteristics. These curets represent an important breakthrough in instrument design and have unique design characteristics (Fig. 19-2 and Table 19-1).
   A. A *face that is tilted in relation to the lower shank*
      1. The face of an area-specific curet tilts at approximately a 70-degree angle to the lower shank.
      2. The tilted face causes one cutting edge to be lower than the other cutting edge on each working-end.
   B. *Only one cutting edge per working-end is used for periodontal instrumentation (the lower cutting edge)*
   C. A *long, complex functional shank* that is especially suited for root surface debridement within periodontal pockets
   D. Other design features of an area-specific curet are similar to those of universal curets:
      1. A *rounded back*
      2. A *rounded toe*
      3. A *semicircular cross section.*
3. Examples of Area-Specific Curet Instruments. Some examples of area-specific curets are the Gracey curet series, Kramer-Nevins series, Turgeon series, After Five Gracey curet series, Gracey +3 curet series, Mini Five Gracey curet series, Gracey +3 Deep Pocket series, and Vision Curvette series.

WORKING-END DESIGN

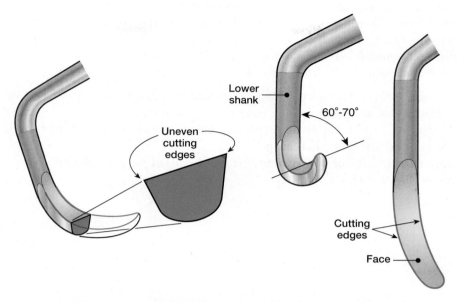

Figure 19-2. Design Characteristics of An Area-Specific Curet.

TABLE 19-1. REFERENCE SHEET: AREA-SPECIFIC CURET	
Cross-Section	Semicircular cross section
Working-End	Rounded back and toe One working cutting edge per working-end
Face	Face tilts at approximately a 70-degree angle to the lower shank; one cutting edge is lower than the other in relation to the lower shank Tilted face means that the lower cutting edge is self-angulated—***the lower cutting edge is automatically at the correct angulation when the lower shank is parallel to the tooth surface to be instrumented***.
Cutting Edges	***Curved cutting edges;*** the curved cutting edges and rounded toe enhance adaptation to rounded root surfaces and root concavities and furcation areas
Application	Each instrument is limited to use on certain teeth and certain surfaces
Primary Functions	***Instrumentation of crown and root surfaces*** Standard curets are used to remove light calculus deposits and deplaquing; rigid Gracey curets can remove medium-sized deposits. Standard area-specific curets have a flexible shank and will bounce over medium-sized calculus deposits whereas rigid Gracey curets have a stronger shank (hence the name rigid) and can be used with more stroke pressure to remove medium- or large-sized deposits.

RELATIONSHIP OF FACE TO LOWER SHANK

A unique design characteristic of an area-specific curet is the relationship of the face of the working-end to the lower shank. Its design differs from that of sickle scalers and universal curets. The face of a sickle scaler or a universal curet meets the lower shank at a 90-degree angle. In contrast—as depicted in Figure 19-3—the face of an area-specific curet is tilted in relationship to the lower shank.

- The tilted face on an area-specific curet causes one cutting edge—the working cutting edge—to be lower than the other cutting edge on each working-end.
- The nonworking cutting edge of an area-specific curet is too close to the lower shank to be used for periodontal instrumentation.
- *Only the lower cutting edge of an area-specific curet is used for periodontal instrumentation* (Fig. 19-4).

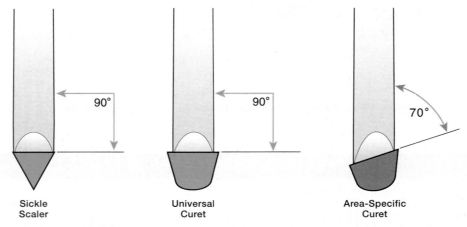

Figure 19-3. Relationship of the Face to the Lower Shank. The face of a sickle scaler or universal curet is at a 90-degree angle to the lower shank. The cutting edges on these instruments are level. The face of an area-specific curet is tilted in relationship to the lower shank. The tilted face causes one cutting edge—the working cutting edge—to be lower than the other cutting edge on each working-end.

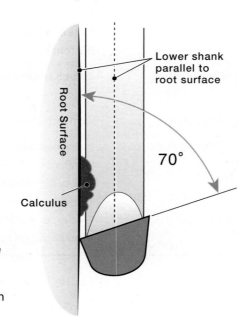

Figure 19-4. Self-Angulated Curet. *The lower cutting edge of an area-specific curet is automatically at the correct angulation for periodontal instrumentation when the lower shank is parallel to the tooth surface to be instrumented.* Instruments with this design characteristic are termed **self-angulated**.

SKILL BUILDING
Identifying the Lower Cutting Edge

Since the face of an area-specific curet is tilted in relationship to the lower shank, one cutting edge is lower than the other cutting edge. The lower cutting edge tilts away from the lower shank.

* Only the lower cutting edge of an area-specific curet is used for periodontal instrumentation.
* The higher cutting edge is angled away from the soft tissue wall of the periodontal pocket to protect the soft tissue and facilitate subgingival instrumentation. The higher cutting edge is not used for periodontal instrumentation.
* The lower cutting edge is identified by holding the instrument with the toe facing the clinician with the *lower shank perpendicular to the floor*. This technique is pictured in Figure 19-5 and described in Box 19-1.

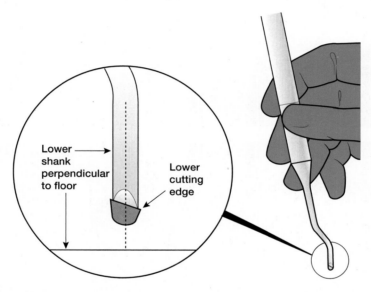

Figure 19-5. Identifying the Lower Cutting Edge. Hold the instrument as pictured here with the toe facing you and the lower shank perpendicular—at a 90-degree angle—to the floor.

Box 19-1 **Identifying the Lower Cutting Edge**

Follow these steps to identify the working cutting edge of an area-specific curet.

1. Hold the instrument so that you are **looking directly at the toe** of the working-end.

2. Raise or lower the instrument handle until the **lower shank is perpendicular (⊥) to the floor**.

3. Look closely at the working-end and note that one of the cutting edges is lower—closer to the floor—than the other cutting edge.

4. The **lower cutting edge is the working cutting edge**—the cutting edge used for instrumentation.

THE GRACEY CURET SERIES

Area-specific curets were developed through the genius of Dr. Clayton Gracey who envisioned a periodontal instrument that would reach root surfaces within deep periodontal pockets without trauma to the pocket epithelium. In the early 1940s, Dr. Gracey worked with Hugo Friedman of Hu-Friedy Manufacturing Company to develop 14 single-ended area-specific Gracey curets (Fig. 19-6). The Gracey instrument series continues to be popular today and is the basis for several other area-specific curets. The Gracey series continues to evolve and is currently available in standard, rigid, extended shanks; and miniature and micro-miniature working-ends.

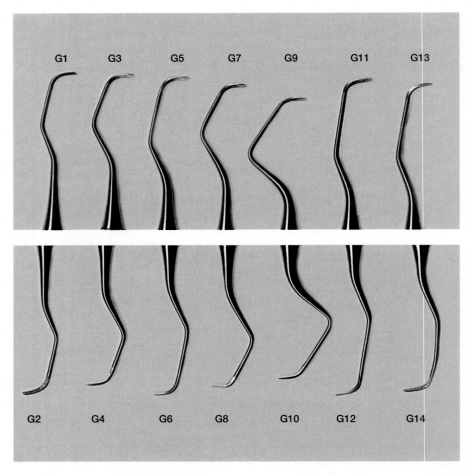

Figure 19-6. The Standard Gracey Curet Series. Depicted above are the 14 Gracey instruments, Gracey 1 to Gracey 14, designed by Dr. Clayton Gracey.

APPLICATION AND COMPARISON OF GRACEY CURET DESIGNS

The original Gracey series contains 14 curets, Gracey 1 to 14 (Table 19-2). In practice, rarely are all 14 curets used on a single patient's mouth. Over the years, clinicians have found that they are able to instrument the mouth using a fewer number of Gracey curets. A set of three or four Gracey curets may be adequate to instrument the entire dentition. Over the years, many modifications have been made to the standard Gracey curet design. Table 19-3 summarizes these design modifications.

TABLE 19-2. THE GRACEY INSTRUMENT SERIES	
Curet	**Area of Application**
Gracey 1 and 2 Gracey 3 and 4	Anterior teeth: all tooth surfaces[G]
Gracey 5 and 6	Anterior teeth: all tooth surfaces[G] Premolar teeth: all tooth surfaces[G] Molar teeth: facial, lingual, and mesial surfaces
Gracey 7 and 8 Gracey 9 and 10	Anterior teeth: all surfaces Premolar teeth: all surfaces Posterior teeth: facial and lingual surfaces[G]
Gracey 11 and 12	Anterior teeth: mesial and distal surfaces Posterior teeth: mesial surfaces only[G] Posterior teeth: facial, lingual, and mesial surfaces
Gracey 13 and 14	Anterior teeth: mesial and distal surfaces Posterior teeth: distal surfaces[G]
Gracey 15 and 16	Posterior teeth: facial, lingual, and mesial surfaces (Not part of the original Gracey series)
Gracey 17 and 18	Posterior teeth: distal surfaces (Not part of the original Gracey series)

The [G] symbol indicates the areas of application as originally designated by Dr. Gracey.

TABLE 19-3. COMPARISON OF GRACEY DESIGNS

Instrument	Design Features
Standard	• Shank Length: standard design • Shank Diameter: standard diameter • Working-End Length: standard length • Working-End Width: standard width
Rigid	• Shank Length: standard length • Shank Diameter: thicker shank • Working-End Length: standard length • Working-End Width: standard width
Extended Lower Shank	• Shank Length: lower shank 3 mm longer than standard • Shank Diameter: standard shank diameter • Working-End Length: standard length • Working-End Width: decreased by 10% compared to standard
Rigid Extended Lower Shank	• Shank Length: lower shank 3 mm longer than standard • Shank Diameter: thicker shank • Working-End Length: standard length • Working-End Width: decreased by 10% compared to standard
Extended Lower Shank and Miniature Working-End	• Shank Length: lower shank 3 mm longer than standard • Shank Diameter: standard shank diameter • Working-End Length: decreased by 50% compared to standard • Working-End Width: decreased by 10% compared to standard
Rigid Extended Lower Shank and Miniature Working-End	• Shank Length: lower shank 3 mm longer than standard • Shank Diameter: thicker shank • Working-End Length: decreased by 50% compared to standard • Working-End Width: decreased by 10% compared to standard
Extended Lower Shank and Micro-Miniature Working-End	• Shank Length: lower shank 3 mm longer than standard • Shank Diameter: thicker functional shank with tapered lower shank • Working-End Length: decreased by 50% compared to standard • Working-End Width: decreased by 20% compared to miniature working-end

Section 2
Technique Practice—Anterior Teeth

SKILL BUILDING
Selecting the Correct Working-End for an Anterior Tooth

Only one cutting edge per working-end of an area-specific curet is used for instrumentation. The clinician observes the face of the working-end as it is adapted to the tooth surface. When the working-end is adapted to the facial (or lingual) surface, the *face* of correct working-end *tilts slightly toward the tooth* and is partially hidden from view.

- Figure 19-7 depicts selection of the correct working-end on an anterior tooth with the face tilting toward the tooth surface.
- Figure 19-8 depicts the incorrect working-end with the face tilted away from the tooth; if used beneath the gingival margin this working-end would traumatize the soft tissue wall of the pocket or sulcus (injure the issue soft tissue lining of the sulcus or pocket).

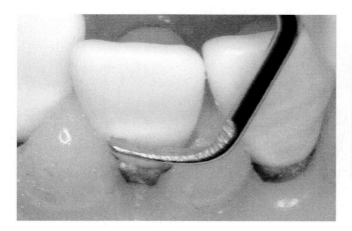

Figure 19-7. Correct Working-End.
- The correct working-end is selected if **the *instrument face* tilts toward the tooth surface** when placed against the midline of the facial (or lingual surface).
- Looking down on the working-end, the face is partially hidden.

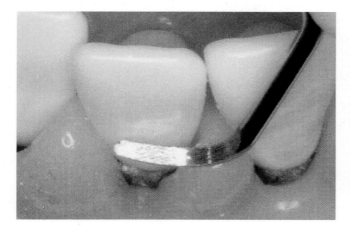

Figure 19-8. Incorrect Working-End.
- The incorrect working-end is selected if **the *instrument face* tilts slightly away from the tooth surface** when placed against the midline of the facial (or lingual surface).
- Looking down on the working-end, the entire face is clearly visible.
This working-end would traumatize the soft tissue if used subgingivally!

APPLICATION OF THE CUTTING EDGES TO ANTERIOR TEETH

Only one cutting edge *per working-end* of an area-specific curet is used for instrumentation of the anterior teeth.

- Figure 19-9 depicts the two cutting edges that are found on a Gracey 1/2 instrument or a Gracey 3/4 curet.
- Figure 19-10 depicts application of the cutting edges of a Gracey 1/2 or a Gracey 3/4 curet to the facial aspect of the maxillary anterior teeth. One cutting edge of the curet adapts to the anterior surfaces toward while the second cutting edge adapts to the anterior surfaces away from the clinician.

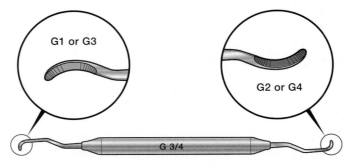

Figure 19-9. Application to Anterior Surfaces. A double-ended area-specific curet has two lower cutting edges that are used on anterior tooth surfaces.

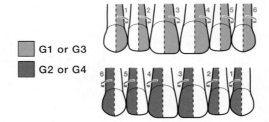

Figure 19-10. Application to Anterior Surfaces. This illustration indicates how the cutting edges of a Gracey 1/2 or Gracey 3/4 are applied to the surfaces toward and surfaces away on the facial aspect of the anterior tooth surfaces.

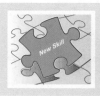

SKILL BUILDING
Step-By-Step Technique on Maxillary Central Incisor

Directions:

- Follow steps 1 to 8 pictured in Figures 19-11 to 19-18 to practice use of an area-specific curet on the maxillary anterior teeth.
- *Use a periodontal typodont* (1–3). *Practice insertion with the gingiva in place, then remove the gingiva to practice making calculus removal strokes on the cervical thirds of the roots.*
- Remember: "Me, My patient, My light, My dominant hand, My nondominant hand, My finger rest, My adaptation."

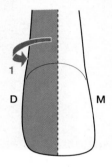

1. **Figure 19-11. Tooth.** As an introduction to using an area-specific curet on the anterior teeth, first practice on the *maxillary right central incisor, facial aspect*.
   Right-handed clinicians—*surface toward.*
   Left-handed clinicians—*surface away.*

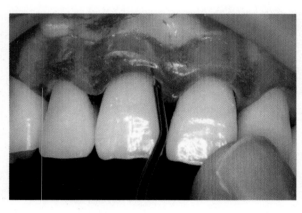

2. **Figure 19-12. Get Ready and Insert.**
   - Select the correct working-end and place it in the Get Ready Zone.
   - The toe of the working-end should aim toward the distal surface.
   - Insert the working-end to the base of the pocket.

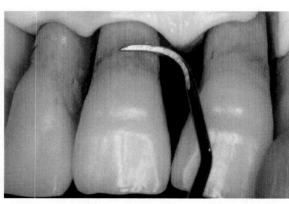

3. **Figure 19-13. Adapt the Toe-Third to the Midline.** Adapt the toe-third to the root surface. *Imagine "locking" the toe-third against the root surface.*

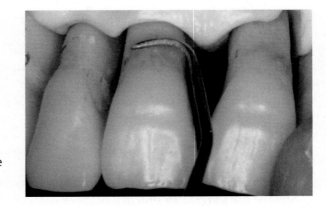

4. **Figure 19-14.** **Work Across Facial Surface.** Make a series of short, precise strokes across the facial surface toward the distofacial line angle.

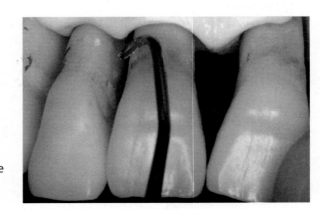

5. **Figure 19-15.** **Roll Handle at Line Angle.** Roll the handle slightly to maintain adaptation of the toe-third at the distofacial line angle.

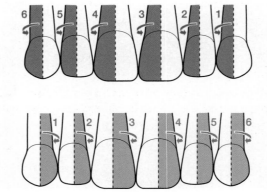

6. **Figure 19-16.** **Distal Surface.** Work at least halfway across the distal surface. The other half of the distal surface will be instrumented from the lingual aspect of the tooth.

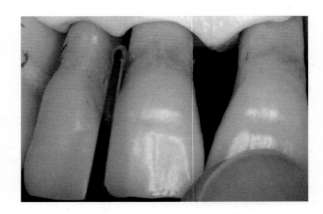

7. **Figure 19-17.** **Sequence.** Next, use the sequence shown in this illustration to instrument the colored tooth surfaces of the facial aspect. Begin with the left canine and end with the right canine.

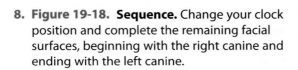

8. **Figure 19-18.** **Sequence.** Change your clock position and complete the remaining facial surfaces, beginning with the right canine and ending with the left canine.

Section 3
Technique Practice—Posterior Teeth

APPLICATION OF THE CUTTING EDGES TO POSTERIOR TEETH

At least two double-ended area-specific instruments are needed for instrumentation of the posterior teeth. Commonly, two to three double-ended Gracey curets are used to instrument the posterior sextants (Fig. 19-19). For example, a clinician might select one of the following combinations of curet working-ends:

- The Gracey 11, 12, 13, and 14 might be selected for the posterior teeth.
- The Gracey 15, 16, 17, and 18 curets could comprise a set of curets for the posterior teeth.
- The Gracey 9, 10 11, 12, 13, and 14 is an example of a set of six curets for the posterior teeth.
- The Gracey 7, 8, 15, 16, 17, and 18 could comprise a set of six curets for the posterior teeth.

Figure 19-19 depicts some of the Gracey curets commonly used on the posterior teeth. Figure 19-20 depicts the application of the curets shown in Figure 19-19 to a posterior sextant.

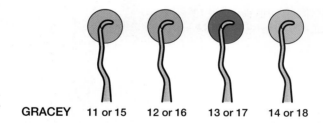

GRACEY   11 or 15   12 or 16   13 or 17   14 or 18

Figure 19-19. Gracey Set for Posterior Teeth. Several Gracey curets are required to instrument a posterior sextant. To instrument a posterior sextant, a clinician might select a set of Gracey curets such as the 11/12 and 13/14 or the 15/16 and 17/18.

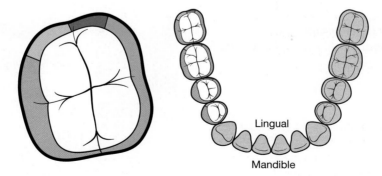

Lingual

Mandible

Figure 19-20. Application of Gracey Cutting Edges to Posterior Surfaces. The illustration indicates how the cutting edges of a Gracey curet are applied to the tooth surfaces of the mandibular right first molar and the mandibular right posterior sextant.

SKILL BUILDING
Selecting the Correct Working-End for a Posterior Tooth

Use the lower shank as the visual clue for selecting the correct working-end for use on a posterior tooth. Think: Posterior = Parallel. Functional shank up and over!

- Figure 19-21 shows selection of the correct working-end for use on the distal surface of the second premolar tooth. Note that the lower shank is parallel to the distal surface.
- Figure 19-22 shows the incorrect working-end for use on the distal surface of the second premolar tooth. Note that the lower shank of this working-end goes "down and around" the facial surface of the premolar.

Figure 19-21. Visual Clue for the Correct Working-End. The correct working-end is selected when:
- The *lower shank is parallel* to the distal surface
- The *functional shank goes "up and over the tooth."*

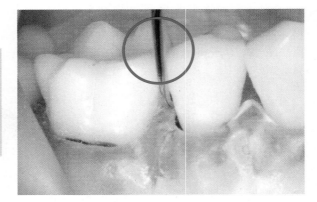

Figure 19-22. Visual Clue for the Incorrect Working-End. The incorrect working-end is selected if the:
- The *lower shank is not parallel*
- The *functional shank is "down and around the tooth."*

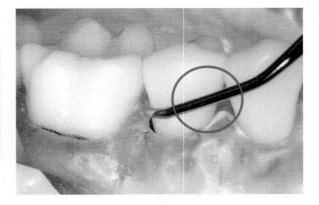

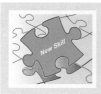

SKILL BUILDING
Step-By-Step Technique on Mandibular First Molar

Directions:

- Follow steps 1 to 18 as shown in Figures 19-23 to 19-40 to practice use of an area-specific curet on the mandibular right posterior sextant.
- *Use a periodontal typodont* (1–3). *Practice insertion with the gingiva in place, then remove the gingiva to practice making calculus removal strokes on the cervical thirds of the roots.*
- Remember: "Me, My patient, My light, My dominant hand, My nondominant hand, My finger rest, My adaptation."

1. **Figure 19-23. Begin With the Distal Surfaces.**
   - As an introduction to the area-specific curet, first practice on the mandibular right first molar.
   - *Use a distal area-specific curet on the distal surface.*

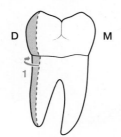

2. **Figure 19-24. Get Ready.**
   - Place the distal curet at the distofacial line angle in the "Get Ready Zone."
   - The toe should aim toward the back of the mouth because this is the direction in which you are working.

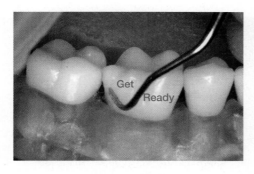

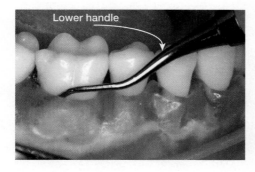

3. **Figure 19-25. Insert.** Lower handle and gently slide the working-end beneath the gingival margin.

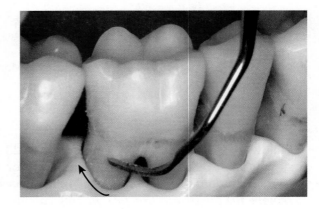

4. **Figure 19-26. Work Across Distal Surface.**
   - Return the handle to an upright position.
   - "Lock" the toe-third against the distofacial line angle.
   - Instrument at least halfway across the distal surface from the facial aspect.

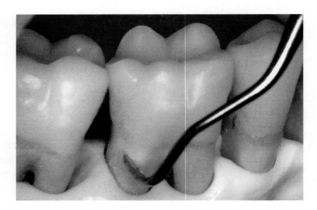

5. **Figure 19-27. Roll the Handle.** Roll the instrument handle to maintain adaptation as you work around the distofacial line angle and on to the distal surface.

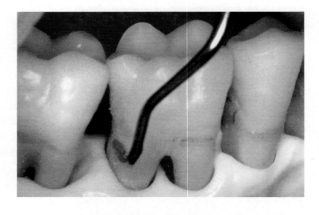

6. **Figure 19-28. Continue Strokes.** Continue making a series of short, precise strokes across the distal surface.

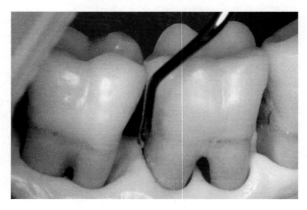

7. **Figure 19-29. Work Across Distal Surface.** Instrument at least halfway across the distal surface from the facial aspect.

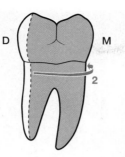

8. **Figure 19-30. Instrument of the Facial and Mesial Surfaces.** Use a facial or mesial curet for the facial surface of the tooth, beginning at the distofacial line angle.

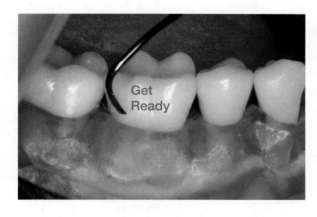

9. **Figure 19-31. Get Ready.** Place the mesial curet in the Get Ready Zone with the toe aiming toward the mesial surface in preparation for insertion.

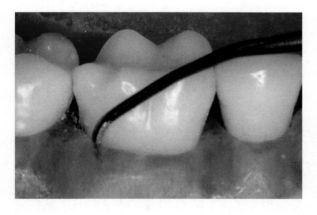

10. **Figure 19-32. Insert.**
    - Lower the instrument handle and gently slide the working-end beneath the gingival margin.
    - Insert the curet to the base of the periodontal pocket.

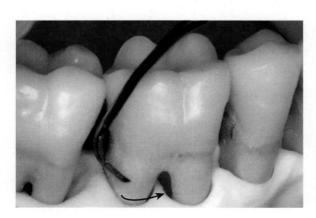

11. **Figure 19-33. Adapt the Toe-Third.**
    - Return the handle to the upright position.
    - "Lock" the toe-third to the root surface at the distofacial line angle.

12. **Figure 19-34. Instrument the Facial Surface.**
Make a series of oblique calculus removal strokes across the facial surface. Maintain the working-end of the curet beneath the gingival margin. Removing the curet from the sulcus or pocket with each stroke will injure the marginal gingival.

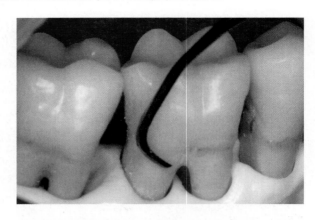

13. **Figure 19-35. Continue Strokes.** Continue making a series of short, precise instrumentation strokes across the facial surface.

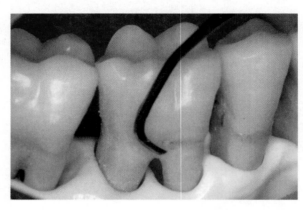

14. **Figure 19-36. Continue Strokes.** Continue strokes across the facial surface.

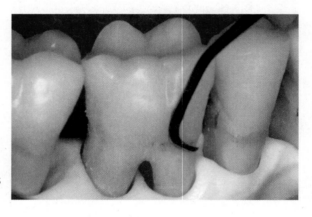

15. **Figure 19-37. Roll the Handle.** As you approach the mesiofacial line angle, roll the handle slightly to maintain adaptation.

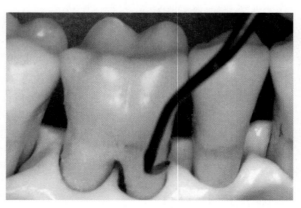

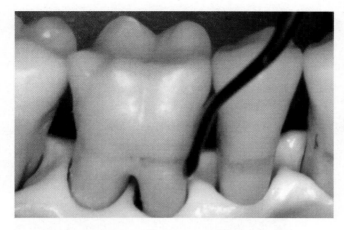

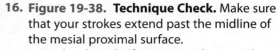

16. **Figure 19-38. Technique Check.** Make sure that your strokes extend past the midline of the mesial proximal surface.
    - Work at least halfway across the mesial surface from the facial aspect.
    - The other half of the mesial surface will be instrumented from the lingual aspect.

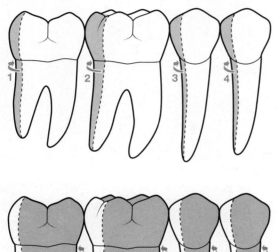

17. **Figure 19-39. Sequence for Distal Surfaces.** Use the sequence shown in this illustration for the distal surfaces in the sextant. It is easier to begin with the posterior-most molar and move forward toward the first premolar because of the pressure exerted against your hand by the patient's cheek.

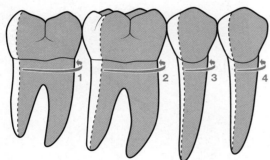

18. **Figure 19-40. Sequence for Facial and Mesial Surfaces.** Use the sequence shown in this illustration to instrument the facial and mesial surfaces in the sextant.

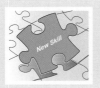

SKILL BUILDING
Use of Horizontal Strokes Below the Gingival Margin

Horizontal strokes are extremely useful in removing calculus deposits that are located (1) near the distofacial or distolingual line angle of posterior teeth and (2) at the midline of the facial or lingual surfaces of anterior teeth. Figures 19-41 to 19-43 depict the use of horizontal strokes on anterior and posterior teeth.

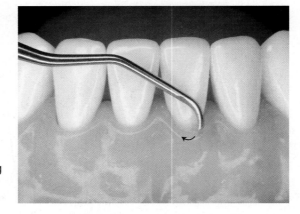

Figure 19-41. Anterior Teeth. The technique for making horizontal strokes with an area-specific curet is similar to that used with a universal curet.

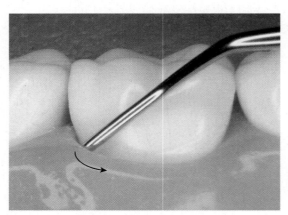

Figure 19-42. Posterior Teeth. Horizontal calculus removal strokes are very effective in removing deposits from the line angle region of posterior teeth.

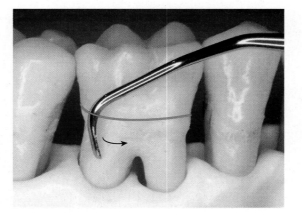

Figure 19-43. Technique Check. The gingiva has been removed from the typodont in this photograph to provide a view of the working-end of an area-specific curet during a horizontal stroke.

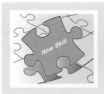

SKILL BUILDING
Step-By-Step Technique on Maxillary First Molar

Directions:

- Follow steps 1 to 10 as pictured in Figures 19-44 to 19-53 to practice use of an area-specific curet on the maxillary left posterior sextant.
- *Use a periodontal typodont (1–3). Practice insertion with the gingiva in place, then remove the gingiva to practice making calculus removal strokes on the cervical thirds of the roots.*
- Remember: "Me, My patient, My light, My dominant hand, My nondominant hand, My finger rest, My adaptation."

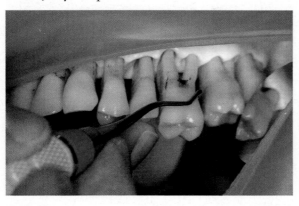

1. **Figure 19-44. Get Ready and Insert.**
   - Turn the toe toward the distal surface. Position the working-end in the Get Ready Zone.
   - Raise the instrument handle and establish a 0-degree angulation.
   - Gently slide the working-end beneath the gingival margin.

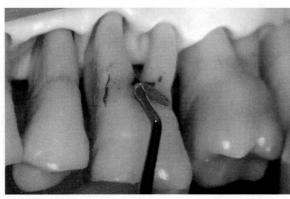

2. **Figure 19-45. Establish Angulation and Lock-Toe Third.**
   - After insertion, return the handle to the correct position.
   - Establish an 80-degree angulation in preparation for a calculus removal stroke.
   - Adapt the toe-third of the working-end to the distofacial line angle. Imagine "locking" the toe-third against the tooth surface.

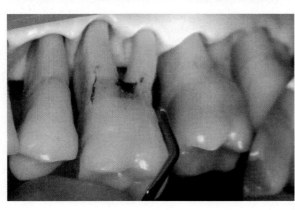

3. **Figure 19-46. Instrument the Distal Surface.**
   Instrument from the distofacial line angle to the midline of the distal surface.

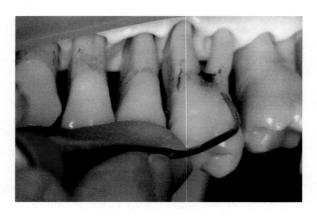

4. **Figure 19-47. Insert on Facial Surface.**
   - Use the facial curet for the facial surface.
   - Place the working-end in the Get Ready Zone on the middle-third of the facial surface near the distofacial line angle.
   - Raise the handle and slide the working-end beneath the gingival margin.

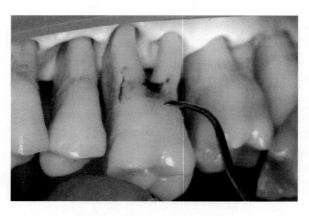

5. **Figure 19-48. Begin at Distofacial Line Angle.**
   Lower the handle to the correct position. Begin instrumentation of the facial surface starting at the distofacial line angle.

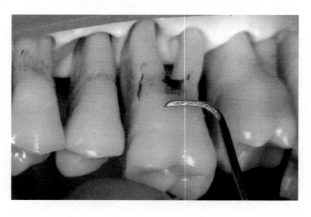

6. **Figure 19-49. Instrument the Facial Surface.**
   Work across the facial surface keeping the toe-third adapted.

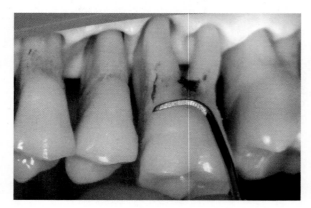

7. **Figure 19-50. Continue Across the Facial Surface.** Make a series of tiny oblique calculus removal strokes across the facial surface.

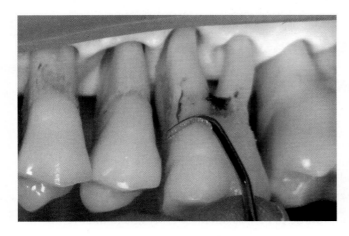

8. **Figure 19-51. Roll the Instrument Handle.** As you approach the mesiofacial line angle, roll the handle slightly to maintain adaptation.

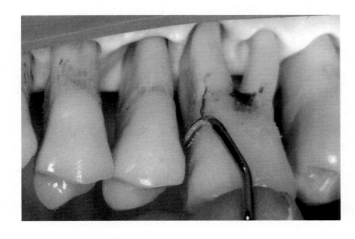

9. **Figure 19-52. Instrument the Mesial Surface.** Work across the mesial surface taking care to assure that the toe-third remains adapted.

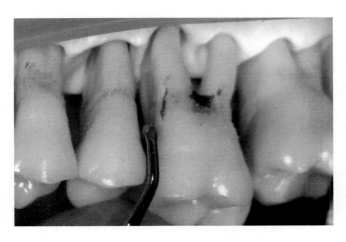

10. **Figure 19-53. Instrument to Midline of Mesial Surface.** Instrument at least halfway across the mesial surface from the facial aspect.

Section 4
Instrumentation Techniques on Root Surfaces

THREE TYPES OF INSTRUMENTATION STROKES FOR ROOT INSTRUMENTATION

Area-specific curets are used to assess characteristics of the root surface, remove biofilm and calculus deposits, and refine root surfaces to facilitate soft tissue healing. Each of these functions requires an instrumentation stroke with unique properties. Although instrumentation strokes are discussed in earlier modules, now is a good time to review their use during periodontal instrumentation. Table 19-4 reviews the characteristics of these instrumentation strokes.

1. Assessment Stroke ("Feeling" Stroke): Evaluation of the Root Surface. During calculus removal, assessment strokes are used with area-specific curets to locate calculus deposits.
   A. When all deposits detectable with a curet have been removed, a definitive evaluation of the root surface should be made using an explorer.
   B. Because the explorer provides superior tactile information, it is common to detect some remaining calculus deposits with an explorer that could not be detected with a curet.
2. Calculus Removal Stroke ("Work" Stroke): Complete Removal of Calculus
   A. Calculus removal strokes are used with area-specific curets to remove calculus deposits from the tooth.
   B. Calculus removal strokes are not used on tooth surfaces that are free of calculus deposits. Periodontal typodonts with flexible "gingiva" are recommended for students learning instrumentation. *Periodontal typodonts allow students to practice insertion into periodontal pockets. Instrumentation practice on periodontal typodonts is ideal since skilled instrumentation of root surfaces is vital to successful dental hygiene therapy* (2,4).
3. Root Debridement Stroke ("Finishing" Stroke): Refines to Facilitate Tissue Healing
   A. Root debridement strokes are used with area-specific curets to remove residual calculus deposits and plaque biofilms from root surfaces exposed due to gingival recession or within deep periodontal pockets. **Residual calculus deposits** are very tiny deposits remaining on the root surface that can be removed using the lighter pressure of a root debridement stroke.
   B. Conservation of cementum is an important goal of instrumentation.
      1. Research studies indicate that complete removal of cementum from the root surface, exposing the ends of dentinal tubules, may allow bacteria to travel from the periodontal pocket into the pulp in some instances (5). In addition, excessive removal of cementum may lead to dentinal sensitivity.
      2. Over the course of many years, overzealous instrumentation can result in removal of all cementum and exposure of the underlying dentin. Within deep periodontal pockets, a plastic "implant" curet or a slim-tipped ultrasonic instrument may be used for biofilm removal when no residual calculus deposits are present.
   C. Conservation of cementum should not be confused with a failure to remove calculus deposits.
      1. The goal of periodontal instrumentation is the *complete* removal of calculus deposits and bacterial products contaminating the tooth surfaces.
      2. Calculus deposits are always covered with living bacterial biofilms that are associated with continuing inflammation if not removed.

TABLE 19-4. STROKE CHARACTERISTICS WITH AREA-SPECIFIC CURETS

	Assessment Stroke	Calculus Removal Stroke	Root Debridement Stroke
Purpose	To assess tooth anatomy; detect calculus and other plaque-retentive factors; the "feeling" stroke	To lift calculus deposits off of the tooth surface	To completely remove all residual (remaining) calculus deposits; disrupt plaque biofilm from root surfaces within deep periodontal pockets
Lateral pressure	Contact with tooth surface, but little pressure	Firm pressure against tooth surface	Moderate pressure against tooth surface
Character	Flowing, feather-light stroke of moderate length	Brief, tiny biting stroke ("bite and release")	Shaving stroke of moderate length
Number	Many overlapping strokes to evaluate the entire root surface	Limited to areas with calculus deposits	Many, multidirectional strokes; covering the entire subgingival root surface

TAILORING STROKE PRESSURE TO THE TASK AT HAND

1. **Three Pressure Forces of the Instrumentation Stroke.** Three types of force are applied during periodontal instrumentation: (1) pinch pressure of the fingers in the modified pen grasp, (2) pressure of the fulcrum to stabilize the hand, and (3) lateral pressure against the tooth during the instrument stroke. These three forces change according to the task—assessment, calculus removal, or root surface debridement. Table 19-5 and Box 19-2 review the correct use of stroke pressure during periodontal instrumentation with an area-specific curet.
2. **The Misuse of Constant Pressure**
   A. Unfortunately, novice clinicians often apply constant firm pressure—with all three forces—in an attempt to control instrumentation strokes. This use of constant pressure is soon stored in the muscle memory and becomes an ongoing bad habit (6–21).
   B. *Researches suggest that use of unnecessary force in a pinch grip is the greatest contributing risk factor in the development of injury among dental hygienists* (10,11).
3. **When to Apply Pressure.** The three most important concepts regarding the use of pressure during periodontal instrumentation are:
   A. **Gauge the Amount of Pressure.** Use as little force as possible to accomplish the task at hand.
   B. **Apply Only Brief Pressure.** *Apply pressure only just prior to and during—NEVER between—instrumentation strokes.*
   C. **Relax After Each Stroke.** PAUSE and RELAX your fingers between each stroke.

TABLE 19-5. BALANCING OF FORCES WITH INSTRUMENTATION STROKES

	Assessment Stroke	Calculus Removal Stroke	Root Surface Debridement Stroke
Pinch Grasp	Relaxed	Firm (but not "death grip")	Moderate
Fulcrum Pressure	Light	Firm	Moderate
Lateral Pressure	Feather light	Firm	Moderate
Character of Stroke	Long, gliding	Short, biting "Bite and release"	Longer, shaving

---

Box 19-2 **Ergonomics of Pressure During Instrumentation**

- **Gauge the Amount of Pressure.** Use as little force as possible to accomplish the task at hand.
- **Apply Only Brief Pressure.** Apply pressure only just prior to and during—NEVER between—instrumentation strokes.
- **Relax After Each Stroke.** PAUSE and RELAX your fingers between each stroke.

Section 5
Production of a Root Debridement Stroke

USE OF MULTIDIRECTIONAL STROKES ON ROOT SURFACES

The use of multidirectional strokes is an important technique for successful instrumentation of root surfaces. Frequently the root surface is hidden beneath the gingival margin within a deep periodontal pocket; thus, the clinician cannot see the deposits. The use of multidirectional strokes assures that every square millimeter of the root surface is assessed for the presence of calculus deposits. Although the concept of multidirectional strokes is presented in earlier modules, it is reviewed here because area-specific curets should be used with multidirectional strokes to assure complete calculus removal beneath the gingival margin within a periodontal pocket (22–26).

1. **Multidirectional strokes** combine the use of three stroke directions: vertical, oblique, and horizontal strokes. Figure 19-54 depicts how these three stroke directions combine to create a multidirectional pattern covering the root surface coronal to the epithelial attachment.
2. The combination of vertical, oblique, and horizontal instrumentation strokes creates a **multidirectional grid** that covers the entire root surface located coronal (above) the soft tissue base of a periodontal pocket.
3. Use of the three stroke directions separately, in sequence, covers the root surface with a grid-like pattern. The clinician covers the root surface using one stroke direction, followed by a second different stroke direction, and finally uses the third stroke direction.
   A. So, for example, the clinician might begin by covering the entire root surface with a series of vertical strokes.
   B. Next the clinician may make a series of strokes in an oblique direction.
   C. Finally, the clinician makes a series of horizontal strokes over the root surface. *It is important to note that the working-end should not come in contact with the soft tissue base of the pocket when using a horizontal stroke.*

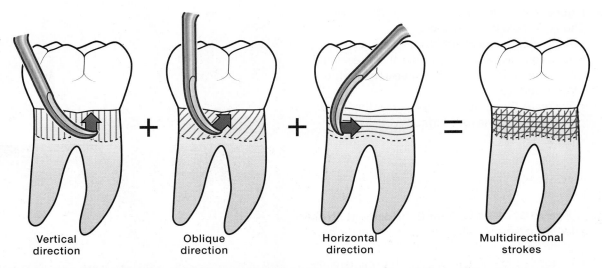

| Vertical direction | Oblique direction | Horizontal direction | Multidirectional strokes |

Figure 19-54. Multidirectional Strokes for Root Instrumentation. Use of three stroke directions, one-by-one in sequence, creates a grid pattern of multidirectional strokes on the root surface. For example as depicted here, the clinician begins with vertical strokes, then oblique strokes, finally horizontal strokes. These strokes combine to create a grid of strokes that cover the entire root surface coronal to the soft tissue base of the periodontal pocket.

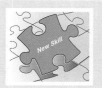

SKILL BUILDING
Root Debridement Strokes

Directions: Follow steps 1 to 3 as shown in Figures 19-55 to 19-57.

- *Right-handed clinicians* work on the mandibular right first molar, facial aspect: *Left-handed clinicians* work on the mandibular left first molar, facial aspect.
- Use a *periodontal typodont with flexible "gingiva"* so that you can practice as if working in a deep periodontal pocket (Fig. 19-56). Use an *area-specific curet* such as a *Gracey curet* for this technique practice.

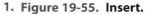

1. **Figure 19-55. Insert.**
   - Insert at a 0-degree angulation with the lower shank close to the tooth surface.
   - Gently slide the working-end beneath the gingival margin and onto the facial surface of the root.
   - *Imagine the face sliding along the facial surface all the way to the base of the pocket.*

2. **Figure 19-56. Prepare for Stroke: Tilt Lower Shank Toward Root Surface.**
   - A root debridement stroke is a shaving stroke.
   - To accomplish a shaving stroke, the face should be approximately at a 60-degree angle to the tooth surface.
   - To create, this angulation, simply tilt the lower shank toward the root surface.

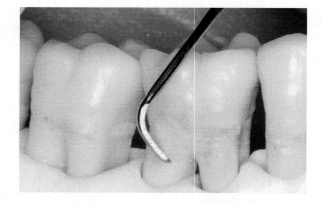

3. **Figure 19-57. Make a Root Debridement Stroke.**
   - Initiate *a light, shaving stroke away from the base of the pocket.*
   - A root debridement stroke is a *lighter* and *longer stroke* than a calculus removal stroke.
   - Practice making a series of strokes to create a multidirectional grid of strokes over the root surface.

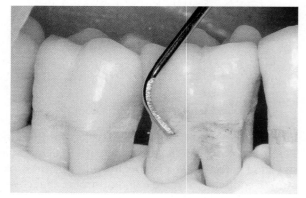

Section 6
Design Overview: Scalers and Curets

TABLE 19-6. SUMMARY SHEET: DESIGN ANALYSIS OF SICKLES AND CURETS

Characteristic	Instrument	Critique
Back pointed	Sickle	Advantage = strong, "bulky" working-end Disadvantage = not recommended for use on root surfaces
Back rounded	Universal and area-specific	Advantage = used subgingivally without tissue trauma Disadvantage = none
Tip (pointed)	Sickle	Advantage = provides good access to proximal surfaces on anterior crowns and enamel surfaces apical to contact areas of posterior teeth Disadvantage = sharp point can gouge cemental surfaces
Toe (rounded)	Universal and area-specific	Advantage = adapts well to convex, rounded root surfaces and root concavities Disadvantage = is wider than a pointed tip and, therefore, more difficult to adapt to proximal surfaces of anterior crowns
Curved cutting edge	Area-specific	Advantage = enhances adaptation to rounded root surfaces and root concavities Disadvantage = none
Face perpendicular to lower shank; Level cutting edges	Sickle and universal	Advantage = efficient, two cutting-edges per working-end both of which can be used for calculus removal Disadvantage = level cutting edges mean that the lower shank must be tilted slightly toward the tooth for correct angulation
Face tilts in relation to lower shank; Uneven cutting edges	Area-specific	Advantage = working cutting edge is self-angulated Disadvantage = only one working cutting edge per working-end means frequent instrument changes

References

1. Dufour LA, Bissell HS. Periodontal attachment loss induced by mechanical subgingival instrumentation in shallow sulci. *J Dent Hyg.* 2002;76(3):207–212.

2. Ruhling A, Konig J, Rolf H, Kocher T, Schwahn C, Plagmann HC. Learning root debridement with curettes and power-driven instruments. Part II: Clinical results following mechanical, nonsurgical therapy. *J Clin Periodontol.* 2003;30(7):611–615.

3. Alves RV, Machion L, Casati MZ, Nociti Junior FH, Sallum AW, Sallum EA. Attachment loss after scaling and root planing with different instruments. A clinical study. *J Clin Periodontol.* 2004;31(1):12–15.

4. Rucker LM, Gibson G, McGregor C. Getting the "feel" of it: the non-visual component of dimensional accuracy during operative tooth preparation. *J Can Dent Assoc.* 1990;56(10):937–941.

5. Berutti E. Microleakage of human saliva through dentinal tubules exposed at the cervical level in teeth treated endodontically. *J Endod.* 1996;22(11):579–582. .

6. Bernard BP. Musculoskeletal disorders and workplace factors. In: *U.S. Department of Health and Human Services,* ed. Cincinnati, OH: NIOSH (National Institute for Occupational Safety); 1997.

7. Kao SY. Carpal tunnel syndrome as an occupational disease. *J Am Board Fam Pract.* 2003;16(6):533–542.

8. Nathan PA, Istvan JA, Meadows KD. A longitudinal study of predictors of research-defined carpal tunnel syndrome in industrial workers: findings at 17 years. *J Hand Surg.* 2005;30(6):593–598.

9. Nathan PA, Meadows KD, Istvan JA. Predictors of carpal tunnel syndrome: an 11-year study of industrial workers. *J Hand Surg Am.* 2002;27(4):644–651.

10. Sanders MA, Turcotte CM. Strategies to reduce work-related musculoskeletal disorders in dental hygienists: two case studies. *J Hand Ther.* 2002;15(4):363–374.

11. Sanders MJ, Turcotte CA. Ergonomic strategies for dental professionals. *Work.* 1997;8(1):55–72.

12. Graham C. Ergonomics in dentistry, Part 1. *Dent Today.* 2002;21(4):98–103.

13. Hayes M, Cockrell D, Smith DR. A systematic review of musculoskeletal disorders among dental professionals. *Int J Dent Hyg.* 2009;7(3):159–165.

14. Hayes MJ, Smith DR, Cockrell D. Prevalence and correlates of musculoskeletal disorders among Australian dental hygiene students. *Int J Dent Hyg.* 2009;7(3):176–181.

15. Hayes MJ, Smith DR, Cockrell D. An international review of musculoskeletal disorders in the dental hygiene profession. *Int Dent J.* 2010;60(5):343–352.

16. Hayes MJ, Smith DR, Taylor JA. Musculoskeletal disorders and symptom severity among Australian dental hygienists. *BMC Res Notes.* 2013;6:250.

17. Hayes MJ, Smith DR, Taylor JA. Musculoskeletal disorders in a 3 year longitudinal cohort of dental hygiene students. *J Dent Hyg.* 2014;88(1):36–41.

18. Hayes MJ, Taylor JA, Smith DR. Predictors of work-related musculoskeletal disorders among dental hygienists. *Int J Dent Hyg.* 2012;10(4):265–269.

19. Kanteshwari K, Sridhar R, Mishra AK, Shirahatti R, Maru R, Bhusari P. Correlation of awareness and practice of working postures with prevalence of musculoskeletal disorders among dental professionals. *Gen Dent.* 2011;59(6):476–483; quiz 84–85.

20. Khan SA, Chew KY. Effect of working characteristics and taught ergonomics on the prevalence of musculoskeletal disorders amongst dental students. *BMC Musculoskelet Disord.* 2013;14:118.

21. Roquelaure Y, Mechali S, Dano C, et al. Occupational and personal risk factors for carpal tunnel syndrome in industrial workers. *Scand J Work Environ Health.* 1997;23(5):364–369.

22. Checchi L, Montevecchi M, Checchi V, Zappulla F. The relationship between bleeding on probing and subgingival deposits. An endoscopical evaluation. *Open Dent J.* 2009;3:154–160.

23. Hodges K. Revisiting instrumentation in anterior segments. *Dimensi Dent Hyg.* 2007;5(2):30–33.

24. Hodges K. Channeling for success. Part 1. *Dimens Dent Hyg.* 2014;11(5):34–37.

25. Stambaugh RV. A clinician's 3-year experience with perioscopy. *Compend Contin Educ Dent.* 2002;23(11A):1061–1070.

26. Wilson TG, Harrel SK, Nunn ME, Francis B, Webb K. The relationship between the presence of tooth-borne subgingival deposits and inflammation found with a dental endoscope. *J Periodontol.* 2008;79(11):2029–2035.

Section 7
Skill Application

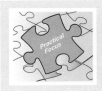

PRACTICAL FOCUS
Fictitious Patient Case

Directions: Refer to Figures 19-58 to 19-60 and the patient assessment data for Mr. Smithfield. Using this information to answer questions 1 to 6 regarding Mr. Smithfield's case.

Periodontal Debridement Case: Mr. Smithfield

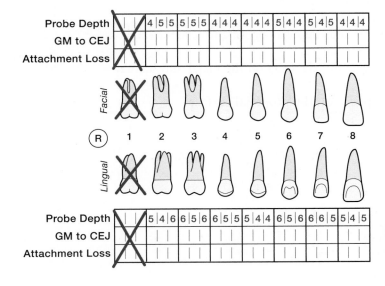

Figure 19-58. Mr. Smithfield: Intraoral Photograph.

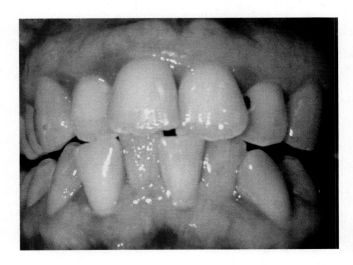

Figure 19-59. Mr. Smithfield: Periodontal Chart for Maxillary Right Quadrant.

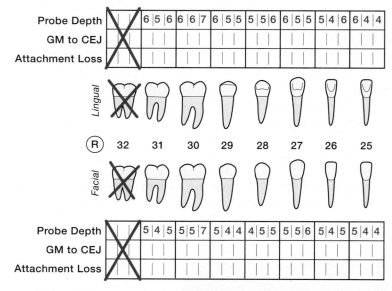

Figure 19-60. Mr. Smithfield: Periodontal Chart for Mandibular Right Quadrant.

Mr. Smithfield: Assessment Data

1. Tissue
   A. Gingival margin of all teeth in this quadrant is level with the CEJ. Probing depths are noted on the chart.
   B. Generalized bleeding upon probing.
2. Deposits
   A. Plaque Biofilm:
      1. Moderate *supra*gingival plaque biofilm on all teeth.
      2. Light subgingival plaque biofilm on all surfaces with moderate *sub*gingival plaque biofilm on the proximal surfaces on all teeth.
   B. Calculus Deposits:
      1. Anterior teeth: light subgingival calculus deposits on all surfaces (facial, lingual, mesial, and distal).
      2. Posterior teeth: light subgingival calculus deposits on the facial and lingual surfaces
      3. Posterior teeth: medium-sized deposits on the proximal surfaces

Mr. Smithfield: Case Questions 1 to 6

1. Does the assessment data indicate healthy sulci or periodontal pockets in this quadrant? Explain which data you used to determine the presence of sulci or pockets?
2. How effective is Mr. Smithfield's self-care (daily plaque control)? Explain which data helped you evaluate the effectiveness of his self-care?
3. After obtaining the probing depths, which type of explorer would you select to explore the teeth in this quadrant?
4. Which of the following instruments would you select for calculus removal on the anterior teeth in this quadrant: sickle scalers, universal curets, and/or area-specific curets? Explain your rationale for instrument selection.
5. Which of the following instruments would you select for calculus removal on the posterior teeth in this quadrant: sickle scalers, universal curets, and/or area-specific curets? Explain your rationale for instrument selection.
6. What anatomical characteristics present a challenge for Dr. Smithfield in his daily self-care and to the hygienist for instrumentation?

- Please refer to Module 20 for content on the design and use of periodontal files.
- Refer to Module 20, for content on Langer curets, Gracey designs with extended shanks and miniature working-ends, Curvettes, and debridement curets.
- Refer to Module 21 for content on the anatomy of root surfaces/root concavities and instrumentation of bi- and trifurcated roots.
- Refer to Module 22 for fictitious patient cases relating to calculus removal.

REFERENCE SHEET—AREA-SPECIFIC CURETS

Use of Area-specific Curets:

An area-specific curet is a periodontal instrument used to remove light to moderate calculus deposits from the crowns and roots of the teeth and to deplaque (remove plaque biofilm from) the root surfaces.

Basic Concepts:

- Insert the working-end beneath the gingival margin at a 0- to 40-degree angulation.
- Maintain adaptation of the toe-third of the cutting edge to the tooth surface.
- Before initiating a calculus removal stroke, press down with your fulcrum finger and apply pressure against the instrument handle with the index finger and thumb to create lateral pressure against the tooth surface.
- Activate the calculus removal stroke using wrist motion activation. Use digital activation in areas where movement is restricted, such as furcation areas and narrow, deep pockets.
- Relax your fingers between each calculus removal stroke.

Anterior Teeth:

- Select the correct working-end:
  - Use only the lower cutting edges for periodontal instrumentation.
  - The lower shank is parallel to the tooth surface being instrumented.
- Sequence: Begin with the surfaces toward your nondominant hand. Start on the canine on opposite side of the mouth and work toward yourself. (Right-Handed clinicians start with the left canine, mesial surface; Left-Handed clinicians start with the right canine, mesial surface.)

Posterior Teeth:

- Select the correct working-end:
  - Use only the lower cutting edges for periodontal instrumentation.
  - The lower shank is parallel to the tooth surface.
- Use a distal curet (G13, G14, G17, G18) for distal surfaces. Use a mesial curet (G11, G12, G15, G16) for mesial surfaces. For facial and lingual surfaces, a mesial curet or the G7, G8, G9, G10 curets may be used.
- Sequence: Complete all distal surfaces first; next instrument the facial and mesial surfaces (or the lingual and mesial surfaces).

Student Self Evaluation Module 19: Area-Specific Curets

Student: _____   Area 1 = _____

Date: _____   Area 2 = _____

Area 3 = _____

Area 4 = _____

DIRECTIONS: Self-evaluate your skill level in each treatment area as: **S** (satisfactory) or **U** (unsatisfactory).

Criteria				
Positioning/Ergonomics	**Area 1**	**Area 2**	**Area 3**	**Area 4**
Adjusts clinician chair correctly				
Reclines patient chair and assures that patient's head is even with top of headrest				
Positions instrument tray within easy reach for front, side, or rear delivery as appropriate for operatory configuration				
Positions unit light at arm's length or dons dental headlight and adjusts it for use				
Assumes the recommended clock position				
Positions backrest of patient chair for the specified arch and adjusts height of patient chair so that clinician's elbows remain at waist level when accessing the specified treatment area				
Asks patient to assume the head position that facilitates the clinician's view of the specified treatment area.				
Maintains neutral position				
Directs light to illuminate the specified treatment area				
Instrument Grasp: Dominant Hand	**Area 1**	**Area 2**	**Area 3**	**Area 4**
Grasps handle with tips of finger pads of index finger and thumb so that these fingers are opposite each other on the handle, but do NOT touch or overlap				
Rests pad of middle finger lightly on instrument shank; middle finger makes contact with ring finger				
Positions the thumb, index, and middle fingers in the "knuckles up" convex position; hyper-extended joint position is avoided				
Holds ring finger straight so that it supports the weight of hand and instrument; ring finger position is "advanced ahead of" the other fingers in the grasp				
Keeps index, middle, ring, and little fingers in contact; "like fingers inside a mitten"				
Maintains a relaxed grasp; fingers are NOT blanched in grasp				
Finger Rest: Dominant Hand	**Area 1**	**Area 2**	**Area 3**	**Area 4**
Establishes secure finger rest that is appropriate for tooth to be treated				
Once finger rest is established, pauses to self-evaluate finger placement in the grasp, verbalizes to evaluator his/her self-assessment of grasp, and corrects finger placement if necessary				

Self Evaluation continues on the next page

Student Self Evaluation Module 19: Area-Specific Curets (*continued*)

Criteria				
Prepare for Instrumentation ("Get Ready")	**Area 1**	**Area 2**	**Area 3**	**Area 4**
Selects correct working-end for tooth surface to be instrumented				
Places the working-end in the "Get Ready Zone" while using a correct finger rest for the treatment area				
Insertion	**Area 1**	**Area 2**	**Area 3**	**Area 4**
Establishes 0-degree angulation (face hugs tooth surface) in preparation for insertion				
Gently inserts curet toe beneath the gingival margin to base of sulcus or pocket				
Adaptation, Angulation, Calculus Removal Stroke	**Area 1**	**Area 2**	**Area 3**	**Area 4**
Assesses the root surface using light, sweeping assessment strokes away from the junctional epithelium				
Correctly orients the lower shank to the tooth surface to be instrumented				
Initiates a stroke away from the junctional epithelium by positioning the working-end beneath a calculus deposit, "locking the toe" against tooth surface and using an angulation between 45 and 80 degrees				
Uses rotating motion to make a short, biting stroke in a coronal direction to snap a deposit from the tooth; does NOT close face toward tooth surface during activation; uses whole hand as a unit, does NOT pull with thumb and index finger				
Maintains appropriate lateral pressure against the tooth throughout the stroke while maintaining control of the working-end				
Precisely stops each individual stroke and pauses briefly (at least 3 seconds) to relax grasp before repositioning working-end beneath calculus deposit; strokes should be short and working-end remains beneath the gingival margin (to avoid trauma to gingival margin): does NOT remove working-end from the pocket with each stroke				
Maintains neutral wrist position throughout motion activation				
Maintains correct adaptation as instrument strokes progress around tooth surface; pivots and rolls instrument handle as needed				
Thoroughly instruments proximal surface under each contact area				
Uses appropriate sequence for the specified sextant				
Demonstrates horizontal strokes at the midlines of anterior teeth and the line angles of posterior teeth				
Keeps hands steady and controlled during instrumentation so that working-end moves with precision, regardless of nervousness				
Root Debridement Stroke	**Area 1**	**Area 2**	**Area 3**	**Area 4**
Establishes a 60-degree angle to the tooth surface				
Demonstrates a series of lighter, longer, shaving strokes away from the base of the periodontal pocket				
Ethics and Professionalism				
Punctuality, appearance, demeanor, attitude, composure, honesty				

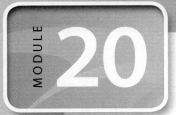
Specialized Periodontal Instruments

Module Overview

In addition to the periodontal instruments discussed in previous modules, the dental hygienist may choose to add other unique instrument designs to his or her instrument set. Specialized instruments include periodontal files, furcation curets, diamond-coated instruments, and universal and area-specific curets with extended shanks, area-specific curets with tiny working-ends.

Module Outline

Section 1   **Periodontal Files**   **489**
General Design Characteristics
Working-End Design
File Selection
Adaptation: Two-Point Contact
Skill Building. Step-By-Step Technique on Posterior Teeth, p. 492
Skill Building. Step-By-Step Technique on Central Incisor, p. 495

Section 2   **Modified Langer Curets**   **497**
General Design Characteristics
Application of Langer Curets

Section 3   **Modified Gracey Curets for Advanced Root Instrumentation**   **499**
Introduction to Modified Gracey Curets Designs
Availability and Application of Gracey Designs
Modified Gracey Curets with Extended Shanks
Modified Gracey Curets with Miniature Working-Ends
Modified Gracey Curets with Micro-Miniature Working-Ends
Vision Curvette Miniature Curets

Section 4   **Quétin, O'Hehir, DeMarco Curets and Diamond-Coated Instruments**   **507**
Quétin Furcation Curets
O'Hehir Debridement Curets/DeMarco Curets
Diamond-Coated Instruments

Section 5   **Subgingival Dental Endoscope**   **513**

Skill Application

Practical Focus: Fictitious Patient Mrs. Jefferson

Advanced techniques for instrumentation of root surfaces are covered in Module 21. Module 21 covers topics such as instrumentation of root concavities and furcation areas and advanced fulcruming techniques.

Key Terms

Periodontal file

Two-point contact

Extended shanks

Miniature working-ends

Micro-miniature working-ends

Diamond-coated instruments

Dental endoscope

Learning Objectives

- Identify instruments that are appropriate for instrumentation of root surfaces within deep periodontal pockets.

- Discuss the advantages and limitations of the design characteristics of periodontal files.

- Demonstrate or describe what is meant by a "two-point contact" when using a periodontal file.

- Compare and contrast standard curets, extended shank curets, miniature curets, and micro-miniature curets.

- Given any instrument, identify where and how it may be used on the dentition.

Section 1
Periodontal Files

GENERAL DESIGN CHARACTERISTICS

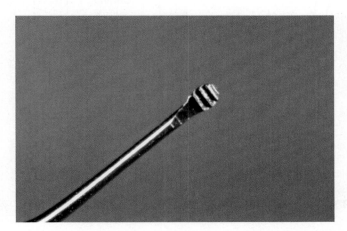

Figure 20-1. The Working-End of a Periodontal File.

1. Functions of Periodontal Files
   A. A periodontal file is a periodontal instrument that is used to prepare calculus deposits before removal with another instrument (Fig. 20-1). A periodontal file is used to crush or roughen a heavy calculus deposit so that it can be removed with a sickle scaler or curet.
   B. Periodontal files are restricted in use, serving only as a supplement to sickle scalers or curets.
   C. Files are limited to use on enamel surfaces or the outer surface of a calculus deposit. The flat base and straight cutting edges do not adapt well to curved root surfaces.
   D. They are used to crush large, tenacious subgingival calculus deposits that are not accessible to the sickle scalers that are usually used to remove heavy calculus deposits. Once the deposit has been crushed, it is then removed by a curet.
   E. Files are used to roughen the surface of burnished calculus deposits to facilitate removal of these deposits with a curet.
   F. Periodontal files can be used to smooth overhanging amalgam restorations.
   G. Because of its design limitations, periodontal files have been replaced to a great extent by ultrasonic instruments. Ultrasonic instruments are very effective at removing large calculus deposits.
2. Design Characteristics. The working-end of a periodontal file has several unique design characteristics (Fig. 20-2 and Table 20-1).
   A. A *series of cutting edges lined up on a base*
   B. *Cutting edges at a 90- to 105-degree angle to the base*
   C. A *rectangular, round, or oblong base*
   D. A *rounded back* to permit subgingival use
   E. A *rigid shank* that transmits limited tactile information to the clinician's fingers
   F. *Area-Specific Use.* Each file is designed for use only on certain tooth surfaces; therefore a set of files is needed to instrument the entire mouth.
3. Examples of Periodontal File Instruments. Some examples of periodontal files include the Hirschfeld 3/7, 5/11, 9/10 files and the Orban 10/11, 12/13 files.

WORKING-END DESIGN

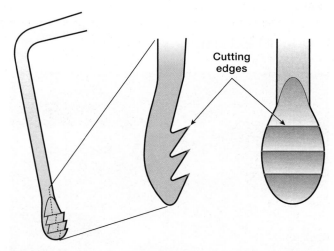

Figure 20-2. Design Characteristics. The working-end of a file has multiple, straight cutting edges.

TABLE 20-1. REFERENCE SHEET: PERIODONTAL FILE	
Working-End	Thin in width and round, rectangular, or oblong in shape
Face	Has a series of cutting edges lined up on a base
Cutting Edges	Multiple edges, at a 90- to 105-degree angulation to the base
Application	Each working-end is designed for single-surface use; a set of files is required to instrument the entire mouth
Primary Functions	• Crush large calculus deposit • Roughen burnished calculus deposit • Smooth overhanging amalgam restoration • Limited to use on enamel surfaces or the outer surface of a calculus deposit; the flat base does not adapt well to curved root surfaces

FILE SELECTION

Each periodontal file is designed for use only on certain tooth surfaces; therefore a set of files is needed to instrument the entire mouth. One of the most versatile series of files is the Hirschfeld series (Table 20-2). A set of Hirschfeld periodontal files includes the Hirschfeld 9/10, 3/7, and 5/11 files. Another common file series is the Orban series. There are two Orban files, the Orban 10/11 and 12/13.

TABLE 20-2. APPLICATION OF PERIODONTAL FILES

Instrument	Area of Application
Hirschfeld 9/10	Facial and lingual surfaces of the anterior teeth
Hirschfeld 3/7	Facial and lingual surfaces of the posterior teeth
Hirschfeld 5/11	Mesial and distal surfaces of the posterior teeth
Orban 10/11	Facial and lingual surfaces of the posterior teeth
Orban 12/13	Mesial and distal surfaces of the posterior teeth

ADAPTATION: TWO-POINT CONTACT

1. Two-point contact with a periodontal file involves adaptation of the working-end to a calculus deposit while resting the lower shank against the tooth (Fig. 20-3). This two-point contact provides the additional stability and leverage needed when making an instrumentation stroke with a file.
2. The *entire face* of the working-end should be flat against the calculus deposit (parallel to the root surface). The face should not be applied at an angle to the tooth surface; in this position the sharp corners on one side of the cutting edges can gouge the cementum while the sharp corners on the opposite end can traumatize the soft tissue.

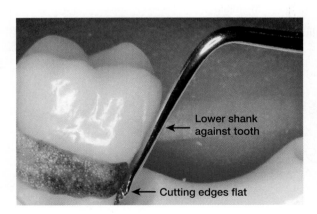

Lower shank against tooth

Cutting edges flat

Figure 20-3. Two-Point Contact.
- Point One: the face of the working-end should be flat against the calculus deposit so that the corners of the straight cutting edges do not gouge the root surface or the soft tissue.
- Point Two: The lower shank should rest against the tooth surface.

APPLICATION OF THE CUTTING EDGES TO POSTERIOR TEETH

A minimum of two double-ended periodontal files is required to instrument the tooth surfaces of the posterior teeth (Figs. 20-4 and 20-5).

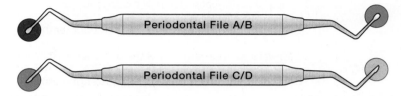

Figure 20-4. Application of Hirschfeld Files to Posterior Surfaces. Two files are used on the posterior teeth. The H 3/7 for facial and lingual surfaces and the H5/11 for the proximal surfaces.

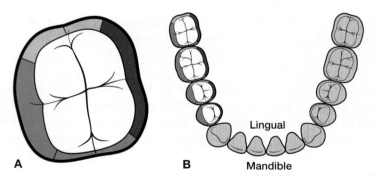

Figure 20-5. Application to Posterior Surfaces. This illustration indicates how the Hirschfeld files are applied to the posterior tooth surfaces.

Skill Building Directions:

- Follow steps 1 to 7 in Figures 20-6 to 20-12 to practice the use of a set of periodontal files.
- Remember: "Me, My patient, My light, My dominant hand, My nondominant hand, My finger rest, My adaptation."

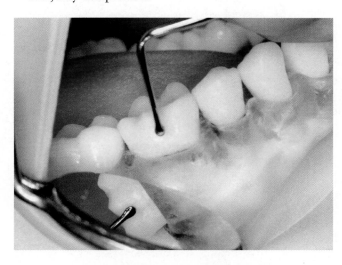

1. **Figure 20-6. Get Ready.** Select the correct file for use on the facial aspect of the mandibular right first molar. In preparation for insertion, place the working-end against the facial surface in the Get Ready Zone.

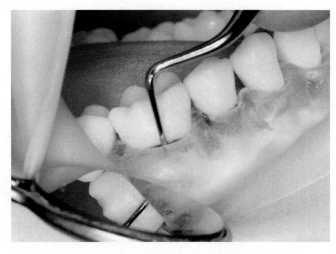

2. **Figure 20-7. Insert.** Gently insert the working-end beneath the gingival margin.

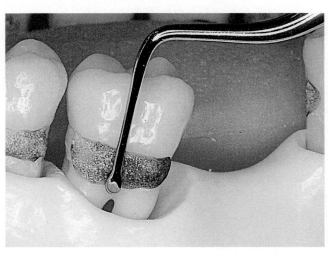

3. **Figure 20-8. Adapt to the Calculus Deposit.** Move the file along the root surface until it is adapted to the calculus deposit.
    - *Remember to establish a two-point contact with the working-end and the lower shank.*
    - Activate pull strokes in a vertical direction.

4. **Figure 20-9. Lingual Surface.** Select the correct file for use on the lingual surface. Gently slip the working-end beneath the gingival margin. Establish two-point contact. Use indirect vision to check the placement of the periodontal file.

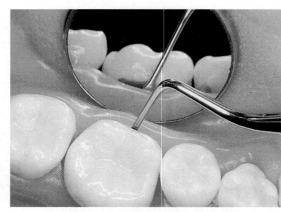

5. **Figure 20-10. Lingual Surface: Adapt to the Calculus Deposit.** Move the file along the root surface until it is adapted to the calculus deposit. Activate pull strokes in a vertical direction.

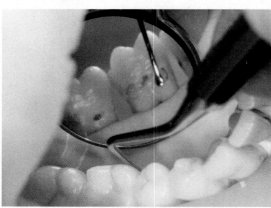

6. **Figure 20-11. Distal Surface.** Select the correct file for the distal surface. Insert the file beneath the gingival margin and position it on the calculus deposit. Activate pull strokes in a vertical direction.

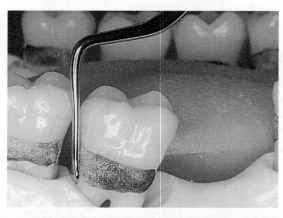

7. **Figure 20-12. Mesial Surface.** Using the correct file for the mesial surface, position the working-end on the calculus deposit. Remember to maintain two-point contact. Activate pull strokes in a vertical direction.

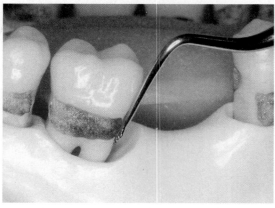

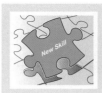

APPLICATION OF THE CUTTING EDGES TO ANTERIOR TEETH

A minimum of one double-ended periodontal file is required to instrument the facial and lingual surfaces of anterior teeth (Figs. 20-13 and 20-14).

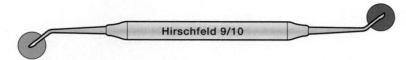

Figure 20-13. Application of a Hirschfeld File to Anterior Teeth. The Hirschfeld 9/10 periodontal file is used to instrument the anterior teeth.

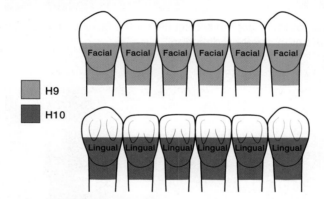

Figure 20-14. Application to Anterior Surfaces. This illustration indicates how the 9/10 Hirschfeld file is applied to the anterior tooth surfaces.

Skill Building Directions:

- Follow steps 1 and 2 to practice use of a periodontal file on the facial and lingual tooth surfaces of anterior teeth (Figs. 20-15 and 20-16).
- Remember: "Me, My patient, My light, My dominant hand, My nondominant hand, My finger rest, My adaptation."

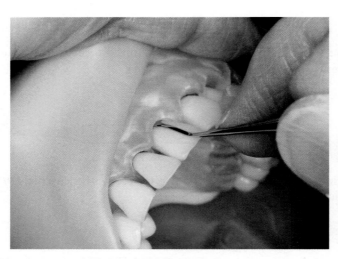

1. **Figure 20-15. Facial Surfaces.** Select the correct file for the facial surface and place it on the calculus deposit. Activate pull strokes in a vertical direction.

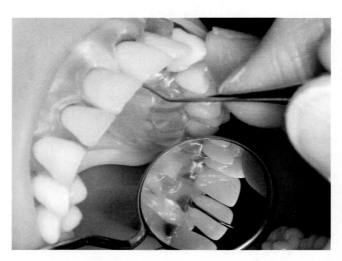

2. **Figure 20-16. Lingual Surfaces.** Insert the correct file beneath the gingival margin. Adapt to the calculus deposit and activate a series of pull strokes in a vertical direction.

Section 2
Modified Langer Curets

GENERAL DESIGN CHARACTERISTICS

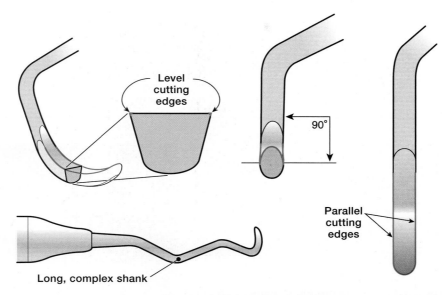

Figure 20-17. **Miniature Langer Curet.**

Langer curets with extended shanks and miniature working-ends are universal curets that have been modified to increase their effectiveness on root surfaces (Fig. 20-17). *The Langer curet may be thought of as a hybrid design that combines features of a universal curet with features typical of an area-specific curet.* This combination of design features allows an instrument to be used on all surfaces of a tooth and provides improved access to root surfaces through the shank design (1).

1. Design Characteristics of a Miniature Langer Curet
    A. **Longer Lower Shank.** The extended lower shank is designed for instrumenting pockets greater than 4 mm in depth.
    B. **Smaller Working-End.** A miniature working-end designed for access into deep narrow pockets.
2. Use
    A. Each curet is limited to use only on certain teeth and certain tooth surfaces. For this reason several Langer curets are required to instrument the entire mouth. Table 20-3 lists the recommended area of use for each curet in the Langer series.
    B. A Langer curet has a long complex functional shank design similar to that of a Gracey curet. Figures 20-18 to 20-20 depict the use of a miniature Langer curets.
    C. A set of three Langer curets—the Langer 5/6, 1/2, 3/4—is needed to instrument the entire dentition. The Langer 17/18—which facilitates access to the posterior teeth—may be used on molar teeth.
3. **Availability.** Langer curets are available in standard, rigid, extended shank, and miniature curet designs.

APPLICATION OF LANGER CURETS

TABLE 20-3. LANGER CURET APPLICATION	
Curet	**Area of Use**
Langer 5/6	Anterior teeth
Langer 1/2	Mandibular posterior teeth
Langer 3/4	Maxillary posterior teeth
Langer 17/18	Posterior teeth

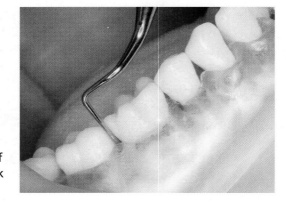

Figure 20-18. **Langer 17/18.** The modified shank design of the Langer 17/18 makes it easier to position the lower shank parallel to the distal surfaces of molar teeth.

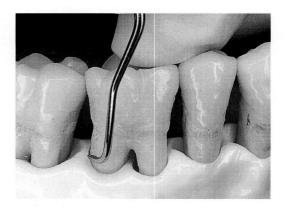

Figure 20-19. **Adaptation to Line Angles.** *Within its recommended area of use, each Langer curet is used like any other universal curet.* The extended shank and miniature working-end of the Langer 1/2 miniature curet facilitate adaptation to the distofacial line angle.

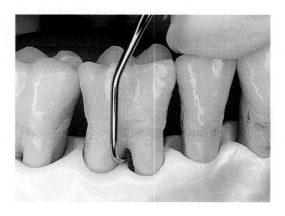

Figure 20-20. **Adaptation to Furcation Area.** The miniature working-end of this miniature Langer curet facilitates adaptation to the furcation area.

Section 3
Modified Gracey Curets for Advanced Root Instrumentation

INTRODUCTION TO MODIFIED GRACEY CURET DESIGNS

Modified designs of Gracey curets are a relatively recent development intended to facilitate treatment effectiveness on root surfaces in periodontal pockets greater than 4 mm in depth. Periodontitis causes alveolar bone loss that exposes the teeth roots to dental plaque biofilm. The effectiveness of instrumentation decreases with increasing probing depths, especially when probing depths exceed 5 mm (2–5). Two research studies conclude that root instrumentation causes an attachment loss (trauma to the base of the pocket from 0.76 mm to 1.06 mm (6,7)). Treatment of periodontally involved patients may be facilitated with the use of specialized instruments with longer shank lengths and miniature working-ends for instrumentation of root concavities and furcation areas.

Table 20-4 summarizes the design modifications of curets designed for use in deep periodontal pockets.

- Modified curet designs with extended shanks are designed to debride root surfaces within deep pockets over 4 mm in depth (Fig. 20-21).
- Modified curets with miniature working-ends and micro-miniature working-ends are designed for use in narrow deep pockets over 4 mm in depth to instrument root branches, line angles, midlines of anterior roots, root concavities, and furcation areas.
- Figures 20-22 to 20-24 demonstrate some of the design modifications.

TABLE 20-4. COMPARISON OF STANDARD AND MODIFIED GRACEY CURET DESIGNS

Instrument	Shank Design	Working-End Length	Working-End Width
Extended shank curet	Lower shank is 3 mm longer than that of a standard Gracey curet	Same length as a standard Gracey curet	10% thinner than a standard Gracey curet
Miniature working-end curet	Lower shank is 3 mm longer than that of a standard Gracey curet	Half the length of a standard Gracey curet	10% thinner than a standard Gracey curet
Micro-miniature working-end curet	Lower shank is 3 mm longer than that of a standard Gracey curet	Half the length of a standard Gracey curet	20% thinner than a standard Gracey curet

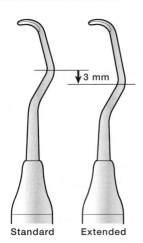

Figure 20-21. Comparison of Standard and Extended Shank Gracey Curets.
- The instrument on the left has a standard shank.
- The instrument on the right has a lower shank that is 3 mm longer. The overall shank length, however, for the instrument on the right is the same as that of a standard Gracey curet.

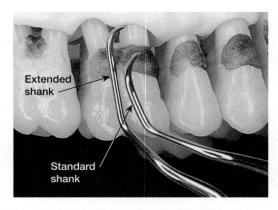

Figure 20-22. Comparison of Extended and Standard Lower Shanks.
- The curet on the left has an extended lower shank. Instruments with extended shanks are used to instrument root surfaces in periodontal pockets over 4 mm in depth.
- The curet on the right has a standard lower shank. It is recommended for use in normal sulci and periodontal pockets that are less than 4 mm in depth.

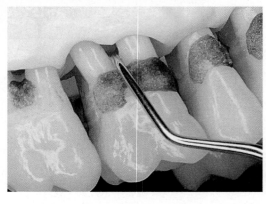

Figure 20-23. Extended Shank Length. The extended lower shank of this modified curet facilitates access to the furcation area of this molar.

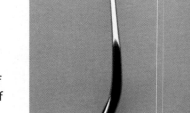
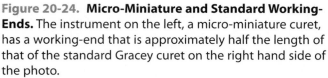

Figure 20-24. Micro-Miniature and Standard Working-Ends. The instrument on the left, a micro-miniature curet, has a working-end that is approximately half the length of that of the standard Gracey curet on the right hand side of the photo.

AVAILABILITY AND APPLICATION OF GRACEY DESIGNS

Area-specific curets with extended shanks and miniature working-ends are modifications of the standard Gracey series. The modified Gracey curets can be applied to the same tooth surfaces and used with the same instrumentation techniques as with the original Gracey series. Table 20-5 lists the availability of the various curet series in standard and modified designs and their area of application.

TABLE 20-5. GRACEY CURET AVAILABILITY AND APPLICATION

Curet	Curet Availability	Tooth Application
Curets 1/2 Curets 3/4	• Standard Gracey series • Extended shank Gracey series • Miniature Gracey series • Micro-miniature series: Gracey 1/2 curet only	• Anterior teeth: all tooth surfaces
Curets 5/6	• Standard Gracey series • Extended shank Gracey series • Miniature Gracey series	• Anterior teeth: all tooth surfaces • Premolar teeth: all tooth surfaces • Molar teeth: facial, lingual, mesial surfaces
Curets 7/8 Curets 9/10	• Standard Gracey series • Extended shank Gracey series • Miniature Gracey series • Micro-miniature series: Gracey 7/8 curet only	• Anterior teeth: all surfaces • Premolar teeth: all surfaces • Posterior teeth: facial and lingual surfaces
Curets 11/12	• Standard Gracey series • Extended shank Gracey series • Miniature Gracey series • Micro-miniature series	• Anterior teeth: mesial and distal surfaces • Posterior teeth: mesial surfaces • Posterior teeth: facial, lingual, and mesial surfaces
Curets 13/14	• Standard Gracey series • Extended shank Gracey series • Miniature Gracey series • Micro-miniature series	• Anterior teeth: mesial and distal surfaces • Posterior teeth: distal surfaces
Curets 15/16	• Standard Gracey series • Extended shank Gracey series	• Posterior teeth: facial, lingual, mesial surfaces
Curets 17/18	• Standard Gracey series	• Posterior teeth: distal surfaces

MODIFIED GRACEY CURETS WITH EXTENDED SHANKS

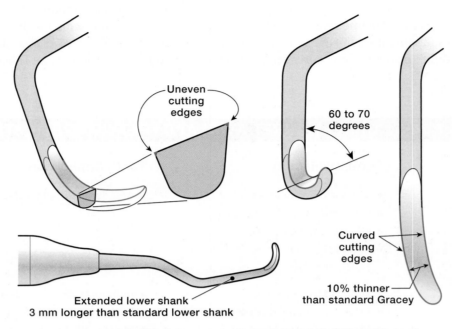

Uneven cutting edges

60 to 70 degrees

Curved cutting edges

Extended lower shank
3 mm longer than standard lower shank

10% thinner than standard Gracey

Figure 20-25. Modified Gracey Curet with Extended Shank Length.

1. **Design Modifications.** The design characteristics of the extended shank curets differ from those of standard Gracey curets in two important respects (Fig. 20-25):
   A. **Longer Lower Shank.**
      1. The extended lower shank is 3-mm longer than the lower shank of a standard Gracey curet.
      2. The longer lower shank permits access to root surfaces within periodontal pockets greater than 4 mm in depth.
   B. **Thinner Working-End.**
      1. The working-end is 10% thinner than that of a standard Gracey curet.
      2. The thinner working-end facilitates insertion beneath the gingival margin and reduces tissue distention away from the root surface.
2. **Use.** Modified Gracey curets with extended shanks are designed for instrumentation of root surfaces within deep pockets over 4 mm in depth.
3. **Examples.** Examples of extended shank Gracey curets include the Hu-Friedy Manufacturing Company's After Five curets, American Eagle Instruments' Gracey +3 Deep Pocket curets, and G. Hartzell's Extended Gracey Curettes.

MODIFIED GRACEY CURETS WITH MINIATURE WORKING-ENDS

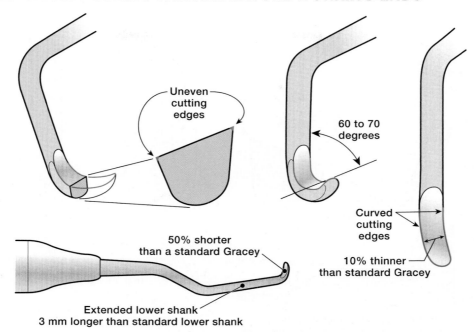

Uneven cutting edges

60 to 70 degrees

Curved cutting edges

50% shorter than a standard Gracey

10% thinner than standard Gracey

Extended lower shank
3 mm longer than standard lower shank

Figure 20-26. Miniature Gracey Curet.

1. **Design Modifications.** The design characteristics of the miniature curets differ from those of standard Gracey curets in three important respects (Fig. 20-26):
   A. **Extended Shank Length**
      1. The extended lower shank is 3-mm longer than the lower shank of a standard Gracey curet.
      2. The longer lower shank permits access to root surfaces within periodontal pockets greater than 4 mm in depth.
   B. **Thinner Working-End**
      1. The working-end is 10% thinner than that of a standard Gracey curet.
      2. The thinner working-end facilitates insertion beneath the gingival margin and reduces tissue distention away from the root surface.
   C. **Shorter Working-End.** The miniature working-end is half the length of a standard Gracey curet. The working-end does not curve up (8). Compare this design to that of the Vision Curvette discussed later in this chapter.
2. **Uses**
   A. Miniature Gracey curets are designed for use in narrow deep pockets over 4 mm in depth for instrumentation of root branches, midlines of anterior roots, root concavities, and furcation areas.
   B. *The miniature curets are not intended to replace either the standard or extended shank Gracey curets for routine instrumentation of all tooth surfaces.* Rather, miniature curets are used instead of standard curets for instrumentation of areas that are extremely difficult to reach with standard working-ends such as furcation areas, line angles, and deep narrow pockets.
   C. Adapt well to narrow facial and lingual surfaces of anterior teeth, furcation areas, and root surfaces in narrow and deep periodontal pockets.
3. **Examples:** Hu-Friedy Mini Five; American Eagle Instruments' Gracey +3 Access curets; G. Hartzell Slim Gracey Curettes

MODIFIED GRACEY CURETS WITH MICRO-MINIATURE WORKING-ENDS

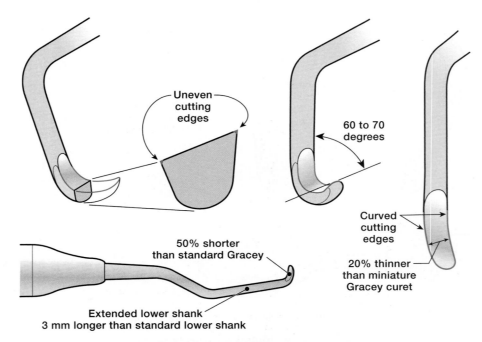

Figure 20-27. Micro-Miniature Gracey Curet.

1. **Design Modifications.** The design characteristics of the micro-miniature curets differ from those of standard Gracey curets in three important respects (Fig. 20-27):
   A. **Longer Shank Length**
      1. The extended lower shank is 3-mm longer than the lower shank of a standard Gracey curet.
      2. The shank has slightly increased rigidity compared to miniature curets.
   B. **Thinner Working-End**
      1. The working-end is 20% thinner than that of a miniature Gracey curet.
      2. The thinner working-end facilitates insertion beneath the gingival margin and reduces tissue distention away from the root surface.
   C. **Shorter Working-End.** The miniature working-end is half the length of a standard Gracey curet.
   D. **Availability.** The micro-miniature set includes four instruments: 1/2, 7/8, 11/12, 13/14
2. **Uses**
   A. Facilitate insertion and adaptation into very tight, deep, or narrow pockets. They facilitate access to narrow furcations; developmental depressions; line angles; and deep pockets on facial, lingual, or palatal surfaces, especially when the tissue is tight and/or thin.
   B. ***Micro-miniature curets are not used routinely instead of the standard Gracey curets, but rather, in special areas of difficult access.*** These curets are ideal for fine deposit removal following instrumentation with other curets.
   C. Vertical or oblique strokes work well with these instruments. Horizontal strokes might not extend far enough subgingivally and may gouge the root surface.
3. **Examples.** Hu-Friedy Micro Mini Fives

VISION CURVETTE MINIATURE CURETS

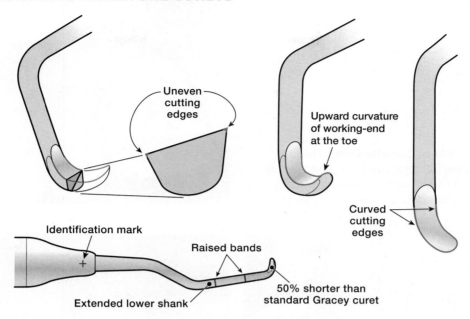

Figure 20-28. **The Vision Curvette Curet.**

1. **Design Modifications.** The design characteristics of Vision Curvette area-specific curets (Hu-Friedy Manufacturing) differ from those of standard Gracey curets in several important respects (Fig. 20-28):
   A. **Extended Shank Design**
      1. Extended lower shank on the Vision Curvette 11/12 and 13/14 curets allows access to root surfaces within periodontal pockets greater than 4 mm in depth.
      2. The lower shank has two *raised bands* at 5 and 10 mm. These raised bands provide a means to visually estimate the pocket depth during instrumentation.
   B. **Shorter Working-End.** The Vision Curvette working-end is shortened to half the length of a standard Gracey curet.
      1. The shorter working-end allows the entire length of the working-end to be adapted to the root surface. The very short cutting edge may "slip" if not well engaged with the tooth surface and strokes must be very close together.
      2. As depicted in Figures 20-29 and 20-30, the miniature working-end provides improved access to root concavities, furcation areas of posterior teeth, and midlines of anterior teeth.
   C. **Working-end Curvature.** The working-end has a slight upward curvature at the toe. This curvature facilitates adaptation to curved root surfaces, particularly at line angles.
   D. **Working-Cutting Edge Identification Mark.** An identification mark ("+") on the handle near the junction of the shank indicates the lower cutting edge. Application of these curets is summarized in Table 20-6.
2. **Uses**
   A. The Vision Curvette series facilitates access to areas that are extremely difficult to reach with standard curets such as narrow deep pockets over 4 mm in depth, root branches, midlines of anterior roots, root concavities, and furcation areas and are very effective for the palatal surfaces of maxillary anterior teeth.
   B. *Vision Curvette curets are not used routinely instead of the standard Gracey curets, but rather, in special areas of difficult access.*

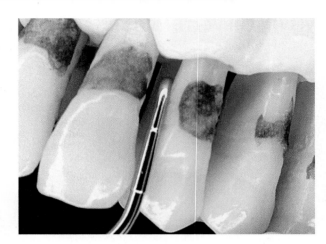

Figure 20-29. Vision Curvette Curet. The lower shank on a Vision Curvette curet has raised bands at 5 and 10 mm that provide a means to visually estimate the pocket depth during instrumentation.

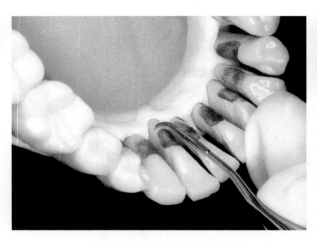

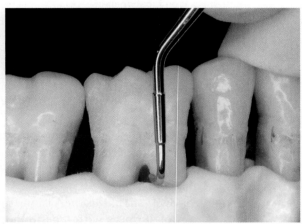

Figure 20-30. Vision Curvette Working-End. The shorter working-end of a Vision Curvette curet facilitates adaptation to narrow anterior root surfaces and the furcation areas of molar teeth.

TABLE 20-6. VISION CURVETTE CURET APPLICATION

Curet	Area of Use
Vision Curvette Sub-Zero	Anterior teeth
Vision Curvette 1/2	Anterior and premolar teeth
Vision Curvette 11/12	Mesial, facial, and lingual surfaces of molars
Vision Curvette 13/14	Distal surfaces of molar teeth

Section 4
Quétin, O'Hehir, DeMarco Curets and Diamond-Coated Instruments

QUÉTIN FURCATION CURETS

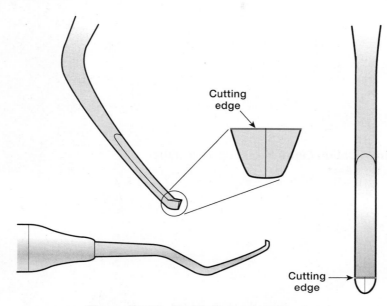

Figure 20-31. Quétin Furcation Curet.

1. **Design Modifications.** The Quétin (kee-tan) furcation curets have very unique design characteristics (Fig. 20-31).
   A. **Working-End Design**
      1. As shown in Figure 20-32, each miniature working-end is a miniature hoe with a single, semicircular cutting edge.
      2. The corners of the cutting edges and back of the working-end are rounded to minimize the potential for gouging the tooth surface.
   B. **Working-End Size.** Each working-end is available in either the 0.9 or 1.3 mm size.
2. **Uses.** Quétin furcation curets are specialized instruments used to debride furcation areas and developmental depressions on the inner aspects of the roots (Figs. 20-33 and 20-34).
3. **Availability.** Quétin curets are available in facial–lingual and mesial–distal instruments. Application of these curets is summarized in Table 20-7.
   A. The shallow semicircular cutting edge fits into the roof or floor of furcation areas. The curvature of the tip also fits into developmental depressions on the inner aspects of the roots.
   B. These instruments remove calculus from recessed areas of the furcation where other curets, even Graceys with miniature working-ends can be too large to gain access.

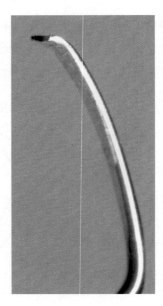

Figure 20-32. Quétin Furcation Curet. A close up view of the working-end of a Quétin curet.

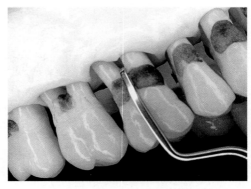

Figure 20-33. Quétin Curet in Furcation. The Quétin 1 curet used on the furcation roof of a maxillary first molar.

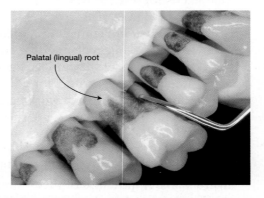

Palatal (lingual) root

Figure 20-34. Quétin Curet in the Mesial Furcation. The Quétin 2 curet used in the mesial furcation of a maxillary first molar. The mesial furcation is accessed from the lingual aspect of the molar.

TABLE 20-7. QUÉTIN CURET APPLICATION

Curet	Area of Use
Quétin 1	Facial and lingual surfaces of posterior teeth
Quétin 2	Mesial and distal surfaces of posterior teeth
Quétin 3	Facial and lingual of anterior teeth

O'HEHIR DEBRIDEMENT CURETS/DEMARCO CURETS

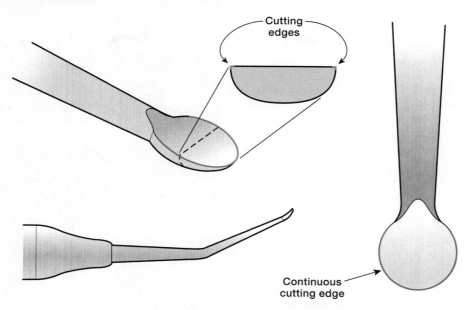

Figure 20-35. The O'Hehir Curet.

1. **Design Modifications.** The O'Hehir Debridement curets and DeMarco curets are examples of a new type of area-specific curet.
   A. **Shape of Working-End.** As shown in Figures 20-35 and 20-36, the working-end of an O'Hehir or DeMarco curet is a tiny circular disk.
   B. **Cutting Edge**
      1. The entire circumference of the working-end is one continuous cutting edge. This design allows the instrument to be used with a push or pull stroke in any direction: vertical, horizontal, or oblique.
      2. The working-end curves into the tooth for easy adaptation in furcations, developmental grooves, and line angles. Figures 20-37 to 20-39 depict use of the O'Hehir curets. Table 20-8 lists areas of use.
   C. **Shank Design.** These curets have extended lower shanks for easy access into deep periodontal pockets.
2. **Uses.** These curets are designed to smooth root surfaces and remove small residual deposits after instrumentation with curets. They are ideal for furcations, developmental grooves, and line angles.
3. **Examples.** O'Hehir Debridement Curets and DeMarco curets.

TABLE 20-8. O'HEHIR DEBRIDEMENT CURET APPLICATION

Curet	Area of Use
O'Hehir 1/2	Facial and lingual surfaces of posterior teeth
O'Hehir 3/4	Mesial and distal surfaces of posterior teeth
O'Hehir 5/6	Anterior teeth
O'Hehir 7/8	Anterior teeth with deep pockets

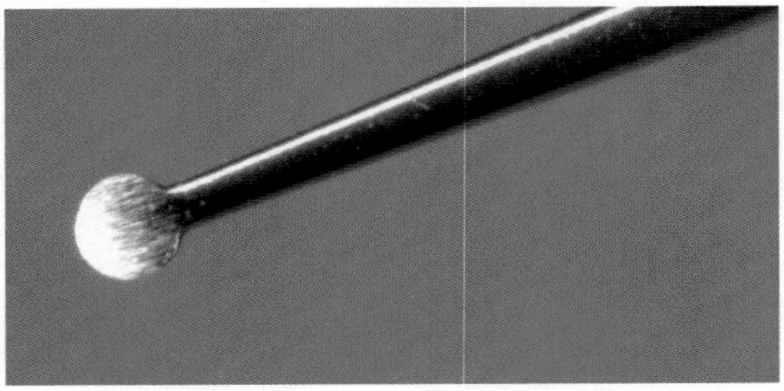

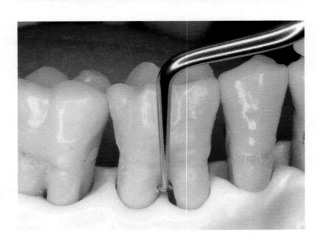

Figure 20-36. O'Hehir Debridement Curet. Close-up view of the disk-shaped working-end of an O'Hehir debridement curet.

Figure 20-37. Adaptation to a Furcation Area. The tiny disk-shaped working-end of the debridement curet curves toward the tooth surface to adapt to the furcation.

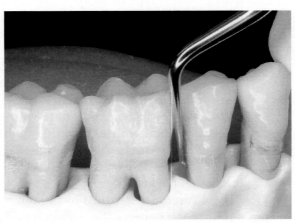

Figure 20-38. Adaptation to a Distal Concavity. The disk-shaped working-end of a debridement curet adapts well to the distal root concavity on the mandibular second premolar.

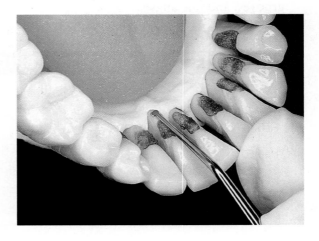

Figure 20-39. Access to the Lingual Surfaces of the Mandibular Anteriors. The O'Hehir 7/8 curet is excellent for adaptation to the lingual surfaces of the mandibular anterior teeth. This instrument features a 15-mm long shank that provides access to the base of even the deepest periodontal pocket.

DIAMOND-COATED INSTRUMENTS

1. **Design Modifications.** The design characteristics of diamond-coated instruments is truly unique:
   A. **No cutting edges.** Diamond-coated instruments have no cutting edges, instead the working-end is coated with a very fine diamond grit. The diamond-coated instruments from Hu-Friedy Manufacturing Co, Inc. have diamond coating placed 360 degrees around the tip. On the Brasseler USA, G. Hartzell & Son instruments the diamond coating is placed 180 degrees around the tip, the back of the 180-degree instrument is smooth for placement against the tissue.
   B. **Pronounced Working-End Curvature.** The working-end design is similar to that of a Nabers furcation probe for easy insertion between the roots of bifurcated and trifurcated teeth (Fig. 20-40).
2. **Uses.** Diamond instruments are used like an emery board to remove small, embedded remnants of calculus that remain on the root surface after instrumentation.
   A. Diamond-coated instruments are finishing instruments for use after deposit removal with other instruments in narrow, inaccessible areas, like furcation areas.
   B. Used for final instrumentation and polishing of root surfaces and furcation areas, not designed for heavy calculus removal.
   C. Should be used with very light pressure and multidirectional strokes to achieve a clean, smooth, even root surface. Caution is indicated since these instruments have the potential to cause over-instrumentation of the root surfaces.
   D. Light strokes in various directions remove the last bits of embedded/burnished calculus from roots in developmental depressions, deep pockets, and furcation areas. Activation of the instrument is with both a push and pull stroke with very light pressure in a multidirectional fashion.
   E. Ideal for Class III furcation areas and root surfaces on both sides of the furcation area and for instrumentation of a Class IV furcation between the mesiobuccal and distobuccal roots and the furcation roof.
3. **Examples:** Hu-Friedy diamond instruments are the Nabors and the MD (mesial–distal) DiamondTec Scalers; the Brasseler Diamond Files F (fine) series includes the F1/F2 (buccal–lingual) instruments and F3/F4 (mesial–distal) instruments.

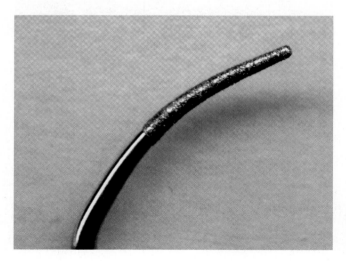

Figure 20-40. Diamond-Coated Instrument. A close-up view of a working-end on a DiamondTEc MD scaler. Note the textured coating on the working-end.

Figures 20-41 and 20-42 depict a diamond-coated instrument in use on a trifurcated maxillary fist molar tooth.

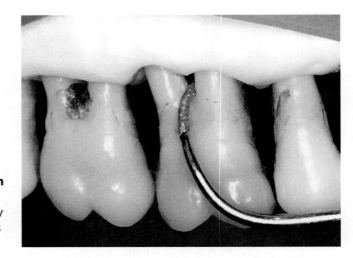

Figure 20-41. Diamond-Coated Instrument in Facial Furcation. The thin, curved working-end of this diamond-coated instrument inserts easily between the distobuccal and mesiobuccal roots of this maxillary first molar.

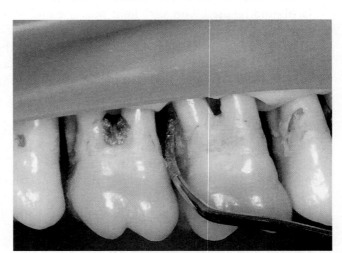

Figure 20-42. Diamond-Coated instrument. A mesial–distal diamond-coated instrument adapted to the distal root concavity of a maxillary first molar.

Section 5
Subgingival Dental Endoscope

A **dental endoscope** is a long, flexible tubular device that has a fiber optic light and video camera attached. The endoscope is used to view and examine inside a periodontal pocket. Once inserted in a periodontal pocket, images of the root are transmitted from the endoscope and projected on a flat screen monitor. First introduced by DentalView, Inc., ownership of the dental endoscope has recently been acquired by Perioscopy Incorporated, Oakland, California.

1. **Description of Dental Endoscope.** The dental endoscope is about 1 meter in length and 0.99 mm in diameter (Fig. 20-43). To maintain sterility, a disposable sterile sheath is placed around the endoscope for each patient use.
   A. The dental endoscope allows for subgingival visualization of the root surface at magnifications of 20× to 40× (9,10).
   B. The endoscope is attached to a flat screen monitor (Figs. 20-44 and 20-45) that provides a highly magnified picture of subgingival conditions. With the dental endoscope, clinicians actually can see subgingival deposits instead of only detecting deposits with an explorer.

2. **Technique**
   A. A limitation of the dental endoscope is that the technique takes time and effort to master (9,11). In his article, *Enhanced Periodontal Debridement with the Use of Micro Ultrasonic, Periodontal Endoscopy* (9), Dr. John Y. Kwan, President/CEO of Perioscopy Incorporated describes mastery of the dental endoscope as "*a difficult task to master. It requires a desire to learn, focused attention, lots of practice, and much patience.*"
   B. Dr. Kwan recommends a two-handed technique for use of the dental endoscope (9). ***For the two-handed technique, the clinician holds the endoscope in the nondominant hand and an instrument in the dominant hand.*** With this technique, the root surface is viewed and instrumented at the same time (Fig. 20-46).

3. **Recommended Use.** ***The dental endoscope is not recommended for routine subgingival instrumentation because this process would be too time consuming.*** Candidates for endoscopy include patients being treated for sites that did not respond to traditional periodontal instrumentation, patients in whom periodontal surgical therapy is contraindicated, and patients receiving maintenance for chronically inflamed or increasing pockets (9).

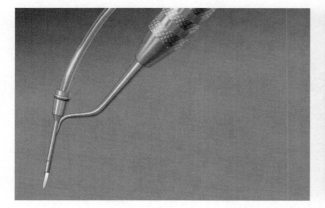
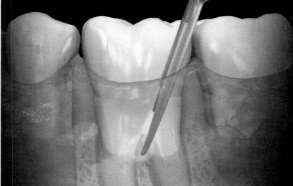

Figure 20-43. Modified Endoscopic Instruments. A modified periodontal instrument is used to guide the endoscope subgingivally. The modified periodontal instruments are of about the size of a periodontal probe and are easily inserted into a periodontal pocket.

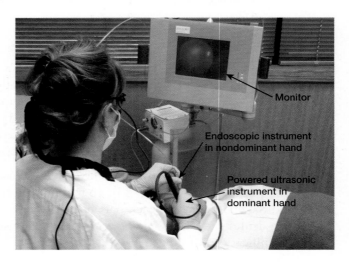

Figure 20-44. Dental Endoscopic System.
- The clinician holds the endoscopic instrument in her nondominant hand.
- In this photo, the clinician uses a powered calculus removal instrument (ultrasonic tip) in her dominant hand.
- Note that the clinician indirectly views the root surface in the monitor, rather than looking in the oral cavity. (Courtesy of John Y. Kwan.)

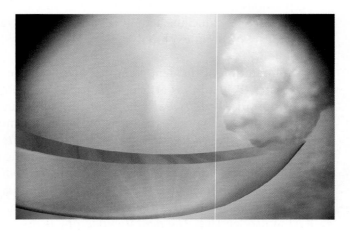

Figure 20-45. Tooth Surface as Seen on Monitor Screen. The endoscope is attached to a flat screen monitor that provides a highly magnified picture of subgingival conditions. Real-time images of the actual subgingival conditions are displayed on the monitor.

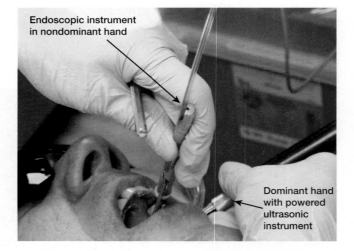

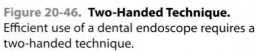

Figure 20-46. Two-Handed Technique.
Efficient use of a dental endoscope requires a two-handed technique.
- The clinician uses the dental endoscope with the nondominant hand.
- The periodontal instrument is held in the dominant hand. (Courtesy of John Y. Kwan.)

References

1. Scaramucci M. The versatility of the universal curet. A review of a hand instrumentation staple. *Dimens Dent Hyg.* 2010;8(2):32, 6, 8.
2. Cobb CM. Clinical significance of non-surgical periodontal therapy: an evidence-based perspective of scaling and root planing. *J Clin Periodontol.* 2002;29(Suppl 2):6–16.
3. Hodges K. Expanding your instrument armamentarium. *Dimens Dent Hyg.* 2009;7(5):31–33.
4. Kunselman B, Scaramucci MK. Make the most out of your modified Gracey curets. *Dimens Dent Hyg.* 2010;8(11):42–44.
5. Nagy RJ, Otomo-Corgel J, Stambaugh R. The effectiveness of scaling and root planing with curets designed for deep pockets. *J Periodontol.* 1992;63(12):954–959.
6. Alves R, Machion L, Casati MZ, Nociti Junior FH, Sallum EA, Sallum WA. Clinical attachment loss produced by curettes and periodontal files. *J Int Acad Periodontol.* 2004;6(3):76–80.
7. Alves RV, Machion L, Casati MZ, Nociti Junior FH, Sallum AW, Sallum EA. Attachment loss after scaling and root planing with different instruments. A clinical study. *J Clin Periodontol.* 2004;31(1):12–15.
8. Long B. Hand instrumentation: What are our options? Part 2. *Access.* 2010(December):35–36.
9. Kwan JY. Enhanced periodontal debridement with the use of micro ultrasonic, periodontal endoscopy. *J Calif Dent Assoc.* 2005;33(3):241–248.
10. Stambaugh RV, Myers G, Ebling W, Beckman B, Stambaugh K. Endoscopic visualization of the submarginal gingiva dental sulcus and tooth root surfaces. *J Periodontol.* 2002;73(4):374–382.
11. Stambaugh R. A clinician's three year experience with perioscopy. *Compend Contin Educ Dent.* 2002;23:1061–1070.

Section 6
Skill Application

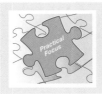

PRACTICAL FOCUS
Fictitious Patient Mrs. Jefferson

Directions: Use the information for Mrs. Jefferson provided in Figures 20-47 and 20-48 and the assessment data to answer the case questions on the following page.

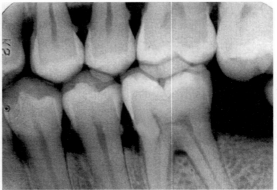

Figure 20-47. Intraoral Photo and Radiograph for Mrs. Jefferson.

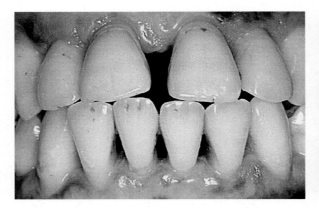

3	3	3	3	2	3	3	2	3	5	6	6	6	6	6	7	6	6							Probe Depth
+1	+1	+1	+2	+2	+2	+2	+4	+2	+1	0	0	0	0	0	0	0	0							GM to CEJ
																								Attachment Loss

Lingual

24 23 22 21 20 19 18 17 (L)

Facial

3	2	3	2	2	2	2	1	3	4	5	5	5	5	5	6	5	5							Probe Depth
+1	+1	+1	+2	+2	+2	+2	+4	+2	+1	0	0	0	0	0	0	0	0							GM to CEJ
																								Attachment Loss
																								Mobility

Figure 20-48. Periodontal Chart for Mrs. Jefferson.

Mrs. Jefferson: Assessment Data

1. Generalized bleeding upon probing.
2. Deposits
   A. Moderate supragingival plaque on all teeth.
   B. Supragingival calculus deposits—light calculus on lingual surfaces of the mandibular anteriors and molar teeth.
   C. Subgingival calculus deposits—small-sized deposits on all teeth; medium-sized deposits on all proximal surfaces.

Mrs. Jefferson: Case Questions

1. *Use the information recorded on Mrs. Jefferson's periodontal chart to calculate the clinical attachment loss on the facial and lingual aspects for teeth 19 to 24 and enter this information on her periodontal chart in Figure 20-24.*
2. Is there mobility or furcation involvement present on Mrs. Jefferson's periodontal chart? If so, which teeth are involved and what is the extent of the mobility and/or furcation involvement.
3. Does the assessment data indicate normal bone levels or bone loss in this quadrant? Does the assessment data indicate healthy sulci or periodontal pockets in this quadrant? Explain which data you used to make these determinations?
4. The gingival margin is located at the CEJ for teeth 19 and 20. There is no gingival recession present on these teeth. Does the location of the gingival margin make the instrumentation of these teeth more difficult or less difficult?
5. Do you expect to encounter any root concavities or furcation involvement while instrumenting the teeth in this quadrant? If so, indicate which teeth will probably have root concavities and/or furcation areas to be instrumented.
6. Based on the assessment information, select explorer(s), probe(s), and calculus removal instruments that would be appropriate for instrumentation of this quadrant. List the instruments you would select and explain your rationale for instrument selection.

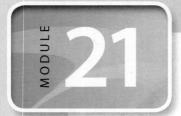

Advanced Techniques for Root Instrumentation

Module Overview

Instrumentation of root surfaces within deep periodontal pockets is complicated by root surface anatomy including root concavities, fissures, and furcation areas. Treating root surfaces located within deep periodontal pockets is challenging especially on maxillary posterior teeth. This module presents strategies and techniques for successful instrumentation of root surfaces for patients with periodontitis.

Module Outline

Section 1   **Anatomical Features that Complicate Instrumentation of Root Surfaces**   **521**

Root Concavities, Furcation Areas, and Grooves
Incorrect Technique Leads to Missed Deposits in Concavities
Skill Building. Exploration of Root Concavities and Furcation Areas, p. 525
Maxillary First Premolar—Proximal Concavity
Mandibular First Molar—Concavities and Furcation Area
Maxillary First Molar—Concavities and Furcation Areas

Section 2   **Introduction to Root Instrumentation**   **529**

Skill Building. Instrumentation of Multirooted Teeth with Area-Specific Curets, p. 529
Instrumentation Sequence
Skill Building. Technique with Area-Specific Curets on Multirooted Teeth, p. 530
Skill Building. Selecting Area-Specific Curets for Applying Horizontal Strokes to Root Surfaces, p. 532

Section 3   **Advanced Intraoral Techniques for Root Instrumentation**   **533**

Cross Arch and Opposite Arch Fulcrums
Finger-on-Finger Fulcrum

Section 4 **Advanced Extraoral Fulcruming Techniques** **536**
Basic Extraoral Fulcruming Techniques: Right-Handed Clinicians
Basic Extraoral Fulcruming Techniques: Left-Handed Clinicians
Criteria for an Effective Extraoral Fulcrum
Modifications to Basic Extraoral Fulcrums: Instrumentation Stroke with
  a Finger Assist

Section 5 **Technique Practice: Extraoral Finger Rests for Right-Handed Clinicians** **542**
Skill Building. "Palm Facing Out" Extraoral Fulcrum: Maxillary
  Right Posterior Sextants, p. 542
Skill Building. "Chin-Cup" Extraoral Fulcrum: Maxillary Right
  Posterior Sextants, p. 545
Skill Building. Maxillary Anterior Teeth, p. 548

Section 6 **Technique Practice: Horizontal Strokes for Right-Handed Clinicians** **549**
Skill Building. Horizontal Strokes on Maxillary Teeth. Curet in
  Toe-Up Orientation, p. 549

Section 7 **Technique Practice: Extraoral Finger Rests for Left-Handed Clinicians** **552**
Skill Building. "Palm Facing Out" Extraoral Fulcrum: Maxillary
  Right Posterior Sextants, p. 552
Skill Building. "Chin-Cup" Extraoral Fulcrum: Maxillary Right
  Posterior Sextants, p. 555
Skill Building. Maxillary Anterior Teeth, p. 558

Section 8 **Technique Practice: Horizontal Strokes for Left-Handed Clinicians** **559**
Skill Building. Horizontal Strokes on Maxillary Teeth. Curet in
  Toe-up Orientation, p. 559

Section 9 **Skill Application** **563**
Student Self Evaluation Module 21: Advanced Techniques for Root
  Surface Instrumentation

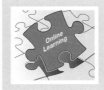

Online resources for this module:
- Advanced fulcrums on the mandibular arch
- Advanced fulcrums on the maxillary arch

Available online at: http://thepoint.lww.com/GehrigFundamentals8e

Key Terms

Cross arch fulcrum
Opposite arch fulcrum
Finger-on-finger fulcrum

Palm facing out technique
Chin-cup technique

Instrumentation stroke with
  a finger assist

Learning Objectives

- Discuss anatomical features that complicate the instrumentation of root surfaces in the presence of attachment loss.

- Demonstrate the use of an explorer on extracted or acrylic teeth including exploration of root concavities and the furcation areas of multirooted teeth.

- Select calculus removal instruments that are appropriate for root instrumentation in the presence of attachment loss.

- Demonstrate the correct sequence for instrumentation of a multirooted tooth with area-specific curets, including the root trunk and individual roots of the tooth.

- Select the correct working-end of an area-specific curet for use with horizontal strokes in mesial and distal root concavities (toe-down or toe-up position).

- Demonstrate each of the following advanced intraoral fulcrums on a periodontal typodont in an appropriate sextant of the dentition for the fulcrum: finger-on-finger intraoral, cross arch, and opposite arch, and instrumentation strokes with a finger assist technique.

- Demonstrate each of the following extraoral fulcrums on a periodontal typodont in an appropriate sextant of the dentition for the fulcrum: extraoral "palm-out" technique, extraoral "chin-cup" technique, and instrumentation strokes with a finger assist technique.

- Demonstrate horizontal strokes in a proximal root concavity on an acrylic tooth or periodontal typodont and explain the rationale for using horizontal strokes in concavities.

- Demonstrate horizontal strokes in the facial concavity located between the CEJ and furcation area of multirooted teeth and explain the rationale for using horizontal strokes in this area.

- Demonstrate horizontal strokes at the distofacial and distolingual line angles on acrylic teeth or periodontal typodont and explain the rational for using horizontal strokes at line angles.

- Demonstrate instrumentation of the furcation area on a mandibular first molar on an acrylic tooth or periodontal typodont.

- Demonstrate instrumentation of the furcations on a maxillary first molar from the facial aspect. Instrument only those furcations that are best accessed from the facial aspect.

- Demonstrate instrumentation of the furcations on a maxillary first molar from the lingual aspect. Instrument only those furcations that are best accessed from the lingual aspect.

Section 1
Anatomical Features that Complicate Instrumentation of Root Surfaces

Instrumentation of a periodontally involved patient requires advanced instrumentation skills because of the concavities found on the roots of most teeth and the furcation areas exposed on some posterior teeth. In health, most of the tooth root is surrounded by alveolar bone. In disease, bone support is lost exposing the root to dental plaque biofilm and requiring instrumentation of these surfaces. Effective instrumentation of the root surfaces requires the clinician to have a complete knowledge of root morphology. *The majority of instrumentation on roots is performed on surfaces that are hidden beneath the gingival margin. A clear mental picture of root anatomy and a keen tactile sense are necessary for subgingival instrumentation to be successful.*

1. A **root concavity** is a linear developmental depression in the root surface. Two examples of root concavities are pictured in Figure 21-1A and B. Figure 21-2 demonstrates the cross section of a root showing the concavity. Root concavities commonly occur on the:
    A. Proximal surfaces of anterior and posterior teeth
    B. Facial and lingual surfaces of molar teeth
2. In health, root concavities are covered with alveolar bone and help to secure the tooth in the bone.
3. In periodontitis, bone loss exposes the root concavities.
    A. If the gingival margin has receded, these concavities can be seen in the mouth.
    B. If the gingival margin is near the CEJ, the root concavities remain hidden beneath the tissue in a periodontal pocket.
    C. Gher and Vernino (1–3) demonstrated that furcations could be located at as little as 3 mm from the cementoenamel junction.
4. It is difficult for a patient to successfully remove biofilm from root surface concavities. Likewise, instrumentation of these areas by a clinician requires skill and an attention to root anatomy (3–5).

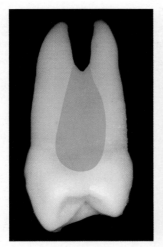
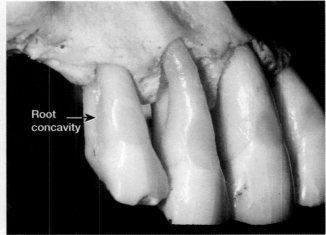

Figure 21-1. Concavity on the Mesial Surface of a Maxillary Premolar Tooth. The photograph on the left shows the linear root concavity—indicated by the *green shading*—on a maxillary right first premolar. The photograph on the right shows the distal root concavity on a maxillary first premolar.

ROOT CONCAVITIES, FURCATION AREAS, AND GROOVES

Root surface morphology can greatly complicate instrumentation, especially when the roots are hidden from view within deep periodontal pockets. These anatomical features depicted in Figure 21-2 include root concavities and depressions, and occasionally, root fissures. Figures 21-3 and 21-4 show root concavities and calculus deposits on extracted teeth.

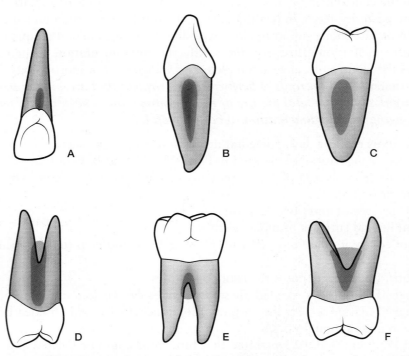

Figure 21-2. Root Concavities, Depressions, and Grooves. Examples of root surface morphology (*shaded areas*) that can hinder instrumentation of root surfaces.

A. *Palatal groove* on maxillary lateral incisor that extends onto the cervical third of the root surface.

B. *Deep linear root concavities* on the proximal surfaces of mandibular canine.

C. *Wide shallow root concavity* on the mesial surface of mandibular molar.

D. *Deep linear proximal root concavities* and *furcation* on maxillary first premolar.

E. *Deep depression on root trunk* and *furcation* on mandibular molar.

F. *Proximal concavities* extending from the furcation to CEJ on maxillary molar.

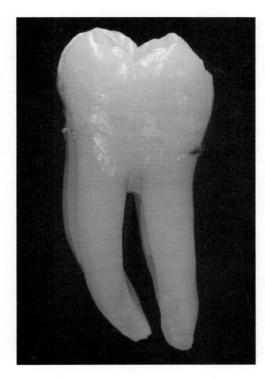

Figure 21-3. Concavities on a Mandibular First Molar.
Concavities—*shaded in green*—on a mandibular first molar include concavities on the:
- distal surface of the distal root.
- distal (interior, furcal) aspect of the mesial root.
- root trunk just coronal to the furcation area. (Adapted with permission from Scheid RC, Weiss G. *Woelfel's Dental Anatomy*. 8th ed. Philadelphia, PA: Lippincott Williams & Wilkins; 2012.)

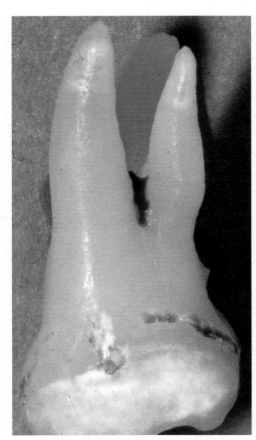

Figure 21-4. Calculus in Furcation Area. Instrumentation is complicated on molar teeth when furcation areas are exposed due to bone loss. This photo shows calculus in the buccal furcation area of a maxillary molar. (Used with permission from Scheid RC, Weiss G. *Woelfel's Dental Anatomy*. 8th ed. Philadelphia, PA: Lippincott Williams & Wilkins; 2012.)

INCORRECT TECHNIQUE LEADS TO MISSED DEPOSITS IN CONCAVITIES

Figures 21-5 to 21-7 illustrate how incorrect instrumentation technique results in failure to remove calculus deposits from a root concavity.

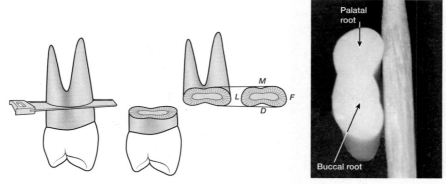

Figure 21-5. Root Concavity in Cross Section. The illustration on the left depicts a premolar tooth cut in half to expose the cross section of the root. The photo, on the right, shows the cross section of the root of a maxillary first premolar. In the photo, a toothpick spans the depression of the mesial root concavity.

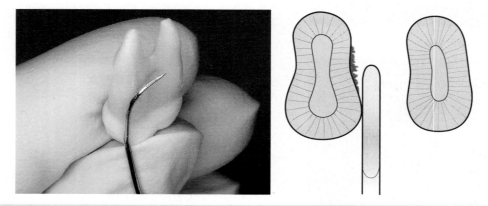

Figure 21-6. Incorrect Technique Causes the Working-End to Span the Concavity. A problem can occur during instrumentation when the clinician does not consider root morphology. The length of the working-end will span the depression, leaving the concavity untouched.

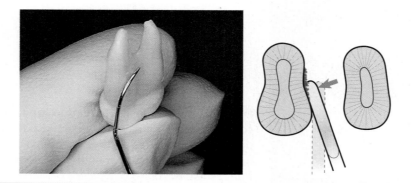

Figure 21-7. Correct Technique for Adaptation to the Concavity. Correct instrumentation technique involves rolling the handle to direct the leading-third of the explorer tip into the root concavity. Note that the middle- and heel-thirds of the working-end are rotated toward the adjacent tooth.

SKILL BUILDING
Exploration of Root Concavities and Furcation Areas

Directions: For this technique practice, you will need the following items:

- An appropriate explorer for root exploration such as a 11/12-type explorer with an extended shank.
- The following acrylic or extracted teeth: maxillary first premolar, maxillary first molar, and mandibular first molar.
- Follow steps as pictured in Figures 21-8 to 21-20.

Note to Course Instructor: A source of acrylic teeth with anatomically correct roots is Kilgore International, Inc., (800) 892-9999 or online at http://www.kilgoreinternational.com.

MAXILLARY FIRST PREMOLAR—PROXIMAL CONCAVITY

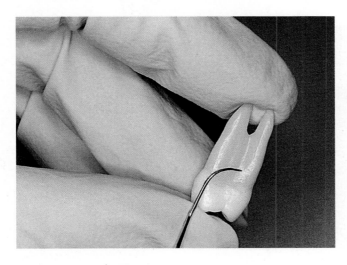

Figure 21-8. Explore the Mesial Surface from Facial Aspect.
- It is important to explore the mesial surface from both the facial and lingual aspects. First, practice exploring the mesial surface from the facial aspect as pictured here.
- *As you explore the concavity, note how difficult it is to completely adapt the explorer tip to the concavity using the basic instrumentation technique used for exploring tooth crowns.*

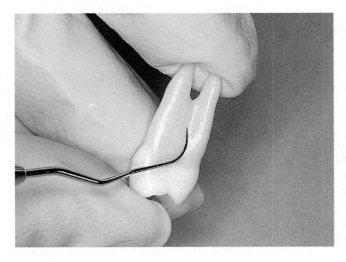

Figure 21-9. Advanced Working-End Position from the Mesial Aspect.
- Proximal root concavities can be more effectively explored by positioning the working-end in a tip-up position.
- Use horizontal strokes to explore the concavity taking care not to touch the soft tissue base of the pocket with the pointed tip of the explorer.

MANDIBULAR FIRST MOLAR—CONCAVITIES AND FURCATION AREA

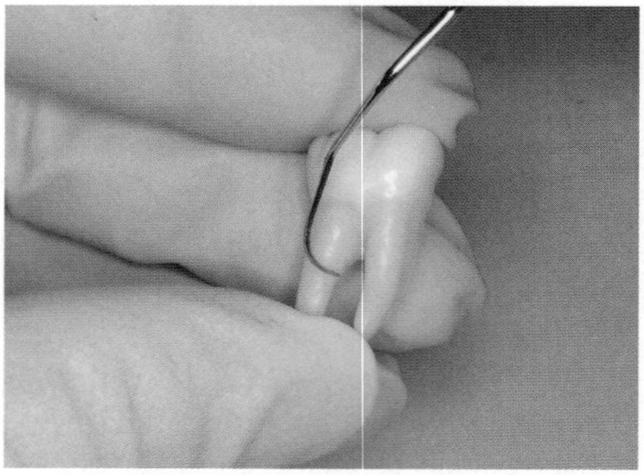

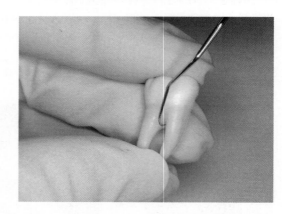

Figure 21-10. Furcation—Mesial Portion of Distal Root. Use the leading-third of the tip to explore the mesial portion of the distal root.

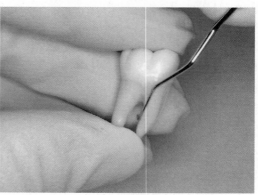

Figure 21-11. Roof of the Furcation. Use the explorer tip to explore the roof of the furcation.

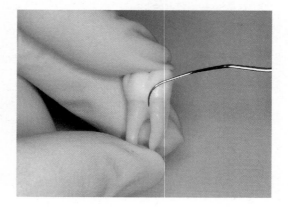

Figure 21-12. Furcation—Distal Portion of Mesial Root. Explore the distal portion of the mesial root.

Figure 21-13. Facial Depression. Most mandibular molars have a deep depression on the root trunk that extends from cervical line to the bifurcation. A tip-down position of the explorer is most effective for exploring this depression. As you explore, note that the depression deepens near the furcation. Take care not to touch the soft tissue base of the pocket with the pointed tip of the explorer.

MAXILLARY FIRST MOLAR—CONCAVITIES AND FURCATION AREAS

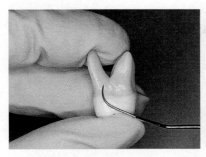 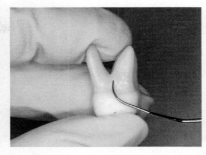 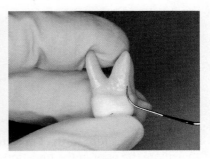

Figure 21-14. Concavity—Advanced Technique. Practice using the explorer in a tip-up position with a series of short horizontal strokes to assess the distal surface of the maxillary first molar. This is the most effective approach for adapting to the concavity below the furcation. Take care not to touch the soft tissue base of the pocket with the pointed tip of the explorer.

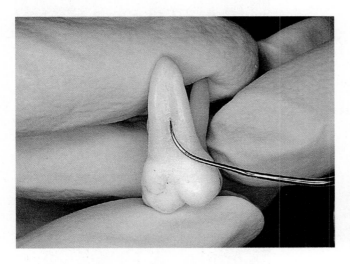

Figure 21-15. Palatal Root Depression. A tip-up approach with horizontal strokes is most effective when exploring the narrow linear depression on the palatal (lingual) root of a maxillary molar.

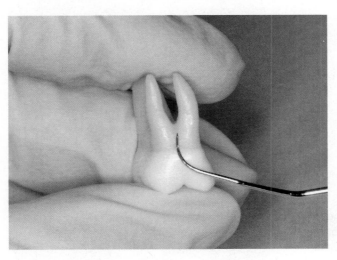

Figure 21-16. Facial Depression. Most maxillary molars have a deep depression on the root trunk that extends from cervical line to the bifurcation. Use a tip-up position and horizontal strokes to explore this area of the molar.

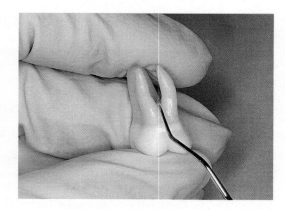

Figure 21-17. Floor of the Furcation. Use the explorer tip to explore the floor of the furcation.

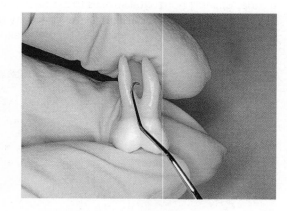

Figure 21-18. Furcation—Mesial Portion of Distal Root. Use the leading-third of the tip to explore the mesial portion of the distal root.

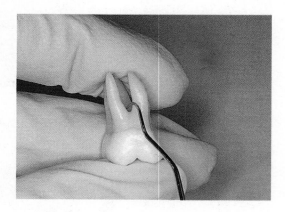

Figure 21-19. Furcation—Distal Portion of Mesial Root. Explore the distal portion of the mesial root.

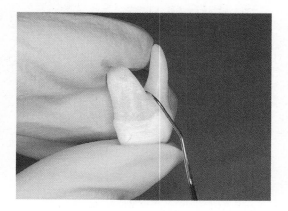

Figure 21-20. Furcation—Mesial Surface. The mesial furcation between the mesiobuccal and palatal roots is located more toward the lingual surface. Therefore, the mesial furcation is explored more easily from the lingual aspect. The distal furcation is located near the center of the tooth and may be explored from either the facial or lingual approach.

Section 2
Introduction to Root Instrumentation

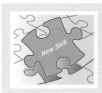

SKILL BUILDING
Instrumentation of Multirooted Teeth with Area-Specific Curets

INSTRUMENTATION SEQUENCE

Successful instrumentation of a multirooted tooth is dependent on a systematic approach to instrumentation. A recommended approach is illustrated in Figures 21-21 to 21-23.

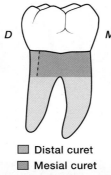

☐ Distal curet
☐ Mesial curet

Figure 21-21. Begin with the Root Trunk. With an area-specific curet use the distal curet on the distal surface of the root trunk and mesial curet on the facial and mesial surfaces of the root trunk.

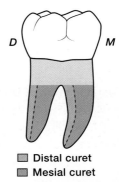

☐ Distal curet
☐ Mesial curet

Figure 21-22. Instrument the Root Branches. First, use the distal curet on the distal aspect of both roots. Second, use the mesial curet on the mesial aspect of the roots.

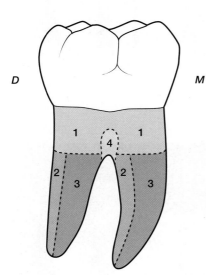

Figure 21-23. Curet Selection of Root Surface by Area.
Area 1. Instrument the root trunk, using the distal curet followed by the mesial curet.
Area 2. Treat each root as a separate tooth. Use the distal curet on the distal portion of each root.
Area 3. Use the mesial curet on the mesial portions of each root.
Area 4. Treat the roof of the furcation and the concavity coronal to the furcation entrance with the mesial curet.
  • Use the toe of the curet against the roof of the furcation on a mandibular tooth.
  • Position the curet and use horizontal strokes in the concavity.

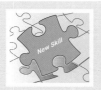

SKILL BUILDING
Technique with Area-Specific Curets on Multirooted Teeth

Directions: To practice instrumentation of the surfaces of multirooted teeth, you will need a set of area-specific curets and a periodontal typodont or an acrylic model of a mandibular first molar. Follow the steps as pictured in Figures 21-24 to 21-28.

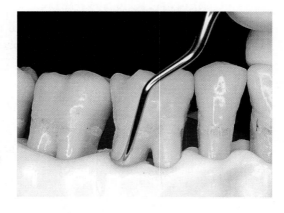

Figure 21-24. Distal Portion of Distal Root. Use the *distal* curet to instrument the distal portion of the distal root, beginning at the line angle.

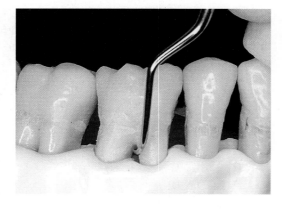

Figure 21-25. Distal Portion of Mesial Root. Using the *distal* curet, instrument the distal portion of the mesial root.

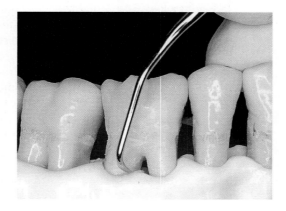

Figure 21-26. Mesial Portion of Distal Root. Beginning at the line angle, use the *mesial* curet to instrument the mesial portion of the distal root.

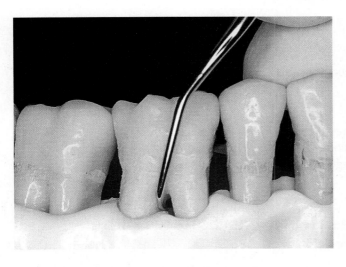

Figure 21-27. Furcation. Instrument the mesial side of the furcation using the *mesial* curet.

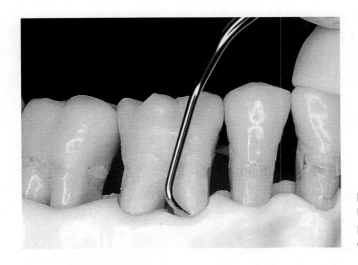

Figure 21-28. Mesial Portion of Mesial Root. Use the *mesial* curet to instrument the mesial portion of the mesial root and the mesial surface of the root.

SKILL BUILDING
Selecting Area-Specific Curets for Applying Horizontal Strokes to Root Surfaces

When using an area-specific curet, the working-end selection for a horizontal stroke requires some thought on the part of the clinician (Box 21-1). It is important to consider that there is only one cutting edge per working-end of the area-specific curet.

Box 21-1 | ## Horizontal Strokes on Proximal Surfaces with Area-Specific Curets

- For distal surfaces, if the G13 is used for vertical strokes, use the G14 for horizontal strokes.
- For mesial surfaces, if the G11 is used for vertical strokes, use the G12 for horizontal strokes.

Switch working-ends of an area-specific curet for horizontal strokes on proximal surfaces.

Directions: Follow the photographs in Figures 21-29 and 21-30 to select the correct area-specific curet for vertical and horizontal strokes on the mesial surface of a molar tooth.

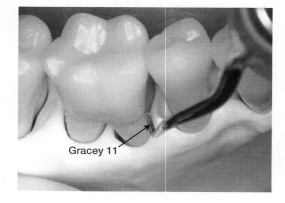

Figure 21-29. Vertical Strokes on Mesial. Root Surface.
- *Adapt the Gracey 11 curet to the mesial surface of a mandibular right molar in position for a VERTICAL stroke.*
- Note that the lower cutting edge with the nail polish is adapted against the mesial surface.
- *The Gracey 11 is the correct working-end for making vertical strokes on the mesial surface.*

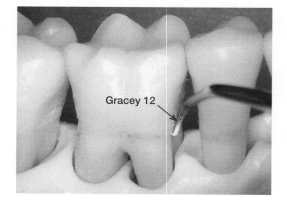

Figure 21-30. Horizontal Strokes on the Mesial Proximal Surface.
- *Next, position the Gracey 12 in a toe-down position for a HORIZONTAL stroke and adapt it to the mesial surface.*
- *The correct working-end is the Gracey 12 when making horizontal strokes on the mesial proximal surface of the mandibular right molar from the facial aspect.*

Section 3
Advanced Intraoral Techniques for Root Instrumentation

Advanced intraoral fulcruming techniques include the (1) cross arch fulcrum, (2) opposite arch fulcrum, and (3) finger-on-finger fulcrum. Advanced fulcruming techniques facilitate access to root surfaces and may reduce stress to the clinician's fingers and wrist when working within deep periodontal pockets (6–10).

CROSS ARCH AND OPPOSITE ARCH FULCRUMS

1. Cross Arch Intraoral Fulcrum
   A. The cross arch fulcrum is accomplished by resting the ring finger on a tooth on the opposite side of the arch from the teeth being instrumented (Fig. 21-31). For example, resting on the left side of the mandible to instrument a mandibular right molar.
   B. *Cross arch fulcrums are most useful when using horizontal strokes in proximal root concavities with curet in either a toe-up or toe-down position.*
2. Opposite Arch Intraoral Fulcrum
   A. The opposite arch fulcrum is an advanced fulcrum used to improve access to deep pockets and to facilitate parallelism to proximal root surfaces (Fig. 21-32).
   B. It is accomplished by resting the ring finger on the opposite arch from the treatment area (for example, resting on the mandibular arch to instrument maxillary teeth).

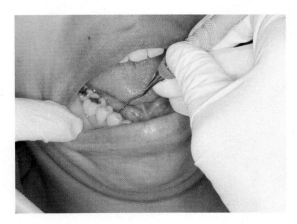

Figure 21-31. Cross Arch Fulcrum. The photograph shows a cross arch fulcrum demonstrated by a right-handed clinician. The clinician fulcrums on the mandibular left premolars while instrumenting the lingual aspect of the mandibular right posteriors.

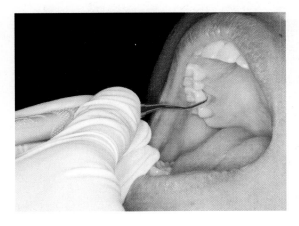

Figure 21-32. Opposite Arch Fulcrum. In this example, an opposite arch fulcrum is being used on the mandibular anterior teeth to instrument a maxillary molar.

FINGER-ON-FINGER FULCRUM

The finger-on-finger fulcrum is accomplished by resting the ring finger of the dominant hand on a finger of the *nondominant* hand.

- This technique allows the clinician to fulcrum in line with the long axis of the tooth to improve parallelism of the lower shank to the tooth surface.
- The nondominant index finger provides a stable rest for the clinician's dominant hand and provides improved access to deep periodontal pockets.
- Figures 21-33 to 21-35, on this page and the next, depict a finger-on-finger fulcrum for the maxillary right and left posterior teeth and mandibular left posterior teeth.

Example 1: Maxillary Right Posteriors, Facial Aspect

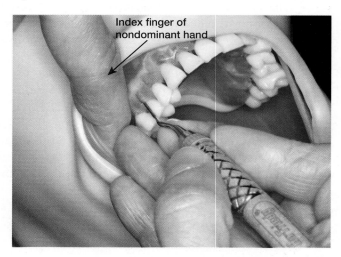

Figure 21-33A. Finger-on-Finger Fulcrum for the Maxillary Right Posteriors, Facial Aspect.
- In this example, the *right-handed clinician* establishes a finger rest on the index finger of the nondominant hand.
- The index finger of the nondominant hand is positioned in the mucobuccal fold, resting against the attached gingiva, alveolar mucosa, and underlying alveolar bone.

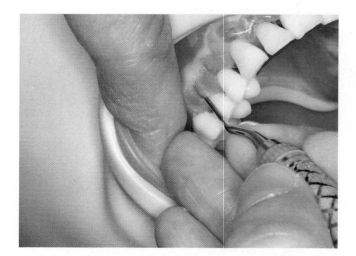

Figure 21-33B. Close-Up View: Finger-on-Finger Fulcrum for the Maxillary Right Posteriors, Facial Aspect. This photograph provides a closer view of the finger-on-finger fulcrum shown above in Figure 21-33A.

Example 2: Maxillary Left Posteriors, Facial Aspect

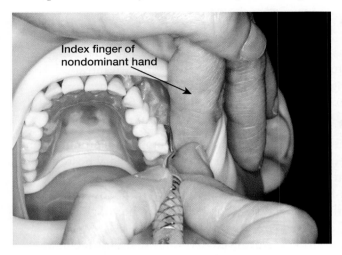

Figure 21-34A. Finger-on-Finger Fulcrum for the Maxillary Left Posteriors, Facial Aspect.
- In this example, the *right-handed clinician* establishes a finger rest on the index finger of the nondominant hand.
- The index finger of the nondominant hand is positioned in the mucobuccal fold, resting against the attached gingiva, alveolar mucosa, and underlying alveolar bone.

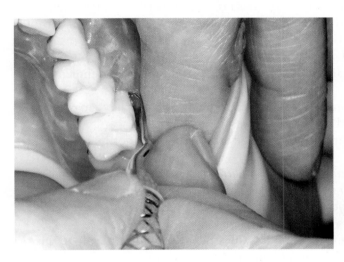

Figure 21-34B. Close-Up View: Finger-on-Finger Fulcrum for the Maxillary Right Posteriors, Facial Aspect. This photograph provides a closer view of the finger-on-finger fulcrum shown above in Figure 21-34A.

Example 3: Mandibular Left Posteriors, Facial Aspect

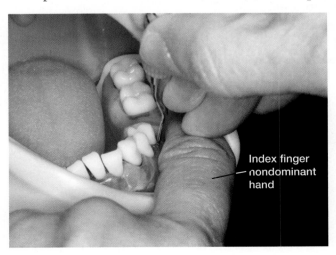

Figure 21-35. Finger-on-Finger Fulcrum for the Mandibular Left Posteriors, Facial Aspect.
- In this example, the *right-handed clinician* establishes a finger rest on the index finger of the nondominant hand.
- The index finger of the nondominant hand is positioned in the mucobuccal fold, resting against the attached gingiva, alveolar mucosa, and underlying alveolar bone.

Section 4
Advanced Extraoral Fulcruming Techniques

There are times when it is difficult to obtain parallelism with the lower shank or to adapt the cutting edge when using a standard intraoral fulcrum. In instances when a standard intraoral fulcrum does not seem to work well, an advanced extraoral fulcruming technique can improve access to the tooth surface and reduce stress on the clinician's fingers and wrist (6–10). Table 21-1 summarizes the advantages and disadvantages of extraoral fulcruming techniques.

1. **When to Use an Advanced Extraoral Fulcrum.** Advanced extraoral fulcrums are required when working in a deep periodontal pocket, especially when instrumenting the maxillary posterior teeth. Advanced extraoral fulcrums facilitate:
    A. **Proper Adaptation.** Advanced extraoral fulcrums facilitate positioning of the lower shank of a Gracey extended shank curet so that the extended shank is parallel to the root surface to be instrumented.
    B. **Complete Coverage with Instrumentation Strokes.** Advanced extraoral fulcrums facilitate insertion of the curet working-end all the way to the base of a deep periodontal pocket. Insert to the base of a deep pocket allows the clinician to cover every millimeter of the root surface with instrumentation strokes.
2. **Considerations and Cautions for use of Advanced Extraoral Fulcrums**
    A. **Clinician Skill Level.** Advanced extraoral fulcruming techniques require greater clinician skill and psychomotor control.
        1. Before attempting advanced fulcruming techniques, the clinician should have mastered the fundamentals of neutral position and standard fulcruming technique.
            a. Bad habits with fundamental techniques and intraoral fulcrums cannot be corrected by the use of advanced fulcrums.
            b. *A clinician with poor skill attainment of fundamental techniques will compound his or her problems by attempting to use advanced fulcrums. Unorthodox methods of instrumentation may serve as a quick fix for achieving an end product, but usually at the expense of the clinician's musculoskeletal system.*
        2. Before attempting advanced fulcruming techniques, the student should self-evaluate his or her skill level with a standard intraoral fulcrum and request a critique from an instructor.
    B. **Selective Use of Advanced Extraoral Fulcrums.** *Advanced fulcruming techniques are NOT intended to replace the intraoral fulcrum.* Intraoral fulcrums provide the best stability for instrumentation. Advanced fulcrums should be used selectively in areas of limited access, and/or in order to maintain neutral body position.

TABLE 21-1. BENEFITS AND DRAWBACKS OF EXTRAORAL FULCRUMING TECHNIQUES

Advantages	Disadvantages
Easier access to maxillary molars	Require a greater degree of muscle coordination and instrumentation skill to achieve calculus removal
Easier access to deep pockets on molar teeth	Greater risk for instrument stick
Improved parallelism of the lower shank to molar teeth	Reduce tactile information to the fingers
Facilitate neutral wrist position for molar teeth	Not well tolerated by patients with TMJ problems

BASIC EXTRAORAL FULCRUMING TECHNIQUES: RIGHT-HANDED CLINICIANS

Basic extraoral fulcruming technique involves resting the fingers or palm of the hand against the patient's chin or cheeks and underlying bone of the mandible.

1. **Resting the Fingers Against the Patient's Chin to Stabilize the Hand**
   - When working on the maxillary *right* posterior sextants, the clinician stabilizes his or her hand by resting the fingers against the patient's chin as shown in Figure 21-36.
   - This "**palm facing out technique**" involves resting the front surfaces of the middle, ring, and little fingers against the skin and underlying bone of the mandible. The fingers should remain straight—not curved like a fist—and together in the grasp. As much of the length of the fingers, as possible, should be kept in contact with the mandible.
2. **Cupping the Patient's Chin to Stabilize the Hand**
   - When working on the maxillary *left* posterior sextants, the clinician stabilizes the hand by cupping the palm of the hand around the patient's chin and mandible as shown in Figure 21-37.
   - This basic extraoral technique is known as the "**chin-cup technique.**"

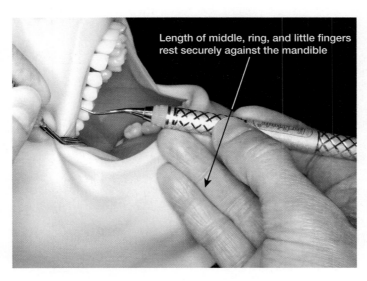

Length of middle, ring, and little fingers rest securely against the mandible

Figure 21-36. Palm Facing Out Technique for Maxillary Right Posterior Sextants.
- For the maxillary right posterior sextants, the clinician rests the fingers of the middle, ring, and little fingers against the skin and underlying bone of the mandibular arch.
- Note that the palm is facing out, away from the patient's face.

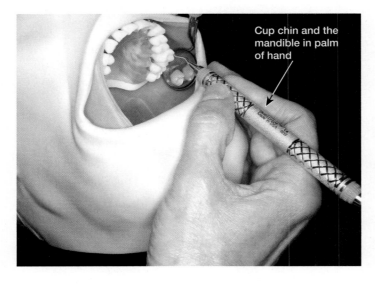

Cup chin and the mandible in palm of hand

Figure 21-37. Chin-Cup Technique for Maxillary Left Posterior Sextants.
- For the maxillary left posterior sextants, the clinician cups the patient's chin and mandible with the palm of his or her hand.
- Note that the palm of the hand is against—toward—the patient's mandible.

RIGHT-HANDED CLINICIAN

BASIC EXTRAORAL FULCRUMING TECHNIQUES: LEFT-HANDED CLINICIANS

Basic extraoral fulcruming technique involves resting the fingers or palm of the hand against the patient's chin or cheeks and underlying bone of the mandible.

1. Resting the Fingers Against the Patient's Chin to Stabilize the Hand
   - When working on the maxillary *left* posterior sextants, the clinician stabilizes his or her hand by resting the fingers against the patient's chin as shown in Figure 21-38.
   - This "**palm facing out technique**" involves resting the front surfaces of the middle, ring, and little fingers against the skin and underlying bone of the mandible. The fingers should remain straight—not curved like a fist—and together in the grasp. As much of the length of the fingers, as possible, should be kept in contact with the mandible.
2. Cupping the Patient's Chin to Stabilize the Hand
   - When working on the maxillary *right* posterior sextants, the clinician stabilizes the hand by cupping the palm of the hand around the patient's chin and mandible as shown in Figure 21-39.
   - This basic extraoral technique is known as the "**chin-cup technique**."

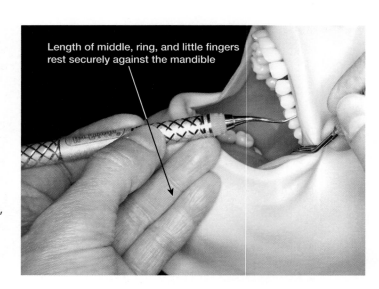

Length of middle, ring, and little fingers rest securely against the mandible

Figure 21-38. Palm-Up Technique for Maxillary Left Posterior Sextants.
- For the maxillary left posterior sextants, the clinician rests the fingers of the middle, ring, and little fingers against the skin and underlying bone of the mandibular arch.
- Note that the palm is facing out, away from the patient's face.

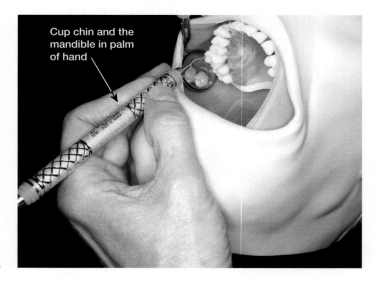

Cup chin and the mandible in palm of hand

Figure 21-39. Chin-Cup Technique for Maxillary Right Posterior Sextants.
- For the maxillary right posterior sextants, the clinician cups the patient's chin and mandible with the palm of his or her hand.
- Note that the palm of the hand is against—toward—the patient's mandible.

CRITERIA FOR AN EFFECTIVE EXTRAORAL FULCRUM

Effective technique for an extraoral fulcrum differs from that of an intraoral fulcrum in two important ways. These technique differences involve the instrument grasp and the technique employed to stabilize the hand. Table 21-2 summarizes the techniques employed for each type of finger rest. Figure 21-40 shows the modified grasp used with an extraoral fulcrum.

TABLE 21-2. TECHNIQUE COMPARISON FOR INTRAORAL AND EXTRAORAL FULCRUMS		
	Intraoral Fulcrum	**Extraoral Fulcrum**
Grasp	• Handle held in a modified pen grasp near the junction of the handle and the shank, close to the working-end	• Handle grasped lower on the handle, farther away from the working-end
Stabilization	• Pad of ring finger rests securely on a stable tooth • Ring finger acts as a "support beam" for the hand • Middle, ring, and little fingers are in contact acting as a unit	• Length of middle, ring, and little fingers rest securely against the skin and underlying bone of the mandible • All three fingers press against the mandible; one finger contact is not effective • Middle, ring, and little fingers are in contact acting as a unit

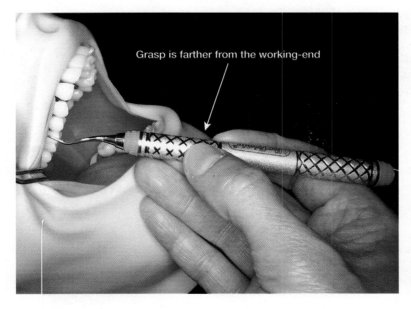

Grasp is farther from the working-end

Figure 21-40. Grasp for Extraoral Fulcrum. The clinician should: (1) grasp the instrument handle farther away from the working-end and (2) stabilize the hand against the underlying bone of the patient's jaw for an effective extraoral fulcruming technique.

MODIFICATIONS TO BASIC EXTRAORAL FULCRUMS: INSTRUMENTATION STROKE WITH A FINGER ASSIST

An instrumentation stroke with a finger assist is accomplished by using the index finger of the nondominant hand *against the shank of a periodontal instrument to assist in the instrumentation stroke* (Figs. 21-41 to 21-43).

- For this advanced technique, the index finger of the nondominant hand is placed against the instrument shank to: (1) concentrate lateral pressure against the tooth surface and (2) help control the working-end throughout the instrumentation stroke.
- The *instrumentation stroke with a finger assist* can be combined with a basic intraoral or extraoral fulcrum.
- The *instrumentation stroke with finger assist* is an extremely effective technique for removing calculus deposits from root surfaces located within deep periodontal pockets.
- *For this technique, the clinician applies pressure against the shank of the instrument. The index finger of the nondominant hand moves with the instrument shank throughout a short, controlled instrumentation stroke.* As long as the nondominant finger remains securely against the shank, the risk of an instrument stick is limited.

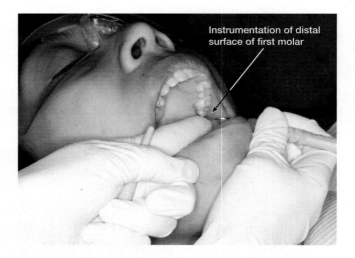

Figure 21-41A. Finger Assist on the Distal Surface.
- The photograph shows a right-handed clinician applying a finger assist behind the instrument shank.
- In this case the clinician is instrumenting the **distal surface** of the maxillary first molar.
- The clinician is using an extraoral arch fulcrum on the mandibular arch.

Instrumentation of distal surface of first molar

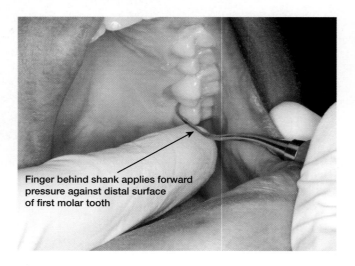

Figure 21-41B. Closer View of Finger Assist on the Distal Surface.
- This photograph is a closer view of the finger assist shown above in Figure 21-42A.
- The clinician is using the index finger of the left hand to apply pressure behind the shank, **thus concentrating lateral pressure with the cutting edge forward against the distal surface of the first molar**.

Finger behind shank applies forward pressure against distal surface of first molar tooth

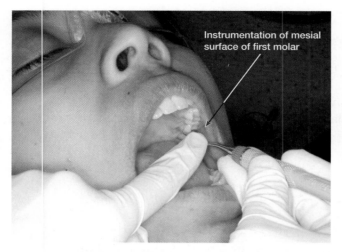

Instrumentation of mesial surface of first molar

Figure 21-42A. Finger Assist on the Mesial Surface.
- The photograph shows a right-handed clinician applying a finger assist against the instrument shank.
- In this case the clinician is instrumenting the *mesial surface* of the maxillary first molar.
- The clinician is using an extraoral arch fulcrum on the mandibular arch.

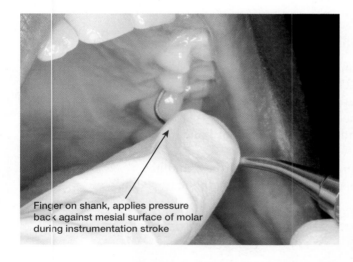

Finger on shank, applies pressure back against mesial surface of molar during instrumentation stroke

Figure 21-42B. Closer View of Finger Assist on the Distal Surface.
- This photograph is a closer view of the finger assist pictured in Figure 21-42A.
- The clinician is using the index finger of the left hand to apply pressure against the shank, *thus concentrating lateral pressure with the cutting edge backward against the mesial surface of the first molar.*

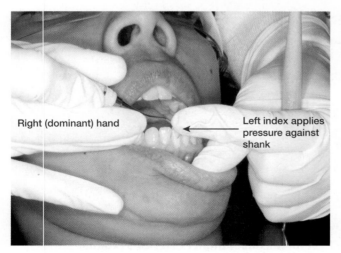

Right (dominant) hand

Left index applies pressure against shank

Figure 21-43. Finger Assist on Mandibular Arch.
- The right-handed clinician—seated behind the patient—positions the left index finger on the shank to stabilize a short horizontal stroke.
- The finger assist helps the clinician to control a short horizontal stroke by concentrating pressure precisely on the cutting edge.

Section 5
Technique Practice: Extraoral Finger Rests for Right-Handed Clinicians

Directions: A set of area-specific curets is recommended for this technique practice. This technique practice is best accomplished on a dental manikin with a periodontal typodont. Follow the directions and photographs in Figures 21-44 to 21-51 to practice the "palm facing out" technique.

SKILL BUILDING
"Palm Facing Out" Extraoral Fulcrum: Maxillary Right Posterior Sextants

Basic Extraoral Finger Rest for Maxillary Right Posterior Sextants

- Rest the front surfaces of the middle, ring, and little fingers against the skin and underlying bone of the mandible as depicted in Figure 21-44.
- Keep the fingers straight and together in the grasp; as much of the length of the fingers, as possible, should be kept in contact with the mandible.
- Apply pressure against the bone of the mandible to stabilize your hand and the instrument during instrumentation.
  - Note that the hand is not simply "hovering over" the skin of the mandible.
  - Rather, the clinician must apply pressure against the underlying bone to stabilize the grasp.

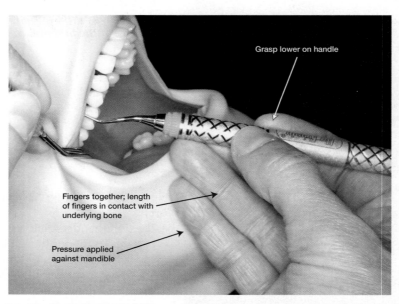

Grasp lower on handle

Fingers together; length of fingers in contact with underlying bone

Pressure applied against mandible

Figure 21-44. Basic Extraoral Finger Rest for Maxillary Right Posterior Sextants.

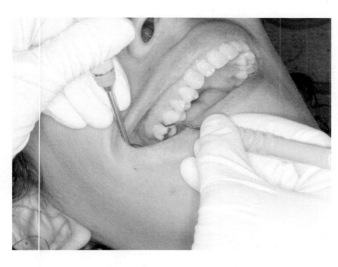

Figure 21-45. Technique Summary for Distal Surfaces of Facial Aspect.
- Extraoral "palm-out" fulcrum
- Vertical and oblique strokes

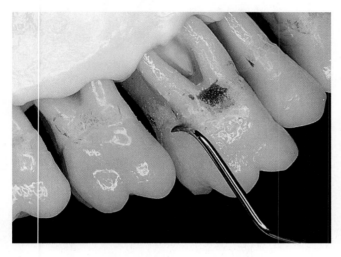

Figure 21-46. Distal Concavity of First Molar.
- Use the *distal curet*.
- Rotate the handle slightly to adapt the toe-third of the cutting edge to the distal concavity.

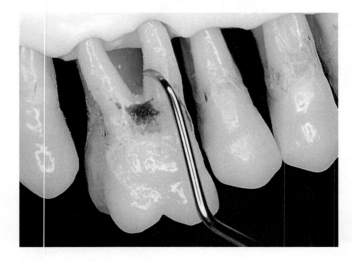

Figure 21-47. Distal Portion of the Mesial Root. Use the *distal curet* on the distal portion of the mesial root.

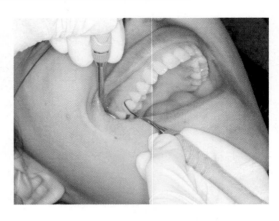

Figure 21-48. Technique Summary for Mesial Surfaces of Facial Aspect.
- Extraoral "palm-out" fulcrum
- Vertical and oblique strokes

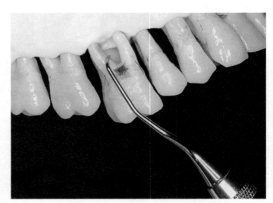

Figure 21-49. Mesial Portion of the Distal Root. Use the *mesial curet* on the mesial portion of the distal root.

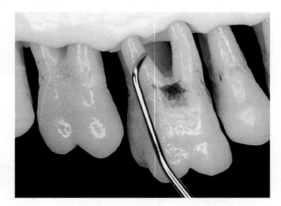

Figure 21-50. Mesial Portion of the Distal Root—Close-up View. The *mesial curet* is used to debride the mesial portion of the distal root and the "roof" of the furcation.

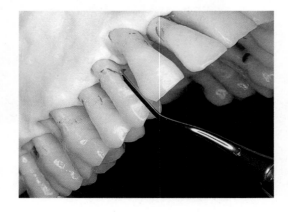

Figure 21-51. Mesial Surface of the First Premolar.
- The maxillary first premolar has the deepest concavity in the entire dentition.
- Use the mesial curet to debride the mesial concavity.
- ***Rotate the toe-third of the cutting edge toward the root surface to adapt to the concavity.***

SKILL BUILDING
"Chin-Cup" Extraoral Fulcrum: Maxillary Right Posterior Sextants

Directions: When working on the maxillary left posterior sextants, the patient's chin and mandible is cupped with the palm of the clinician's hand. Follow the directions and photographs in Figures 21-52 to 21-59 to practice the "chin-cup" technique.

Basic Extraoral Finger Rest for Maxillary Left Posterior Sextants

- Cup the patient's chin and mandible in the palm of the hand.
- Rest the palm of the hand and the palmer surfaces of the middle, ring, and little fingers against the skin and underlying bone of the mandible.
- Keep the fingers straight and together in the grasp; as much of the length of the fingers, as possible, should be kept in contact with the mandible.
- Apply pressure against the bone of the mandible to stabilize your hand and the instrument during instrumentation.
  - Note that the hand is not simply "hovering over" the skin of the mandible.
  - Rather, the clinician must apply pressure against the underlying bone to stabilize the grasp.

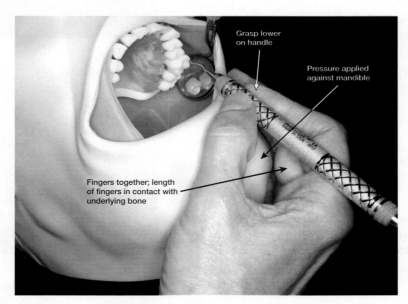

Figure 21-52. Basic Extraoral Finger Rest for Maxillary Left Posterior Sextants.

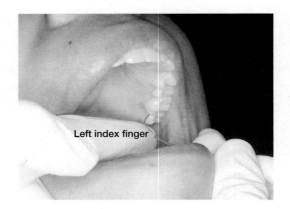

Figure 21-53. Technique Summary for Distal Surfaces.
- Extraoral "chin-cup" fulcrum with a finger assist
- Vertical strokes

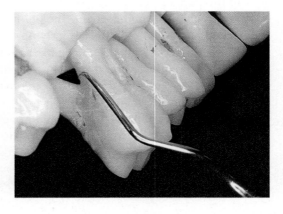

Figure 21-54. Distal Concavity.
- Use a ***distal curet*** to debride the distal concavity with vertical strokes. ***It is important to rotate the toe-third of the curet to adapt to the concavity.***
- Use the index finger of your nondominant hand to apply pressure behind the shank, thus ***concentrating pressure with the cutting edge forward against the distal surface*** of the first molar.

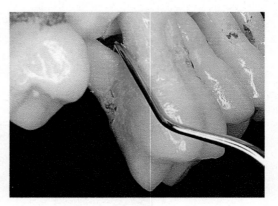

Figure 21-55. Distal Furcation.
- The distal furcation entrance is located near the midline of the tooth and therefore, can be instrumented from both the facial and lingual aspects.
- Use the ***distal curet*** to instrument the distal furcation.

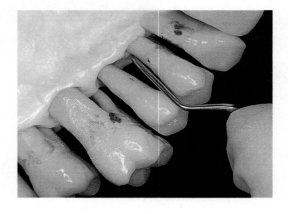

Figure 21-56. Distal Surface of Premolar.
- Use the ***distal curet*** on the distal surface of the premolar.
- Use the index finger of your nondominant hand to apply pressure behind the shank, thus ***concentrating pressure with the cutting edge forward against the distal surface*** of the premolar.

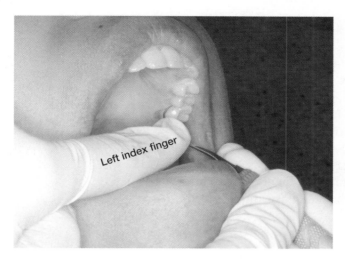

Figure 21-57. Technique Summary for Mesial Surfaces.
- Extraoral "chin-cup" fulcrum with a finger assist
- Index finger of nondominant hand provides lateral pressure back against mesial surface
- Vertical strokes

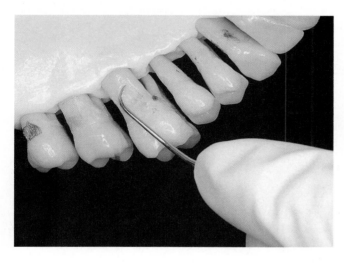

Figure 21-58. Lingual Surface of Palatal Root.
- The palatal root commonly has a deep depression.
- Use the *mesial curet*.
- Use the index finger of your nondominant hand to apply pressure against the shank, thus *concentrating pressure with the cutting edge against the lingual surface* of the first molar (Fig. 21-43).

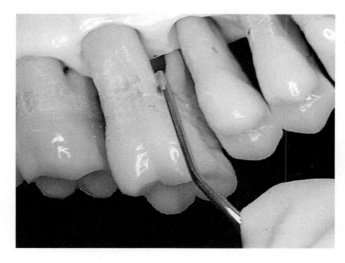

Figure 21-59. Mesial Furcation.
- The entrance to the mesial furcation is located toward the lingual aspect—rather than being located at the midline of the mesial surface.
- Due to its location the entrance is best accessed from the lingual aspect using a mesial curet.

RIGHT-HANDED CLINICIAN

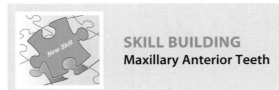

SKILL BUILDING
Maxillary Anterior Teeth

Due to the narrow roots, subgingival instrumentation of anterior teeth is challenging for the clinician (11–12).

Directions: Follow the directions and photographs in Figures 21-60 and 21-61 to practice advanced fulcruming techniques on the maxillary anterior teeth.

Maxillary Anteriors, Lingual Aspect

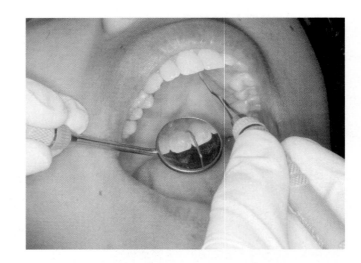

Figure 21-60. Technique Summary for Lingual Aspect Using Vertical Strokes.
• Extraoral fulcrum
• Vertical strokes

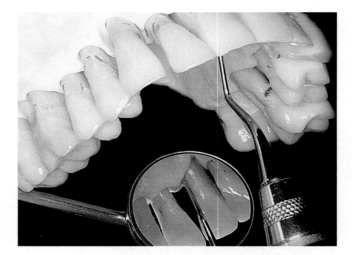

Figure 21-61. Lingual and Mesial Surfaces.
• Note that the root tapers toward the lingual.
• Use the index finger of your nondominant hand to apply pressure against the shank.

RIGHT-HANDED CLINICIAN

Section 6
Technique Practice: Horizontal Strokes for Right-Handed Clinicians

SKILL BUILDING
Horizontal Strokes on Maxillary Teeth. Curet in Toe-up Orientation

Horizontal instrumentation strokes—made with the curet in either a toe-up or toe-down position—are very effective for instrumenting root concavities (13).

Directions: Follow the directions and photographs in Figures 21-62 to 21-71 to practice horizontal strokes in the toe-up position on the maxillary posterior teeth.

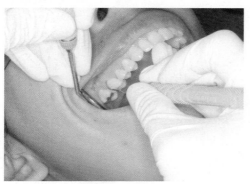

Figure 21-62. Technique Summary for Distal Concavities.
- Intraoral fulcrum
- Working-end in the toe-up position with Gracey miniature 7 or 13 curets
- Very short, controlled horizontal strokes

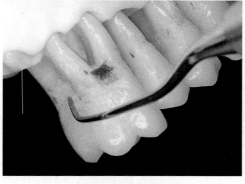

Figure 21-63. Distal Concavity of First Molar.
- The Gracey miniature 7/8 works well in this area.
- Use the opposite working-end from the one that you used to make vertical strokes on the distal.
- Use the curet in a toe-up position, adapt the lower cutting edge, and make a series of horizontal strokes. This technique facilitates calculus removal from the concavity.

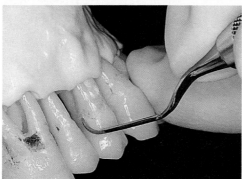

Figure 21-64. Distal Concavity of First Premolar. Use the curet in a toe-up position to make a series of short controlled horizontal strokes in the distal concavity.

RIGHT-HANDED CLINICIAN

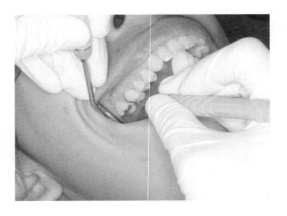

Figure 21-65. Technique Summary for Facial and Mesial Concavities.

- Intraoral fulcrum
- Working-end in the toe-up position
- Short horizontal strokes

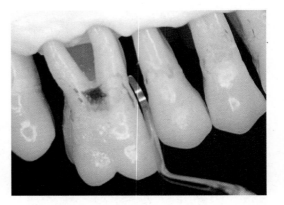

Figure 21-66. Facial Concavity.

- A common area for missed calculus deposits is the broad concavity that extends from the furcation to the CEJ on molar teeth.
- Use the Gracey miniature 12 curet in a toe-up position to make short horizontal strokes in the depression.

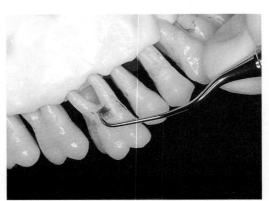

Figure 21-67. Mesial Concavity of Molar.

- Use the Gracey miniature 11 curet in a toe-up position to make horizontal strokes in the concavity.
- This is the opposite working-end from the one you would use to make vertical strokes on the mesial surface.

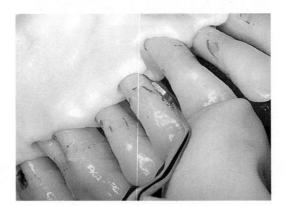

Figure 21-68. Mesial Concavity of Premolar. Use the Gracey miniature 11 curet in a toe-up position to make horizontal strokes in the concavity.

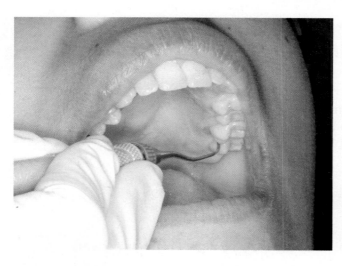

Figure 21-69. Technique Summary for Mesial Concavities.
- Cross arch fulcrum
- Working-end in the toe-up position
- Short horizontal strokes

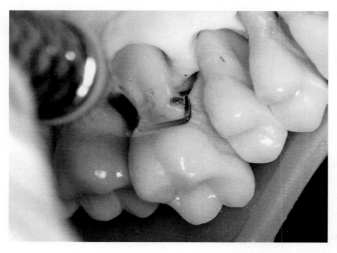

Figure 21-70. Mesial Concavity of Molar.
- The linear concavities often are difficult to debride using vertical strokes.
- Use the miniature curet in a toe-up position (toward the palate) with horizontal strokes to debride the concavity. This is the opposite working-end from the one you would use to make vertical strokes on the mesial surface.

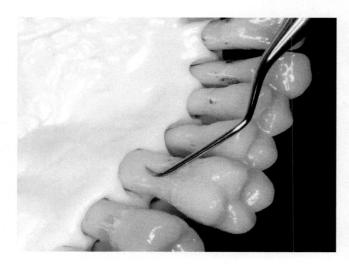

Figure 21-71. Palatal Root Depression.
- The palatal root has a narrow root depression that is difficult to instrument using vertical strokes.
- Use a miniature curet in a toe-up position with a series of short horizontal strokes. Begin making strokes at the base of the pocket, then move coronally slightly, and repeat the process.

RIGHT-HANDED CLINICIAN

Section 7
Technique Practice: Extraoral Finger Rests for Left-Handed Clinicians

Directions: A set of area-specific curets is recommended for this technique practice. This technique practice is best accomplished on a dental manikin with a periodontal typodont. Follow the directions and photographs in Figures 21-72 to 21-79 to practice the "palm facing out" technique.

SKILL BUILDING
"Palm Facing Out" Extraoral Fulcrum: Maxillary Right Posterior Sextants

Basic Extraoral Finger Rest for Maxillary Left Posterior Sextants
Rest the front surfaces of the middle, ring, and little fingers against the skin and underlying bone of the mandible as depicted in Figure 21-72.

- Keep the fingers straight and together in the grasp; as much of the length of the fingers, as possible, should be kept in contact with the mandible.
- Apply pressure against the bone of the mandible to stabilize your hand and the instrument during instrumentation.
  - Note that the hand is not simply "hovering over" the skin of the mandible.
  - Rather, the clinician must apply pressure against the underlying bone to stabilize the grasp.

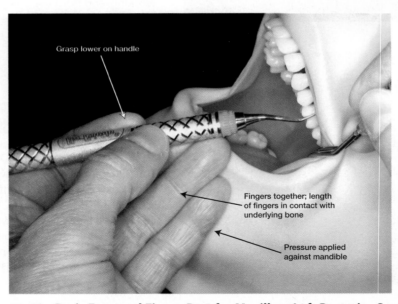

Grasp lower on handle

Fingers together; length of fingers in contact with underlying bone

Pressure applied against mandible

Figure 21-72. **Basic Extraoral Finger Rest for Maxillary Left Posterior Sextants.**

LEFT-HANDED CLINICIAN

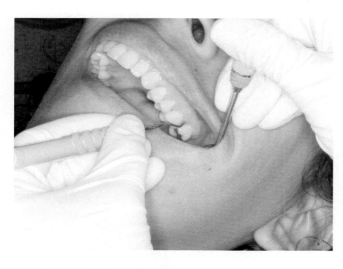

Figure 21-73. Technique Summary for Distal Surfaces of Facial Aspect.
- Extraoral "palm-out" fulcrum
- Vertical and oblique strokes

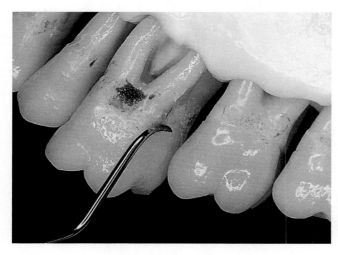

Figure 21-74. Distal Concavity of First Molar.
- Use the *distal curet*.
- Rotate the handle slightly to adapt the toe-third of the cutting edge to the distal concavity.

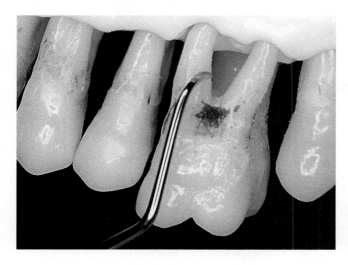

Figure 21-75. Distal Portion of the Mesial Root. Use the *distal curet* on the distal portion of the mesial root.

LEFT-HANDED CLINICIAN

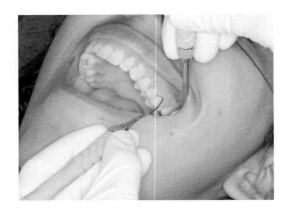

Figure 21-76. Technique Summary for Mesial Surfaces of Facial Aspect.
- Extraoral "palm-out" fulcrum
- Vertical and oblique strokes

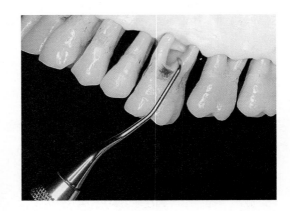

Figure 21-77. Mesial Portion of the Distal Root. Use the *mesial curet* on the mesial portion of the distal root.

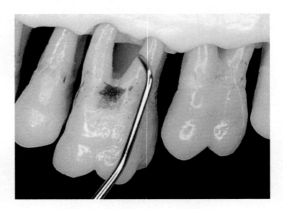

Figure 21-78. Mesial Portion of the Distal Root—Close-up View. The *mesial curet* is used to debride the mesial portion of the distal root and the "roof" of the furcation.

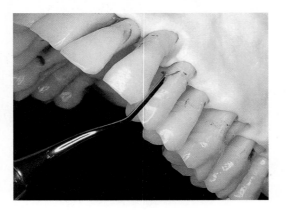

Figure 21-79. Mesial Surface of the First Premolar.
- The maxillary first premolar has the deepest concavity in the entire dentition.
- Use the mesial curet to debride the mesial concavity.
- ***Rotate the toe-third of the cutting edge toward the root surface to adapt to the concavity.***

SKILL BUILDING
"Chin-Cup" Extraoral Fulcrum: Maxillary Right Posterior Sextants

Directions: When working on the maxillary right posterior sextants, the patient's chin and mandible is cupped with the palm of the clinician's hand. Follow the directions and photographs in Figures 21-80 to 21-87 to practice the "chin-cup" technique.

Basic Extraoral Finger Rest for Maxillary Right Posterior Sextants

- Cup the patient's chin and mandible in the palm of the hand.
- Rest the palm of the hand and the palmer surfaces of the middle, ring, and little fingers against the skin and underlying bone of the mandible.
- Keep the fingers straight and together in the grasp; as much of the length of the fingers, as possible, should be kept in contact with the mandible.
- Apply pressure against the bone of the mandible to stabilize your hand and the instrument during instrumentation.
  - Note that the hand is not simply "hovering over" the skin of the mandible.
  - Rather, the clinician must apply pressure against the underlying bone to stabilize the grasp.

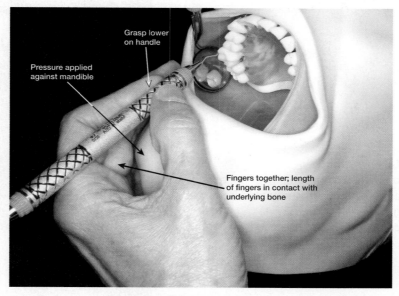

Figure 21-80. Basic Extraoral Finger Rest for Maxillary Right Posterior Sextants.

LEFT-HANDED CLINICIAN

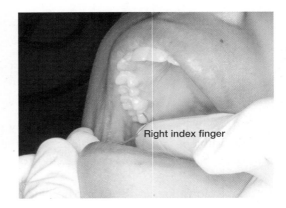

Figure 21-81. Technique Summary for Distal Surfaces.
- Extraoral "chin-cup" fulcrum with a finger assist
- Vertical strokes

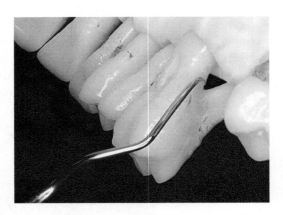

Figure 21-82. Distal Concavity.
- Use a ***distal curet*** to debride the distal concavity with vertical strokes. ***It is important to rotate the toe-third of the curet to adapt to the concavity.***
- Use the index finger of your nondominant hand to apply pressure behind the shank, thus ***concentrating pressure with the cutting edge forward against the distal surface*** of the first molar.

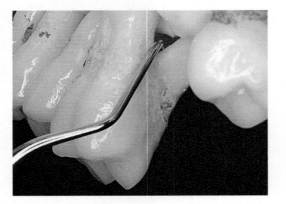

Figure 21-83. Distal Furcation.
- The distal furcation entrance is located near the midline of the tooth and therefore, can be instrumented from both the facial and lingual aspects.
- Use the ***distal curet*** to instrument the distal furcation.

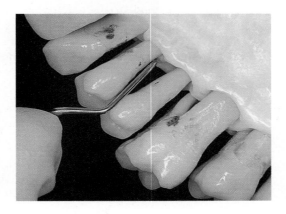

Figure 21-84. Distal Surface of Premolar.
- Use the ***distal curet*** on the distal surface of the premolar.
- Use the index finger of your nondominant hand to apply pressure behind the shank, thus ***concentrating pressure with the cutting edge forward against the distal surface*** of the premolar.

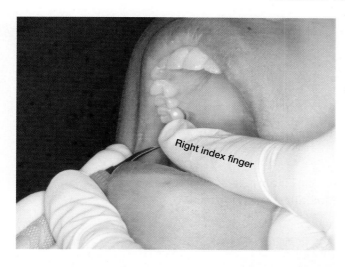

Figure 21-85. Technique Summary for Mesial Surfaces.
- Extraoral "chin-cup" fulcrum with a finger assist
- Index finger of nondominant hand provides lateral pressure back against mesial surface
- Vertical strokes

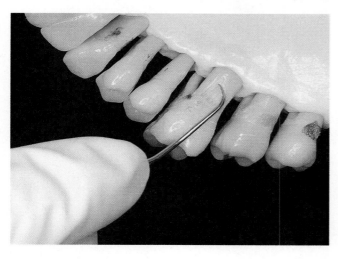

Figure 21-86. Lingual Surface of Palatal Root.
- The palatal root commonly has a deep depression.
- Use the *mesial curet*.
- Use the index finger of your nondominant hand to apply pressure against the shank, thus *concentrating pressure with the cutting edge against the lingual surface* of the first molar.

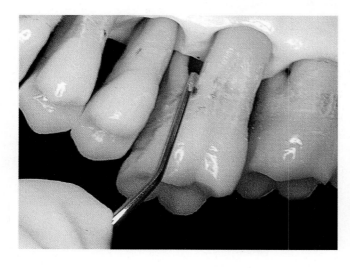

Figure 21-87. Mesial Furcation.
- The entrance to the mesial furcation is located toward the lingual aspect—rather than being located at the midline of the mesial surface.
- Due to its location the entrance is best accessed from the lingual aspect using a mesial curet.

LEFT-HANDED CLINICIAN

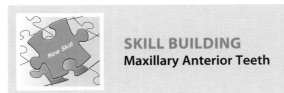

SKILL BUILDING
Maxillary Anterior Teeth

Due to the narrow roots, subgingival instrumentation of anterior teeth is challenging for the clinician (11,12).

Directions: Follow the directions and photographs in Figures 21-88 and 21-89 to practice advanced fulcruming techniques on the maxillary anterior teeth.

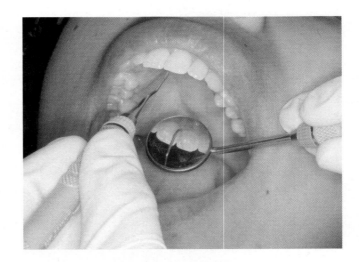

Figure 21-88. Technique Summary for Lingual Aspect Using Vertical Strokes.
- Extraoral fulcrum
- Vertical strokes

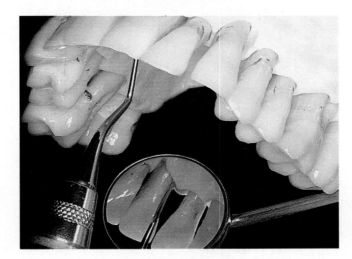

Figure 21-89. Lingual and Mesial Surfaces.
- Note that the root tapers toward the lingual.
- Use the index finger of your nondominant hand to apply pressure against the shank.

Section 8
Technique Practice: Horizontal Strokes for Left-Handed Clinicians

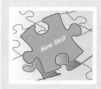

SKILL BUILDING
Horizontal Strokes on Maxillary Teeth. Curet in Toe-up Orientation

Horizontal instrumentation strokes—made with the curet in either a toe-up or toe-down position—are very effective for instrumenting root concavities (13).

Directions: Follow the directions and photographs in Figures 21-90 to 21-99, to practice horizontal strokes in the toe-up position on the maxillary posterior teeth.

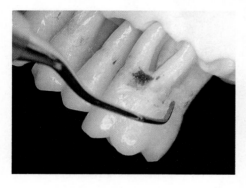

Figure 21-90. Technique Summary for Distal Concavities.
- Intraoral fulcrum
- Working-end in the toe-up position with Gracey miniature 7 or 13 curets
- Very short, controlled horizontal strokes

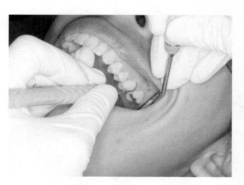

Figure 21-91. Distal Concavity of First Molar.
- The Gracey miniature 7/8 works well in this area.
- Use the opposite working-end from the one that you used to make vertical strokes on the distal.
- Use the curet in a toe-up position, adapt the lower cutting edge, and make a series of horizontal strokes. This technique facilitates calculus removal from the concavity.

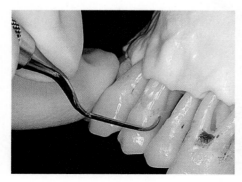

Figure 21-92. Distal Concavity of First Premolar. Use the curet in a toe-up position to make a series of short controlled horizontal strokes in the distal concavity.

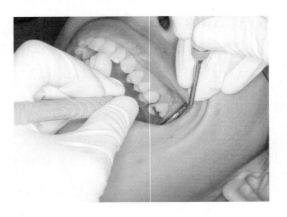

Figure 21-93. Technique Summary for Facial and Mesial Concavities.
- Intraoral fulcrum
- Working-end in the toe-up position
- Short horizontal strokes

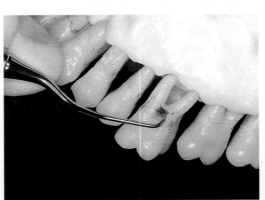

Figure 21-94. Facial Concavity.
- A common area for missed calculus deposits is the broad concavity that extends from the furcation to the CEJ on molar teeth.
- Use the Gracey miniature 12 curet in a toe-up position to make short horizontal strokes in the depression.

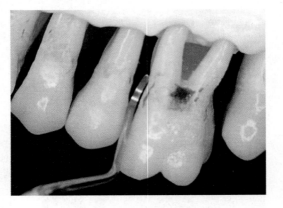

Figure 21-95. Mesial Concavity of Molar.
- Use the Gracey miniature 11 curet in a toe-up position to make horizontal strokes in the concavity.
- This is the opposite working-end from the one you would use to make vertical strokes on the mesial surface.

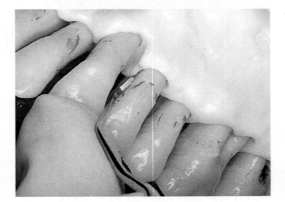

Figure 21-96. Mesial Concavity of Premolar. Use the Gracey miniature 11 curet in a toe-up position to make horizontal strokes in the concavity.

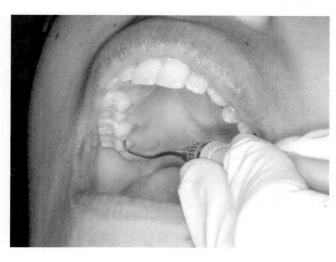

Figure 21-97. Technique Summary for Mesial Concavities.
- Cross arch fulcrum
- Working-end in the toe-up position
- Short horizontal strokes

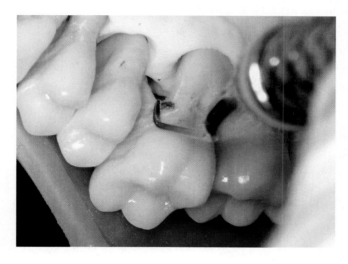

Figure 21-98. Mesial Concavity of Molar.
- The linear concavities often are difficult to debride using vertical strokes.
- Use the miniature curet in a toe-up position (toward the palate) with horizontal strokes to debride the concavity. This is the opposite working-end from the one you would use to make vertical strokes on the mesial surface.

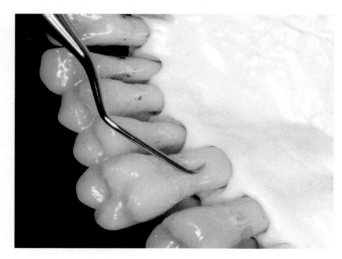

Figure 21-99. Palatal Root Depression.
- The palatal root has a narrow root depression that is difficult to instrument using vertical strokes.
- Use a miniature curet in a toe-up position with a series of short horizontal strokes. Begin making strokes at the base of the pocket, then move coronally slightly, and repeat the process.

References

1. Bower RC. Furcation morphology relative to periodontal treatment. Furcation root surface anatomy. *J Periodontol.* 1979;50(7):366–374.
2. Bower RC. Furcation morphology relative to periodontal treatment. Furcation entrance architecture. *J Periodontol.* 1979;50(1):23–27.
3. Gher ME, Vernino AR. Root morphology–clinical significance in pathogenesis and treatment of periodontal disease. *J Am Dent Assoc.* 1980;101(4):627–633.
4. Alves RV, Machion L, Casati MZ, Nociti Junior FH, Sallum AW, Sallum EA. Attachment loss after scaling and root planing with different instruments. A clinical study. *J Clin Periodontol.* 2004;31(1):12–15.
5. Gher ME, Jr., Vernino AR. Root anatomy: A local factor in inflammatory periodontal disease. *Int J Periodontics Restorative Dent.* 1981;1(5):52–63.
6. Chismark AM, Millar D. Scaling and exercise strategies to prevent hand, wrist, and arm injuries. *RDH Magazine.* 2014;34(5):48–49.
7. Cosaboom-FitzSimons ME, Tolle SL, Darby ML, Walker ML. Effects of 5 different finger rest positions on arm muscle activity during scaling by dental hygiene students. *J Dent Hyg.* 2008;82(4):34.
8. Dong H, Barr A, Loomer P, Rempel D. The effects of finger rest positions on hand muscle load and pinch force in simulated dental hygiene work. *J Dent Educ.* 2005;69(4):453–460.
9. Millar D. Reinforced periodontal instrumentation and ergonomics. *J CDHA.* 2009;24(3):8–16.
10. Nguygen M, Pattison A. Activate alternative fulcrums. Part 2. *Dimens Dent Hyg.* 2014;12(5):24–28.
11. Hodges K. Revisiting instrumentation in anterior segments. *Dimens Dent Hyg.* 2007;5(2):30–33.
12. Kiehl N. Instrumenting periodontally involved anterior teeth. *Dimens Dent Hyg.* 2012;10(11):26–29.
13. Costley SM. Mastering apical orientation of the tip. *Dimens Dent Hyg.* 2013;11(2):38–39, 43–44.

Section 9
Skill Application

Student Self Evaluation Module 21: Advanced Techniques for Root Surface Debridement

Student: _____   Date: _____

DIRECTIONS FOR STUDENT: Evaluate your skill level as: **S** (satisfactory) or **U** (unsatisfactory).

CRITERIA	
Right-Handed Clinicians—Maxillary Right Posteriors, Facial Aspect **Left-Handed Clinicians—Maxillary Left Posteriors, Facial Aspect** Selects an appropriate curet and demonstrates a palm-out fulcrum for this sextant	
Selects an appropriate curet and demonstrates instrumentation of the broad facial concavity adjacent to the furcation area on the facial aspect	
Selects an appropriate curet and demonstrates the toe-up technique for the instrumentation of the mesial concavity on the first premolar	
Right-Handed Clinicians—Maxillary Left Posteriors, Lingual Aspect **Left-Handed Clinicians—Maxillary Right Posteriors, Lingual Aspect** Selects an appropriate curet and demonstrates a chin-cup fulcrum with a finger assist for the distal surface of the first molar	
Selects an appropriate curet and demonstrates instrumentation of the mesial surface of the first molar	
Selects an appropriate curet and demonstrates instrumentation of the distal furcation on the first molar tooth	
Selects an appropriate curet and demonstrates instrumentation of the mesial furcation on the first molar tooth. States whether the mesial furcation should be accessed from the facial or lingual aspect and explains the rationale	
Right-Handed Clinicians—Maxillary Left Posteriors, Lingual Aspect **Left-Handed Clinicians—Maxillary Right Posteriors, Lingual Aspect** Selects an appropriate curet and demonstrates a cross arch fulcrum for this sextant	
Selects an appropriate curet and demonstrates the toe-up technique for the instrumentation of the distal root concavity on the first molar	
Selects an appropriate curet and demonstrates and demonstrates the toe-up technique for the instrumentation of the palatal root depression.	
Mandibular Anteriors, Lingual Aspect Selects an appropriate curet and using an extraoral fulcrum, instruments the lingual aspect	

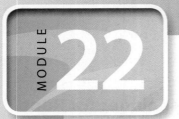

MODULE

22

Fictitious Patient Cases: Communication and Planning for Success

Module Overview

Periodontal instrumentation for the removal of plaque biofilm and dental calculus is an important component of nonsurgical periodontal therapy. This module begins with a discussion of the objective and rationale for periodontal instrumentation and word choices for explaining periodontal instrumentation to the patient. The second part of the module presents information on appointment planning and instrument sequencing for calculus removal. Section 3 contains six fictitious patient cases for practice in appointment planning and word choice when communicating with patients about periodontal instrumentation.

Module Outline

Section 1   **Understanding and Explaining Instrumentation**   566

Objectives and Rationale for Periodontal Instrumentation
Word Choice When Communicating with Patients
Informed Consent for Periodontal Instrumentation

Section 2   **Planning for Calculus Removal**   571

Complete Calculus Removal—The Gold Standard for Care
Instrument Selection for Calculus Removal
Strategies for Calculus Removal

Section 3   **Practical Focus—Fictitious Patient Cases**   574

Skill Building. Communication and Planning for Periodontal
    Instrumentation
Fictitious Patient Case 1
Fictitious Patient Case 2
Fictitious Patient Case 3
Fictitious Patient Case 4
Fictitious Patient Case 5
Fictitious Patient Case 6

Key Terms

Periodontal maintenance
Informed consent
Capacity for consent

Written consent
Verbal consent

Implied consent
Informed refusal

Learning Objectives

- List two objectives of periodontal instrumentation.

- Discuss the rational for periodontal instrumentation in the treatment of patients.

- Discuss the ways in which a clinician's choice of words can facilitate or hinder communication with patients regarding dental hygiene care and periodontal instrumentation.

- Define and discuss the terms informed consent, capacity for consent, written consent, and informed refusal as these terms apply to periodontal instrumentation.

- Given a fictitious patient case, plan appointments for periodontal instrumentation and develop communication strategies for clarifying periodontal instrumentation to the patient.

Section 1
Understanding and Explaining Instrumentation

OBJECTIVE AND RATIONALE FOR PERIODONTAL INSTRUMENTATION

1. Objective of Periodontal Instrumentation
   A. The objective of periodontal instrumentation is the mechanical removal of microorganisms and their products for the prevention and treatment of periodontal diseases.
      1. *Because of the structure of biofilms, physical removal of bacterial plaque biofilm is the most effective mechanism of control.*
      2. Most subgingival plaque biofilm located within periodontal pockets cannot be reached by the patient using toothbrushes, floss, or mouth rinses.
         a. For this reason, frequent periodontal debridement of subgingival root surfaces to remove or disrupt bacterial plaque mechanically is an essential component of the treatment of periodontitis.
         b. In fact, periodontal instrumentation is likely to remain the most important component of nonsurgical periodontal therapy for the foreseeable future.
   B. The removal of calculus deposits from tooth surfaces is a critical step in any plan for nonsurgical periodontal therapy.
      1. Calculus deposits harbor living bacterial biofilms; thus, if the calculus remains, so do the pathogenic bacteria, making it impossible to re-establish periodontal health (1–3).
      2. *In order to re-establish periodontal health, root surfaces must be free of plaque biofilm and all calculus deposits.* Periodontal instrumentation must cover every square millimeter of the root surface.
      3. Calculus removal is always a fundamental part of periodontal therapy.
2. Rationale for Periodontal Instrumentation. The scientific basis for performing periodontal instrumentation includes all points listed below.
   A. To arrest the progress of periodontal disease by removing plaque biofilms and plaque biofilm retentive calculus deposits.
   B. To induce positive changes in the subgingival bacterial flora (count and content).
   C. To create an environment that assists in maintaining tissue health and/or permits the gingival tissue to heal, thus, eliminating inflammation in the periodontium.
   D. To increase the effectiveness of patient self-care by eliminating areas of plaque biofilm retention that are difficult or impossible for the patient to clean.
   E. To prevent recurrence of disease during periodontal maintenance. Periodontal maintenance refers to continuing patient care provided by the dental team to help the periodontitis patient maintain periodontal health following complete nonsurgical or surgical periodontal therapy.

WORD CHOICE WHEN COMMUNICATING WITH PATIENTS

Precise dental terminology is important when recording treatment performed in the patient record or when communicating with other healthcare professionals. Unfortunatley, that same dental terminology often confuses patients and causes them to miss the message that the hygienist is trying to convey. The hygienist's goal should be to convey information in a clear, easily-understood manner that builds trust in the hygienist and what he or she advises. Hygienists cannot be successful in helping patients maintain and improve their periodontal health if they cannot communicate in a clear manner using words that do not confuse, bore, or alarm patients.

There are several aspects relating to word choice—or terminology—to consider when talking with patients about dental hygiene care and periodontal instrumentation.

1. **Word Choice Creates a Mental Image in the Patient's Mind**
   A. Upon hearing a word, most listeners picture an image of the word in his or her mind. For example, when the listener hears the word "toothbrush" he pictues the image of a toothbrush in his mind. Most individuals do not picture the letters T.O.O.T.H.B.R.U.S.H. in their minds.
   B. Some words may create a negative or frightening image in the patient's mind. For some individuals the words "deep scaling" might produce a disturbing mental image. A dental hygienist must be aware of the mental pictures that he or she creates in the patient's mind as he or she speaks.
2. **Word Choice Pertaining to Dental Hygiene Services.** Dental hygienists hope that patients will value the care that they provide. The value a patient perceives may be influenced by the way that the hygienist refers to planned dental hygiene services.
   A. Using words such as "dental cleaning" or "prophy" minimizes the perceived value of hygiene care. Hygienists do not simply shine the teeth as the phrase "clean the teeth" implies.
   B. Word choices such as "dental hygiene services" or "dental hygiene therapies" better convey the complex, therapeutic nature of dental hygiene care.
   C. Instead of saying, "Can we set up your next cleaning appointment?" consider a statement such as "Let's customize the timing for your next visit. Setting the correct interval between care visits helps to maintain the health of your mouth."
3. **Word Choice Pertaining to Periodontal Instrumentation.** In most cases, an individual who has periodontal disease is an adult who will appreciate clear, informative communication about his or her periodontal health status. Listed below are some examples of word choices that may not help communicate the indended message and some suggestions for alternate word choices that produce clear, acceptance-building pictures in the minds of patients.
   A. **"Gum Disease" Versus "Active Infection"**
      1. The words "gum disease" do not clearly convey the situation to the patient, but these words could create a pretty frightening picture in the patient's mind or cause the patient to believe that the situation is hopeless.
      2. An alternative choice of words might be "an active infection." All adults know that an infection is something serious that needs to be treated, but also the word "infection" implies a condition that can be treated.
   B. **"Scale and Root Plane" Versus "Bring the Infection Under Control"**
      1. Words such as "scale" and "root plane" do not clarify the treatment procedure for the patient, but they may conjure up very negative mental pictures. For example, hearing that his teeth are going to be "root planed" might cause a patient to picture layers of his teeth being shaved away the manner that a wood worker shaves off layers of wood. The terms "scale and root plane your teeth" might cause the patient to envision the planned treatment as something very aggressive and uncomfortable.
      2. Even the phase "instrument the teeth" does nothing to explain the procedure to the patient. On the positive side, "instrument" does not produce the negative mental images that the aggressive sounding terms "scale and root planing" elicit.
      3. The ideal solution to word use when explaining periodontal instrumentation is simply to EXPLAIN in everyday words how the patient will benefit from the procedure. An explanation—such as "bring the infection under control

by removing bacteria and hard deposits from the roots of your teeth"—helps patients to understand the intent and significance of periodontal instrumentation.

   C. **"Bone Loss" Versus "Permanent Bone Damage"**
1. Although the term "bone loss" is very accurate it might not create an accurate mental image for the patient. A patient might not know that bone loss is permanent or understand precisely why this loss is significant.
2. An alternative phrase to consider is "permanent damage to the bone that supports your teeth." Permanent bone damage clearly conveys that bone is not healthy and that this problem is serious.

   D. **"Recall Appointment" Versus "Customized Interval for Dental Health Care"**
1. To the patient the phrase "recall appointment" may create the image of an endless string of dates in a calendar. The phase does nothing to convey the significance of returning for care.
2. Instead, the words "customized interval for your dental health care" are a phrase that is both acceptance-building and conveys that ongoing care is important.

INFORMED CONSENT FOR PERIODONTAL INSTRUMENTATION

The core value of "Individual Autonomy and Respect for Human Beings" within the Code of Ethics for the American Dental Hygienists' Association discusses informed consent (4). According to this core value, "People...have the right to full disclosure of all relevant information so they can make informed choices about their care."

1. **Informed Consent for Periodontal Instrumentation**
   A. It is the responsibility of the dental hygienist to provide complete and comprehensive information about the recommended plan for periodontal instrumentation so that the patient can make a well-informed decision about either accepting or rejecting the proposed treatment (5,6).
   B. Informed consent involves not only informing the patient about the expected successful outcomes of periodontal instrumentation, but the possible risks, unanticipated outcomes and alternative treatments as well. The patient should be made aware of the costs for each of the options involved, which may influence the patient's ultimate decision. Box 22-1 summarizes some of the ethical considerations for informed consent.
2. **Capacity for Consent.** A patient must also have the capacity to consent.
   A. Capacity for consent—the ability of a patient to fully understand the proposed treatment, possible risks, unanticipated outcomes and alternative treatments—takes into account the patient's age, mental capacity and language comprehension.
   B. The patient would expect that the dental hygienist would carry out the proposed periodontal instrumentation according to the proper standard of care, or that of the "reasonably prudent hygienist", and perform the services in a manner that "any hygienist would do in the same or similar situation."
   C. Two-way communication between the patient and the hygienist is the best way to initiate the informed consent process.
3. **Documenting Consent**
   A. Once the patient is satisfied and agrees to the proposed plan for periodontal instrumentation, it is best if it is written in the patient's chart and signed by the patient and hygienist. This is an example of written consent. Written consent is legally binding and will hold up in a court of law.

B. Both verbal consent (verbally agreeing to a proposed treatment without any formal written documentation) and implied consent (sitting in a dental chair and opening one's mouth for the hygienist), although acceptable for certain procedures, is not as legally sound as written consent.

4. **Informed Refusal.** Despite being informed of the proposed treatments, risks and alternatives, the patient may decide to refuse the treatment plan. This is called "informed refusal."

A. Autonomy, as defined by the ADHA Code of Ethics, guarantees "self-determination" of the patient, and is linked to informed consent (4).

B. Only after the patient has received informed consent can a decision be made to either accept or reject the proposed treatment.

C. Although refusal may not be the optimal choice of the treating hygienist, the patient has a right to make any decision about his/her treatments that only affects him/her personally and does not pose a threat to others. Radiographs, fluoride treatments and sealants are a few services for which patients have exercised informed refusal.

D. As a result, each dental office should include an informed consent/refusal form as part of the patient treatment record to insure proper documentation.

E. Figure 22-1 shows an example of an informed consent/informed refusal form.

Box 22-1 | **Ethical Considerations for Informed Consent for the Patient**

- Reasoning/importance of proposed periodontal instrumentation
- Expected outcomes of the proposed periodontal instrumentation
- Risks involved in the proposed periodontal instrumentation
- Possible unexpected results of periodontal instrumentation
- Alternative approaches to periodontal instrumentation, such as hand or ultrasonic instrumentation; four 1-hour treatment sessions or two 2-hour treatment sessions
- Possible consequences of refusal of treatment
- Costs of proposed treatment and alternatives
- Patient's capacity to consent (age, mental, language comprehension)
- Written consent by patient

Informed Consent/Informed Refusal Form

1. I _____ , (name) agree to the proposed dental treatment by
_____ , (name) RDH.

2. I fully understand the importance of the proposed treatment.___Yes ___No

3. I understand that _____ is the expected outcome of the proposed treatment.

4. I understand that the possible risks/and or unanticipated outcomes of the proposed
treatment are_____ .

5. The possible treatment alternatives to the proposed treatment are_____ .

6. I have been informed of the costs of the proposed and alternative treatments.__Yes ___No

7. I understand the possible consequence(s) of refusal of the proposed treatment
is/are _____ .

8. I have the capacity to consent to the proposed treatment. ___Yes ___No

9. I refuse the proposed treatment. ___Yes ___No

10. Please list the treatment you are refusing. _____

_____   _____   _____
Patient Signature   Date   RDH Signature

Figure 22-1. Sample Informed Consent/Informed Refusal Form.

Section 2
Planning for Calculus Removal

Frequently, it is not possible to remove calculus deposits from all the teeth in a single appointment. In this instance, calculus removal is completed in a series of treatment sessions.

1. *The multiple appointment approach to calculus removal is based on the concept of complete calculus removal from any tooth treated at a single appointment.*
   A. The hygienist begins instrumentation on a tooth with the goal of completely removing all calculus deposits from that tooth before moving on to a second tooth.
   B. Incomplete periodontal instrumentation leaves behind calculus deposits that are rough, irregular, and covered with bacterial plaque biofilm. Between the current dental appointment and the next, microorganisms in the biofilm continue to multiply.
2. *At each appointment the clinician should treat only as many teeth, sextants, or quadrants as he or she can render calculus-free at that appointment.* For example, the clinician may complete a single sextant (facial and lingual aspects) on a patient with periodontitis or complete two quadrants (half the mouth) on a patient with gingivitis.

COMPLETE CALCULUS REMOVAL—THE GOLD STANDARD FOR CARE

When multiple appointments are needed for calculus removal, the clinician must decide how to divide up the work.

1. Complete Several Teeth
   A. With extremely difficult cases, the student clinician only may complete a few teeth (both facial and lingual aspects).
   B. In most instances, however, the clinician will be able to complete the facial and lingual aspects of a sextant or quadrant.
2. Complete One Sextant or Quadrant
   A. Usually, it is possible for student clinicians to complete one sextant or quadrant at an appointment—for example, the mandibular right posterior sextant.
   B. For example, the clinician might begin by treating the facial and lingual aspects of a posterior sextant. Treatment can end here for the appointment, or if time permits, the adjacent anterior teeth are completed to the midline of the arch (resulting in completion of the quadrant—for example, the mandibular right quadrant).
3. Complete Two Quadrants on the Same Side of the Mouth
   A. When two quadrants are completed at one appointment, treatment of *a maxillary and mandibular quadrant on the same side of the mouth* is recommended (versus treating the entire maxillary arch or the entire mandibular arch).
   B. Completing a maxillary and mandibular quadrant on one side of the mouth is preferred for several reasons.
      1. This approach gives the patient an untreated side on which to chew comfortably.
      2. Completing quadrants on one side of the mouth usually divides the work more evenly since the maxillary arch is more difficult for most clinicians.
      3. When local anesthesia is indicated for two quadrants, it is recommended that a maxillary and mandibular quadrant on the same side of the mouth be selected.

INSTRUMENT SELECTION FOR CALCULUS REMOMAL

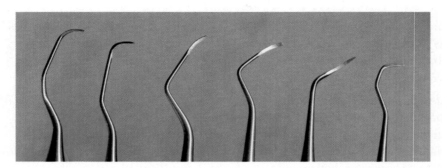

Figure 22-2. Calculus Removal Instruments. An important component of periodontal debridement is selecting the correct instrument for the task.

For calculus removal, periodontal instruments, such as those pictured in Figure 22-2, are selected based on the size and location of the calculus deposits. Table 22-1 summarizes strategies for instrumentation selection when working with hand instruments.

1. Large-sized calculus deposits most commonly are located above the gingival margin and can be removed using sickle scalers. Future modules discuss the use of powered instruments for removal of large-sized deposits.
2. Small- or medium-sized calculus deposits are located below the gingival margin and can be removed using either universal or area-specific curets.
   - Small or medium-sized deposits on root surfaces located within sulci or shallow periodontal pockets can be removed with a universal curet.
   - Small or medium-sized deposits located on root surfaces within deep periodontal pockets can be removed with area-specific curets.
   - Tenacious and large-sized deposits can be removed with rigid curets.

TABLE 22-1. GENERAL GUIDE FOR SELECTION OF CALCULUS REMOVAL INSTRUMENTS

Type of Deposit	Location of Deposit	Instrument
Large-sized deposits	Above the gingival margin	Sickle scalers
Medium-sized deposits	Above and below the gingival margin	Universal curets
		Area-specific curets with rigid shanks
Small-sized deposits	Above the gingival margin	Universal curets
Small-sized deposits	On cervical-third of root	Universal curets
Small-sized deposits	On middle or apical-third of root	Area-specific curets

STRATEGIES FOR CALCULUS REMOVAL

Box 22-2 shows patient assessment data for a fictitious patient. *Although it is critical for the clinician to develop an individualized calculus removal plan to meet the unique needs of each patient, beginning clinicians often find it helpful to review an example of a typical plan for calculus removal (Table 22-2).* The calculus removal plan shown in Table 22-2 simply provides an example of one approach to calculus removal; other acceptable plans for calculus removal could be developed. A plan for calculus removal is individualized based on the periodontal condition of the patient and the skill level of the clinician providing the care.

Box 22-2   **Fictitious Patient Example**

Patient Assessment Data:

- 28 teeth (third molars have not erupted)
- Gingival margin is at the CEJ on all teeth; probing depths vary between 4 and 5 mm
- **Supragingival deposits**—heavy deposits above the gingival margin on the lingual surface of the mandibular anterior teeth and the facial aspect of the maxillary molars.
- **Subgingival deposits**—medium-sized deposits on the cervical-third of the roots of all teeth; small-sized deposits generalized on all teeth.

TABLE 22-2. TYPICAL CALCULUS REMOVAL PLAN FOR EXAMPLE PATIENT

Treatment Area	Instrument(s)—Listed in the Order of Use
Appt. 1: Mandibular anterior sextant	1. Anterior sickle for supragingival deposits 2. Universal curet for small/medium-sized deposits 3. Area-specific curets for small-sized deposits; esp. deposits located within pockets
Appt. 2: Mandibular right posterior sextant	1. Universal curet for small/medium-sized deposits 2. Area-specific curets for small-sized deposits; esp. deposits located within pockets
Appt. 3: Maxillary right posterior sextant	1. Posterior sickle for supragingival deposits on molar teeth 2. Universal curet for small/medium-sized deposits 3. Area-specific curets for small-sized deposits; esp. deposits located within pockets
Appt. 4: Maxillary anterior sextant	1. Universal curet for small/medium-sized deposits 2. Area-specific curets for small-sized deposits; esp. deposits located within pockets
Appt. 5: Maxillary left posterior sextant	1. Posterior sickle for supragingival deposits on molar teeth 2. Universal curet for small/medium-sized deposits 3. Area-specific curets for small-sized deposits; esp. deposits located within pockets
Appt. 6: Mandibular left posterior sextant	1. Universal curet for small/medium-sized deposits 2. Area-specific curets for small-sized deposits; esp. deposits located within pockets

Section 3
Practical Focus—Fictitious Patient Cases

SKILL BUILDING
Communication and Planning for Periodontal Instrumentation

This section presents six fictitious patients. These patients allow practice with communication skills and planning for periodontal instrumentation.

Directions: Photocopy the **Calculus Removal Plan** form in Figure 22-3 (or create a similar form yourself on tablet paper).

For each fictitious patient case:

1. *Use the information recorded on the periodontal chart to calculate the clinical attachment loss on the facial and lingual aspects and enter this information on the patient's periodontal chart.*
2. Determine how many appointments you will need for calculus removal.
3. List the treatment area(s) to be completed at each appointment. For example at a single appointment, can you complete (1) the entire mouth, (2) the maxillary and mandibular right quadrants (half the mouth), (3) the mandibular right quadrant (half the mandibular arch), (4) the mandibular right sextant, or (5) the mandibular anterior sextant?
4. Select appropriate instruments for use at each appointment. Indicate the sequence the instruments will be used in and the use of each instrument. Select calculus removal instruments from (1) your school's instrument kit or (2) any of the instruments found in Modules of this book. Refer to the example in Table 22-2 for ideas on how to plan instrumentation.
5. *On the back of the form:*
   - *Explain your rationale for instrument selection and sequence.*
   - *Write your response to the communication scenario.*

Calculus Removal Plan	
Treatment Area	**Instrument(s) - Listed in the order of use**
Appointment #1:	
Appointment #2 (if needed):	
Appointment #3 (if needed):	
Appointment #4 (if needed):	
Appointment #5 (if needed):	
Appointment #6 (if needed):	

Figure 22-3. **Calculus Removal Plan.**

FICTITIOUS PATIENT CASE 1: Mrs. Braithwaite

Refer to Figures 22-4A to G and Box 22-3 for information on Fictitious Patient Case 1.

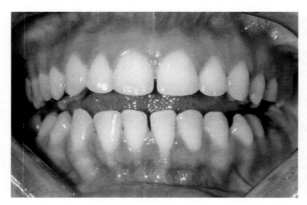

Figure 22-4A

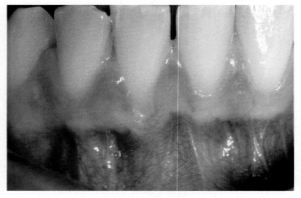

Figure 22-4B

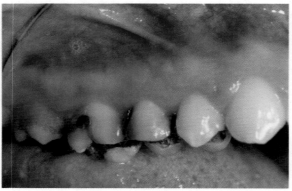

Figure 22-4. C and D: Facial Aspects of the Maxillary Posterior Sextants.

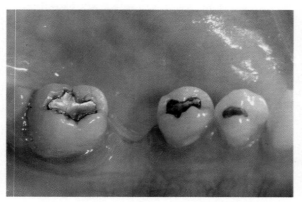

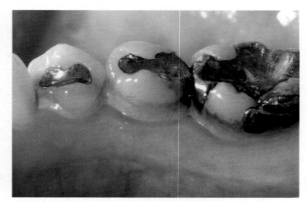

Figure 22-4. E and F: Lingual Aspects of the Mandibular Posterior Sextants.

2	1	2	2	2	2	2	2	2	2	3	3	3	3	4	4	4	4	4	4	5			Probe Depth
0	+3	0	0	+3	0	0	+3	0	+1	+1	+1	+1	+1	+1	+1	+1	+1	+1	+2	+1			GM to CEJ
																							Attachment Loss

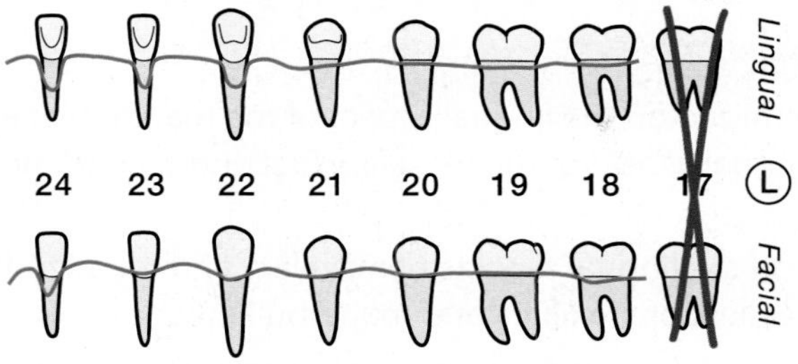

Lingual
24 23 22 21 20 19 18 17 (L)
Facial

2	1	2	2	2	2	2	2	3	3	2	3	3	2	3	3	3	4	2	2	2			Probe Depth
0	+2	0	0	0	0	0	0	0	0	0	0	0	0	0	0	0	0	+2	+2	+2			GM to CEJ
																							Attachment Loss
																							Mobility

Figure 22-4. G: Partial Periodontal Chart for Patient 1.

Box 22-3 **Fictitious Patient Case 1**

Assessment Data

1. **Supragingival Calculus Deposits:**
   - Moderate deposits generalized on the lingual aspect of the mandibular arch
   - Moderate deposits on lingual aspect of the maxillary first and second molars

2. **Subgingival Calculus Deposits:**
   - Medium-sized deposits on the lingual aspects of maxillary and mandibular arches
   - Light deposits on facial aspect of maxillary and mandibular arches

Communication Scenario

You are a recent graduate of a dental hygiene program and have just started working in a new dental office. You learn that the other dental hygienist in the practice, Samantha, believes that forceful, scraping calculus removal strokes should cover all tooth and root surfaces. Samantha states she has been practicing for 20 years and forceful stokes is what she learned in school. You feel a little intimidated since you just graduated 5 months ago, nevertheless, you mention to her that you were taught that biting strokes are initiated directly under a calculus deposit followed by relaxed assessment strokes until the clinician encounters the next calculus deposit. This technique helps prevent musculoskeletal damage to the clinician, is more time-efficient, and more comfortable for the patient.

For a while you accept that you and she have a difference of opinion about calculus removal work strokes, but you and Samantha see the same patients and it is not unusual for a patient to question you about your instrumentation. For example, Mrs. Braithwaite asked: "Why don't you use a lot of pressure against my teeth and scrape, scrape, scrape over and over on each tooth like Samantha always does? Are you getting my teeth clean?"

- How would you answer Mrs. Braithwaite?
- In addition, these patient questions make you feel that you should discuss calculus removal technique for periodontal instrumentation with Samantha.
- How would you approach this issue with Samantha?

FICTITIOUS PATIENT CASE 2: Mr. Riveras

Refer to Figures 22-5A to F and Box 22-4 for information on Fictitious Patient Case 2.

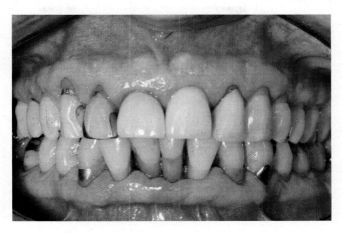

Figure 22-5A

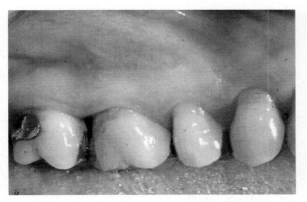 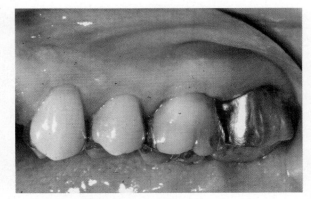

Figure 22-5. B and C: Facial Aspects of Maxillary Posterior Sextants.

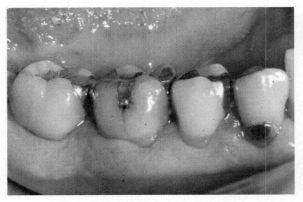 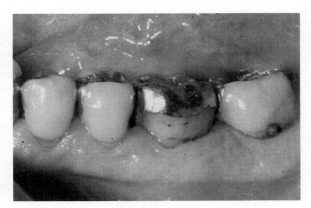

Figure 22-5. D and E: Facial Aspects of Mandibular Posterior Sextants.

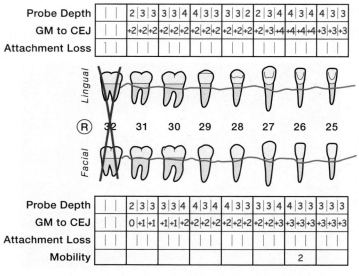

Probe Depth			2	3	3	3	3	4	4	3	3	3	3	2	2	3	4	4	3	4	4	3	3
GM to CEJ			+2	+2	+2	+2	+2	+2	+2	+2	+2	+2	+2	+2	+3	+4	+4	+4	+4	+3	+3	+3
Attachment Loss																								

Lingual

(R) 32   31   30   29   28   27   26   25

Facial

Probe Depth			2	3	3	3	3	4	4	3	4	4	3	3	3	3	4	4	3	3	3	3	3
GM to CEJ			0	+1	+1	+1	+1	+2	+2	+2	+2	+2	+2	+2	+2	+3	+3	+3	+3	+3	+3	+3	+3
Attachment Loss																								
Mobility														2										

Figure 22-5. F: Partial Periodontal Chart for Patient 2.

| Box 22-4 | **Fictitious Patient Case 2** |

Assessment Data

1. **Supragingival Calculus Deposits:**
   - No supragingival calculus present; patient self-care is excellent

2. **Subgingival Calculus Deposits:**
   - Light deposits on root surfaces of molar teeth

Communication Scenario

Your patient, Mr. Riveras, has had excellent self-care for the past several years. As a result, today you find little biofilm and scattered light calculus deposits in his mouth. In the past, Mr. Rivera suffered some bone loss.

  Mr. Riveras states that he knows he has been doing a great job with his routine self-care at home and is certain that you will not even need to use any instruments today on his teeth.

- If you ask Mr. Riveras about his daily self-care routine, how would you expect him to reply?
- Will you need to perform periodontal instrumentation on this patient? If so, how will you explain this treatment need to Mr. Riveras without making him feel that you are not pleased with how well he is doing with his at home self-care?
- If you plan to instrument the root surfaces, how would you explain this to the patient? Of the instruments you can select from, which might cause damage to the root surfaces or soft tissue? Which instrument(s) would be ideal for removing light deposits and plaque biofilm from root surfaces?
- What special consideration would you give to tooth #26 during periodontal instrumentation?

FICTITIOUS PATIENT CASE 3: Mr. Sconyers

Refer to Figures 22-6A to G and Box 22-5 for information on Fictitious Patient Case 3.

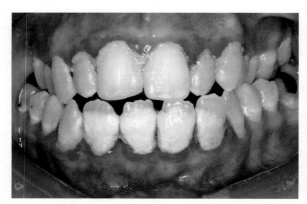
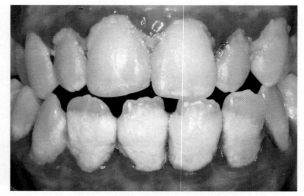

Figure 22-6A and B

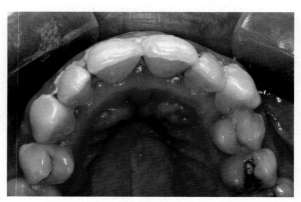
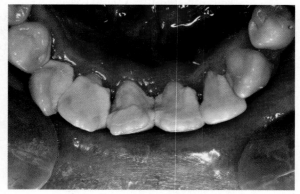

Figure 22-6. **C and D:** Lingual Aspects of the Maxillary and Mandibular Anterior Sextants.

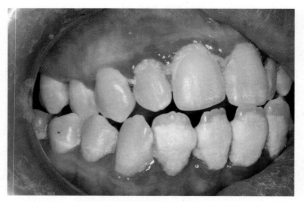
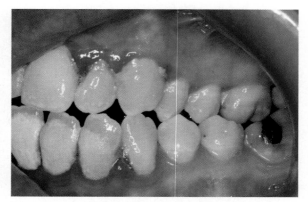

Figure 22-6. **E and F:** Right and Left Sides of Mouth. (Courtesy of Dr. Richard Foster, Guilford Technical Community College, Jamestown, NC.)

																								Mobility
4	3	4	4	3	4	4	3	4	4	3	4	4	3	3	3	3	3	3	3	3			Probe Depth
-1	-1	-1	-1	-1	-1	-2	-1	-1	-1	-1	-1	0	0	0	-1	-1	-1	-1	-1	-1			GM to CEJ
																							Attachment Loss

9	10	11	12	13	14	15	16	Ⓛ		Facial / Lingual

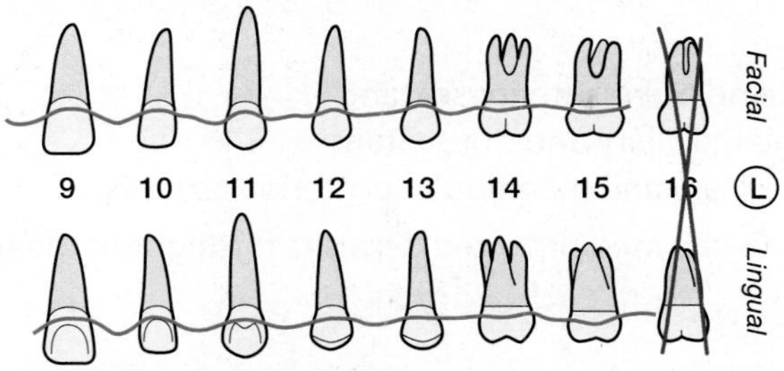

5	4	5	5	4	5	5	4	5	5	5	5	5	5	5	6	5	5	5	5	5			Probe Depth
-2	-2	-2	-2	-2	-2	-2	-2	-2	-2	-2	-2	-2	-2	-2	-2	-2	-2	-2	-3	-2			GM to CEJ
																							Attachment Loss

Figure 22-6. G: Partial Periodontal Chart for Patient 3.

Box 22-5 **Fictitious Patient Case 3**

Assessment Data

1. **Supragingival Calculus Deposits:**
   - Heavy deposits on the mandibular anterior sextant
   - Moderate deposits on the maxillary anterior sextant
   - Light deposits on the maxillary and mandibular posterior sextants

2. **Subgingival Calculus Deposits:** Medium-sized deposits throughout the mouth

Communication Scenario

Mr. David Sconyers just returned from a tour of duty in Afghanistan. For the last 9 months, he was in a classified combat zone and did not have access to clean water for brushing his teeth. His visit to your office was prompted when he noticed a foul taste in his mouth.

- Using a mirror, you point out the dark red line at the gingival margin to Mr. Sconyers. How would you explain the cause of this "red line"? What is the significance of this inflammation to Mr. Sconyer's oral and systemic health? How would you explain the significance of inflammation to the patient?
- How would you explain the significance of daily self-care to Mr. Sconyers?
- When planning treatment which sextant would you treat first? What words will you use to explain your ideal treatment plan to Mr. Sconyers?
- How would you describe the tissue improvement that you expect to occur after treatment?

FICTITIOUS PATIENT CASE 4: Ms. Ashton

Refer to Figures 22-7A to F and Box 22-6 for information on Fictitious Patient Case 4.

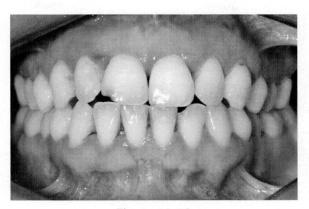

Figure 22-7A

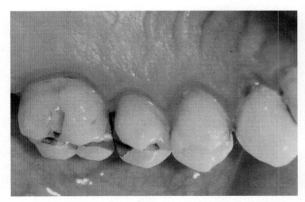 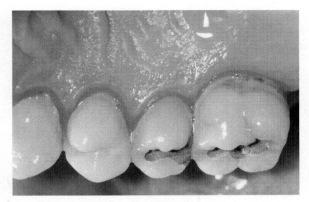

Figure 22-7. **B and C:** Lingual Aspects of the Maxillary Posterior Sextants.

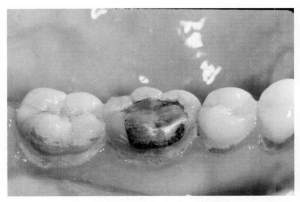 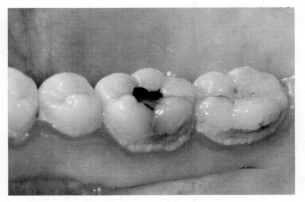

Figure 22-7. **D and E:** Lingual Aspects of the Mandibular Posterior Sextants.

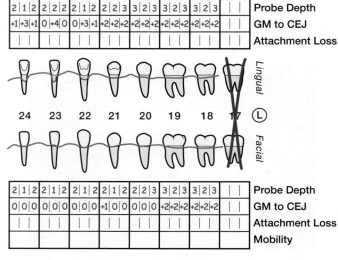

Figure 22-7. F: Partial Periodontal Chart for Patient 4.

| Box 22-6 | **Fictitious Patient Case 4** |

Assessment Data

1. **Supragingival Calculus Deposits:**
   - Light to moderate deposits on lingual aspect throughout the entire mouth

2. **Subgingival Calculus Deposits:** Medium-sized deposits throughout the entire mouth

Communication Scenario

You have accepted a full time dental hygiene position in a general dental practice and are completing your first month of employment. You thoroughly enjoy all the office personnel and respect the clinical work of the dentist, Dr. Stuart.

You review the chart of your last patient for the day, Allie Ashton who is 35 years old. She has been a patient of the practice for the last 10 years. Ms. Ashton is a lawyer. There is nothing eventful about her chart or medical/dental history.

After you seat Ms. Ashton and review her medical history, she mentions in passing that you are not to treat any of her 1st molars, as they are extremely sensitive. She says that every hygienist in the office has abided by her wishes, to simply "skip" those teeth when performing their dental hygiene services.

You see no mention or documentation in the dental record by the previous hygienists. Furthermore, upon probing Ms. Ashton's mouth, you note that on numerous locations on the first molar teeth, attachment loss gradually has increased over the years. The bitewings that were taken today also show generalized horizontal bone loss in those areas.

- How should you treat Allie Ashton?
- What are her alternatives in her dental hygiene therapies?
- Does her profession play a role in your decision making process?
- How can you document that Ms. Ashton is aware of her treatment options?
- What discussion, if any, would you have with her about the previous dental care she received in the office?

FICTITIOUS PATIENT CASE 5: Mr. Pilgrim

Refer to Figures 22-8A to F and Box 22-7 for information on Fictitious Patient Case 5.

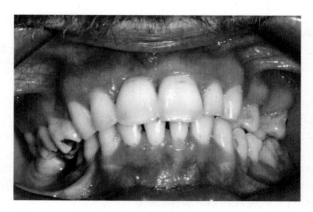

Figure 22-8A

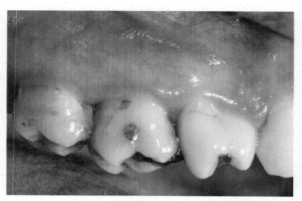

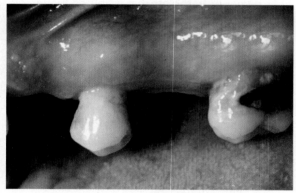

Figure 22-8. B and C: Facial Aspect of Maxillary Posterior Sextants.

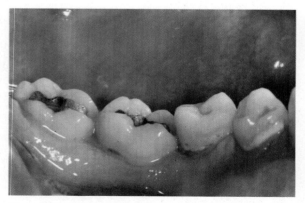

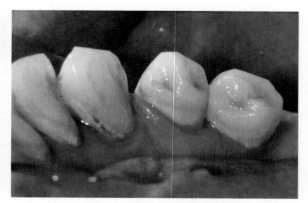

Figure 22-8. D and E: Mandibular right posterior sextant and mandibular left incisors, canine, and premolar teeth.

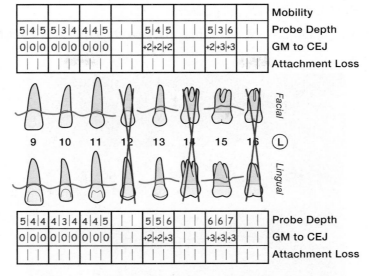

Figure 22-8. F: Partial Periodontal Chart for Patient 5.

Box 22-7 **Fictitious Patient Case 5**

Assessment Data

1. **Supragingival Calculus Deposits:**
   - Moderate deposits generalized on the lingual aspect throughout the mouth

2. **Subgingival Calculus Deposits:**
   - Medium-sized deposits on the lingual aspects of maxillary and mandibular arches
   - Light deposits on facial aspect of maxillary and mandibular arches

Communication Scenario

Mr. Richard Pilgrim is a personal trainer who was referred to your dental office by one of his clients. New to your practice, his chief complaint is "brown spots that show when I smile."

- In examining Mr. Pilgrim's teeth, you note that the brown spots are calculus deposits that are stained (superficial, extrinsic stain).
- In recommending treatment, how would you explain the importance of removing calculus deposits and biofilm—over removing brown spots—to Mr. Pilgrim?
- What words would you use to inquire if Mr. Pilgrim has concerns about his missing teeth?
- How would you communicate the significance of missing teeth to the health of his periodontium?

FICTITIOUS PATIENT CASE 6: Mrs. Piccolo

Refer to Figures 22-9A to B and Box 22-8 for information on Fictitious Patient Case 6.

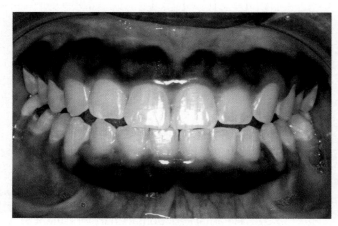

Figure 22-9A

Probe Depth			2	2	2	2	2	2	2	1	2	2	1	2	3	4	3	3	3	3	3	3	3
GM to CEJ			0	0	0	0	0	0	0	0	0	0	0	0	-3	-2	-1	-2	-2	-2	-2	-3	-3
Attachment Loss																							

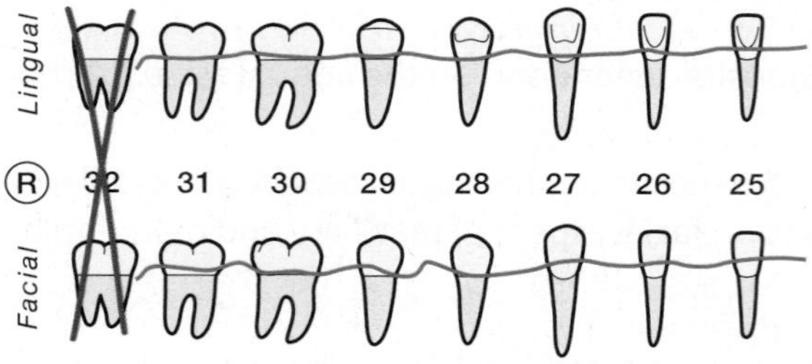

Lingual

(R)   32   31   30   29   28   27   26   25

Facial

Probe Depth			2	1	2	2	2	2	2	1	2	2	1	2	3	3	3	3	3	3	3	3	3
GM to CEJ			0	0	0	0	0	0	0	0	0	0	0	0	-3	-3	-3	-3	-3	-3	-3	-3	-3
Attachment Loss																							
Mobility																							

Figure 22-9. B: Partial Periodontal Chart for Patient 6.

> **Box 22-8** | **Fictitious Patient Case 6**
>
> **Assessment Data**
> 1. **Supragingival Calculus Deposits:**
>   - Light deposits on lingual aspect of mandibular anteriors
> 2. **Subgingival Calculus Deposits:**
>   - Light deposits on the proximal tooth surfaces of the posterior sextants throughout the mouth
>
> **Communication Scenario**
> Jacqueline Piccolo has just been accepted to the school of nursing at a local community college and states that she is 4 months pregnant with her first child. As one of her admission requirements for nursing school, she is required to receive a through dental examination and complete any needed dental treatment prior to beginning her training next fall. "Jay," as she prefers to be called, is very excited about nursing school and happily told you about earning an "A" in the microbiology course that is a prerequisite for the nursing program.
>
> - How will Jay's knowledge of microbiology enter into your choice of words during patient education?
> - Is it important to educate Jay about gingival enlargement during pregnancy due to pregnancy hormones and the presence of plaque biofilm? If so, how would you explain this information to the patient?

References

1. Checchi L, Montevecchi M, Checchi V, Zappulla F. The relationship between bleeding on probing and subgingival deposits. An endoscopical evaluation. *Open Dent J.* 2009;3:154–160.
2. Fujikawa K, O'Leary TJ, Kafrawy AH. The effect of retained subgingival calculus on healing after flap surgery. *J Periodontol.* 1988;59(3):170–175.
3. Wilson TG, Harrel SK, Nunn ME, Francis B, Webb K. The relationship between the presence of tooth-borne subgingival deposits and inflammation found with a dental endoscope. *J Periodontol.* 2008;79(11):2029–2035.
4. *Bylaws and Code of Ethics.* Chicago, IL: American Dental Hygienists' Association; 2009.
5. McCombs G. Protect yourself with informed consent. *Dimensions Dent Hyg.* 2010;8(11):60–63.
6. Sfikas PM. A duty to disclose. Issues to consider in securing informed consent. *J Am Den Assoc.* 2003;134(10):1329–1333.

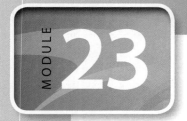

Concepts for Instrument Sharpening

Module Overview

This module discusses the importance and advantages of using calculus removal instruments with sharp cutting edges. Topics include methods for evaluating sharpness and reestablishing sharp cutting edges without altering the original design characteristics of the working-end.

Module Outline

Section 1   **Introduction to Sharpening Concepts**   594
Advantages of Sharp Instruments
Design Characteristics of a Sharp Cutting Edge
The Working-End in Cross Section
The Dull Cutting Edge
Evaluating Sharpness

Section 2   **Preserving Working-End Design**   599
The Lateral Surfaces and Tip or Toe
Common Sharpening Errors
Instrument Replacement
Instrument Tip Breakage

Section 3   **Planning for Instrument Maintenance**   604
When to Sharpen

Section 4   **Sharpening Armamentarium**   605
Work Area and Equipment
Sharpening Stones
Lubrication and Care of Stones
Restoration of a Sharp Edge and Sharpening Techniques

Section 5   **Skill Application**   609
Practical Focus

Key Terms

Sharp cutting edge   Straight cutting edges   Sharpening stone
Dull cutting edge   Curved cutting edges   Lubricant

Learning Objectives

- List the benefits of using instruments with sharp cutting edges for periodontal instrumentation.

- Define and differentiate the terms "sharp cutting edge" and "dull cutting edge."

- Given a variety of periodontal instruments, distinguish between those with sharp cutting edges and those with dull cutting edges.

- Demonstrate two methods for determining if a cutting edge is sharp.

- Describe important design characteristics to be maintained when sickle scalers, universal and area-specific curets are sharpened.

- Differentiate the following sharpening stones according to grain, recommended use, and preferred lubricant: composition synthetic stone, India stone, Arkansas stone, and ceramic stone.

- Demonstrate the correct care of a sharpening stone.

- Describe common sharpening errors.

- Value the practice of sharpening at the first sign of dullness.

Section 1
Introduction to Sharpening Concepts

ADVANTAGES OF SHARP INSTRUMENTS

Effective periodontal instrumentation with hand-activated instruments is possible only with properly maintained sharp cutting edges. *It is impossible to overemphasize the importance of mastering the techniques for instrument sharpening.* In 1908, one of the founders of modern dentistry, G. V. Black stated that "*Nothing in the technical procedures of dental practice is more important than the care of the cutting edges of instruments… The student who can not, or will not learn this should abandon the study of dentistry*" (1). Instrument sharpening is a skill needed on a daily basis. Effective periodontal instrumentation cannot be achieved with dull periodontal instruments.

A sharp cutting edge allows:

1. **Easier Calculus Removal**
   A. A sharp cutting edge "bites into" the calculus deposit, removing it in an efficient manner.
   B. A dull cutting edge will slide over the calculus deposit and may burnish it.
2. **Improved Stroke Control**
   A. A sharp cutting edge grabs a calculus deposit, making it easier to detect and remove.
   B. A dull cutting edge tends to slide over the tooth surface.
      1. A dull cutting edge is likely to burnish a calculus deposit, removing only the outer layer of calculus rather than the entire deposit.
      2. A dull cutting edge must be pressed with greater force against a deposit to achieve calculus removal.
      3. Excessive force used with a dull cutting edge increases the likelihood of losing control of the stroke. The clinician is more likely to slip or sustain an instrument stick (cut) to his or her fingers when using a dull instrument.
3. **Reduced Number of Strokes/Working Efficiency**
   A. It takes fewer strokes to remove a calculus deposit with a sharp cutting edge.
   B. Sharp instruments reduce the overall treatment time.
   C. Sharp instruments decrease the likelihood of burnished calculus deposits.
4. **Increased Patient Comfort and Satisfaction**
   A. More lateral pressure must be exerted against the tooth when using a dull instrument. A sharp instrument allows the clinician to use less force, making the instrumentation process more comfortable for the patient.
   B. A sharp cutting edge permits the clinician to make fewer, better-controlled instrument strokes. Therefore, sharp instruments decrease the time required for calculus removal. Patients appreciate shorter appointments.
5. **Reduced Clinician Fatigue**
   A. A dull cutting edge requires greater stroke pressure and more instrumentation strokes for calculus removal.
   B. The excessive lateral pressure and extra number of strokes needed with a dull instrument places unnecessary strain on the clinician's musculoskeletal system (2).

DESIGN CHARACTERISTIC OF A SHARP CUTTING EDGE

Calculus removal involves the use of lateral pressure and a biting stroke against the tooth surface. Dulling of the sharp cutting edge is an inevitable outcome of periodontal instrumentation. As an instrument is used, minute particles of metal are worn away from the working-end. Studies indicate that the cutting edges of curets probably should be sharpened after 15 to 40 calculus removal strokes (3–8). *Loss of metal from the working-end changes the cutting edge from a fine line to a rounded surface resulting in a dull, ineffective cutting edge.*

The outcome of the evolution of periodontal instruments, over the years, is a cutting edge design with precise characteristics that allow the instrument to be effective and safe for calculus removal. Correct sharpening technique requires knowledge of the design characteristics of sickle scalers and curets. It is important to understand the cross-sectional design of sickle scalers and curets and to recognize that the relationship of the face to the lateral surface is the same for all these instruments. On all sickle scalers and curets, a sharp cutting edge (Figs. 23-1 and 23-2) is a fine line formed by the pointed junction of the instrument face and lateral surface. Figures 23-3 to 23-5 depict the cross section of the working-end.

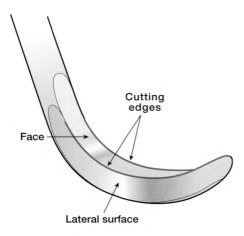

Figure 23-1. The Sharp Cutting Edge. A sharp cutting edge is a line. It has length, but no width.

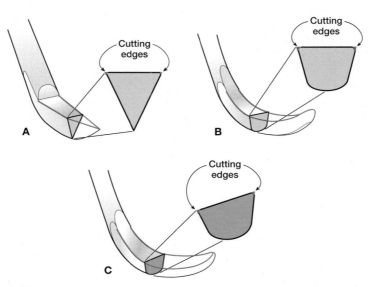

Figure 23-2. Cutting Edges on Sickle Scalers and Curets. For all sickle scalers and curets, the cutting edge is formed by the junction of the instrument face and lateral surface. The illustrations depict the following instruments in cross section: **A.** Sickle scaler. **B.** Universal curet. **C.** Area-specific curet.

THE WORKING-END IN CROSS SECTION

When sharpening, it is vital to maintain the relationship between the instrument face and lateral surfaces (Figs. 23-3 to 23-5). *For sickle scalers, universal curets, and area-specific curets, the internal angle formed between the face and a lateral surface is an angle between 70 and 80 degrees.*

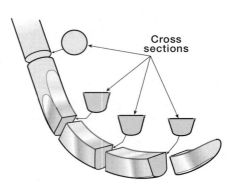

Figure 23-3. The Working-End in Cross Section. The key to understanding the cutting edge of an instrument is the ability to visualize the working-end in cross section.

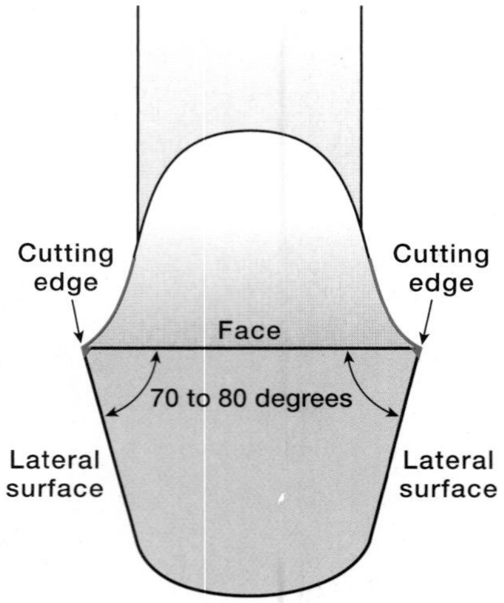

Figure 23-4. A Sharp Cutting Edge on a Universal Curet. The internal angle formed by the junction of the face and the lateral surface of a universal curet is between 70 and 80 degrees.

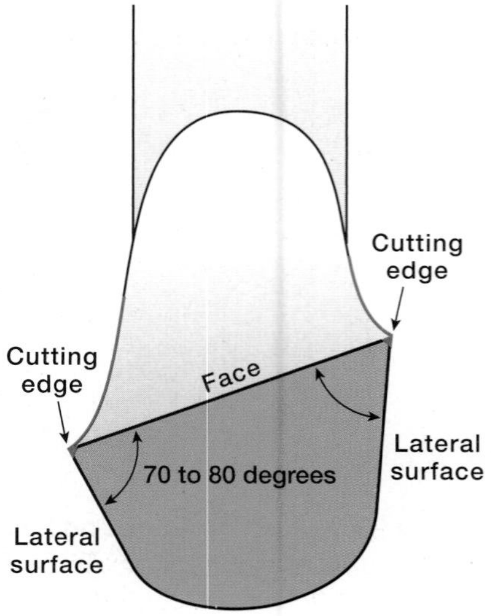

Figure 23-5. A Sharp Cutting Edge on an Area-Specific Curet. The relationship of the face to the lower shank is unique for area-specific curets. Just as for a universal curet, however, the internal angle formed by the junction of the face and the lateral surface of an area-specific curet is between 70 and 80 degrees.

THE DULL CUTTING EDGE

As the working-end is used against the tooth surface, over time, the metal of the cutting edge is worn away. A dull cutting edge results when metal is worn away from the cutting edge until the junction between the face and lateral surface becomes a rounded surface instead of a fine line (Fig. 23-6).

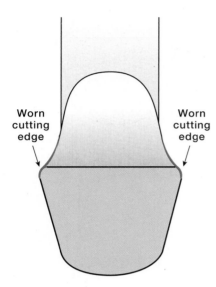

Worn cutting edge

Worn cutting edge

Figure 23-6. A Dull Cutting Edge. With use against the tooth surface, metal is worn away from the cutting edge until it becomes a **rounded surface** instead of a fine line. A dull cutting edge is a rounded junction between the instrument face and the lateral surface.

EVALUATING SHARPNESS

A dull cutting edge can be detected by visual or tactile evaluation.

1. **Visual Evaluation.** A cutting edge is evaluated visually by holding the working-end under a bright light source, such as the dental light or a high-intensity lamp. Figures 23-7 and 23-8 depict cutting edges examined under a strong light source. In this method, the instrument face is held approximately perpendicular to the light beams. The working-end is slowly rotated while looking at the junction of the face and the lateral surface.
   A. A dull cutting edge will reflect light because it is rounded and thick. The reflected light appears as a bright line running along the edge of the face.
   B. A sharp cutting edge is a line—with no thickness—and does not reflect the light.
2. **Tactile Evaluation with a Test Stick.**
   A. **Plastic Test Stick.** Another method of evaluating sharpness is with tactile means by testing the cutting edge against a plastic or acrylic rod known as a **sharpening test stick.** Test sticks are designed specifically for use in evaluating sharpness (Fig. 23-9).
      1. A dull cutting edge will slide over the surface of the stick.
      2. A sharp cutting edge will bite into—grab—the surface of the test stick.
   B. **Technique.** A plastic test stick is an effective means for evaluating sharpness when used with correct technique.
      1. The cutting edge is evaluated using the same technique as that used for calculus removal—that is: (1) a finger rest is established on the stick, (2) the cutting edge is applied at a face-to-stick angulation of 70 to 80 degrees, and (3) a short, biting stroke activated upward against the plastic.
      2. All areas of the cutting edge must be tested for sharpness—the heel-, middle-, and toe- or tip-thirds.

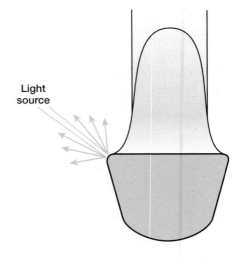

Figure 23-7. Visual Detection of a Dull Cutting Edge. The rounded surface of a dull cutting edge has thickness and thus, will reflect light back to the viewer.

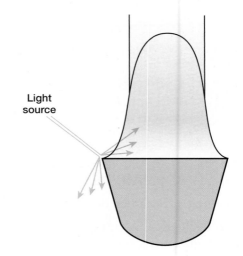

Figure 23-8. Visual Detection of a Sharp Cutting Edge. A sharp cutting edge has no thickness and therefore does not reflect light.

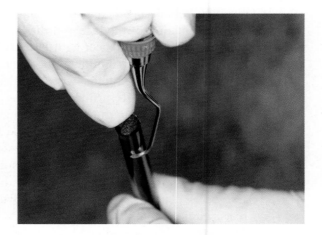

Figure 23-9. Tactile Detection with a Sharpening Test Stick. Sharpness can be evaluated using a test stick. A test stick is a cylindrical rod made of plastic or acrylic. Sharpening test sticks are autoclavable. Note that the clinician establishes a finger rest and adapts the working-end at a 70- to 80-degree face-to-plastic angulation.

Section 2
Preserving Working-End Design

Preserving the original design characteristics of the working-end is an essential goal of instrument sharpening. In addition to the 70- to 80-degree internal angle of the working-end, the design of the lateral surfaces, back, toe, and tip must be maintained.

THE LATERAL SURFACES AND TIP OR TOE

The working-ends of some periodontal instruments have curved lateral surfaces while others have straight lateral surfaces. Figure 23-10 depicts a variety of instrument working-ends, some with straight cutting edges and others with curved cutting edges; some with rounded toes, others with pointed tips.

- *Sharpening the cutting edges in sections is a strategy that preserves the design characteristics of any working-end regardless of whether it has straight or curved cutting edges.*
- If you make a habit of consistently sharpening the cutting edge in sections, you will never destroy a curved cutting edge by flattening the lateral surface (Figs. 23-11 and 23-12).
- On the other hand, sharpening a straight cutting edge in sections still results in a straight cutting edge.

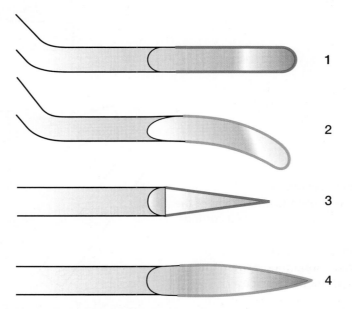

Figure 23-10. Straight Versus Curved Cutting Edges. The working-end may have **straight cutting edges** or **curved cutting edges**.

This design feature refers to the lateral surfaces being either straight or curved in design—not to whether the instrument has a rounded toe or pointed tip. To determine if the cutting edges are straight or curved, look down at the working-end from a bird's-eye view.

1. Instrument 1 is a universal curet with straight, parallel cutting edges.
2. Instrument 2 is an area-specific curet with curved working and nonworking cutting edges.
3. Instrument 3 is a sickle scaler with straight cutting edges.
4. Instrument 4 is a sickle scaler with curved cutting edges. This type of sickle scaler often is referred to as a flame-shaped sickle scaler.

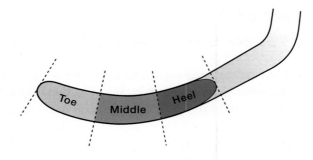

Figure 23-11. Cutting Edge Sections. Divide the cutting edge into three imaginary sections for sharpening: the heel-third, middle-third, and tip- or toe-third.

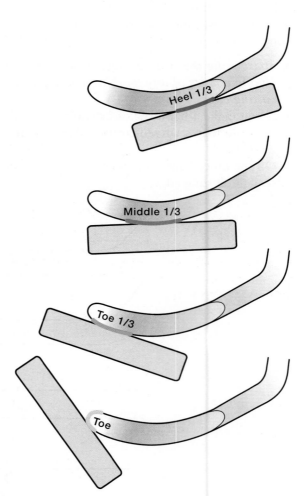

Figure 23-12. Sharpen in Sections.
- The sharpening stone is applied to only a third of the cutting edge at a time to maintain a curved cutting edge.
- Sharpen the (1) heel-third, (2) middle-third, and (3) the toe- or tip-third of the cutting edge. If the instrument is a curet, (4) sharpen the toe.

COMMON SHARPENING ERRORS

- Preserving the original design characteristics of the working-end is an essential goal of instrument sharpening.
- In addition to the 70- to 80-degree internal angle of the working-end, the design of the lateral surfaces, back, toe, and tip must be maintained.
- A clinician who is not knowledgeable about working-end design can radically alter an instrument's design characteristics with incorrect sharpening technique.
- An incorrectly sharpened instrument will be ineffective for calculus removal and may fracture easily. Figures 23-13 to 23-16 depict how the original design characteristics of the working-end can be altered through incorrect sharpening technique.

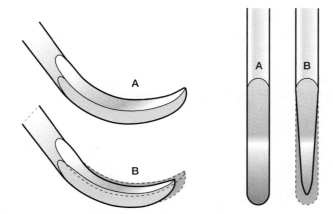

Figure 23-13. Alteration of Working-End Design. A: A new universal curet. Note that curet A has straight lateral surfaces and a rounded toe. **B:** In sharpening the curet shown in A, the clinician has altered its design characteristics. It is thinner and shorter than the original and the curet toe has been sharpened to a point.

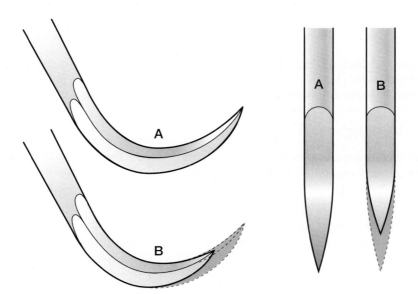

Figure 23-14. Unnecessary Metal Removal. A: A new sickle scaler. **B:** The working-end of this scaler has been excessively shorted in length by sharpening.

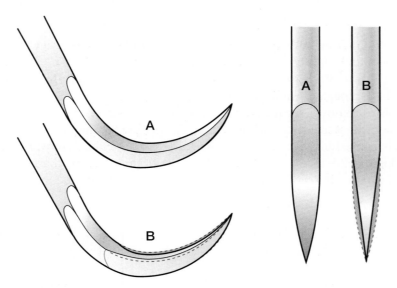

Figure 23-15. **Altered Shape. A:** A new sickle scaler. **B:** In this example, incorrect sharpening technique resulted in straight cutting edges while the cutting edges on the original sickle were curved (flame shaped).

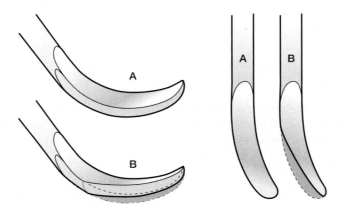

Figure 23-16. **Flattened Cutting Edge. A:** A new area-specific curet with curved cutting edges. **B:** In this example, incorrect sharpening technique created a straight lateral surface and a pointed tip. The original design characteristics of the instrument were curved lateral surfaces and a rounded toe.

INSTRUMENT REPLACEMENT

It is important to recognize that sickle scalers and curets have a limited use-life and must eventually be discarded. Frequent sharpening that preserves the working-end design combined with care during handling and sterilization will prolong an instrument's use-life. Eventually, every instrument will need to be replaced. When a working-end becomes thin from use and sharpening, the instrument should be discarded. One research study reports that a 20% reduction in size results in a significant reduction in working-end strength (9).

INSTRUMENT TIP BREAKAGE

A broken instrument tip is a serious situation that all hygienists hope not to encounter. When a working-end breaks in the patient's mouth, the remnant of the working-end must be located.

1. **Maintenance for Prevention of Breakage.** The instrument's working-ends should be carefully inspected under magnification after each use.
   A. Thin or improperly sharpened working-ends can break during calculus removal.
   B. Frequent sharpening, correct sharpening technique, and discarding of instruments with thin or poorly sharpened working-ends minimizes the possibility of a broken tip.
2. **Management of a Broken Working-End.** Breaking a working-end during instrumentation creates a serious problem.
   A. If not removed the metal fragment can cause tissue inflammation and abscess formation. If the tip is aspirated (inhaled) into the lungs, a serious infection is likely to develop. If swallowed, the tip probably will pass harmlessly through the gastrointestinal system.
   B. If the tip cannot be located in the mouth, the patient should be referred for a chest x-ray to assure that the tip has not been aspirated into a lung.
   C. Refer to Box 23-1 for the procedure for finding and retrieving a broken working-end.

Box 23-1   Retrieving a Broken Working-End

1. Stop instrumentation immediately, remain calm, and inform the patient of the problem.

2. Maintain retraction and patient head position.
   A. Do NOT use compressed air to attempt to locate the metal fragment. Compressed air could move the metal fragment around the mouth or drive it into the soft tissues.
   B. Do NOT use suction to attempt to remove the metal fragment. Suction could remove the tip but also eliminates the ability to confirm that the metal fragment has been removed.

3. Examine the location where the fracture occurred, mucobuccal fold, and the floor of the mouth. If the metal fragment is located on the surface of the tissue, blot the area with a gauze square. The metal fragment will catch in the gauze material for easy removal.

4. If the fragment cannot be located on the outer surfaces of the tissues, examine the sulci or pockets in the area.
   A. Insert a curet into the sulcus or pocket at the distofacial or distolingual line angle and move slowly forward until the fragment is located.
   B. Once located, use the curet like a scoop to remove the tip from beneath the gingival margin and catch it with a gauze square.

5. If the fragment cannot be located, take a periapical radiograph of the area. If located, use a curet as described above to remove the tip. If this fails, refer the patient to a periodontist for surgical removal of the metal fragment.

6. If the fragment still cannot be located in the mouth, the patient should be referred for a chest x-ray to assure that the tip has not been aspirated into a lung. After referral, it is important to follow-up with the patient to confirm that a chest x-ray was obtained.

Section 3
Planning for Instrument Maintenance

WHEN TO SHARPEN

Sickle scalers, curets, and periodontal files should be sharpened after each use and as needed during periodontal instrumentation. Instruments should be sharpened lightly after each use. Neglected cutting edges require extensive sharpening increasing the likelihood of damaging the working-end. Table 23-1 summarizes the consequences of sharpening frequency.

1. Sharpening Following Instrument Use
   A. Each sickle scaler or curet used during the appointment should be sharpened.
   B. Instruments that were not used do not need to be sharpened; modern stainless steel instruments are not dulled by autoclaving or other sterilization methods.
   C. Ideally, instruments used for treatment should be sterilized before sharpening to decrease the risk for disease transmission (10). Sterilized instruments are sharpened and sterilized a second time prior to use.

2. Sharpening During Treatment
   A. Depending on the extent of calculus deposits present, instruments may have to be sharpened during treatment.
   B. Sharpening contaminated instruments presents an increased risk for disease transmission through an instrument stick. Ideally, it is best to have a variety of individually wrapped, sterilized sharp instruments to replace instruments dulled during treatment.
   C. If contaminated instruments must be sharpened, take steps to diminish risk for disease transmission.
      1. Sharpening stones should be a part of each instrument cassette so that sterile sharpening stones are always available. If instrument cassette tray setups are not used, sharpening stones should be kept in sealed sterilized packages until needed.
      2. Use safe sharpening techniques: gloves, good lighting, stabilize hand on flat, stable working surface.
      3. The work area should be disinfected and covered with a barrier such as plastic wrap or an impervious-backed paper. The barrier should cover both the top and edge of the countertop.
      4. Any sharpening aid or device used at chairside must be dissembled and sterilized after each use.
      5. A natural stone is not recommended for sharpening during treatment, as these stones require lubrication with oil. Oil lubricants cannot under go sterilization. Ceramic stones are best for chairside sharpening since water can be used as a lubricant with these stones.

TABLE 23-1. CONSEQUENCES RELATIVE TO FREQUENCY OF SHARPENING

Immediate Sharpening ("Good Habit")	Infrequent Sharpening ("Bad Habit")
• Maintained cutting edges need only a few light sharpening strokes and minor recontouring to restore the sharp edge	• Dull neglected cutting edges require many, firm sharpening strokes and extensive recontouring
• Calculus removal is easier for both the clinician and patient	• Calculus removal is difficult and tiring for both the clinician and patient
• Instruments have a long use-life	• Instruments have a short use-life

Section 4
Sharpening Armamentarium

WORK AREA AND EQUIPMENT

A sharpening work area must be a part of every treatment room so that periodontal instruments can be sharpened at the first sign of dullness. The right work area is important in assuring an efficient and safe sharpening procedure.

1. A stable, flat work surface is essential for good sharpening technique. A countertop in the treatment room makes a good surface. A bracket table or other unstable surface is not appropriate for the sharpening procedure.
2. A good light source, such as the dental unit light or a high-intensity lamp should illuminate the sharpening work area.
3. All equipment required for sharpening should be assembled and ready for use in the treatment room (Fig. 23-17).

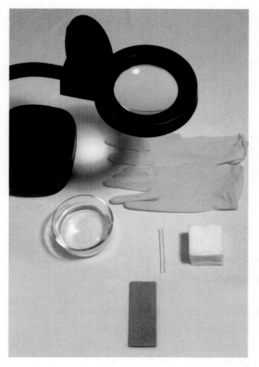

Figure 23-17. Sharpening Equipment.
- Sharpening stone(s)
- Plastic sharpening test stick
- Magnifying light, lens, or loops
- Gauze
- Lubricant
- Gloves
- Safety glasses

SHARPENING STONES

A sharpening stone is used to remove metal from the lateral surfaces to restore a sharp, fine cutting edge. Sharpening stones are made of abrasive particles that are harder than the metal of the instruments to be sharpened.

- Sharpening stones may be made from natural stone or synthetic, man-made materials (4,5,11).
- The grain—or abrasiveness—is an important characteristic of a sharpening stone.
- Fine grain stones—400 grit or higher—produce significantly sharper cutting edges that will stay sharper longer (12).
- Table 23-2 summarizes information on various types and uses of sharpening stones.

TABLE 23-2. SHARPENING STONES AND TOOLS

Type	Grit	Use	Lubricant	Sterilization[a]
Ceramic synthetic stone	Fine	• Routine sharpening of metal and some plastic implant instruments	Water	All methods
Arkansas natural stone	Fine	• Routine sharpening of metal instruments	Mineral oil	All methods[b]
Neivert Whittler	—	• Routine sharpening of metal instruments	Water	All methods
India synthetic stone	Medium	• Sharpening of metal instruments that are dull	Water or oil	All methods
Composition synthetic stone	Coarse	• Sharpening of metal instruments that are extremely dull or that need reshaping	Water	All methods
Power devices and honing machines	Varies	• Routine sharpening and sharpening of instruments that are extremely dull	As directed by maker	As directed by maker
Test stick	Smooth	• Evaluate sharpness	None	All methods

[a]Includes autoclave, dry heat, or chemical sterilization.
[b]Natural stones become brittle over time with heat exposure.

LUBRICATION AND CARE OF STONES

1. **Lubrication of Sharpening Stone**
   A. A lubricant is a substance, such as water or oil, applied to the surface of a sharpening stone to reduce friction between the stone and the instrument (Fig. 23-18).
   B. Lubrication helps to prevent the metal shavings from sticking to the surface of the stone. These metal shavings can become embedded in the surface of the sharpening stone and reduce its effectiveness.
   C. Lubrication reduces frictional heat between the metal instrument and the stone. Stones that are used without lubrication will need to be replaced more frequently than stones used with lubricant.
   D. A synthetic stone that can be lubricated with water is recommended for use when sharpening instruments during patient treatment.
   E. A natural stone that must be lubricated with oil is not recommended for use when sharpening during patient treatment because the oil cannot be effectively sterilized.
2. **Care of Sharpening Stone**
   A. The sharpening stone should be cleaned in an ultrasonic cleaner or scrubbed with a brush and hot water to remove metal particles from the surface of the stone.
   B. After cleaning, the stone should be dried on a paper towel and placed in an autoclave bag or on an instrument cassette to be sterilized.

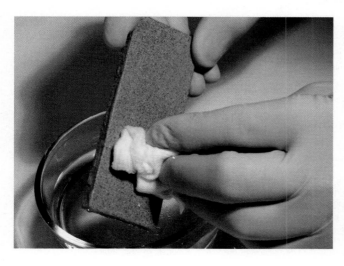

Figure 23-18. Lubrication of Sharpening Stone. The sharpening stone is lubricated with water or oil to help prevent metal shavings from becoming embedded in the surface of the stone.

RESTORATION OF A SHARP EDGE AND SHARPENING TECHNIQUES

1. Approaches to Metal Recontouring
   A. **Effective Approach.** The recommended sharpening method for reestablishing a fine, sharp cutting edge is to remove metal from the lateral surfaces of the working-end. Removing metal from the lateral surfaces restores the sharp edge while preserving the strength of the working-end. The darker green shading shown in Figure 23-19 indicates the area of metal to be removed from a universal curet to restore fine, sharp cutting edges.
   B. **Ineffective Approach.** Removing metal from the instrument's face is not recommended. Although this method may result in a sharp cutting edge, removing metal from the face weakens the working-end making it more likely to break (3,4,13,14).
2. **Techniques for Instrument Sharpening.** There are many different sharpening techniques. Two of the most common approaches to restoring a sharp cutting edge include sharpening using (1) the moving stone technique and (2) the moving instrument technique. Sharpening techniques are presented in the next module of the book.

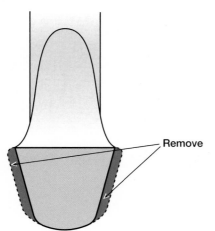

Remove

Figure 23-19. Remove Metal from the Lateral Surfaces to Restore a Sharp Cutting Edge. The recommended sharpening method for reestablishing the fine cutting edge is to remove metal from the lateral surfaces of the working-end. This illustration shows a universal curet; the portion of the working-end shaded in *dark green* would be removed from the lateral surfaces during sharpening.

References

1. Black G. *A Work on Operative Dentistry: The Technical Procedures in Filling Teeth*. Chicago, IL: Medico-Dental Publishing Company; 1908.
2. Michalak-Turcotte C. Controlling dental hygiene work-related musculoskeletal disorders: The ergonomic process. *J Dent Hyg*. 2000;74(1):41–48.
3. Balevi B. Engineering specifics of the periodontal curet's cutting edge. *J Periodontol*. 1996;67(4):374–378.
4. Huang CC, Tseng CC. Effect of different sharpening stones on periodontal curettes evaluated by scanning electron microscopy. *J Formos Med Assoc*. 1991;90(8):782–787.
5. Tal H, Panno JM, Vaidyanathan TK. Scanning electron microscope evaluation of wear of dental curettes during standardized root planing. *J Periodontol*. 1985;56(9):532–536.
6. Scaramucci MK. Sharpening 101. *Dimen Dent Hyg*. 2007;5(5):18–20.
7. Scaramucci MK. Back to basics. Refresh your skills with the review of sharpening fundamentals. *Dimen Den Hyg*. 2011;9(9):40–42.
8. Hodges K. On the cutting edge. *Dimen Den Hyg*. 2004;2(4):16, 8, 20.
9. Murray GH, Lubow RM, Mayhew RB, Summitt JB, Usseglio RJ. The effects of two sharpening methods on the strength of a periodontal scaling instrument. *J Periodontol*. 1984;55(7):410–413.
10. Marquam B. Keep eye on sharpening techniques to prevent disease transmission. *RDH*. 1992;12(8):20–21, 23.
11. Andrade Acevedo RA, Cardozo AK, Sampaio JE. Scanning electron microscopic and profilometric study of different sharpening stones. *Braz Dent J*. 2006;17(3):237–242.
12. Rossi R, Smukler H. A scanning electron microscope study comparing the effectiveness of different types of sharpening stones and curets. *J Periodontol*. 1995;66(11):956–961.
13. Marquam BJ. Strategies to improve instrument sharpening. *Dent Hyg (Chic)*. 1988;62(7):334–338.
14. Paquette OE, Levin MP. The sharpening of scaling instruments: II. A preferred technique. *J Periodontol*. 1977;48(3):169–172.

Section 5
Skill Application

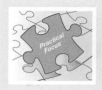

PRACTICAL FOCUS

Nola has asked you to evaluate her instrumentation technique because she says that all her patients complain that she is "so rough." Nola hopes that you can tell her what she is doing wrong. Nola is about to begin periodontal instrumentation on a patient with medium-sized supragingival and subgingival calculus deposits. The working-ends of her instruments are pictured below.

- Evaluate each working-ends shown in Figures 23-20 to 23-25 and if problems are found, identify them.
- How efficient and effective do you think calculus removal will be using these instruments?
- What recommendations would your give Nola?

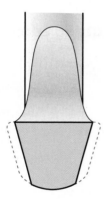

Figure 23-20. Universal Curet.

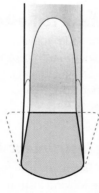

Figure 23-21. Universal Curet.

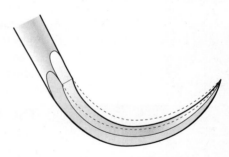

Figure 23-22. Sickle Scaler.

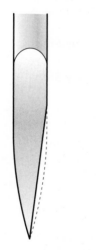

Figure 23-23. Sickle Scaler.

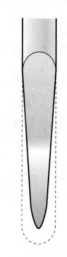

Figure 23-24. Universal Curet.

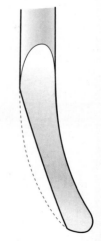

Figure 23-25. Area-Specific Curet.

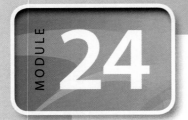

MODULE 24

Instrument Sharpening Techniques

Module Overview

This module discusses two commonly used methods for sharpening periodontal instruments: the moving stone technique and the moving instrument technique.

Skill practice sections provide experience in positioning the instrument and sharpening stone. Step-by-step instructions are provided in the moving stone and moving instrument techniques. *Module 23 should be completed before beginning this module.*

Module Outline

Section 1   **Removing Metal to Restore a Sharp Cutting Edge**   **612**
Goal of Instrument Sharpening
Reestablishing a Sharp Cutting Edge
How to Restore a Sharp Cutting Edge
Sharpen the Cutting Edge in Sections
Contour the Curet Toe
Contour the Back of a Curet

Section 2   **The Moving *Instrument* Technique**   **616**
Overview of the Moving Instrument Technique
Innovations in the Moving Instrument Technique
Effectiveness of the Moving Instrument Technique
Essential Skill Components of the Moving Instrument Technique
Sharpening Horse Set-Up
Skill Building. Moving Instrument Technique: Step-by-Step for Curets, p. 620
Skill Building. Moving Instrument Technique: Step-by-Step for Sickle Scalers, p. 623

Section 3   **The Moving *Stone* Technique**   **624**
Overview of the Moving Stone Technique
Essential Skill Components of the Moving Stone Technique
Skill Building. Establishing Correct Angulation, p. 627
Basic Principles with Curets and Sickle Scalers
Sharpening Guide R
Sharpening Guide L
Skill Building. Moving Instrument Technique for Curets and Sickle Scalers, p. 633

| Section 4 | **Evaluating Sharpness** | **636** |

Skill Building. Evaluating Sharpness of Cutting a Edge, p. 636

| Section 5 | **Sharpening a Periodontal File** | **637** |

| Section 6 | **Skill Application** | **639** |

Student Self Evaluation Module 24: Instrument Sharpening

Key Terms

Moving stone technique
Moving instrument
   technique

Metal burs
Wire edge
Tanged file

Learning Objectives

- Compare and contrast the moving stone and the moving instrument techniques for instrument sharpening.

- Describe and demonstrate the proper relationship of the instrument's working-end to the sharpening stone.

- Demonstrate the correct grasp for both the instrument and the sharpening stone when using the moving stone technique.

- Demonstrate the correct finger rest and grasp when using the moving instrument technique.

- Describe and demonstrate the sharpening procedure for sickle scalers, universal curets, and area-specific curets using the moving stone technique.

- Describe and demonstrate the sharpening procedure for sickle scalers, universal curets, and area-specific curets using the moving instrument technique.

- Sharpen a dull sickle scaler, universal curet, and area-specific curet to produce a sharp, fine cutting edge while preserving all the original design characteristics of the working-ends.

- If applicable, sharpen a dull periodontal file with a tanged file to restore sharp cutting edges while preserving all the original design characteristics of the working-end.

- Demonstrate the procedure for using a plastic sharpening stick to determine if the entire length of a cutting edge is sharp.

- Value sharp instruments and the practice of sharpening at the first sign of dullness or after each use of an instrument.

611

Section 1
Removing Metal to Restore a Sharp Cutting Edge

GOAL OF INSTRUMENT SHARPENING

The goal of instrument sharpening is to restore a fine sharp cutting edge to a dull working-end. To be successful, a sharpening technique should remove a minimum amount of metal from the instrument and maintain the original design characteristics of the working-end.

A review of the literature reveals a variety of techniques for sharpening periodontal instruments (1–14). Various authors have described the criteria of an ideal sharpening method:

- Is easy to learn
- Relies on inexpensive equipment
- Employs a technique that provides good visibility of the working-end and good control during the sharpening process
- Removes a minimum amount of metal from the instrument's working-end
- Maintains the original design characteristics of the working-end

This module presents two commonly used sharpening techniques:

1. The moving stone technique that involves holding the instrument stationary and moving a sharpening stone over a lateral surface of the working-end.
2. The moving instrument technique that involves moving the working-end of the periodontal instrument across a stationary sharpening stone.

REESTABLISHING A SHARP CUTTING EDGE

Regardless of the sharpening method used, the process of restoring a sharp cutting edge involves removing metal from the lateral surfaces of the working-end.

- Metal is removed from a lateral surface until the junction with the face is restored to a fine line with no width (7,15–17).
- Figure 24-1 indicates the metal (shaded in dark green) that would be removed from a universal curet to restore sharp cutting edges.

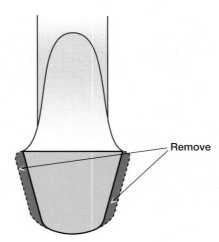

Figure 24-1. Metal is Removed from the Lateral Surfaces to Restore a Sharp Cutting Edge. Sharp cutting edges are restored on a universal curet by removing the portion of the lateral surfaces shaded in *dark green* from the working-end. Removing this metal restores sharp cutting edges to the working-end.

HOW TO RESTORE A SHARP CUTTING EDGE

It is vital to retain the original design characteristics of the working-end when removing metal from the lateral surfaces during sharpening. *A sharp cutting edge is restored by removing metal from the lateral surface while maintaining the 70- to 80-degree internal junction between the face and the lateral surface.* Figures 24-2 and 24-3 illustrate the consequences of correct and incorrect angulation between the instrument face and the sharpening stone.

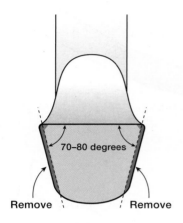

Figure 24-2. Correct Approach to Restoring a Sharp Cutting Edge.
- The *dark green shading* in this illustration indicates the portions of the working-end to be removed during sharpening.
- By placing the sharpening stone at a 70- to 80-degree angle to the face, the ideal design characteristics of the working-end will be maintained after sharpening.

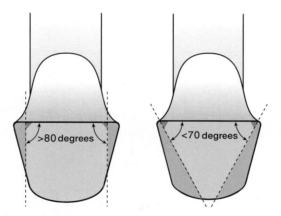

Figure 24-3. Incorrect Approach to Restoring a Sharp Cutting Edge. The *red shading* in these illustrations indicates the portions of the working-end removed during incorrect sharpening technique.
- If the stone contacts the lateral surface at an angle greater than 80 degrees, the end result is a bulky working-end that is difficult to adapt to the tooth surface. Heavy lateral pressure would be needed to remove any calculus deposits with this working-end.
- If the sharpening stone contacts the lateral surface at an angulation less than 70 degrees, the end result is a working-end that is weakened due to excessive removal of metal. Such a working-end would dull quickly and could break during calculus removal.

SHARPEN THE CUTTING EDGE IN SECTIONS

Regardless of the sharpening method used, the cutting edges should be sharpened in sections to preserve the original design characteristics of the cutting edge. Figures 24-4 and 24-5 depict the concept of sharpening the cutting edge in sections.

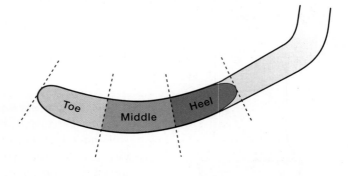

Figure 24-4. Cutting Edge Sections. Divide the cutting edge into three imaginary sections for sharpening: the heel-third, middle-third, and tip- or toe-third.

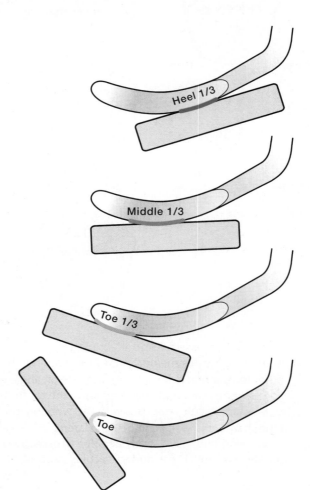

Figure 24-5. Sharpen the Cutting Edge in Sections.
- The sharpening stone is applied to only a third of the cutting edge at a time to maintain a curved cutting edge.
- Sharpen (1) the heel-third, (2) the middle-third, and (3) the toe- or tip-third of the cutting edge. If the instrument is a curet, (4) sharpen the toe.

CONTOUR THE CURET TOE

Contouring is the process of removing metal from the toe and back to maintain the original design characteristics of these curved surfaces. Contouring the toe of a curet with the sharpening stone is necessary to maintain its rounded contour.

- Note the three divisions of the curet toe as labeled in Figure 24-6.
- Sections 1 and 3 tend to be used more often in instrumentation than section 2. Therefore, sections 1 and 3 may require more shaping with the sharpening stone than section 2.
- Sharpening the toe involves moving the stone from the lateral surface and around the toe as depicted in Figure 24-7.

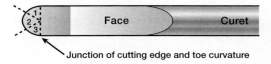

Junction of cutting edge and toe curvature

Figure 24-6. Divisions of the Curet Toe. The three divisions of the toe of a curet working-end.

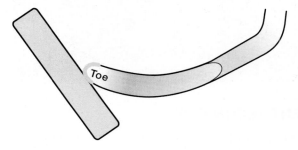

Figure 24-7. Contouring of the Curet Toe. Instead of stopping at the junction of the lateral surface and the curvature of the toe, the clinician continues the sharpening stroke to move around the toe.

CONTOUR THE BACK OF A CURET

Without contouring the junction between the back of a curet and its lateral surfaces eventually becomes pointed (Fig. 24-8). Occasional sharpening of the back is performed to maintain the original design of the curet.

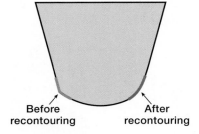

Before recontouring   After recontouring

Figure 24-8. Recontouring the Back. The back of a curet must be contoured slightly with the sharpening stone to maintain a smooth rounded back.

Section 2
The Moving *Instrument* Technique

OVERVIEW OF THE MOVING INSTRUMENT TECHNIQUE

As the name suggests, the **moving instrument technique** involves removing metal from the lateral surface by moving the working-end across the surface of a stabilized sharpening stone (Fig. 24-9).

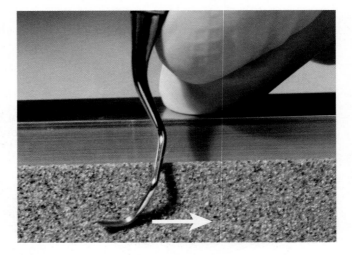

Figure 24-9. Moving Instrument Technique. For the moving instrument technique the working-end is moved across a stationary sharpening stone.

INNOVATIONS IN THE MOVING INSTRUMENT TECHNIQUE

- For many years, the moving *stone* technique has been the most common method of instrument sharpening taught in dental hygiene programs. The fact that it is easy to see the angle formed between the face and the stone probably accounts for the popularity of the moving *stone* method.
- Until recently, the moving *instrument* method used the technique of placing the sharpening stone on a flat countertop. In this position it is not possible to view the angle between the stone and the instrument face. The inability to see the face-to-stone angulation made the moving instrument technique difficult to teach to novice clinicians.
- A new sharpening tool, called the Sharpening Horse, is changing the way that clinicians regard the moving instrument technique (Fig. 24-10). *The Sharpening Horse allows the clinician to see the face-to-stone angulation while using the moving instrument technique* (8).

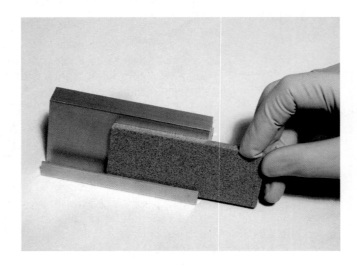

Figure 24-10. Sharpening Horse. The Sharpening Horse is a device for holding the sharpening stone in a fixed position.

- The Sharpening Horse allows the clinician to view the face-to-stone angulation.
- This tool facilitates use of the moving instrument technique.
- Information on the Sharpening Horse tool is available at www.dhmethed.com.

EFFECTIVENESS OF THE MOVING INSTRUMENT TECHNIQUE

A recent study examined the results of many different sharpening methods. *Researchers found that the technique that produces the most precise cutting edge without wire edges and irregularities is the moving instrument technique* (1). For the study, experienced clinicians sharpened instruments using nine different sharpening techniques including moving stone, moving instrument, Neivert Whittler, and powered sharpening techniques. Figures 24-11 and 24-12 compare the results obtained with the moving instrument and the moving stone techniques.

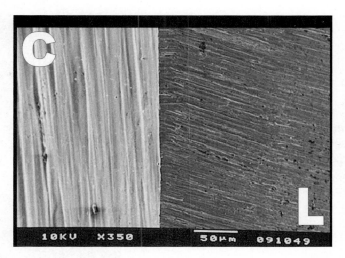

Figure 24-11. Moving Instrument Technique. A scanning electron microscopy (SEM) image shows that the moving *instrument* technique produced a precise, defined cutting edge with an exact junction between the coronal (C)—instrument face—and the lateral surface (L). (Used with permission from Acevedo R, Sampaio J, Shibli J. Scanning electron microscope assessment of several resharpening techniques on the cutting edges of Gracey curettes. *J Contemp Dent Pract.* 2007;8(7):70–77.)

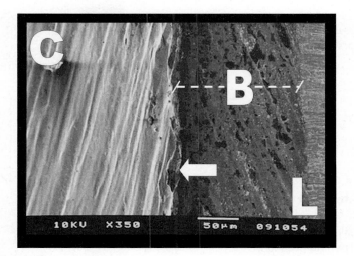

Figure 24-12. Moving Stone Technique. A scanning electron microscopy (SEM) image shows that the moving *stone* technique produced a bevel and wire edges between the coronal (C)—instrument face— and the lateral surface (L). (Used with permission from Acevedo R, Sampaio J, Shibli J. Scanning electron microscope assessment of several resharpening techniques on the cutting edges of Gracey curettes. *J Contemp Dent Pract.* 2007;8(7):70–77.)

ESSENTIAL SKILL COMPONENTS OF THE MOVING INSTRUMENT TECHNIQUE

Essential skill components of the moving instrument technique are: (1) using a modified pen grasp, (2) using the ring finger as a support beam for the hand, and (3) sliding the ring finger along the top of the Sharpening Horse tool during sharpening (Figs. 24-13 to 24-15).

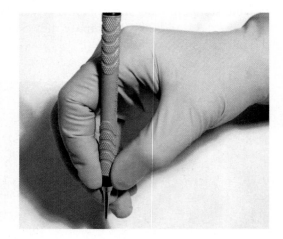

Figure 24-13. Skill Component 1: Instrument Grasp. A modified pen grasp is used to hold the instrument for the moving instrument sharpening technique.

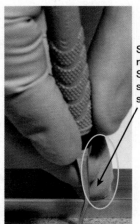

Straight fulcrum finger rests on top of the Sharpening Horse to support the hand during sharpening

Figure 24-14. Skill Component 2: Ring Finger as Support Beam.
- The ring finger is a critical element for use of the Sharpening Horse.
- *The ring finger acts as a support beam and rests on top of the Sharpening Horse tool throughout the sharpening process.*

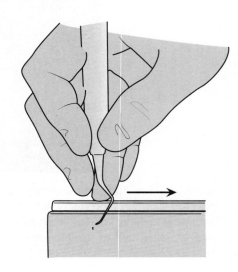

Figure 24-15. Skill Component 3: Slide on Fulcrum as You Work.
- The ring finger slides along the beam of the Sharpening Horse during the sharpening procedure.
- *Right-handed clinicians* move from left to right along the beam, sharpening the heel-third, then middle-third, and finally the toe/tip-third of the cutting edge.
- *Left-handed clinicians* move from right to left along the beam, sharpening from heel to toe/tip-third.

SHARPENING HORSE SET-UP

The two photos in Figure 24-16 show the components of the Sharpening Horse system and the assembled Sharpening Horse. Figure 24-17 shows a simple way to adjust the height of the sharpening stone in the horse by using a sharpening stick to elevate the height of the stone in the holder.

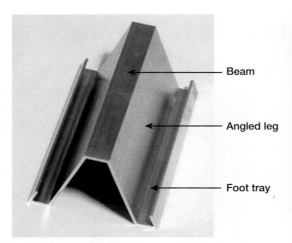
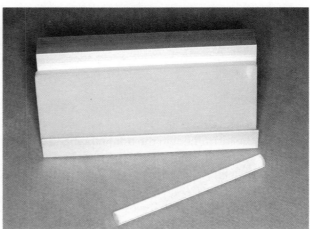

Figure 24-16. Components of the Sharpening Horse System. The Sharpening Horse system consists of a metal device that holds a sharpening stone at a fixed angle, a ceramic sharpening stone, and an acrylic test stick.

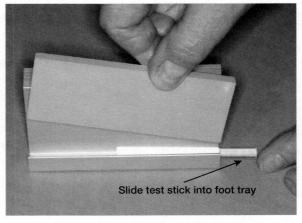

Figure 24-17. Modifying Stone Height. For most clinicians the sharpening stone is at an ideal height as it rests in the foot tray.
- Clinicians with petite hands or short fingers may find it helpful to raise the height of the stone in the holder.
- Sliding a test stick into the foot tray and resting the stone on top of the test stick easily raises the height of the stone in the holder.

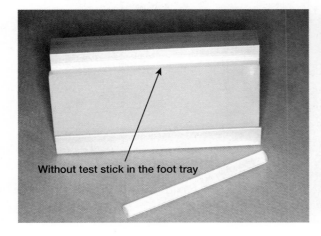
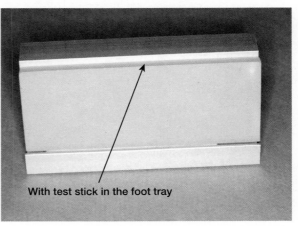

SKILL BUILDING
Moving Instrument Technique: Step-by-Step for Curets

Directions: Lubricate the stone with water and place it in the holder. Follow the steps depicted in Figures 24-18 to 24-26 to practice sharpening a curet.

1. **Figure 24-18. Grasp and Finger Rest.**
   - Grasp the instrument in the dominant hand using a modified pen grasp.
   - Establish a finger rest on the top of the beam of the Sharpening Horse.
   - Stabilize the horse with the nondominant hand.
   - ***Hold the ring finger straight and use it as a support beam for the hand throughout the entire sharpening procedure.***

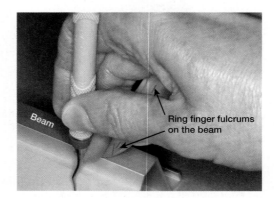

2. **Figure 24-19. Face-to-Stone Angulation.**
   - ***Position the instrument face parallel to the tabletop.***
   - With the face in this position, the Sharpening Horse device holds the stone at the correct angulation for sharpening.
   - Note that the position of the face is the same—parallel to the tabletop—when sharpening both sickle scalers and curets.

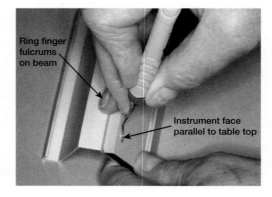

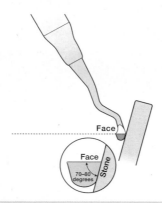

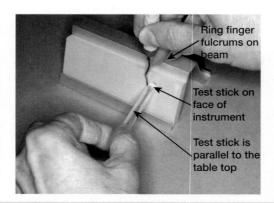

Figure 24-20. Technique Check. For all sickle scalers and curets, the working-end is properly positioned if ***the face is parallel to the table top.*** One technique for checking for parallelism is to place a sharpening stick on the face and verify that the stick is parallel to the table top.

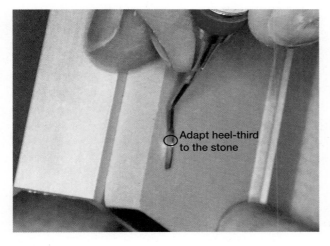

Adapt heel-third to the stone

3. **Figure 24-21. Begin with Heel-Third.**
   - Holding the ring finger straight, position the heel-third of the cutting edge against the sharpening stone.
   - *Slide both the finger rest and instrument a short distance along the stone to sharpen the heel-third of the cutting edge.*

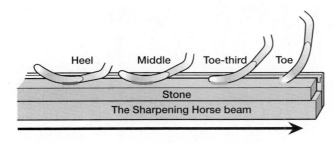

Heel   Middle   Toe-third   Toe

Stone
The Sharpening Horse beam

4. **Figure 24-22. Sharpen Cutting Edge in Sections.**
   - Start at one end of the stone. Adapt the *heel-third* of the cutting edge to the stone.
   - *Slide the finger rest and instrument a short distance along the beam to sharpen the heel-third of the cutting edge.*

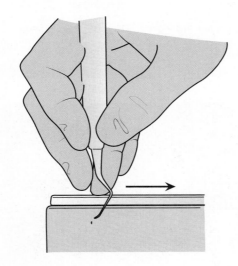

5. **Figure 24-23. Slide the Fulcrum along the Beam.**
   - Throughout the sharpening process, slide the fulcrum finger along the beam of the Sharpening Horse.
   - As the cutting edge moves along the stone, pivot the working-end to sharpen the middle-third and toe-third of the cutting edge.

(The steps for sharpening a curet continue on the next page.)

6. **Figure 24-24. Pivot the Working-End.**
   - Keeping the finger rest in place, pivot the working-end slightly so that the ***middle-third*** of the cutting edge is against the stone.
   - Slide both the finger rest and instrument a short distance along the stone to sharpen the middle-third of the cutting edge.

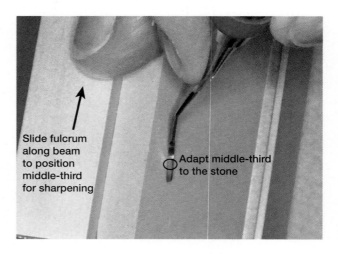

Slide fulcrum along beam to position middle-third for sharpening

Adapt middle-third to the stone

7. **Figure 24-25. Pivot the Working-End.**
   - Keeping the finger rest in place, pivot the working-end slightly so that the ***toe-third*** of the cutting edge is against the stone.
   - Slide both the finger rest and instrument a short distance along the stone to sharpen the toe-third of the cutting edge.

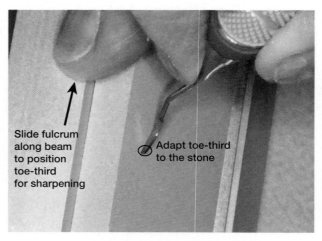

Slide fulcrum along beam to position toe-third for sharpening

Adapt toe-third to the stone

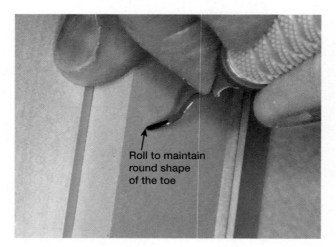

Roll to maintain round shape of the toe

8. **Figure 24-26. Pivot onto the Toe.** Pivot to sharpen and round the ***toe*** of the working-end.

9. Complete the Sharpening Process:
   - Complete the sharpening process by recontouring the back of the working-end on the top edge of the sharpening stone.
   - Turn the Sharpening Horse around to sharpen the opposite cutting edge of a universal curet or sickle scaler.
   - *After sharpening turn to Section 4 of this module to evaluate sharpness.*

SKILL BUILDING
Moving Instrument Technique: Step-by-Step for Sickle Scalers

The sharpening technique for a sickle scaler is essentially the same as that used with a curet (Figs. 24-27 and 24-28). The cutting edges of a sickle scaler meet in a point; therefore, on a sickle scaler there is no rounded toe to contour.

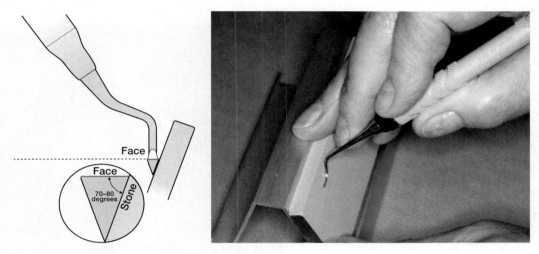

Figure 24-27. Sharpening Technique for a Sickle Scaler.

- **Adapt Sickle to Stone.** Establish the correct face-to-stone angulation by positioning the face parallel to the countertop.
- **Establish Fulcrum.** The complex shank bend of some posterior sickles—such as the Nevi sickle pictured here—means that the clinician lowers the hand to obtain parallelism of the face to the tabletop.
- **Sharpen.** Slide the finger rest along the top of the Sharpening Horse while moving the working-end across the stone.

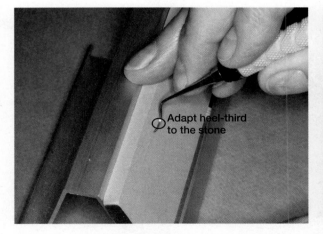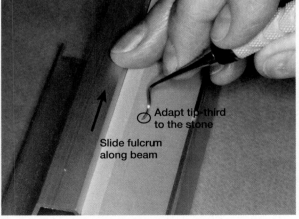

Figure 24-28. Sharpen Cutting Edge of a Sickle in Thirds. Using a similar technique to that used for a curet, sharpen the heel-third, middle-third, and tip-third of a sickle scaler.

Section 3
The Moving *Stone* Technique

OVERVIEW OF THE MOVING STONE TECHNIQUE

As the name suggests, the **moving stone technique** involves removing metal from the working-end by moving a sharpening stone over a lateral surface of a stabilized instrument (Figs. 24-29 and 24-30). The moving stone technique is one of the oldest methods for instrumentation sharpening (16).

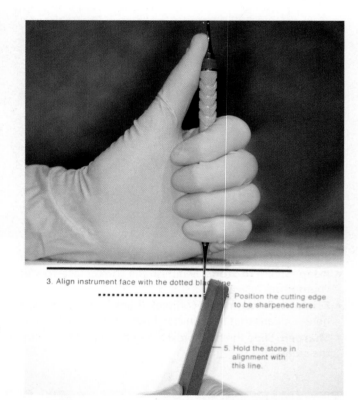

Figure 24-29. Moving Stone Technique.
- The moving stone technique involves grasping the instrument and stabilizing it against a countertop.
- The sharpening stone is held in the clinician's other hand and is moved over the lateral surface of the working-end.

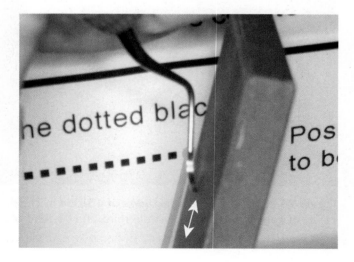

Figure 24-30. Movement of Stone. The sharpening stone is positioned against the lateral surface and moved up and down to remove metal from the working-end.

ESSENTIAL SKILL COMPONENTS OF THE MOVING STONE TECHNIQUE

The moving stone technique is one of the most complex methods of instrument sharpening, involving many steps to obtain a sharp cutting edge. The steps in the moving stone technique build upon one another. If the first step is incorrect, then all steps that follow will be incorrect.

Skill Component 1: Positioning the Instrument against a Stable Surface

An important component of correct sharpening technique is the position of the instrument face.

The instrument face is positioned parallel to the countertop for sharpening. Position the working-end of a sickle scaler, universal curet, or area-specific curet so that the face is parallel (=) to the countertop. Figures 24-31 and 24-32 depict the face of a sickle scaler, universal curet, and area-specific curet positioned with the instrument face parallel to the countertop.

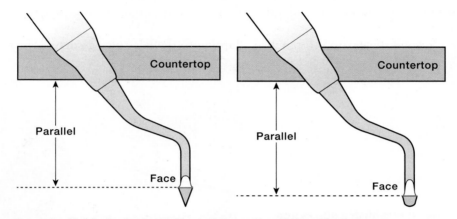

Figure 24-31. Face of a Sickle Scaler or Universal Curet Parallel to Countertop.
- For sharpening, a sickle scaler or a universal curet, position the instrument face parallel (=) to the countertop.
- When positioned with the face parallel to the countertop, the lower shanks of these instruments are perpendicular (⊥) to the countertop.
- *Two cutting edges are sharpened on each working-end of a sickle scaler or a universal curet.*

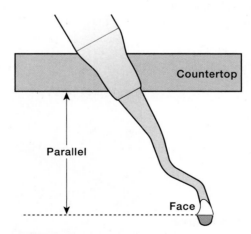

Figure 24-32. Face of an Area-Specific Curet Parallel to Countertop.
- For sharpening, an area-specific curet, position the instrument face parallel (=) to the countertop.
- When positioned with the face parallel to the countertop, the lower shank of an area-specific is NOT perpendicular to the countertop.
- *One cutting edge, the working cutting edge, is sharpened on each area-specific curet.*

Skill Component 2: Establishing Angulation of the Stone to the Instrument Face

To maintain the original design characteristics of the working-end *the angulation between the instrument face and the sharpening stone should be between 70 and 80 degrees.*

- Beginning clinicians often experience difficulty in visualizing the 70- to 80-degree angle used in instrument sharpening.
- Follow the directions in Figures 24-33 and 24-34 on this page to gain experience in establishing the correct angulation between the sharpening stone and the instrument face.

Directions

- For this Skill Practice you will need a rectangular sharpening stone and the *illustrations*— Figures 24-35 and 24-36 located on the next page of this module.
- Use the first illustration to practice adapting the stone to the right cutting edge of a universal curet.
- Next, use the second illustration to practice adapting to the left cutting edge.

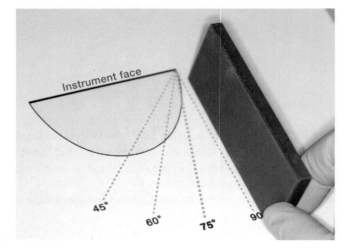

Figure 24-33. Step 1: Establish a 90-Degree Angle.
- Place your sharpening stone on the *dotted line* labeled as a 90-degree angle. Your sharpening stone is now positioned at a 90-degree angle to the instrument face.
- This position gives you a visual starting point from which to establish the correct angulation.

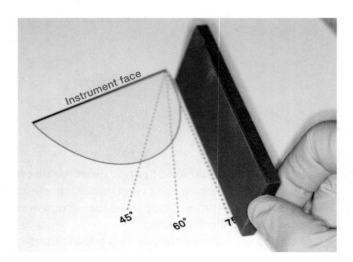

Figure 24-34. Step 2: Establish a 75-Degree Angle.
- Swing the lower end of the sharpening stone toward the instrument back.
- Align your stone with the *dotted line* labeled as a 75-degree angle. Your sharpening stone is now at the proper angle to the face.

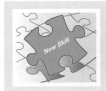

SKILL BUILDING
Establishing Correct Angulation

Use Figures 24-35 and 24-36 below to practice establishing correct angulation of a sharpening stone to the instrument face.

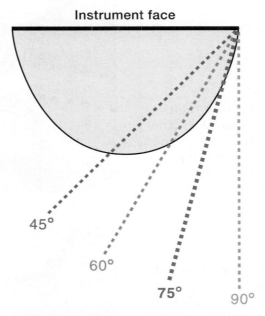

Figure 24-35. Angle for Right Cutting Edge.

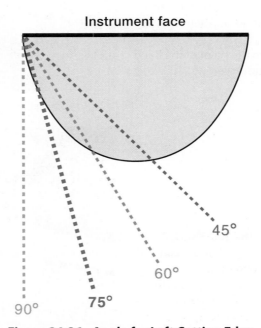

Figure 24-36. Angle for Left Cutting Edge.

Skill Component 3: Sharpen the Cutting Edge in Sections

A technique of rotating the sharpening stone is used to sharpen the cutting edge in sections (Figs. 24-37 to 24-39). First the stone is adapted to the heel-third of the cutting edge. Next the middle-third is sharpened. After sharpening the middle-third, the stone is rotated again to adapt to the toe- or tip-third of the cutting edge. For this technique, the stone is rotated away from the palm of the hand *while maintaining correct angulation of the stone to the instrument face.*

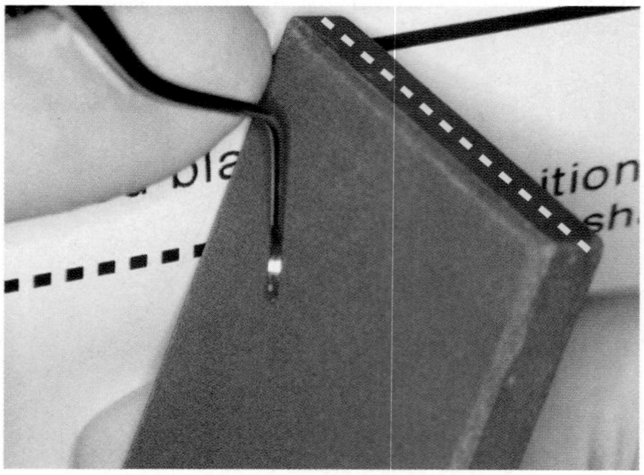

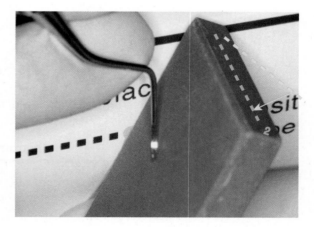

Figure 24-37. Step 1: Sharpen the Heel-Third.
Begin by adapting the stone to the heel-third of the cutting edge. Note that the middle and toe-thirds of the cutting edge are not in contact with the sharpening stone. Use a Sharpening Guide to establish a 75-degree angle with the sharpening stone.

Figure 24-38. Step 2: Sharpen the Middle-Third.
While maintaining correct angulation, rotate the stone away from the palm of your hand slightly. The stone is now positioned to sharpen the middle-third of the cutting edge.

- The *yellow dotted line* on the photograph indicates the position of the sharpening stone when sharpening the *heel-third*.
- The stone is rotated away from the palm of the hand to the position indicated by the *orange dotted line* for sharpening the *middle-third*.

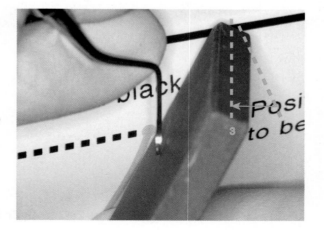

Figure 24-39. Step 3: Sharpen the Toe-Third. Rotate the stone away from the palm of your hand again. Sharpen the toe-third of the cutting edge.

- The *green dotted line* on the photograph indicates the position of the sharpening stone when sharpening the *toe-third*.
- Continue to Figure 24-40 to contour the curet toe.

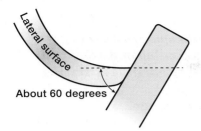

Lateral surface

About 60 degrees

Figure 24-40. Contouring the Toe. Occasional sharpening of the toe maintains the original design characteristics of a curet. With a curet, sharpening continues around the toe to maintain the rounded contour.

Skill Component 4: Removing Metal Burs from the Cutting Edge

Sharpening can produce minute **metal burs** that project from the cutting edge (Fig. 24-41).

1. A cutting edge with metal burs is sometimes termed a **wire edge** because the metal burs are like tiny wire projections. The use of a wire edge on the root surfaces can result in gouging of the cementum.
2. The metal burs are impossible to see with the naked eye but can be seen using magnification.
3. Burs can be avoided by finishing with a down stroke toward the cutting edge as depicted below.
4. Burs can easily be seen under magnification and removed using a light stroke with a cylindrical sharpening stone.

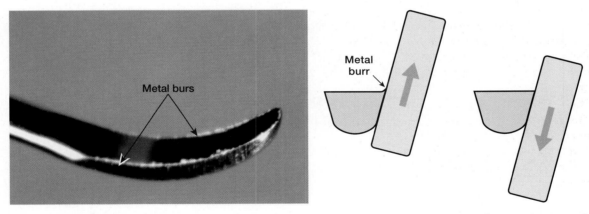

Metal burs

Metal burr

Figure 24-41. Metal Burs. As shown in the photograph on the left, sharpening can produce minute metal burs that project from the cutting edge. Burs can be prevented by finishing with a down stroke of the sharpening stone toward the cutting edge as depicted in the drawing above.

BASIC PRINCIPLES WITH CURETS AND SICKLE SCALERS

1. **Consistent Basic Principles.** *The basic steps in the moving stone technique are the same for all area-specific curets, universal curets, and sickle scalers. The relationship of the face of the working-end to the countertop is the same for all area-specific curets, universal curets, and sickle scalers.*
   - The working-end is positioned so that the face is parallel to the countertop.
   - Once the face is parallel to the countertop, the stone positioned at a 70- to 80-degree angle to the face (Fig. 24-42).
2. **Minor Differences.** Only a few differences apply to the techniques used with these three instruments.
   - Two sharpening edges per working-end are sharpened for universal curets and sickle scalers.
   - Only one cutting edge per working-end—the lower cutting edge—is sharpened on an area-specific curet.
   - The rounded toe and back should be contoured on area-specific and universal curets.

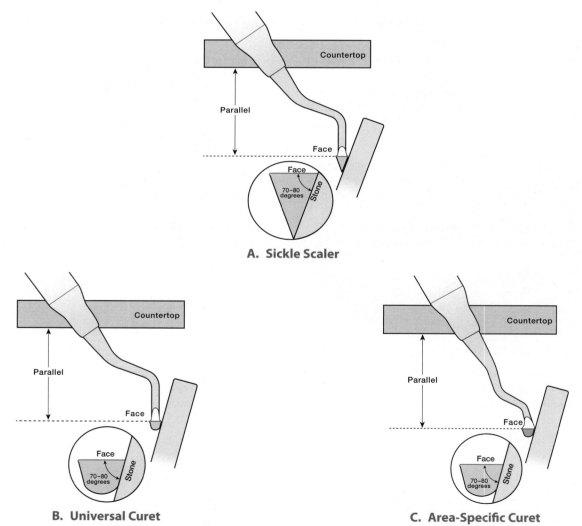

A. Sickle Scaler

B. Universal Curet

C. Area-Specific Curet

Figure 24-42. Basic Principles for Moving Stone Technique. Preparation for the moving stone technique includes: (1) positioning the face parallel to the countertop and (2) establishing a 70- to 80-degree angle between the face and the stone. These principles apply to all sickle scalers, universal curets, and area-specific curets.

SHARPENING GUIDE R

Directions for Use of Sharpening Guides: Photocopy **Sharpening Guide R** (Fig. 24-43) and **Sharpening Guide L** (Fig. 24-44) and place them back-to-back in a single plastic page protector or have them laminated. Another way to use a photocopied Sharpening Guide is to tape it to the countertop and cover it with a piece of plastic wrap.

Use Sharpening Guide R for:

- The right cutting edge of a universal curet or sickle scaler
- For ODD numbered Gracey curets, such as a G11 and G13

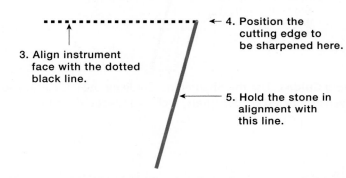

Sharpening Guide R

1. Fold this page in half along the solid black line.
2. Place the folded edge on a countertop so that the black line is aligned along the edge of the counter.

3. Align instrument face with the dotted black line.

4. Position the cutting edge to be sharpened here.

5. Hold the stone in alignment with this line.

Figure 24-43. Sharpening Guide R. Use this Sharpening Guide for the right cutting edge of a universal curet or sickle scaler and for odd numbered Gracey curets, such as a Gracey 11 or 13.

SHARPENING GUIDE L

Use Sharpening Guide L for:

- The left cutting edge of a universal curet or sickle scaler
- For EVEN numbered Gracey curets, such as a G12 and G14

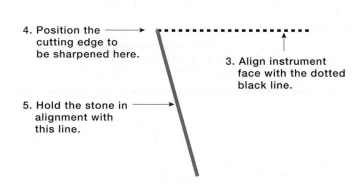

Sharpening Guide L

1. Fold this page in half along the solid black line.
2. Place the folded edge on a countertop so that the black line is aligned along the edge of the counter.

4. Position the cutting edge to be sharpened here.

3. Align instrument face with the dotted black line.

5. Hold the stone in alignment with this line.

Figure 24-44. Sharpening Guide L. Use this Sharpening Guide for the left cutting edge of a universal curet or sickle scaler and for even numbered Gracey curets, such as a Gracey 12 or 14.

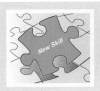

SKILL BUILDING
Moving Instrument Technique for Curets and Sickle Scalers

Directions:

- Cover the top and front surfaces of the counter with a barrier such as plastic wrap. Secure the barrier to the countertop with autoclave or masking tape.
- Place *Sharpening Guide R* on the counter so that the heavy black line falls along the edge of the counter. Secure the guide to the countertop with autoclave or masking tape. *Begin by sharpening the right cutting edge of a universal curet.*
- Follow the steps shown in Figures 24-45 to 24-54 to practice the moving stone sharpening technique.
- Lubricate the stone. If the stone is synthetic, lubricate it on both sides with a few drops of water. Synthetic stones are recommended for sharpening during treatment. If the stone is natural, lubricate it on both sides with a few drops of oil.

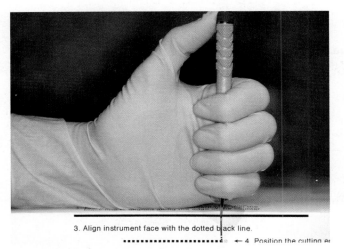

1. **Figure 24-45. Grasp the Instrument.** *Grasp the instrument handle in the palm of your nondominant hand.* Rest your hand and arm on the countertop. Stabilize the instrument handle with your thumb.

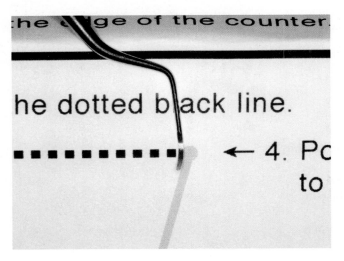

2. **Figure 24-46. Position the Instrument Face.**
   - Align the instrument face with the *dotted line* on the Sharpening Guide. This will position the working-end so that the face is parallel (=) to the countertop.
   - Keeping the face aligned with the *dotted line,* slide your nondominant hand over until the cutting edge to be sharpened is positioned *at the far right-hand side* of the dotted line.

3. **Figure 24-47.** **Grasp the Sharpening Stone.**
   - *Grasp the sharpening stone with your dominant hand.*
   - Hold the stone on the edges so that your fingers do not get in the way when sharpening.

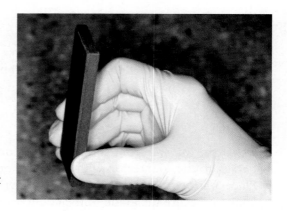

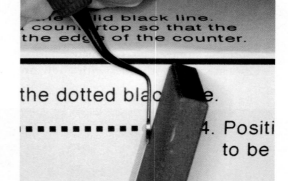

4. **Figure 24-48.** **Position the Sharpening Stone.** Align the sharpening stone with the *solid line*. This is the correct angulation for sharpening.

5. **Figure 24-49.** **Adapt the Stone to the Heel-Third of the Cutting Edge.**
   - The photographs show a bird's-eye view looking down at the instrument face.
   - Make several short up and down strokes to sharpen this section of the cutting edge. If a metal sludge forms on the working-end, wipe it with a gauze square.

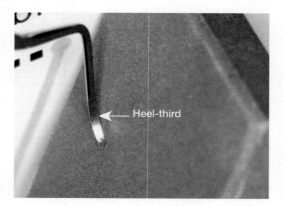

Heel-third

6. **Figure 24-50.** **Sharpen the Middle-Third of the Cutting Edge.**
   - When the heel section is sharp, rotate the stone so that it is in contact with the middle-third of the cutting edge.
   - Make several short up and down strokes to sharpen this section of the cutting edge.

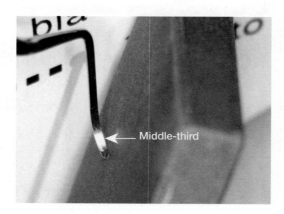

Middle-third

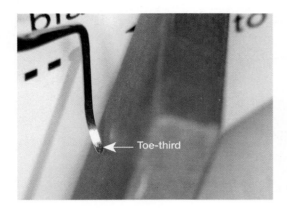

7. **Figure 24-51. Sharpen the Toe-Third of the Cutting Edge.**
   - Rotate the stone so that it is in contact with the toe-third of the cutting edge.
   - Make several short up and down strokes to sharpen this section of the cutting edge.

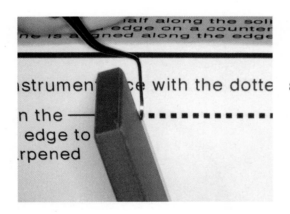

8. **Figure 24-52.** *For Universal Curets and Sickle Scalers Only—Reposition the Stone to Sharpen the Left Cutting Edge.*
   - Use **Sharpening Guide L** to position the stone for sharpening the left cutting edge on a universal curet or sickle scaler.
   - Sharpen the left cutting edge using the same technique as for the right cutting edge.

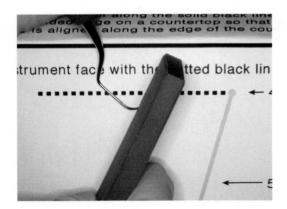

9. **Figure 24-53.** *For Curets Only—Sharpen the Curet Toe.*
   - To recontour the curet toe, make a series of sharpening strokes around the toe. Be careful to keep the face parallel (=) to the countertop.
   - Move the stone in up and down strokes as you work your way around the toe.

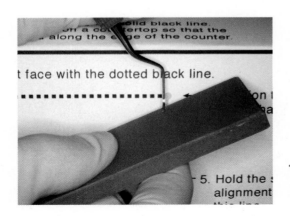

10. **Figure 24-54.** *For Curets Only—Recontour the Back.*
    To recontour the back, use semicircular strokes around the back of the curet.

Section 4
Evaluating Sharpness

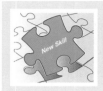

SKILL BUILDING
Evaluating Sharpness of a Cutting Edge

After sharpening follow steps 1 to 3 shown in Figures 24-55 to 24-57 to evaluate the sharpening process.

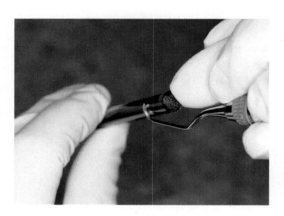

Figure 24-55. Step 1: Grasp a Sharpening Test Stick in Your Nondominant Hand.
- Position the stick so that you are looking down on the top. Establish a finger rest on the flat, top surface of the stick and adapt the cutting edge at a 70- to 80-degree angle to the stick.
- *The cutting edge must be adapted to the stick at the same angulation that you would use against a tooth surface.*

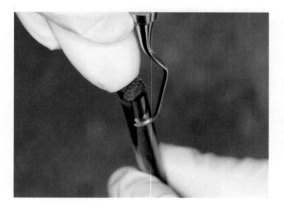

Figure 24-56. Step 2: Evaluate Cutting Edge.
- If the cutting edge is sharp, it will scratch or "grab" the surface of the test stick. A dull edge will slide over the surface of the test stick.
- Test the heel-third, middle-third, toe-third, and toe for sharpness. Note that it is possible for one section of the cutting edge to be sharp while other sections are dull.

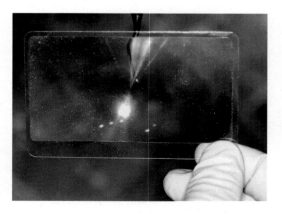

Figure 24-57. Step 3: Examine Under Magnification.
- Use a magnifying lens or loupes to examine the working-end.
- Evaluate the working-end to assure that its original design has been preserved.
- Inspect the cutting edges for wire edges.

Section 5
Sharpening a Periodontal File

The working-end of a periodontal file is difficult to sharpen due to the multiple cutting edges. For this reason, many clinicians send files to professional instrument sharpening services to be sharpened. To sharpen a file, the clinician will need to use a metal file known as a tanged file.

- Use your nondominant hand to stabilize the file on a countertop. Grasp the tanged file with your dominant hand.
- Lay the tanged file in a horizontal position against the first cutting edge. Move the file back and forth across the cutting edge (Fig. 24-58).
- Repeat the same procedure for each of the cutting edges. Use a sharpening test stick to evaluate the sharpness of the cutting edges.

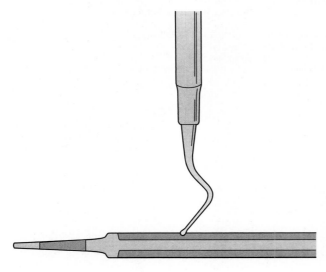

Figure 24-58. Sharpening a Periodontal File. A tanged file is used to sharpen the cutting edges of a periodontal file. Since files are difficult to sharpen, many clinicians rely on a professional sharpening service to sharpen these instruments.

References

1. Acevedo R, Sampaio J, Shibli J. Scanning electron microscope assessment of several resharpening techniques on the cutting edges of Gracey curettes. *J Contemp Dent Pract.* 2007;8(7):70–77.

2. Andrade Acevedo RA, Cardozo AK, Sampaio JE. Scanning electron microscopic and profilometric study of different sharpening stones. *Braz Dent J.* 2006;17(3):237–242.

3. Daniel SJ, Harfst SA. *Mosby's Dental Hygiene: Concepts, Cases, and Competencies.* St. Louis, MO: Mosby; 2004:xxvii, 858 pp.

4. Darby ML. *Mosby's Comprehensive Review of Dental Hygiene.* 6th ed. St. Louis, MO: Mosby; 2010:xi, 864 pp.

5. Darby ML, Walsh MM. *Dental Hygiene : Theory and Practice.* 3rd ed. St. Louis, MO: Saunders/Elsevier; 2010:xviii, 1276 pp.

6. Hodges K. On the cutting edge. *Dimen Den Hyg.* 2004;2(4):16,8,20.

7. Huang CC, Tseng CC. Effect of different sharpening stones on periodontal curettes evaluated by scanning electron microscopy. *J Formos Med Assoc.* 1991;90(8):782–787.

8. Di Fiore A, Mazzoleni S, Fantin F, Favero L, De Francesco M, Stellini E. Evaluation of three different manual techniques of sharpening curettes through a scanning electron microscope: A randomized controlled experimental study. *Int J Dent Hyg.* 2015;13(2):145–150.

9. Moses O, Tal H, Artzi Z, Sperling A, Zohar R, Nemcovsky CE. Scanning electron microscope evaluation of two methods of resharpening periodontal curets: A comparative study. *J Periodontol.* 2003;74(7):1032–1037.

10. Rossi R, Smukler H. A scanning electron microscope study comparing the effectiveness of different types of sharpening stones and curets. *J Periodontol.* 1995;66(11):956–961.

11. Scaramucci MK. Sharpening 101. *Dimen Den Hyg.* 2007;5(5):18–20.

12. Scaramucci MK. Back to basics. Refresh your skills with the review of sharpening fundamentals. *Dimen Den Hyg.* 2011;9(9):40–42.

13. Silva MV, Gomes DA, Leite FR, Sampaio JE, de Toledo BE, Mendes AJ. Sharpening of periodontal instruments with different sharpening stones and its influence upon root debridement–scanning electronic microscopy assessment. *J Int Acad Periodontol.* 2006;8(1):17–22.

14. Wilkins EM. *Clinical practice of the Dental Hygienist.* 9th ed. Philadelphia, PA: Lippincott Williams & Wilkins; 2009.

15. Balevi B. Engineering specifics of the periodontal curet's cutting edge. *J Periodontol.* 1996;67(4):374–378.

16. Marquam BJ. Strategies to improve instrument sharpening. *Dent Hyg (Chic).* 1988;62(7):334–338.

17. Paquette OE, Levin MP. The sharpening of scaling instruments: II. A preferred technique. *J Periodontol.* 1977;48(3):169–172.

Section 6
Skill Application

Student Self Evaluation Module 24: Instrument Sharpening

Student: _____

Date: _____

Instrument 1 = _____

Instrument 2 = _____

Instrument 3 = _____

Instrument 4 = _____

DIRECTIONS: Evaluate your skill level as: **S** (satisfactory) or **U** (unsatisfactory).

CRITERIA:	1	2	3	4
Before sharpening assesses the design characteristics of the working-end to be sharpened and describes these characteristics				
Selects an appropriate location for sharpening process (stable surface, good light source), prepares area for sharpening, and assembles armamentarium; maintains sterile technique				
Lubricates the sharpening stone				
Holds the instrument handle in a stable grasp				
Identifies the cutting edge to be sharpened				
Establishes a face-to-stone angulation between 70 to 80 degrees				
Sharpens the cutting edge in sections: heel-, middle-, and toe-thirds				
Evaluates sharpness of entire length of cutting edge and if necessary, sharpens any remaining dull sections of the cutting edge				
Uses magnification to evaluate the sharpened working-end and indicates if the design has been preserved successfully				

Pain Control During Periodontal Instrumentation

Module Overview

This module discusses aspects of pain control during periodontal instrumentation including: (1) pain control within the scope of dental hygiene care, (2) strategies that can be employed by hygienists to allay patient fear, and (3) pain control modalities that can be useful for routine periodontal instrumentation.

Module Outline

Section 1 | **Pain Control During Dental Hygiene Care** | **642**

Introduction to Pain Control During Periodontal Instrumentation
Pain Control Within the Scope of Dental Hygiene Care

Section 2 | **Strategies to Allay the Fear of Pain During Periodontal Instrumentation** | **644**

Dealing With Fear of Pain in Dental Hygiene Patients
Use of Nitrous Oxide and Oxygen Inhalation Sedation During
    Periodontal Instrumentation
Distraction Technique to Reduce Anxiety During Periodontal
    Instrumentation
Relaxation Technique to Reduce Anxiety During Periodontal
    Instrumentation

Section 3 | **Using Local Anesthesia for Pain Control During Periodontal Instrumentation** | **647**

Local Anesthetics Administered Through Injection
Guidelines for Selection of Local Anesthetic Agents for Periodontal
    Instrumentation
Types of Injections of Local Anesthetic Agents
Topical Application of Local Anesthetics
Intrapocket Local Anesthesia
Transmucosal Anesthesia Patches
Reversal of Local Anesthetic Effects
Failure of Local Anesthetic Agents
Technologies Designed to Reduce Pain from Dental Injections

Key Terms

Topical anesthesia
Infiltration injection
Regional nerve block
 injection
Nitrous oxide/oxygen
 inhalation sedation

Distraction technique
Relaxation technique
Vasodilation
Vasoconstrictors
Potency of the anesthetic
 agent

Protein binding
Intrapocket local anesthesia
Transmucosal anesthesia
 patches
Computer-controlled
 anesthetic delivery

Learning Objectives

- Explain the terms topical anesthesia, infiltration injections, and regional nerve block injections.

- Explain the need for pain control during periodontal instrumentation.

- Explain the relationship between anxiety and perception of pain.

- List strategies that can be useful to the dental hygienist to allay fear of pain.

- List local anesthetic agents that are commonly used to control pain during periodontal instrumentation.

- Explain the factors to consider when selecting local anesthetic agents for use during periodontal instrumentation.

- Explain the term intrapocket local anesthesia.

- List some reasons for failure of local anesthetic agents.

- List some technologies designed to reduce pain from dental injections.

Section 1
Pain Control During Dental Hygiene Care

INTRODUCTION TO PAIN CONTROL DURING PERIODONTAL INSTRUMENTATION

1. It is common for patients to be fearful of experiencing pain while undergoing dental procedures including those procedures performed by a dental hygienist.
   A. Fear of pain has often been cited as one of the primary reasons patients fail to comply with recommendations for dental care of all types.
   B. It is critical that members of the dental team employ strategies both to help patients deal with fear of pain and to understand methods of controlling pain during therapeutic procedures.

2. Most patients with chronic periodontitis will require thorough periodontal instrumentation as part of nonsurgical therapy.
   A. For many patients periodontal instrumentation may indeed cause pain without proper patient management.
   B. Pain can arise during periodontal instrumentation from both the use of hand instruments and the use of ultrasonic powered instruments.
   C. The most reliable means of providing painless periodontal instrumentation is the careful injection of local anesthetic agents.
   D. Complicating care for many patients is the fact that the mere thought of an injection of local anesthetic can also cause fear in patients (i.e., fear of pain from the "shot").

3. For many patients pain control with injections of local anesthetic agents is an important aspect of periodontal instrumentation whether the dental hygienist or the dentist performs the injections.
   A. Local anesthesia agents can provide pain control when the drug is deposited close to a nerve by injecting an anesthetic drug or placing the drug topically on the mucosa or gingiva or in a periodontal pocket.
   B. Local anesthetic agents cause a temporary loss of feeling in an area—the patient remains fully awake but has no feeling at the site.
   C. Local anesthetic agents are the most common drugs used in dentistry, and for the large majority of patients, these agents have been demonstrated to be safe and effective when used correctly.
   D. It should be noted that pain intensity experienced during periodontal instrumentation is dramatically different among patients and that pain intensity can vary between different areas of the mouth in the same patient.

PAIN CONTROL WITHIN THE SCOPE OF DENTAL HYGIENE CARE

1. The scope of dental hygiene practice related to the administration of local anesthetics during periodontal debridement can be confusing since it varies from region to region. Regulations and statutes in different states in the United States or different provinces in Canada determine if dental hygienists are licensed to administer local anesthesia.
   A. Regulations pertaining to the administration of local anesthesia by dental hygienists often are described based upon the intended mode of administration for the local anesthetic agent—that is, the administration of topical applications of anesthetic agents, administration of infiltration injections of anesthetic agents, or administration of regional nerve block injections of anesthetic agents.
   B. These three modes of administration will be discussed later in this chapter in the context of pain control during periodontal instrumentation, but a short orientation to these methods is outlined below.
      1. Topical anesthesia refers to the technique of applying an anesthetic agent to the surface of either the gingiva or mucosa—allowing the anesthetic agent to diffuse through the surface epithelium and block pain impulses from superficial tissues.
      2. Infiltration injection refers to the technique of injecting a local anesthetic agent into the tissues *near the site where anesthesia is needed*—allowing the anesthetic agent to diffuse through tissues near the site of the injection and block pain impulses from the tissues near the site of injection.
      3. Regional nerve block injection refers to the technique of injecting local anesthetic agents *near the site of a particular nerve branch*—allowing the anesthetic agent to reach the nerve branch itself and block pain impulses from the entire nerve branch (thus anesthetizing an entire region of the mouth).
   C. Related to the administration of local anesthesia by injection, regulations governing the practice of dental hygiene usually fall into one of three broad categories:
      1. Some jurisdictions do not allow dental hygienists to administer local anesthetic agent by injection.
      2. Some jurisdictions allow dental hygienists to administer local anesthetic agents by injection but only using infiltration injections.
      3. Some jurisdictions allow dental hygienists to administer local anesthetic agents by injection using both infiltration injections and regional nerve block injections.
2. Because of the variation in statutes and regulations governing the administration of local anesthesia by hygienists, each dental hygienist must become familiar with the rules of the jurisdiction governing the practice of dental hygiene in the individual state or province in which she or he is licensed.

Section 2
Strategies to Allay the Fear of Pain During Periodontal Instrumentation

A few patients with extreme fear of all dental procedures will require special management with antianxiety or sedative-hypnotic drugs; though these agents will not be discussed in this book, the administration of these drugs can include inhalation, oral, intramuscular, and intravenous routes.

DEALING WITH FEAR OF PAIN IN DENTAL HYGIENE PATIENTS

1. Patient anxiety can have an impact on the perception of pain (i.e., in general the higher the level of anxiety, the greater the pain sensitivity experienced by the patient), so minimizing patient anxiety is an important first step in pain control.
   A. Many patients come to a dental appointment with some level of anxiety, whether they show overt signs of anxiety or not.
   B. Patients should be reassured that a certain level of anxiety in a dental setting is normal; helping a patient to realize that anxiety is to be expected may make the patient better able to deal with it.
2. A clinician's chairside manner is one key element in keeping the patient calm during any dental procedure. All patients should be approached with a calm and confident manner.
   A. Patients should be informed about what to expect during a dental appointment to avoid unpleasant surprises during the treatment.
   B. It is frequently helpful to give a patient some sense of control over the dental procedure. For example, instructing the patient how to signal the clinician if he or she experiences discomfort can also be helpful in reducing anxiety. An example of a signal that can be used is having the patient raise a hand if uncomfortable. Allowing the patient to hold the suction device during ultrasonic instrumentation is another example of giving the patient some control over a procedure. The water flow from the ultrasonic tip creates anxiety in some patients.
3. There are numerous other strategies that can allay some patient anxiety and minimize the risk of unnecessary discomfort during periodontal instrumentation; examples of these strategies are listed below and in Box 25-1.
   A. Evaluate the patient's emotional status prior to periodontal instrumentation to identify patients that might need special management.
   B. Use precise and gentle tissue manipulation during periodontal instrumentation to increase patient confidence in your clinical skills.
   C. Monitor the patient for signs of pain or fear (such as facial expressions, pallor, or perspiration) throughout periodontal instrumentation.
   D. Select properly sharpened hand instruments for use during periodontal instrumentation, since dull instruments can inflict unnecessary tissue trauma and can lead to the use of excessive force.
   E. Implement strategies to prevent pain prior to periodontal debridement rather than attempting to deal with patient discomfort after it has already begun.

> **Box 25-1**   ## Strategies to Allay Patient Anxiety or Reduce the Risk of Unnecessary Discomfort During Periodontal Instrumentation
>
> - Evaluate the patient's emotional status.
> - Use precise and gentle tissue manipulation.
> - Monitor the patient for signs of pain or fear.
> - Select properly sharpened periodontal instruments.
> - Implement strategies to prevent pain prior to periodontal instrumentation.

USE OF NITROUS OXIDE AND OXYGEN INHALATION SEDATION DURING PERIODONTAL INSTRUMENTATION

1. **Nitrous oxide/oxygen inhalation sedation** is a technique that uses a blend of two gases—nitrous oxide and oxygen (N_2O-O_2)—to relieve patient anxiety during many clinical dental procedures including periodontal instrumentation. Regulations differ from state to state pertaining to whether the dental hygienist may administer nitrous oxide/oxygen sedation.
   A. A fitted mask is placed over the patient's nose and, as the patient breathes normally, uptake of the gases occurs through the lungs.
   B. At the end of treatment, the gas is eliminated from the lungs after a relatively short period of breathing oxygen and has no lingering effects.
2. Nitrous oxide and oxygen inhalation sedation is one technique that has been used successfully during periodontal instrumentation to allay fear.
   A. Nitrous oxide and oxygen inhalation sedation can produce a state in which a patient is conscious and perfectly able to obey commands, but feels a sense of well-being and remains relaxed.
   B. Nitrous oxide and oxygen inhalation sedation is safe and effective when used appropriately in dealing with patients with mild to moderate anxiety.
3. The use of nitrous oxide and oxygen to allay fear provides several advantages to both the clinician and the patient. These advantages include: quick onset of action, easy regulation of the concentration of the gases delivered, and rapid recovery following administration.
   A. These advantages make this modality ideal for sedating many patients during relatively short procedures such as periodontal instrumentation.
   B. It should be pointed out that though the use of nitrous oxide and oxygen is very effective in allaying mild to moderate patient anxiety, the use of this modality does not control the pain from procedures. Additional pain control measures such as the use of local anesthesia are also necessary.

DISTRACTION TECHNIQUE TO REDUCE ANXIETY DURING PERIODONTAL INSTRUMENTATION

1. One technique that has been used to reduce anxiety and discomfort during periodontal instrumentation is using a distraction technique (i.e., to actively engage a patient's mind at something other than the dental treatment).
2. Since fear or anxiety can lower a patient's threshold for a pain reaction to a stimulus, distraction techniques can alter how a patient's brain interprets a particular stimulus.
3. Examples of how these distraction techniques can be used in a dental setting include allowing the patient to watch a patient-selected television program or listen to patient-selected music using a headset. Both of these types of activities have been demonstrated to be able to take the patient's mind off an actual dental procedure.
4. Though these distraction techniques can be useful in managing selected patients, for some patients they do not appear to be reliable methods of controlling either anxiety or pain during periodontal instrumentation.

RELAXATION TECHNIQUE TO REDUCE ANXIETY DURING PERIODONTAL INSTRUMENTATION

1. Relaxation technique is also a method that can be used to reduce tension and anxiety during a dental procedure.
2. There are several relaxation strategies that have been recommended to elicit a relaxation response in dental patients. Relaxation techniques that have been used include: deep breathing, guided imagery, progressive relaxation, and biofeedback.
3. Used in carefully selected patients, relaxation techniques can indeed decrease heart rate, respiratory rate, and muscle tension.
4. Though relaxation techniques can produce a sense of calmness, in most patients they do not appear to be adequate for the control of the discomfort produced during periodontal instrumentation.

Section 3
Using Local Anesthesia for Pain Control During Periodontal Instrumentation

Using local anesthesia for pain control is a comprehensive topic that cannot be covered in detail in this textbook chapter. However, the information in this section will provide the reader with a handy outline of the topic that can easily be supplemented with any of the outstanding textbooks that are currently available related to this topic.

LOCAL ANESTHETICS ADMINISTERED THROUGH INJECTION

The most effective method for controlling pain during periodontal instrumentation is the administration of a local anesthetic agent by injection. Local anesthesia is any technique—that can be given by injection, spray, or ointment—to induce a temporary loss of sensation in a specific part of the body. In the simplest of terms, local anesthetic agents control pain by blocking pain impulses from reaching the brain.

1. Local anesthetic agents are some of the most important drugs used in all of dentistry; these agents have a long history of safe and effective use in the control of pain that arises during all types of periodontal procedures.
2. Historically, local anesthetic agents have been classified into types of agents that have been described as either esters or amides.
   A. Currently local anesthetic agents available in dental anesthetic cartridges are all of the amide type.
   B. The amide-type local anesthetic agents are believed to produce a lower incidence of allergic reactions in patients.
3. There are a number of local anesthetic agents available for use during periodontal instrumentation. Examples of commonly used local anesthetics agents that can be used for periodontal instrumentation include lidocaine, mepivacaine, prilocaine, articaine, and bupivacaine.
4. Injectable local anesthetic agents used in dentistry produce varying degrees of vasodilation (i.e., dilation of blood vessels) at the site of injection.
   A. This property of vasodilation increases the blood flow at the injection site and facilitates the local anesthetic agent being carried away relatively quickly by the resultant increased blood flow.
   B. This vasodilation effect of local anesthetic agents can *decrease* their duration of action, decrease their effectiveness, increase the blood level of the agent, and increase the amount of bleeding at the site of the injection.
   C. To counteract the natural vasodilation effects of local anesthetic agents, other drugs called vasoconstrictors are often added to injectable local anesthetic agents.
      1. Vasoconstrictors in low concentrations cause the local blood vessels to constrict or narrow down.
      2. By restricting the amount of blood and plasma entering and leaving the site of an injection, vasoconstrictors have the net effect of slowing the vascular absorption of the anesthetic solution. This keeps the anesthetic solution in place longer and prolongs the action of the drug.
   D. In addition to increasing the duration of action of the anesthetic agent, vasoconstrictors can increase the effectiveness of the agent, decrease bleeding at the site, and lower the blood level of the agent. Table 25-1 outlines some common

vasoconstrictors used in local anesthetic agents intended for use during dental procedures such as periodontal instrumentation.

E. Thorough periodontal instrumentation requires manipulation of periodontal tissues and can of course result in hemorrhage (or bleeding) during the procedure. Local anesthetic agents with vasoconstrictors can improve visibility of the site for the clinician by helping to control hemorrhage during the procedure.

5. To increase the safety for the patient, lower doses of vasoconstrictor are normally preferred. Lower doses produce fewer side effects, and using a higher dose of vasoconstrictor does not prolong the duration of action over the lower doses.

6. It should be noted that vasoconstrictors are contraindicated in some patients either because of the patient's health status or because of possible interactions with other medications that the patient is taking. Discussion of these contraindications is beyond the scope of this chapter, but these discussions can be found in any of the excellent textbooks related entirely to pain control.

TABLE 25-1. VASOCONSTRICTORS COMMONLY USED IN DENTAL LOCAL ANESTHETIC AGENTS

Agent	Other Name	Concentrations Available in Dentistry		
Epinephrine	Adrenalin	1:50,000	1:100,000	1:200,000
Levonordephrin	Nordephrin	1:20,000		

GUIDELINES FOR SELECTION OF LOCAL ANESTHETIC AGENTS FOR PERIODONTAL INSTRUMENTATION

1. The selection of a specific injectable local anesthetic agent should be based upon the type of procedure to be performed combined with several other critical factors. Examples of other critical factors for the dental hygienist or dentist to consider when selecting an injectable local anesthetic agent are discussed below and listed in Box 25-2.

A. **Potency of the anesthetic agent** is always an important factor in selection.
   1. Potency of the local anesthetic refers to the lowest concentration of drug that can actually block conduction of the pain impulse.
   2. Potency can be affected by lipid solubility of the drug, its inherent vasodilator effect, and its tissue diffusion properties.

B. **Time of onset** is also a factor to consider in selection.
   1. Time of onset refers to how rapidly the anesthetic effects actually occur.
   2. Time of onset is also affected by lipid solubility of the drug, but other factors affect this property also.

C. **Duration of action** of the agent and the length of time that pain control is needed are other critical factors in selection.
   1. Duration of action is primarily determined by the protein-binding capacity of the anesthetic (the greater the binding the longer the duration).
      a. Protein binding refers to the binding of a drug to proteins in blood plasma. The interaction can also be between the drug and tissue membranes, red blood cells, and other components of the blood.

      b. The amount of drug bound to protein determines how effective the drug is in the body.

         1. The bound drug is kept in the blood stream while the unbound components of the drug may be metabolized or extracted, making them the active part of the drug.

         2. So, if an anesthetic agent is 90% bound to a binding protein and 10% is free, it means that 10% of the drug is active in the system and causing pharmacologic effect (pain control).

    2. Duration of action can also be affected by an agent's inherent vasodilator effect and its tissue diffusion properties.

    3. As already discussed, the duration of action of local anesthetic agents can be increased by combining the anesthetic agent with a vasoconstrictor.

D. The need for pain control following the office procedure is another factor to consider in selection of local anesthetic agent.

    1. When continuing oral pain is expected as a result of a treatment procedure—as it might be following some types of periodontal surgery—it is wise to consider this fact when selecting an anesthetic agent.

    2. Though lingering oral pain from periodontal instrumentation would not normally be expected, in some patients with a history of low tolerance for pain this may be an important factor to consider.

E. Another factor to consider in selection is the health status of the patient, including a history of allergies and current medications being taken by the patient.

Box 25-2   **Examples of Factors to Consider When Selecting a Local Anesthetic Agent**

- Type of procedure to be performed.
- Potency of the anesthetic agent.
- Time of onset of the anesthetic effects.
- Duration of action of the anesthetic agent.
- Need for pain control following the office procedure.
- Health status of the patient including allergies and current medications.

---

2. Table 25-2 provides an overview of common injectable dental local anesthetic agents along with the expected duration of action of each agent.

A. Lidocaine and mepivacaine with vasoconstrictors are excellent choices of anesthetic agents for periodontal instrumentation since their protein binding is intermediate and their lipid solubility is also intermediate resulting in an expected duration of action of a few hours.

B. Bupivacaine would be a less ideal choice for routine periodontal instrumentation since the lipid solubility is high and its protein binding is high resulting in an expected duration of action of anesthesia for 4 to 9 hours. Such a long duration of action might be ideal for some periodontal surgical procedures but is excessive for most periodontal instrumentation procedures.

C. An injectable amide local anesthetic agent, articaine, has been used successfully for periodontal procedures; one advantage to articaine that has been reported is that it can be metabolized quickly thus reducing toxicity associated with repeated injections.

TABLE 25-2. COMMON INJECTABLE LOCAL ANESTHETIC AGENTS WITH THEIR DURATION OF ACTION

Duration	Agent	Duration of Soft Tissue Anesthesia
Short	Lidocaine 2%	1–2 hours
	Mepivacaine 3%	2–3 hours
Intermediate	Lidocaine 2%/1:100,000 epinephrine	3–5 hours
	Mepivacaine 2%/1:20,000 levonordephrin	3–5 hours
	Articaine 4%/1:100,000 epinephrine	3–4 hours
	Prilocaine 4%/1:200,000 epinephrine	3–8 hours
Long	Bupivacaine 0.5%/1:200,000 epinephrine	4–9 hours

TYPES OF INJECTIONS OF LOCAL ANESTHETIC AGENTS

The administration of local anesthetic agents through injection in dentistry is usually described as being either regional nerve block local anesthesia or infiltration local anesthesia.

1. Regional Nerve Block Anesthesia
   A. As discussed in Section 1 of this chapter, regional nerve block local anesthesia refers to injections of local anesthetic agent into sites near nerve branches, allowing the local anesthetic agent to stop the transmission of pain impulses from the entire area of the oral cavity innervated by the nerve branch.
   B. Using regional block local anesthesia for dental procedures can frequently result in fewer penetrations of the oral mucosa with the needle and use of smaller volumes of anesthesia compared with using strictly infiltration anesthesia.
   C. Properly administered regional block local anesthesia can result in profound anesthesia for completely pain-free periodontal instrumentation.
   D. Regional block anesthesia fits in with the standard dental hygiene protocol of performing quadrant or half-mouth procedures during periodontal instrumentation.
   E. Only regional block anesthesia can produce profound anesthesia in mandibular posterior teeth in most patients since the thickness of the cortical plate in the mandible frequently precludes the diffusion of infiltration anesthesia through the thick cortical bone.
   F. Figures 25-1, 25-2 and Table 25-3 provide an overview of nerve branches and the types of injections that might be used to produce anesthesia. Note that for most nerve branches supplying the jaws, nerve block anesthesia is the method of choice.
   G. Specific techniques for administering nerve block anesthesia will not be discussed in this textbook, but there are many excellent textbooks available on this extensive topic.
2. Infiltration Anesthesia
   A. Also as discussed in Section 1 of this chapter, infiltration local anesthesia refers to injections of local anesthetic agent in or near the site to be treated—allowing the local anesthetic agent to diffuse through the tissues and stop the transmission of pain impulses from the site.
   B. Using infiltration local anesthesia would affect nerve impulses from the site while not affecting other areas innervated by a particular nerve branch.
   C. Though there are distinct advantages to regional block anesthesia for most sites in the oral cavity, note that in Table 25-3 there are some sites where infiltration anesthesia is the method of choice.
   D. Specific techniques for administering infiltration anesthesia will not be discussed in this textbook, but there are many excellent textbooks available on this extensive topic.

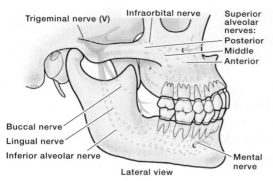

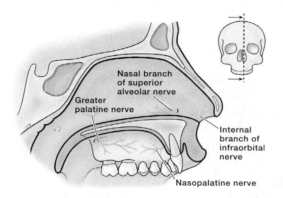

Figure 25-1. Nerve Supply to the Periodontium (Lateral View). The nerve supply to the periodontium is derived from the branches of the trigeminal nerve.

Figure 25-2. Nerve Innervation to the Palate.

TABLE 25-3. PRODUCING ANESTHESIA FOR PERIODONTAL INSTRUMENTATION USING INJECTION LOCAL ANESTHETICS

Nerve Branch	Ideal Type of Local Anesthesia	Structures Affected
Greater palatine	Block anesthesia	Posterior palatal mucosa
Posterior superior alveolar	Block anesthesia	Maxillary posterior teeth Maxillary buccal mucosa
Infraorbital	Block anesthesia	Maxillary anterior mucosa
Anterior superior alveolar	Infiltration anesthesia	Maxillary anterior teeth
Nasopalatine	Block anesthesia	Anterior palatal mucosa
Inferior alveolar	Block anesthesia	Mandibular molars and mandibular premolars
Mental	Block anesthesia	Mandibular buccal mucosa
Incisive	Block anesthesia	Mandibular canine Mandibular incisors
Lingual	Block anesthesia	Mandibular lingual mucosa
Buccal	Infiltration anesthesia	Mandibular buccal mucosa

TOPICAL APPLICATION OF LOCAL ANESTHETICS

1. Topical anesthesia is a condition of temporary numbness caused by applying an anesthetic agent directly to the mucosal and gingival tissues. This technique has been used in dentistry for many years.
2. Application of topical anesthetic agents prior to injection can promote patient comfort during the initial penetration of a needle through the mucosa.
3. There are several topical local anesthetics available for use, and one example is lidocaine in liquid or gel form that can be applied prior to injection of local anesthetic agents. Use of these topical agents prior to injection can minimize patient discomfort during the injection.
4. It should be noted that using topical anesthetic agent applied to surface mucosa or gingiva does not normally result in the profound anesthesia of a site needed when performing periodontal instrumentation.

INTRAPOCKET LOCAL ANESTHESIA

1. Patient anxiety associated with injections of local anesthetic agent is an important concern, and there has long been a need for an effective substitute for injections to produce local anesthesia during periodontal instrumentation.
2. One alternative to injections of local anesthetic agents during periodontal instrumentation is the use of intrapocket local anesthesia. Intrapocket local anesthesia refers to placing a local anesthetic agent into a periodontal pocket where it is allowed to diffuse through adjacent tissues.
   A. An example of intrapocket anesthetic application that has been used is a mixture of lidocaine and prilocaine in a thermosetting gel.
   B. This technique involves placement of the gel into a periodontal pocket and can be useful in pain control during periodontal instrumentation in some adults; the most profound anesthesia following the application of this product occurs between 5 and 20 minutes.
   C. Though intrapocket anesthetic application of lidocaine/prilocaine gel produces less profound anesthesia than injections of local anesthetic agents, these gel applications have reduced the need for anesthetic injections during periodontal instrumentation in selected patients.
   D. For some patients where periodontal instrumentation can be expected to produce moderate to severe pain, these gel applications may not be adequate to control discomfort during these procedures.
3. There have also been attempts to use the anesthetic agent benzocaine as an intrapocket anesthetic agent.
   A. Benzocaine, however, is less effective in controlling pain during periodontal instrumentation than injections of lidocaine.
   B. More investigation is needed in the use of benzocaine as an intrapocket anesthetic agent during periodontal instrumentation.

TRANSMUCOSAL ANESTHESIA PATCHES

1. Another approach to avoiding injections is by using topical anesthesia delivered by patches placed directly to mucosal tissues; these patches are referred to as transmucosal anesthesia patches.

2. In attempts to use transmucosal patches, lidocaine-containing patches have been applied directly to the tissues at the site intended for treatment.

3. Though more research is needed related to the use of these transmucosal patches during periodontal instrumentation, it does appear that this mode of administration of lidocaine may be useful in selected sites in some patients undergoing periodontal instrumentation.

REVERSAL OF LOCAL ANESTHETIC EFFECTS

1. Prolonged soft tissue anesthesia resulting from the use of intraoral local anesthetic agents can result in problems for some patients in the form of self-inflicted injuries and disturbance of oral function.

2. This lingering "numbness" that can result for several hours is an annoying result of dental treatment for many patients.

3. The FDA has approved a drug (*phentolamine mesylate*) for the reversal of soft tissue anesthesia at the end of a dental procedure. Phentolamine mesylate can induce a rapid return of sensation blocked by the local anesthetic by increasing vasodilation in the site and clearing the anesthetic agent from the site of the injection.

4. Of course, the use of phentolamine mesylate to reverse local anesthetic numbness would require additional injections at the end of a clinical dental procedure.

5. Though more study of the use of this drug is needed in the context of dental hygiene procedures as well as other dental procedures, this medication may prove useful in the practice of dentistry at least in selected patients.

FAILURE OF LOCAL ANESTHETIC AGENTS

1. Though administration of local anesthetic agents by injection can be a safe and a very effective mechanism for controlling pain during dental procedures, including periodontal instrumentation, all clinicians should recognize the fact that a few patients present special challenges by failing to develop profound anesthesia in the site intended.

2. The most common site for failure to develop profound anesthesia following injection of an anesthetic agent using recommended techniques is in the region supplied by the *inferior alveolar nerve.*

3. There are a variety of reasons for this apparent failure of the anesthetic agent. Examples include inaccuracy of deposition of the agent at the intended site, variations in anatomy from patient to patient, variation among individuals in response to drugs, and status of the tissues at the site of deposition of the agent.

4. Additional injection techniques have been recommended for use in patients where the normally recommended injection techniques fail to produce profound anesthesia.

5. Though a detailed discussion of these additional techniques is beyond the scope of this book, examples of these methods include techniques such as intraosseous injections, periodontal ligament injections, and intraseptal anesthesia.

TECHNOLOGIES DESIGNED TO REDUCE PAIN FROM DENTAL INJECTIONS

1. Devices that Produce Vibrations
   A. Devices that can produce vibrations in sites to be injected have been developed in ongoing efforts to reduce pain from dental injections.
   B. The use of these devices is based upon the gate control theory of pain management. The gate theory of pain management suggests that pain, such as that produced by injections, can be reduced by the stimulation of nerve fibers through the use of touch or vibration.
   C. At this point research into the efficacy of these devices has resulted in mixed results, and more investigation is needed in this area.
2. Computer-Controlled Local Anesthetic Delivery Systems
   A. Computer-controlled local anesthetic delivery (C-CLAD) systems incorporate computer technology to control the rate of flow of the anesthetic through the needle.
   B. Though most dental anesthetic injections utilize a traditional aspirating syringe, the C-CLAD technology utilizes a lightweight handpiece that allows a clinician to use a grasp that can provide improved tactile sensation and control during the injection.
   C. The improved control of the syringe and the fixed flow rates through syringe have been shown to provide an improved injection experience for the patient for some of these devices.
3. Jet Injectors
   A. Jet injection technology utilizes pressure to create a thin column of anesthetic fluid with enough force to penetrate soft tissue without the need for a needle.
   B. Jet injection devices are thought to provide faster anesthetic absorption with minimal tissue damage and little or no pain.
   C. Though this idea of jet injection seems intriguing, the efficacy of this type of device has been limited in studies; additional research is needed in this area.
4. Buffering Local Anesthetics
   A. Most dental local anesthetics are supplied in sterile carpules and many come with varying concentrations of vasoconstrictors as already discussed in this chapter. Local anesthetics that contain vasoconstrictors in the carpules can have a pH that approaches 3.5 (acidic in chemical nature).
   B. It should be noted that the pH of normal oral tissues is approximately 7.4 and when an acidic chemical is injected into the oral tissues, there is a natural buffering action by the body that raises the pH to the normal body pH. However, because the initial injection material is more acidic than normal tissues, the injection can result in a temporary "burning" sensation.
   C. Buffering refers to processing dental anesthetics in dental anesthesia cartridges to make them more alkaline (or basic in chemical nature) prior to the injection.
   D. The effect of buffering is reported to hasten the onset of anesthesia as well as to reduce the pain from the injection.
   E. Recent technical advances have lead to the marketing of a system for buffering lidocaine 2% epinephrine 1:100,000.
   F. At this point, more clinical trials of this technique are needed, but this novel approach may one day prove useful in some clinical settings.

Suggested Readings

Al-Melh MA, Andersson L. Comparison of topical anesthetics (EMLA/Oraqix vs. benzocaine) on pain experienced during palatal needle injection. *Oral Surg Oral Med Oral Pathol Oral Radiol Endod.* 2007;103(5):e16–e20.

Anderson JM. Use of local anesthesia by dental hygienists who completed a Minnesota CE course. *J Dent Hyg.* 2002;76(1): 35–46.

Antoniazzi RP, Cargnelutti B, Freitas DN, Guimarães MB, Zanatta FB, Feldens CA. Topical intrapocket anesthesia during scaling and root planing: a randomized clinical trial. *Braz Dent J.* 2015;26(1):26–32.

Becker DE, Reed KL. Local anesthetics: review of pharmacological considerations. *Anesth Prog.* 2012;59(2):90–101; quiz 102–103.

Bhalla J, Meechan JG, Lawrence HP, Grad HA, Haas DA. Effect of time on clinical efficacy of topical anesthesia. *Anesth Prog.* 2009;56(2):36–41.

Blanton PL, Jeske AH; ADA Council on Scientific Affairs; ADA Division of Science. Avoiding complications in local anesthesia induction: anatomical considerations. *J Am Dent Assoc.* 2003;134(7):888–893.

Boynes SG, Riley AE, Milbee S, Bastin MR, Price ME, Ladson A. Evaluating complications of local anesthesia administration and reversal with phentolamine mesylate in a portable pediatric dental clinic. *Gen Dent.* 2013;61(5):70–76.

Burns CA, Ferris G, Feng C, Cooper JZ, Brown MD. Decreasing the pain of local anesthesia: a prospective, double-blind comparison of buffered, premixed 1% lidocaine with epinephrine versus 1% lidocaine freshly mixed with epinephrine. *J Am Acad Dermatol.* 2006;54(1):128–131.

Canakçi CF, Canakçi V. Pain experienced by patients undergoing different periodontal therapies. *J Am Dent Assoc.* 2007;138(12): 1563–1573.

Chung JE, Koh SA, Kim TI, et al. Effect of eutectic mixture of local anesthetics on pain perception during scaling by ultrasonic or hand instruments: a masked randomized controlled trial. *J Periodontol.* 2011;82(2):259–266.

Derman SH, Lowden CE, Hellmich M, Noack MJ. Influence of intra-pocket anesthesia gel on treatment outcome in periodontal patients: a randomized controlled trial. *J Clin Periodontol.* 2014;41(5):481–488.

Derman SH, Lowden CE, Kaus P, Noack MJ. Pocket-depths-related effectiveness of an intrapocket anaesthesia gel in periodontal maintenance patients. *Int J Dent Hyg.* 2014;12(2):141–144.

DiMatteo A. Efficacy of an intrapocket anesthetic for scaling and root planing procedures: a review of three multicenter studies. *Compend Contin Educ Dent.* 2005;26(2 suppl 1):6–10.

Donaldson D, Gelskey SC, Landry RG, Matthews DC, Sandhu HS. A placebo-controlled multi-centred evaluation of an anaesthetic gel (Oraqix) for periodontal therapy. *J Clin Periodontol.* 2003;30(3):171–175.

Gunsolley JC. The need for pain control during scaling and root planing. *Compend Contin Educ Dent.* 2005;26(2 suppl 1):3–5.

Haas DA. An update on local anesthetics in dentistry. *J Can Dent Assoc.* 2002;68(9):546–551.

Hersh EV, Lindemeyer RG. Phentolamine mesylate for accelerating recovery from lip and tongue anesthesia. *Dent Clin North Am.* 2010;54(4):631–642.

Hersh EV, Moore PA, Papas AS, et al.; Soft Tissue Anesthesia Recovery Group. Reversal of soft-tissue local anesthesia with phentolamine mesylate in adolescents and adults. *J Am Dent Assoc.* 2008;139(8):1080–1093.

Jeffcoat MK, Geurs NC, Magnusson I, et al. Intrapocket anesthesia for scaling and root planing: results of a double-blind multicenter trial using lidocaine prilocaine dental gel. *J Periodontol.* 2001;72(7):895–900.

Kakroudi SH, Mehta S, Millar BJ. Articaine hydrochloride: is it the solution? *Dent Update.* 2015;42(1):88–90, 92–93.

Kanaa MD, Whitworth JM, Meechan JG. A comparison of the efficacy of 4% articaine with 1:100,000 epinephrine and 2% lidocaine with 1:80,000 epinephrine in achieving pulpal anesthesia in maxillary teeth with irreversible pulpitis. *J Endod.* 2012;38(3):279–282.

Kumar PS, Leblebicioglu B. Pain control during nonsurgical periodontal therapy. *Compend Contin Educ Dent.* 2007;28(12):666–669; quiz 670–671.

Laviola M, McGavin SK, Freer GA, et al. Randomized study of phentolamine mesylate for reversal of local anesthesia. *J Dent Res.* 2008;87(7):635–639.

Loomer PM, Perry DA. Computer-controlled delivery versus syringe delivery of local anesthetic injections for therapeutic scaling and root planing. *J Am Dent Assoc.* 2004;135(3):358–365.

Magnusson I, Geurs NC, Harris PA, et al. Intrapocket anesthesia for scaling and root planing in pain-sensitive patients. *J Periodontol.* 2003;74(5):597–602.

Malamed SF. Local anesthetics: dentistry's most important drugs, clinical update 2006. *J Calif Dent Assoc.* 2006;34(12):971–976.

Malamed SF, Falkel M. Advances in local anesthetics: pH buffering and dissolved CO_2. *Dent Today.* 2012;31(5):88–93; quiz 94–95.

Malamed SF, Gagnon S, Leblanc D. Efficacy of articaine: a new amide local anesthetic. *J Am Dent Assoc.* 2000;131(5):635–42.

Matthews DC, Rocchi A, Gafni A. Factors affecting patients' and potential patients' choices among anaesthetics for periodontal recall visits. *J Dent.* 2001;29(3):173–179.

Mayor-Subirana G, Yagüe-García J, Valmaseda-Castellón E, Arnabat-Domínguez J, Berini-Aytés L, Gay-Escoda C. Anesthetic efficacy of Oraqix® versus Hurricane® and placebo for pain control during non-surgical periodontal treatment. *Med Oral Patol Oral Cir Bucal.* 2014;19(2):e192–e201.

Nanitsos E, Vartuli R, Forte A, Dennison PJ, Peck CC. The effect of vibration on pain during local anaesthesia injections. *Aust Dent J.* 2009;54(2):94–100.

Nasehi A, Bhardwaj S, Kamath AT, Gadicherla S, Pentapati KC. Clinical pain evaluation with intraoral vibration device during local anesthetic injections. *J Clin Exp Dent.* 2015;7(1):e23–e27.

Perry DA, Gansky SA, Loomer PM. Effectiveness of a transmucosal lidocaine delivery system for local anaesthesia during scaling and root planing. *J Clin Periodontol.* 2005;32(6):590–594.

Reed KL, Malamed SF, Fonner AM. Local anesthesia part 2: technical considerations. *Anesth Prog.* 2012;59(3):127–136; quiz 137.

Said Yekta-Michael S, Stein JM, Marioth-Wirtz E. Evaluation of the anesthetic effect of epinephrine-free articaine and mepivacaine through quantitative sensory testing. *Head Face Med.* 2015;11:2.

Saijo M, Ito E, Ichinohe T, Kaneko Y. Lack of pain reduction by a vibrating local anesthetic attachment: a pilot study. *Anesth Prog.* 2005;52(2):62–64.

Saunders TR, Psaltis G, Weston JF, Yanase RR, Rogy SS, Ghalie RG. In-practice evaluation of OraVerse for the reversal of soft-tissue anesthesia after dental procedures. *Compend Contin Educ Dent.* 2011;32(5):58–62.

Saxena P, Gupta SK, Newaskar V, Chandra A. Advances in dental local anesthesia techniques and devices: an update. *Natl J Maxillofac Surg.* 2013;4(1):19–24.

Scarfone RJ, Jasani M, Gracely EJ. Pain of local anesthetics: rate of administration and buffering. *Ann Emerg Med.* 1998;31(1):36–40.

Singh S, Garg A. Comparison of the pain levels of computer controlled and conventional anesthesia techniques in supraperiosteal injections: a randomized controlled clinical trial. *Acta Odontol Scand.* 2013;71(3–4):740–743.

Singla H, Alexander M. Posterior superior alveolar nerve blocks: a randomised controlled, double blind trial. *J Maxillofac Oral Surg.* 2015;14(2):423–431.

Sisty-LePeau N, Boyer EM, Lutjen D. Dental hygiene licensure specifications on pain control procedures. *J Dent Hyg.* 1990;64(4):179–185.

Su N, Liu Y, Yang X, Shi Z, Huang Y. Efficacy and safety of mepivacaine compared with lidocaine in local anaesthesia in dentistry: a meta-analysis of randomised controlled trials. *Int Dent J.* 2014;64(2):96–107.

Tripp DA, Neish NR, Sullivan MJ. What hurts during dental hygiene treatment. *J Dent Hyg.* 1998;72(4):25–30.

Wiswall AT, Bowles WR, Lunos S, McClanahan SB, Harris S. Palatal anesthesia: comparison of four techniques for decreasing injection discomfort. *Northwest Dent.* 2014;93(4):25–29.

Yagiela JA. Recent developments in local anesthesia and oral sedation. *Compend Contin Educ Dent.* 2004;25(9):697–706; quiz 708.

Yagiela JA. What's new with phentolamine mesylate: a reversal agent for local anaesthesia?*SAAD Dig.* 2011;27:3–7.

Yesilyurt C, Bulut G, Taşdemir T. Pain perception during inferior alveolar injection administered with the Wand or conventional syringe. *Br Dent J.* 2008;205(5):E10; discussion 258–259.

Yogesh Kumar TD, John JB, Asokan S, Geetha Priya PR, Punithavathy R, Praburajan V. Behavioral response and pain perception to computer controlled local anesthetic delivery system and cartridge syringe. *J Indian Soc Pedod Prev Dent.* 2015;33(3): 223–238.

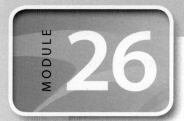

26

Powered Instrument Design and Function

Module Overview

Powered instrumentation devices use the rapid energy vibrations of an electronically powered instrument working-end and fluid irrigation to fracture calculus from the tooth surface and clean the environment of the periodontal pocket. This module presents principles of the design and function of powered instruments and techniques for powered instrumentation.

Module Outline

Section 1 **Introduction to Powered Instrumentation** **660**
Types of Powered Instrumentation Devices
Effectiveness of Powered Ultrasonic Instrumentation
Modes and Mechanisms of Action
Contraindications for Powered Instrumentation
Health Concerns for Powered Instrumentation
Fundamental Skills for Powered Instrumentation
Differing Approaches to Calculus Removal: Hand versus Powered
Instrumentation Stroke with an Ultrasonic Instrument

Section 2 **Powered Working-End Design** **676**
Working-End Selection and Sequence for Instrumentation
Design Characteristics of the Paired Slim Perio Tips
Powered Working-Ends for Use on Dental Implants
Instrument Working-End Wear and Replacement

Section 3 **Adaptation—Orientation of Working-End to Tooth** **682**
Powered Working-Ends Adapt Like a Universal Curet
Orientation of a Powered Working-End to the Tooth Surface

Section 4 **Use of "Universal" Magneto & Piezo Working-Ends** **685**
Use of "Universal" Working-Ends in the Transverse Orientation
Use of "Universal" Working-Ends in the Vertical Orientation

Section 5   **Use of Curved, Paired Magneto Working-Ends**   **687**

Identification of a Curved Working-End as "Right" or "Left"
Efficient Sequence for Use of Paired Magneto Working-Ends in a
    Transverse Orientation on the Posterior Teeth
Use of Paired Magneto Working-Ends in a Transverse Orientation
Efficient Sequence for Use of Paired Magneto Working-Ends in a
    Vertical Orientation on the Posterior Teeth
Use of Paired Magneto Working-Ends in a Vertical Orientation
Use of Paired Magneto Working-Ends in a Vertical Orientation: Cross
    Arch Finger Rest for Lingual Aspects

Section 6   **Use of Curved, Paired Piezo Working-Ends**   **693**

Identification of a Curved Working-End as "Right" or "Left"
Efficient Sequence for Use of Paired Piezo Working-Ends in a
    Transverse Orientation on the Posterior Teeth
Use of Paired Piezo Working-Ends in a Transverse Orientation
Efficient Sequence for Use of Paired Piezo Working-Ends in a Vertical
    Orientation on the Posterior Teeth

Section 7   **Instrumentation Challenges**   **697**

Removing Stubborn Calculus Deposits
Smoothing Defective Margins on Restorations
Instrumenting Furcation Areas of Multi-Rooted Teeth
Skill Building: Accessing Furcation Areas, p. 700

Section 8   **Technique Hints for Powered Instrumentation**   **701**

Patient and Clinician Preparation
Fluid Containment During Instrumentation
Handpiece Cord Management
Ten Secrets for Successful Powered Instrumentation

Section 9   **Set-Up of an Ultrasonic Unit**   **705**

**Skill Building: Steps for Set-Up of a Piezo or Magneto
Ultrasonic Unit, p. 705**

Section 10   **Skill Application**   **708**

Practical Focus: Adaptation of Powered Working-End
Practical Focus: The Lateral Surfaces are "Where the Action Is!"
Fictitious Patient Case: Mr. Burlington
Student Self Evaluation Module 26: Powered Instrumentation

Key Terms

Powered instrumentation
  devices
Sonic powered devices
Ultrasonic powered devices
Piezoelectric ("piezo") devices
Magnetostrictive ("magneto")
  devices

Fluid lavage
Cavitation
Frequency
Amplitude
Cleaning efficiency
Fluid reservoirs
Dental aerosols

Standard working-ends
Slim perio working-ends
Active area of the working-end
Transverse working-end
  orientation
Vertical working-end
  orientation

Learning Objectives

- Discuss the history and technologic advances of powered instrumentation.

- Name the major types of powered instrumentation technology.

- Name the two subtypes of **ultrasonic** powered instrumentation technology.

- Describe the various modes of action of powered instrumentation devices.

- Compare and contrast the advantages and limitations of powered instrumentation.

- Discuss the benefits to the patient when powered instrumentation is integrated into the treatment plan.

- Discuss medical and dental contraindications for powered instrumentation.

- Define the terms "frequency" and "amplitude" and describe how these factors determine the cleaning efficiency of powered instrumentation.

- Compare and contrast the design features of standard and slim perio powered working-ends.

- Discuss criteria for the selection of powered working-ends in relation to the instrumentation task to be performed.

- Demonstrate how to determine powered working-end wear and at what point a working-end should be discarded.

- Define the term "active working-end area" as it pertains to a powered working-end. In a preclinical or clinical setting, demonstrate correct adaptation of the active portion of a powered instrument working-end.

- In a preclinical or clinical setting, demonstrate correct stroke pressure for use with a powered working-end.

- In a preclinical or clinical setting, demonstrate correct working-end adaptation in a (1) transverse orientation and (2) vertical orientation in all sextants of the dentition.

- Given a set of paired, curved working-ends, correctly identify the "right" and "left" working-end.

- On a typodont, demonstrate an efficient sequence for use of curved working-ends in a (2) transverse orientation and (2) vertical orientation on the posterior sextants of the dentition.

- Describe an effective strategy for removing tenacious calculus deposits during powered instrumentation.

- On an extracted tooth, demonstrate the use of a diamond-coated working-end for smoothing a defective margin on a restoration.

- On a typodont, demonstrate how to access and enter a furcation area of a multi-rooted tooth with a ball-tipped powered working-end.

- Identify pre-treatment considerations before the initiation of powered instrumentation.

- Prepare (set-up) a powered instrumentation device for use.

- In a clinical setting, demonstrate correct technique for use of a powered instrumentation device, including: treatment room, clinician and patient preparation; armamentarium selection/set-up and infection control; grasp, finger rest, adjustment of water flow, working-end adaptation and stroke, and fluid control.

- In a clinical setting, select appropriate powered working-ends for a patient case.

- In a clinical setting, use correct technique to effectively remove calculus deposits and plaque biofilm using a powered instrumentation device.

Section 1
Introduction to Powered Instrumentation

Powered instrumentation devices use a rapidly vibrating irrigated working-end to dislodge calculus from the tooth surface, disrupt plaque biofilm and flush out bacteria from the periodontal pocket (Fig. 26-1) (1–3). For example, a powered ultrasonic device may consist of an ultrasonic generator (Fig. 26-2) and a handpiece with interchangeable instrument working-ends or inserts (Fig. 26-3). Initially introduced in the late 1950s, powered instruments were bulky and limited to removing heavy, supragingival calculus deposits (1). Over the years, powered instrument design has evolved to a point that this technology now plays an indispensable role in nonsurgical periodontal instrumentation. Table 26-1 summarizes the evolution of powered instrument design.

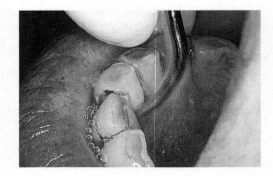

Figure 26-1. Powered Instrument Working-End in Action. This photograph shows an activated powered working-end. A constant stream of water is used to cool the rapidly vibrating working-end. (Courtesy of Parkell, Inc.)

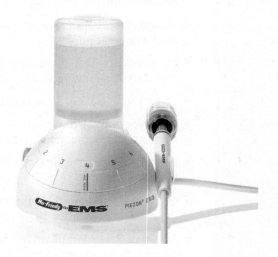

Figure 26-2. Powered Instrumentation Device. One example of an ultrasonic device, this unit consists of an ultrasonic generator, handpiece, and fluid reservoir for ultrasonic instrumentation. (Courtesy of Hu-Friedy Mfg. Co, LLC.)

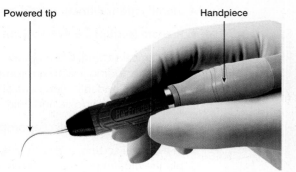

Powered tip   Handpiece

Figure 26-3. Interchangeable Instrument Working-End. An example of an interchangeable instrument working-end that is inserted into the handpiece of a powered instrumentation device.

TABLE 26-1. A TIME LINE FOR THE EVOLUTION OF POWERED INSTRUMENTS	
Date	**Event**
Late 1950s	Development of the first powered instruments.
1960s and 70s	Powered instruments are used to remove heavy calculus deposits. The bulky design of powered working-ends limits use to supragingival instrumentation or sites where the tissue allows easy subgingival insertion. Hand instruments such as Gracey curets are the primary instruments for use within periodontal pockets.
Late 1980s	Slim working-ends are developed for powered devices. Slim working-ends are significantly smaller than the working-end of a standard Gracey curet; however not all powered devices offer slim working-ends.
Today	Modern powered working-ends have been shown to be as effective as hand instruments for removing subgingival calculus deposits, plaque biofilms, and bacterial products from periodontally involved teeth.

TYPES OF POWERED INSTRUMENTATION DEVICES

Powered instruments can be classified into two main groups on the basis of their operating frequencies and method of activation: sonic and ultrasonic (Fig. 26-4).

1. **Sonic powered devices** convert air pressure into high-frequency sound waves that produce vibrations of the powered working-end. Sonic devices operate at a relatively low frequency of 3,000 to 8,000 cycles per second and are driven by compressed air from the dental unit.
2. **Ultrasonic powered devices** convert electrical energy into high-frequency sound waves that produce rapid vibrations of the powered working-end. These devices operate inaudibly at 18,000 to 50,000 cycles per second (kHz). Ultrasonic devices can be further categorized into magnetostrictive and piezoelectric on the basis of the mechanism used to convert the electrical energy into the mechanical energy used to activate the powered working-ends.
   A. **Piezoelectric ("piezo") devices** use electrical energy to activate crystals within the handpiece to produce vibrations of the powered working-end.
   B. **Magnetostrictive ("magneto") devices** transfer electrical energy to metal stacks or a ferrous rod to produce vibrations of the powered working-end.

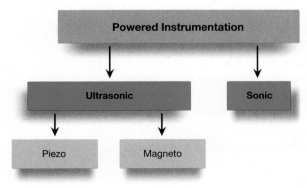

Figure 26-4. Powered Device Classification. The two major types of powered instrumentation devices are ultrasonic and sonic. Ultrasonic devices are subdivided into piezo and magneto devices.

EFFECTIVENESS OF POWERED ULTRASONIC INSTRUMENTATION

This module focuses on powered instrumentation with ultrasonic devices. The advantages of ultrasonic over sonic instrumentation include more rapid vibrations of the powered working-end and in most cases, a wider selection of working-ends for the device. Research investigations indicate that powered ultrasonic instrumentation is as effective as hand instrumentation in removal of calculus deposits, control of subgingival plaque biofilms, and reduction of inflammation when used by a skilled clinician (1,4,5). As with hand instrumentation, the effectiveness of powered instrumentation is determined by the skill of the clinician and the thoroughness of posttreatment evaluation with an explorer of the treatment area. Table 26-2 presents a comparison of powered and hand instrumentation.

1. Strengths of Powered Instrumentation
   A. **Effective Removal of Calculus Deposits and Plaque Biofilms**
      1. When used by skilled clinicians, powered instrumentation has been shown to attain similar results as hand instrumentation for supra- and sub-gingival calculus removal and removal of subgingival plaque biofilms (6).
      2. As with hand instrumentation, an explorer is used to thoroughly re-evaluate the treatment area for residual deposits.
   B. **Pocket Penetration.** Slim working-ends penetrate deeper into periodontal pockets than hand instruments (Fig. 26-5) (7–11).
   C. **Access to Furcation Areas.** Slim working-ends are effective in treating Class II and III furcations when used by experienced clinicians (11–13).
   D. **Irrigation (Lavage).** Water irrigation of the pocket washes toxic products and free-floating bacteria from the pocket and provides better vision during instrumentation by removing blood from the treatment site (14).
   E. **Shorter Instrumentation Time.** Several studies have shown that instrumentation time may be reduced when using powered instruments in conjunction with hand instruments for effective calculus removal and treatment planning (2,4,7,15,16).
   F. **Facilitation of Difficult Instrumentation Tasks**
      1. If a minor amalgam overhang is acting as a biofilm trap, the excess amalgam can be removed using a specialized powered instrument working-end designed for this purpose.
      2. Removal of orthodontic cement or debonding of orthodontic brackets is facilitated by use of a powered standard tip.
2. Limitations of Powered Instrumentation
   A. **Clinician Skill Level.** The skill level of the clinician is the best predictor of the outcome of periodontal instrumentation regardless of whether hand or powered instrument is used.
      1. A powered instrument is ineffective and may even be harmful if the clinician is not skilled in the technique. *Powered instrumentation—whether magneto or piezo—is just as technique-sensitive as is hand instrumentation.*
      2. A complete understanding of root anatomy is the key to successful periodontal instrumentation. Clinicians experience less tactile sensitivity when using powered instruments than with hand instruments.
   B. **Production of Aerosols.** A disadvantage of power-driven scalers is the production of aerosols contaminated with oral microorganisms. For this reason, additional care is required to achieve and maintain good infection control when using powered instrumentation (6).

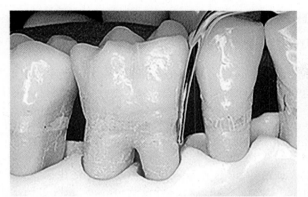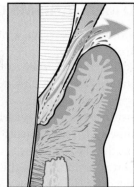

Figure 26-5. Pocket Penetration of Slim Working-End and Fluid Lavage. Slim working-ends penetrate deeper into periodontal pockets and reach the base of the pocket better than hand instruments. The water lavage reaches a depth that is equal to the depth reached by the powered instrument working-end.

TABLE 26-2. COMPARISON OF POWERED AND HAND INSTRUMENTATION

Ultrasonic Instrumentation	Hand Instrumentation
• Several mechanisms of action: mechanical, water irrigation, and cavitation	• One mechanism of action: mechanical calculus removal
• Small size of instrument working-end (0.3–0.55 mm)	• Larger size working-ends (0.76–1.0 mm)
• Easily inserted in pocket with minimal distention (stretching) of pocket wall away from the tooth	• Must be positioned apical to deposit resulting in considerable distention of pocket wall
• Powered working-end can remove calculus deposit from above; working in an apical direction beginning at the gingival margin and moving toward the junctional epithelium	• Curet must be positioned beneath the deposit for removal; working in a coronal direction beginning at the junctional epithelium and moving toward the gingival margin
• Tissue trauma less likely resulting in a faster healing rate	• Larger working-end with sharp cutting edge(s) more likely to cause tissue trauma
• No cutting edges to sharpen	• Frequent sharpening required
• Treatment outcomes dependent on the clinician's skill level with powered instrumentation and knowledge of root anatomy	• Treatment outcomes dependent on the clinician's skill level with hand instrumentation and knowledge of root anatomy
• Aerosol production; moderate to high levels of aerosols	• Low levels of splatter production

MODES AND MECHANISMS OF ACTION

1. **Modes of Action for Powered Instrumentation.** Powered instruments have several modes of action.
   A. **Mechanical Removal.** Very rapid vibrations of the powered working-end create micro-fractures in a calculus deposit that result in gradual removal of the deposit (1).
   B. **Water Irrigation**
      1. A constant stream of water exits near the point of the electronically powered working-end. This constant flushing action within the periodontal pocket is termed the fluid lavage.
      2. The water irrigation to the working-end is needed to dissipate the heat produced by the friction caused by the rapidly moving working-end against the tooth surface.
      3. Water irrigation also plays an important role in periodontal therapy. The water stream of certain powered working-ends penetrates to the base of periodontal pockets and washes toxic products and free-floating bacteria from the pocket. Research indicates that a greater area is cleaned when water is used for power instrumentation compared to power instrumentation without water (1,17,18).
   C. **Cavitation of the Water Stream**
      1. Cavitation is the formation of tiny bubbles when the water stream contacts the vibrating working-end.
      2. When these tiny bubbles collapse, they produce shock waves that may alter or destroy bacteria by tearing the bacterial cell walls (18,19).
2. **Mechanisms of Action of Powered Instrumentation.** How efficiently a powered instrument removes calculus is determined by the powered working-end's frequency (vibration), amplitude (stroke), design in cross section ("geometry"), and the surface of the working-end in contact with the tooth.
   A. **Frequency (Vibration)**
      1. Frequency is the measure of how many times a powered working-end vibrates per second. The frequency of the working-end can be compared to the settings for the windshield wipers on a car (Fig. 26-6).
         a. **Low Frequency.** When the wiper setting is on low, the wipers only go back and forth a few times in a minute. Similarly, when the frequency of the powered device is low, the instrument working-end vibrates fewer times per second.
         b. **High Frequency.** When the wiper setting is on high, the windshield wipers go back and forth many times in a minute. Correspondingly, when the frequency of a powered device is high, the instrument working-end vibrates more times per second.

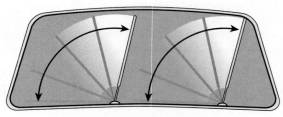

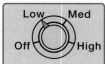

Figure 26-6. Frequency. The speed of the back and forth movements of windshield wipers can be compared to the low and high frequencies of a powered working-end.

B. Amplitude (Stroke Length)
1. Amplitude is a measure of how far the powered working-end moves back and forth during one cycle. Higher amplitude delivers a longer, more powerful stroke; lower amplitude delivers a shorter, less powerful stroke.
2. Power Adjustment. The amplitude of a powered working-end is adjusted using the power setting on an ultrasonic device.
    a. Higher-power settings deliver a longer, more forceful stroke. Lower-power settings deliver a shorter, less powerful stroke.
    b. Higher-power settings deliver a longer, more powerful stroke that may be uncomfortable for the patient. The lowest effective power setting always should be used during powered instrumentation.
    c. A research investigation found no difference in the cleaning efficiency of ultrasonic instruments when operated at high-power levels or medium-power levels (15). *Therefore, to maximize patient comfort and minimize potential damage to the tooth surface, the power setting should rarely be placed above the medium setting.*
    d. *Most slim-diameter working-ends cannot be used at higher-power levels because of the risk of breakage.*
        1. Dentsply Cavitron makes two slim-diameter working-ends, called Thin-Sert inserts that are specially designed to withstand use on high power without danger of breaking.
        2. Parkell makes the Burnett Power Working-end that can be used on high power for removal of tenacious calculus.
3. Understanding Amplitude
    a. Low Amplitude. Using the example of a child on a swing, low amplitude would be a gentle push against the child's back, causing the swing to move forward a short distance before returning to its starting position (Fig. 26-7). Lower amplitude causes the powered working-end to move a shorter distance.
    b. High Amplitude. Higher amplitude causes the powered working-end to move a longer distance. This is similar to a more forceful push against a child's back, causing the swing to travel a longer distance before returning to its original position.

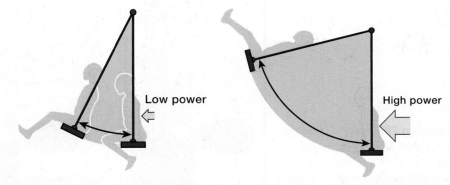

Low power   High power

Figure 26-7. Amplitude. Low amplitude (low power) can be compared to a gentle push against the back of the child on the swing. High amplitude (high power) is comparable to a more forceful push against the child's back.

3. Cleaning Efficiency of Powered Instrumentation (Frequency + Amplitude = Cleaning Efficiency).
   A. The cleaning efficiency of a powered instrument is primarily determined by a combination of frequency and amplitude. Frequency determines the number of vibrations while amplitude determines the length of each stroke.
   B. **Understanding Cleaning Efficiency.** As an aid in understanding cleaning efficiency imagine a boxer who is trapped in a wooden box. In order to escape, the boxer decides to try to punch through the side of the box.
      1. **Low Frequency/ Low Amplitude.** In the first instance shown in Figure 26-8A, the boxer is trapped in a narrow box, so that when he tries to punch the side of the box, his swing is hindered by the size of the box. He hits his elbow on the back of the box as he makes his punches. He is only able to made a few, short thrusts against the side of the box.
         a. This example is similar to low frequency—few vibrations, or punches—combined with low amplitude—short strokes, or limited movement of the boxer's arm.
         b. A combination of low frequency and amplitude is ideal for disruption of plaque biofilm from the root surface (deplaquing).
      2. **High Frequency/High Amplitude.** In the second example shown in Figure 26-8B, the boxer is trapped in a wide box. Now the boxer is able to pull his arm back to make many, long thrusts at the side of the box.
         a. This example is similar to high frequency—many vibrations, or punches—combined with high amplitude—long strokes, or longer thrusts of the boxer's arm.
         b. A combination of a higher frequency combined with higher amplitude is ideal for the removal of tenacious calculus deposits.
4. Pattern of Working-End Movement
   A. The movement of magneto working-end primarily moves in an elliptical motion; however, the motion ranges from nearly linear, to elliptical or circular, depending on the type of unit, and shape and length of the working-end (6,20).
   B. A piezo working-end is activated by dimensional changes in crystals housed within the handpiece as electricity is passed over the surface of the crystals. The resultant vibration produces working-end movement that is primarily linear in direction (6,20,21).

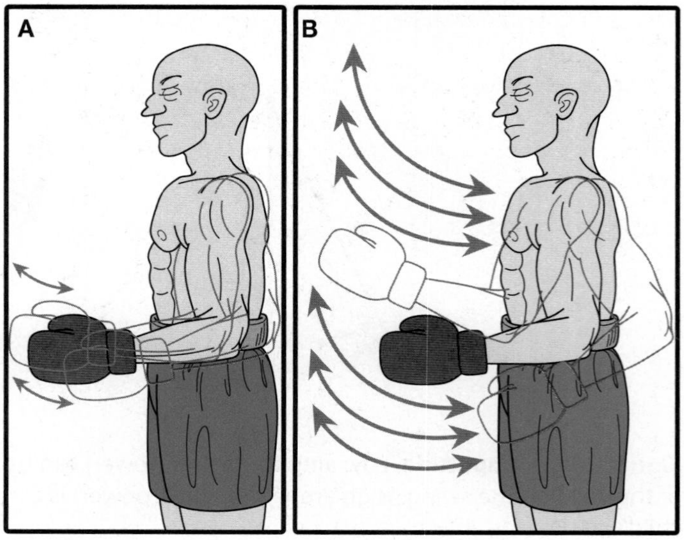

Figure 26-8. Cleaning Efficiency. Cleaning efficiency is determined by a combination of the number of vibrations and the stroke length of the powered working-end. A boxer trapped in a narrow box (**A**) can exert much less force per punch than the same boxer trapped in a wider box (**B**).

5. **Water or Irrigant Flow to the Powered Working-End**
   A. Ultrasonic working-ends should be cooled by fluid to prevent overheating. Fluid—usually water—flowing around or through the working-end is used as a coolant. For piezo devices, only the working-end needs to be cooled with water to prevent overheating. With magneto devices, the handpiece and working-end should be irrigated with water to prevent overheating of the handpiece and working-end.
      1. Fluid constantly flows through or around the powered working-end dispersing in a fine water spray from the working-end.
      2. The clinician can adjust the volume of the water supplied to the instrument working-end.
         a. Too little water flow to the instrument working-end can result in heat damage to the dental pulp. More water flow is recommended for calculus removal (Fig. 26-9A) and a less water flow is needed for deplaquing (Fig. 26-9B).
         b. *One of the most common mistakes made by beginning clinicians is using too little water. A warm handpiece is a sign of inadequate water flowing through the handpiece and instrument working-end.*
      3. Changing from one powered working-end to another during treatment may require adjustment of the water flow (22).
   B. Water is provided to the instrument working-end through either an external or internal fluid flow tubes. Figures 26-10 and 26-11 depict correct water flow adjustment for external and internal fluid flow tubes.

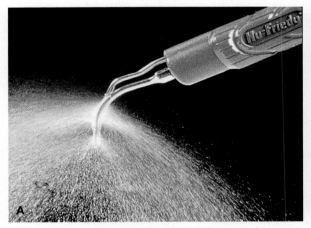
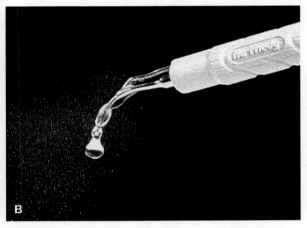

Figure 26-9. **Water Flow. (A) Water Flow for Calculus Removal.** The instrument on the left is adjusted so that the water breaks into a fine mist at the instrument working-end. **(B) Water Flow for Deplaquing.** The instrument working-end on the right is adjusted so that the water halo is smaller and water drips from the instrument working-end. (Courtesy of Hu-Friedy Mfg. Co, LLC.)

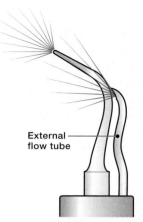

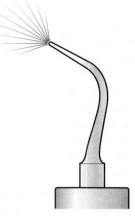

External flow tube

Figure 26-10. Water Adjustment for Working-Ends with External Flow Tubes. For instrument working-ends with external flow tubes, the water flow should be adjusted so that the water breaks into a fine mist near the end of the external flow tube and at the very end of the working-end.

Figure 26-11. Water Adjustment for Working-Ends with Internal Flow Tubes. For instrument working-ends with internal flow systems, the water flow should be adjusted so that the water breaks into a fine mist at the very end of the working-end.

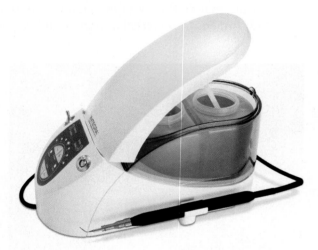

Figure 26-12. Ultrasonic Device with Fluid Reservoir Bottles. Pictured is an ultrasonic device with two fluid reservoirs. Fluid reservoirs may be used to deliver distilled water, or chemotherapeutic agents to a magnetostrictive or piezoelectric powered instrument working-end. (Courtesy of Parkell, Inc.)

6. **Fluid Reservoirs and Powered Instrumentation.** Some ultrasonic devices have fluid reservoirs (bottles) that can be used to deliver distilled water or other fluid solutions to the instrument working-end. Figure 26-12 shows one example of an ultrasonic device with fluid reservoirs.

   A. **Irrigant Solutions.** Solutions commonly used for irrigation include distilled water, sterile saline, and chemotherapeutic agents (antimicrobials), such as chlorhexidine.

   B. **Effectiveness of Chemotherapeutic Agents**

      1. The use of chemotherapeutic agents with ultrasonic instruments has *not* been shown to enhance pocket depth reduction beyond that achieved by hand instrumentation or ultrasonic instrumentation with water. (6,14,23).

      2. Pathogenic microorganisms in plaque biofilms—which are found mainly in deep pockets (equal to or greater than 4 mm)—are highly resistant to antimicrobial agents and systemic antibiotics (24,25). The only way to totally disrupt the biofilm is through mechanical removal. Mechanical removal can be accomplished with hand instruments, powered instruments, or specialized subgingival air polishing tips. Control of bacteria in dental plaque biofilms is best achieved by the physical disruption of the biofilm (26).

CONTRAINDICATIONS FOR POWERED INSTRUMENTATION

The decision to include powered instrumentation in a patient's treatment plan is based on each individual patient's medical and dental histories. A thorough review of the patient's medical history is a must prior to the use of this technology and consultation with the patient's physician may be indicated. Table 26-3 summarizes contraindications for powered instrumentation.

TABLE 26-3. CONTRAINDICATIONS FOR POWERED INSTRUMENTATION

Contraindication	Rationale
Communicable disease	Individual with communicable disease that can be disseminated by aerosols generated during powered instrumentation
Susceptibility to infection	Individual with a high susceptibility to opportunistic infection that can be transmitted by contaminated dental unit water lines or inhaled aerosols generated during powered instrumentation, such as immuno-suppression from disease, chemotherapy, uncontrolled diabetes, organ transplant; debilitated individuals with chronic medical conditions (27,28)
Respiratory risk	Individual with respiratory disease or difficulty in breathing; such an individual is at high risk of infection from aspiration of septic material or microorganisms from biofilms into the lungs (29,30). Examples include: history of emphysema, cystic fibrosis, asthma; history of cardiac disease with secondary pulmonary disease or breathing problem
Cardiac implantable devices	The American Academy of Periodontology recommends consultation with the patient's cardiologist (6,31); some newer devices have protective coverings
Difficulty in swallowing	Individuals with difficulty in swallowing or who are prone to gagging may aspirate liquids into the lungs along with microorganisms from biofilms into the lungs increasing risk of respiratory infection (32). Examples include: history of multiple sclerosis, amyotrophic lateral sclerosis, muscular dystrophy, Parkinson disease, or paralysis
Young age	Primary and newly erupted teeth of young children have large pulp chambers that are more susceptible to thermal (heat) damage to the pulp the powered working-end becomes overheated (1,33)
Dentinal surfaces or demineralized areas	Exposed dentin or the re-mineralizing enamel surface of a demineralized area can be removed; dentinal tubules can be exposed leading to increased or new dentinal sensitivity (1,33)
Restorations or dental implants	Powered instrumentation may result in rough surfaces, such as chips, nicks and scratches on the amalgam, composite and porcelain surfaces (34); powered working-ends will damage titanium surfaces of dental implants unless the working-end is one especially designed for implant surfaces (35)

HEALTH CONCERNS FOR POWERED INSTRUMENTATION

1. **Water Tubing Contamination.** Biofilm forms on the internal surfaces of the waterline tubing found in the dental unit and ultrasonic devices. Microorganisms from waterline tubing can become aerosolized when dental handpieces, powered instruments, or air polishers are used in treatment procedures.

   A. Microbial growth inside waterline tubing poses risks for both dental professionals and their patients (36).

   B. Options to control water tubing contamination of electronically powered devices include a combination of:

   1. **Self-contained reservoirs.** Some ultrasonic units have the ability to use an independent reservoir bottle that requires no waterline hook-up. The reservoir can be used to deliver distilled water or antimicrobial solution to ultrasonic instrument tip.

   2. **Point-of-use filters.** Point-of-use filters, such as the one shown in Figure 26-13, are easily installed in existing dental unit waterlines to physically reduce the numbers of microorganisms in the water flowing over the instrument tip (Fig. 26-49).

   3. **Flushing of the water tubing.** At the beginning of each day, the handpiece water line should be flushed by stepping on the foot pedal and allowing water to flow through the handpiece for at least 2 minutes. To reduce microbial contamination, waterlines should be chemically treated, flushed for 20 to 30 seconds between patients, and flushed for 30 seconds before a sterile working-end or insert is attached/inserted to a powered instrument handpiece (37).

2. **Contaminated Dental Aerosols and Powered Instrumentation**

   A. Overview of Dental Aerosols

   1. Dental aerosols are airborne particles that are composed of debris, microorganisms, and blood propelled into the air from the oral cavities of individuals treated throughout the day in a dental office (38). Dental aerosols are defined as being particles smaller than 50 micrometers, with any particles larger than 50 micrometers being described as splatter (39,40).

   2. The saliva, gingival tissues, nose, throat, and lungs of healthy patients contain large numbers of *streptococci*, *staphylococci*, gram-negative bacteria, and viruses (41). Viruses include the common cold, influenza, and herpetic viruses.

   3. *Aerosols stay airborne and float on office air currents moving some distance from the point of origin (42). Very small particles can remain suspended at the end of the procedure for many hours. Therefore, the risk of contamination continues long after the procedure is over.*

   4. Small aerosolized particles remain airborne and enter the nasal passage and are capable of penetrating deep into the respiratory tree (42–44).

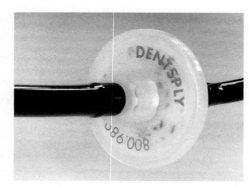

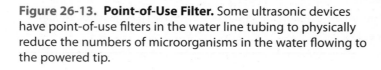

Figure 26-13. Point-of-Use Filter. Some ultrasonic devices have point-of-use filters in the water line tubing to physically reduce the numbers of microorganisms in the water flowing to the powered tip.

B. Dental Aerosols and Powered Instrumentation
1. The use of prophy angles, air-water syringes, and even hand instruments produce some splatter in the form of relatively large droplets.
2. *Powered instruments and air polishers are the greatest producers of small particle aerosol contamination in dentistry* (45–52).
3. Several studies show that blood is found routinely in the aerosols produced by powered instrumentation (46,53,54).
4. One study found a significantly greater prevalence of nasal irritation, running eyes, and itchy skin in a dental hygienist group who often use aerosol generating instruments compared to a control group of clerical staff working in a hospital environment (55).

3. Potential Occupational Risks of Powered Instrumentation
A. Musculoskeletal Damage. Some studies suggest that dental hygienists may be in danger of nerve damage from dental instruments that cause vibration, such as powered instruments.
1. One study found that about one-quarter of dental hygienists who use high-frequency powered instruments will develop a type of nerve damage that blunts the sense of touch and causes weakness (56,57).
2. A reduction in strength and tactile sensitivity was observed in women dentists and dental hygienists when compared to women dental assistants and medical nurses who were not exposed to vibration (58).
B. Hearing Loss
1. Further research is necessary to confirm the effect of powered instrumentation on hearing as there is limited research on this issue and available studies have yielded differing results.
   a. One study reports tinnitus, an early sign of hearing loss, following powered instrumentation use in both clinicians and patients (59).
   b. A study by Wilson, however, found that the hearing ability of dental personnel does not differ from that of nondental controls (individuals not working in the dental office environment). Wilson's study indicates that occupational exposure to powered instruments is not harmful to hearing (60).
2. The use of hearing protection devices has been suggested for dental healthcare providers.
   a. Hearing protection devices, if used, must protect the dental professional from potential noise damage. At the same time, the clinician must be able to hear sufficiently to communicate with the patient.
   b. One option is to purchase custom earplugs, the same type of hearing protection used by many musicians for protection from occupationally induced hearing loss. Garner et al. (61) found that the "musician's style ear plug is perfectly suited to the dental environment and is an affordable and comfortable solution."

4. Magnetic Fields
A. Recently, there has been growing concern regarding the biologic effects of occupational exposure of dental personnel to weak time-varying magnetic fields, such as those produced by ultrasonic instrumentation devices.
B. Bohay found that magnetic field strengths recorded in the dental operatory were comparable to those reported from measurements of common household appliances (62).
C. Scientific evidence on this question is not clear. More studies are needed to clearly understand the effects of electromagnetic fields emitted by ultrasonic devices (62–65).

FUNDAMENTAL SKILLS FOR POWERED INSTRUMENTATION

As with hand-activated instrumentation, powered instrumentation relies on basic fundamental skills that are essential for success. This section discusses fundamental skills and techniques as they apply to powered instrumentation.

Position

- The clinician position used for powered instrumentation is the same as for hand instrumentation.
- Neutral seated or standing position throughout powered instrumentation.
- Position the patient in the normal supine position and with his or her head turned to one side. The patient's head is positioned to the side so the water flow will pool in the corner of the mouth where it can be evacuated.
  - The patient turns toward the clinician for anterior sextants and posterior aspects facing away from the clinician.
  - The patient turns slightly away from the clinician for posterior aspects facing toward the clinician.

Grasp

- A modified pen grasp is recommended for all powered instrumentation.
- Since the powered working-end does all the work of calculus removal, lateral pressure and fulcrum pressure against the tooth are not needed to concentrate the force of instrumentation strokes.

Finger Rests

- Advanced finger rests—extraoral, cross arch, opposite arch—are preferred for use with powered instrumentation since the "work" of calculus removal is accomplished by the powered working-end rather than by activation initiated by the clinician.

Adaptation

- Adapt the few 2 to 3 mm of the lateral surface against the tooth surface. Only the terminal few millimeters of the lateral surface is effective at calculus removal.
- Keep the terminal-third of the lateral surface adapted at all times as it is moved around line angles and tooth curvatures and concavities. Pivoting the wrist is helpful in maintaining adaptation.

Lateral Pressure

- Feather-light lateral pressure is all that is needed with the powered working-end against a calculus deposit or the tooth surface for deplaquing.
- In fact, moderate or firm pressure decreases the effectiveness of the powered working-end and can even stop the vibrations of the working-end completely!
- Effective powered instrumentation requires a light touch.

Assessment/End Point of Instrumentation

- With any instrumentation technique, an explorer is still the instrument of choice to evaluate the final clinical end point of calculus removal.
- If the clinic or dental office has an endoscope, the clinician should consider using endoscopic evaluation of the root surface. The endoscope allows the clinician to observe the subgingival root anatomy and residual calculus following instrumentation.

DIFFERING APPROACHES TO CALCULUS REMOVAL: HAND VERSUS POWERED

The technique used for calculus removal with a powered working-end is very different from that used with hand instruments (66).

1. **Calculus Removal Technique with a Curet.** A curet—such as a Gracey extended shank curet—must be *positioned apical to (below) the calculus deposit*—starting at the base of the pocket and working toward the cementoenamel junction (CEJ).

2. **Calculus Removal with a Powered Ultrasonic Instrument**
   A. A powered working-end works from the *coronal-most region of the deposit*— starting near the CEJ and working apically (toward the base of the pocket).
   B. There is no need to position the working-end beneath the deposit. This is a great advantage when working in deep periodontal pockets. Figure 26-14 shows the differing techniques used with a hand-activated curet and a powered working-end.

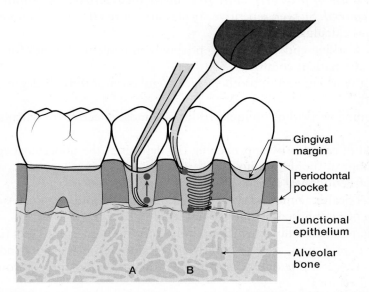

Figure 26-14. Different Techniques with a Hand-Activated Instrument versus a Powered Instrument Working- for Calculus Removal.
A. Subgingival Calculus Removal with a Curet. Calculus removal with a curet takes place from the base of the pocket upward toward the CEJ. Often it is difficult to position the curet under calculus deposits near the base of the pocket.
B. Subgingival Calculus Removal with a Powered Working-End. Calculus removal with a powered working-end takes place from the top of the deposit downward toward the base of the pocket.

INSTRUMENTATION STROKE WITH AN ULTRASONIC INSTRUMENT

1. Strokes for Calculus Removal
    A. Powered working-ends break up heavy calculus deposits by putting little micro-fractures in the deposit. The powered working-end needs to be moved slowly and methodically over the surface of a deposit for *some time* in order to allow the micro-fractures to develop. *A common misconception is that a powered working-end is like a magic wand—beginning clinicians often mistakenly believe that a quick "swipe" of the working-end over the tooth surface will be effective. Rather, correct technique requires many slow, repetitive instrumentation strokes to accomplish calculus removal.*
    B. Only gentle pressure is needed for calculus removal during powered instrumentation.
        1. Firm pressure greatly reduces the effectiveness of the instrument.
        2. *Rather than use of pressure, many slow methodical strokes are required for calculus removal.* Slower, repetitive strokes are more effective in removing large or tenacious calculus deposits.
    C. The powered working-end should be kept slowly moving at all times for effective debridement and patient comfort.
    D. Maintaining a working-end to tooth surface angulation of 0 to 15 degrees is recommended.
    E. Slow, overlapping vertical or oblique strokes are most effective for calculus removal.
    F. Begin removal of calculus by approaching the deposit at the uppermost edge.
2. Strokes for Subgingival Biofilm Removal
    A. Deplaquing of Periodontal Pockets: Why is it important?
        1. Periodontal health cannot be achieved without the periodic removal or disruption of established plaque biofilm (67).
        2. Pathogenic plaque biofilms, which are found mainly in deep pockets (equal to or greater than 4 mm), are highly resistant to antimicrobial agents and systemic antibiotics (24,25). The only way to totally disrupt the biofilm is through mechanical removal.
        3. Control of bacteria in dental plaque biofilms is best achieved by the physical disruption of plaque biofilm. It is critical to cover every square millimeter of the root surface within a periodontal pocket with continuous, closely spaced, methodical overlapping strokes to mechanically disrupt and remove the plaque biofilm colonies. Ultrasonic instrumentation under low power is sufficient to accomplish this task.
    B. Technique for Subgingival Deplaquing
        1. Because only the first 2 to 4 mm of the powered working-end actively removes biofilm, a thorough and systematic approach to subgingival instrumentation is of great importance (66). The overlapping strokes must be very close together to effectively remove plaque biofilm.
        2. The powered working-end should be kept moving at all times for effective debridement and patient comfort. The overlapping strokes can be a little faster than with hand-activated instrumentation because the purpose of debridement in periodontal maintenance therapy is to remove biofilm and lighter newly formed calculus deposits (68).

3. In contrast to techniques for removal of calculus deposits, *biofilm removal within a periodontal pocket* is accomplished using a series of gentle sweeping motions over the root surface (Fig. 26-15). *As with all ultrasonic instrumentation, it is vital to employ slow, methodical strokes over the tooth surface.* Box 26-1 offers suggestions for visualizing correct adaptation of the working-end. For deplaquing, short, over-lapping strokes should cover every millimeter of the root surface using strokes in vertical, oblique, or horizontal directions.

4. For biofilm removal, unnecessary loss of cementum from the root's surface should be avoided as far as possible by applying light force and selecting a lower-power setting (2,66,69,70).

5. *Normal sulci in the absence of inflammation are likely colonized by beneficial flora and need not be deplaqued.*

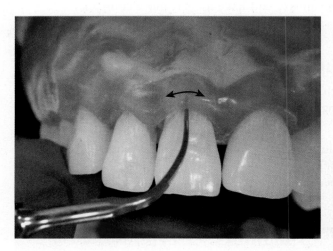

Figure 26-15. Sweeping Motions for Subgingival Deplaquing. For *subgingival deplaquing*, a lateral surface of the working-end is adapted to the root surface and moved in a series of sweeping motions. The stroke motion should be slow and methodical.

Box 26-1 **Using Sweeping Motions for Biofilm Disruption**

During ultrasonic instrumentation, imagine that the working-end is a crayon. The goal is to gently color the entire root surface using the *side of a crayon*—rather than the point of the crayon.

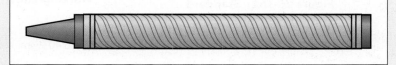

Section 2
Powered Working-End Design

As with the working-ends of hand instruments, there are a wide variety of instrument working-end designs available for ultrasonic devices. At this time, working-ends for sonic devices are more limited in selection. The two basic types of ultrasonic working-ends are standard working-ends (Fig. 26-16A) and slim perio working-ends (Fig. 26-16B). In addition to these two broad classifications of working-ends, there are specialized working-ends for use on titanium surfaces and for smoothing of defective margins on dental restorations. Table 26-4 compares the design features and uses of standard and slim perio working-end designs.

- Standard working-ends are larger in size and have shorter shank lengths than slim perio working-ends. These standard working-ends are comparable to sickle scalers and universal curets in function.
- Slim Perio working-ends are up to 40% smaller in size and have longer, more complex shanks than standard working-ends.

WORKING-END SELECTION AND SEQUENCE FOR INSTRUMENTATION

Powered working-ends vary in shape, size, length, and curvature. Factors to be considered when selecting an instrument working-end for a particular instrumentation task include:

1. The extent and mode of attachment of calculus deposits (small-, medium-, or large-sized deposits?); (lightly adherent?, tenacious?)
2. The location of calculus deposits (deposits located above the gingival margin or below the gingival margin?)

TABLE 26-4. POWERED WORKING-END DESIGN

Size		

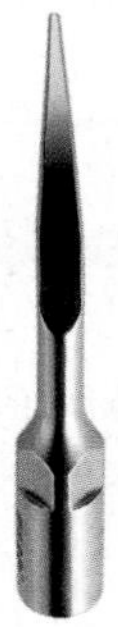

Figure 26-16A. **Standard Working-Ends.**

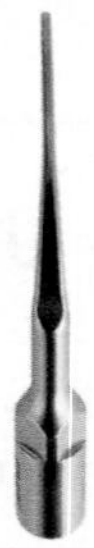

Figure 26-16B. **Slim Perio Working-Ends.**

Characteristics	Standard size	Up to 40% smaller in size
	Shorter shank lengths	Longer shank lengths
Use	Heavy deposit removal: supragingival use and for subgingival deposits easily accessed without undue tissue distension	Light to moderate deposits and deplaquing
		Instrumentation of root concavities and furcation areas

Sequence for Use of Powered Working-Ends

1. A Combination of Inserts
    A. *Powered instrumentation frequently requires a combination of standard and slim perio instrument working-ends.*
    B. In addition to working-end size, clinicians should consider the cross section of the working-end.
        1. Working-ends that have a rectangular, trapezoidal, or beveled cross section are more effective for calculus removal.
        2. Working-ends that are round in cross section are most effective for removal of plaque biofilm (deplaquing).
2. Sequence of Working-Ends
    A. Using the example of a patient with supragingival and subgingival calculus deposits, powered instrumentation begins with standard working-ends and progresses to slim perio working-ends. Figure 26-17 summarizes the approach for working-end selection and sequencing.
        1. Standard working-ends first are used for moderate to heavy supragingival or subgingival calculus deposits.
        2. After instrumentation with standard working-ends, slim perio working-ends are used. Slim perio working-ends work well in removing light subgingival calculus deposits, plaque biofilm, and soft debris. Table 26-5 provides a guide for working-end use.

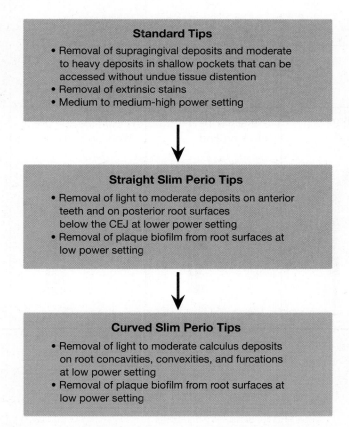

Standard Tips
- Removal of supragingival deposits and moderate to heavy deposits in shallow pockets that can be accessed without undue tissue distention
- Removal of extrinsic stains
- Medium to medium-high power setting

Straight Slim Perio Tips
- Removal of light to moderate deposits on anterior teeth and on posterior root surfaces below the CEJ at lower power setting
- Removal of plaque biofilm from root surfaces at low power setting

Curved Slim Perio Tips
- Removal of light to moderate calculus deposits on root concavities, convexities, and furcations at low power setting
- Removal of plaque biofilm from root surfaces at low power setting

Figure 26-17. Sequence for Instrumentation. Powered instrumentation frequently requires a combination of standard and slim perio instrument working-ends.

TABLE 26-5. WORKING END USE GUIDE[a]

		Enamel Surfaces Flat Tooth Anatomy		Enamel and Root Surfaces	
				Supra/Subgingival	Deep Pockets
Calculus Deposits	Heavy	▓			
	Medium	▓	▓	▓	▓
	Light		▓	▓	▓
Biofilm	Heavy			▓	▓
	Medium			▓	▓
	Light			▓	▓
		Standard, Broad Working-End	Standard, Medium Working-End	Slim Perio, Straight Working-Ends	Slim Perio, Curved Paired Working-Ends

[a]Working-end images courtesy of Hu-Friedy/EMS.

DESIGN CHARACTERISTICS OF THE PAIRED SLIM PERIO TIPS

Certain slim perio tips are used as a set of three; this is similar to using the Gracey 1/2, 11/12, and 13/14 as a set of hand instruments (Figs. 26-18 to 26-20). Use of all three slim perio tips is recommended to ensure that all areas of the root are thoroughly instrumented.

- The straight slim working-end is similar in design to a calibrated probe and may be used "universally" on all tooth surfaces throughout the mouth
- The two curved working-ends are paired—in right-curved and left-curved versions—and similar in design to a furcation probe. These curved working-ends are especially useful for difficult to reach proximal root surfaces, concavities, and furcation areas

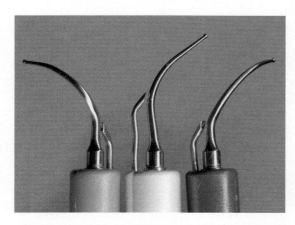

Figure 26-18. Set of Slim-Diameter Tips. Slim-diameter tips come in a set of three tips: a straight tip, a right-curved tip, and a left-curved tip.

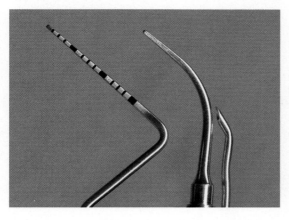

Figure 26-19. Straight Slim-Diameter Tip.
- The photograph shows a periodontal probe and a straight slim-diameter powered tip. Note that the working-ends of these two instruments are very similar in design.
- Straight slim-diameter powered tips are most effective on anterior root surfaces and posterior root surfaces that are 4 mm or less apical to (below) the CEJ.

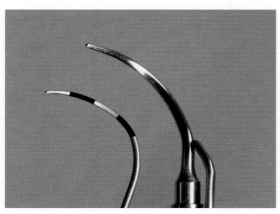

Figure 26-20. Curved Slim-Diameter Tips.
- The photograph shows a curved furcation probe and a curved slim-diameter powered tip.
- Curved slim-diameter tips are designed for use on posterior root surfaces located more than 4 mm apical to the CEJ.
- Curved tips adapt well to root curvatures, concavities, and furcation areas and reach calculus deposits under the contact areas of posterior teeth.

POWERED WORKING-ENDS FOR USE ON DENTAL IMPLANTS

Instruments used for the assessment and debridement of implant teeth should be made of a material that is softer than titanium, since titanium is a soft metal that is easily damaged by metal instruments.

- Metal instruments—whether hand-activated or powered—may scratch the titanium implant surface resulting in increased plaque biofilm retention, which in turn, compromises periodontal health.
- Powered instrument working-ends coated with a nonmetallic plastic or carbon material are appropriate for instrumentation of dental implants (Figs. 26-21 and 26-22). Studies show no damaging effects from the use of plastic or carbon working-ended powered instruments (71–76).
- A study by Sato el al. (76) suggests that ultrasonic instruments fitted with nonmetallic working-ends are more effective than the use of hand-activated plastic scalers in the removal of calculus deposits and plaque biofilms around a dental implant.

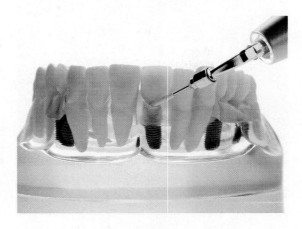

Figure 26-21. A Plastic-Coated Working-End for Instrumentation of Dental Implants. This Hu-Friedy EMS implant piezo working-end features an instrument coating made of a high-tech Polyether Ether Ketone (PEEK) fiber that safely cleans implant abutment surfaces and restorations. (Courtesy of Hu-Friedy Mfg. Co, LLC.)

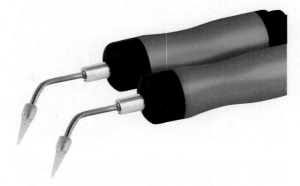

Figure 26-22. Powered Inserts for Instrumentation of Dental Implants. The GentleClean working-ends by Parkell, Inc. are examples of powered working-ends specially designed for use on dental implants. (Courtesy of Parkell, Inc.)

INSTRUMENT WORKING-END WEAR AND REPLACEMENT

The working-end of the powered instrument should be inspected regularly for signs of wear. With use, the instrument working-end is worn down. As an instrument working-end wears, its effectiveness decreases (Fig. 26-23).

1. A rule of thumb is that 1 mm of wear results in approximately 25% loss of efficiency.
2. Approximately 50% loss of efficiency occurs at 2 mm of wear and a working-end with this amount of wear should be discarded.

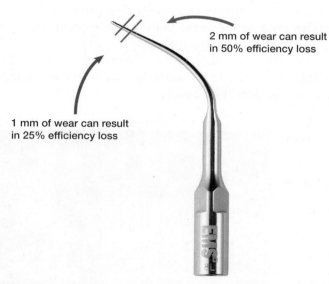

2 mm of wear can result in 50% efficiency loss

1 mm of wear can result in 25% efficiency loss

Figure 26-23. Working-End Wear Guide. Powered instrument working-ends should be evaluated regularly for working-end wear. Working-ends should be discarded after 2 mm of wear. (Courtesy of Hu-Friedy Mfg. Co, LLC.)

Section 3
Adaptation—Orientation of Working-End to Tooth

POWERED WORKING-ENDS ADAPT LIKE A UNIVERSAL CURET

1. Technique is Important for Powered Instrumentation! One of the most common technique errors made by clinicians is the mistaken belief that it is not important how the powered working-end is adapted to the tooth surface.

2. Energy Dispersion by the Surfaces of the Working-End. Powered instrument working-ends disperse energy vibrations from each surface of the working-end (77). By adapting the appropriate working-end surface, the clinician can control energy dispersion.

    A. High-energy vibrations are released at the point of the working-end. *The point of a powered instrument working-end is never adapted directly on a tooth surface due to potential discomfort for the patient and damage to the tooth surface* (Fig. 26-24) (20,68).

    B. *Adaptation of the lateral surfaces of the working-end is recommended for removal of calculus and biofilm* (Fig. 26-25).

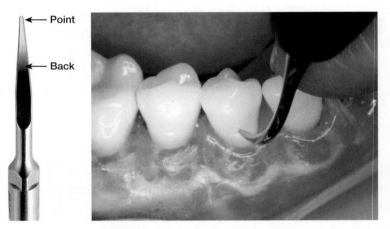

Figure 26-24. Incorrect Adaptation. The point of a powered instrument working-end should *NOT* be placed directly against a tooth surface. The high-energy output of the point could damage the surface of the tooth.

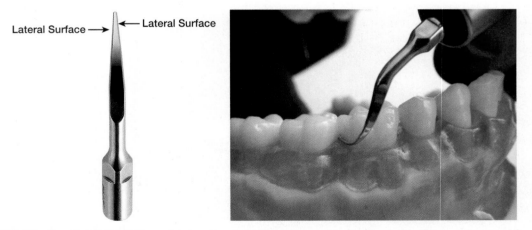

Figure 26-25. Correct Adaptation. A lateral surface of a powered instrument working-end is used for calculus removal and deplaquing of tooth surfaces. The adaptation of the lateral surfaces on a powered working-end is much like the adaptation of a cutting edge with a sickle scaler or universal curet.

3. The Powered Working-End is Adapted Like a Universal Curet
   A. **Hand Instrumentation.** During hand instrumentation, the *cutting edges* of a universal curet are adapted to the tooth surface.
   B. **Powered Instrumentation.** During powered instrumentation, the *lateral surfaces* of the powered working-end are adapted to the tooth (Fig. 26-26). The lateral surfaces of an ultrasonic powered working-end are the most effective for removal of calculus deposits.
4. Adapt the 2 to 3 mm of the Working-End
   A. **Hand Instrumentation.** With a universal curet, the *toe-third* of the cutting edge is adapted to the tooth surface.
   B. **Powered Instrumentation.**
      1. The portion of the instrument working-end that is capable of doing work is called the active area of the working-end. *As illustrated in Figure 26-26, the power to remove calculus is concentrated in the last 2 to 4 mm of the lateral surfaces of the powered instrument working-end*
      2. With a powered working-end, the last 2 to 4 mm of the lateral surface—the active portion—is adapted to the tooth surface. Remember that the point of a powered working-end is never directed toward the tooth surface or against the soft tissue.

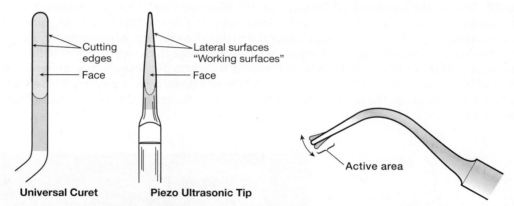

Figure 26-26. Adaptation for Effective Calculus Removal. As depicted in the drawing on the left, universal curets and powered instrument working-ends are adapted in a similar manner, with the curet's cutting edge or the working-end's lateral surface adapted to the tooth surface. The drawing on the right shows the active area of a powered working-end (the last 2 to 4 mm of the working-end). The active area is the portion of the working-end with the concentrated power for calculus removal.

ORIENTATION OF A POWERED WORKING-END TO THE TOOTH SURFACE

There are two basic techniques for adapting a powered working-end to a tooth surface.

1. **Transverse Working-End Orientation.** With the transverse working-end orientation the powered working-end is positioned with the lateral surface in a transverse (crosswise) orientation to the long axis of the tooth. This technique is shown in Figure 26-27. *The transverse working-end orientation can be used when removing calculus deposits above or slightly below the gingival margin.*

2. **Vertical Working-End Orientation.** For the vertical working-end orientation, the powered working-end is positioned with the lateral surface against the tooth surface, in a similar manner to a universal curet in a toe-down position. This technique is shown in Figure 26-28. *The vertical working-end orientation is used for calculus removal and deplaquing when instrumenting shallow or deep periodontal pockets.*

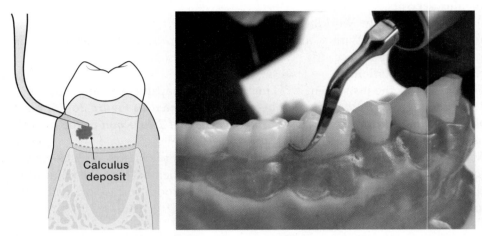

Figure 26-27. Transverse Working-End Orientation. The illustration and photograph depict the lateral surface in a transverse (crosswise) orientation to the long axis of the tooth. This orientation is similar to that used when a cutting edge of a universal curet is adapted to the tooth surface. When removing a deposit from a proximal surface, calculus removal starts at the outermost edge (facial-most region) of the deposit proceeds inward until the entire deposit has been removed. Note on a proximal surface, it often is necessary to remove "half" of the deposit from the facial aspect and the remainder by approaching the deposit from the lingual aspect of the tooth. The photo shows a lateral surface adapted to the distal surface of the mandibular first molar.

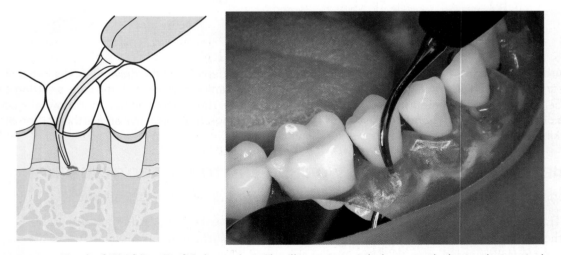

Figure 26-28. Vertical Working-End Orientation. The illustration and photograph depict the vertical orientation with a lateral surface against the root surface; this orientation is similar to a curet in a "toe-down" position.

Section 4
Use of "Universal" Magneto & Piezo Working-Ends

USE OF "UNIVERSAL" WORKING-ENDS IN THE TRANSVERSE ORIENTATION

Box 26-2 | Use of the Transverse Orientation for Powered Instrumentation

- The transverse orientation of a powered working-end is used for removal of calculus deposits from coronal surfaces and for subgingival deposits, slightly below the gingival margin that are easily accessed without undue tissue distention (stretching of the tissue away from the root).
- For example, if a patient has both supragingival and subgingival calculus deposits, the clinician begins placing the working-end in the transverse orientation for supragingival calculus removal. Next, the clinician changes to a vertical working-end orientation for subgingival calculus removal.

A universal curet—with its two level cutting edges—can be used on all tooth surfaces throughout the mouth. Similarly, powered working-end with a universal design can be used on all tooth surfaces. Box 26-2 summarizes use of a powered working-end in the transverse orientation. Figures 26-29 and 26-30 show a transverse orientation of the working-end.

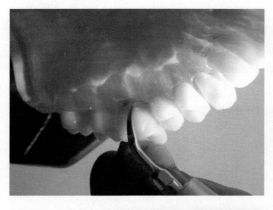

Figure 26-29. The Lateral Surface of a Standard Working-End Adapted to a Proximal Surface.
- A lateral surface of the working-end is adapted to the mesial surface of the molar for removal of a supragingival deposit.
- The transverse orientation is very effective on proximal tooth surfaces for removal of calculus deposits located beneath the contact areas of two adjacent teeth.

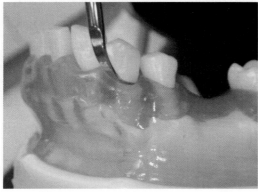

Figure 26-30. Transverse Orientation on a Facial Surface. The picture shows a lateral surface adapted to the facial surface in a similar manner to the adaptation of a universal curet.

USE OF "UNIVERSAL" WORKING-ENDS IN THE VERTICAL ORIENTATION

Box 26-3	Use of the Vertical Orientation for Powered Instrumentation

- The vertical orientation is used in periodontal pockets for calculus removal and deplaquing.
- For example, for a patient with supragingival and subgingival calculus deposits, the clinician begins placing the working-end in the transverse orientation for supragingival calculus removal. Next, the clinician changes to a vertical working-end orientation for subgingival calculus removal.

Box 26-3 summarizes the use of a powered working-end in a vertical orientation. The photographs in Figures 26-31 and 26-32 depict use of a straight slim perio working-end in a vertical orientation.

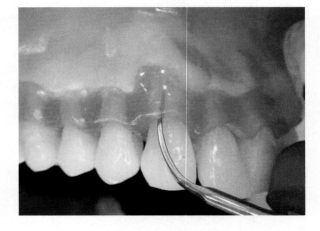

Figure 26-31. Vertical Orientation on an Anterior Tooth. This photograph shows a straight slim working-end with the lateral surface against the root surface in a deep periodontal pocket.

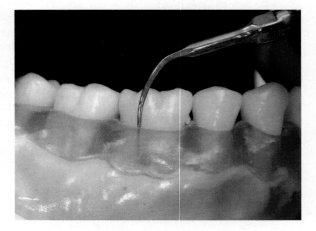

Figure 26-32. Vertical Orientation on a Posterior Tooth. This photograph shows the use of a straight slim perio instrument working-end with the lateral surface against the root surface in a periodontal pocket of a molar tooth.

Section 5
Use of Curved, Paired Magneto Working-Ends

NOTE: This section discusses use of curved, paired **MAGNETO** working-ends. Refer to Section 6 for use of paired **PIEZO** working-ends.

IDENTIFICATION OF A CURVED WORKING-END AS "RIGHT" OR "LEFT"

- Curved powered working-ends come in right and left styles and both working-ends are needed to instrument the entire dentition. This is similar in concept to using two posterior Gracey curets.
- *The identification of a working-end as either "right" or "left" does NOT refer the location that the working-end is used in the mouth. Rather, the "right" or "left" designation refers to the direction of curvature of the working-end, itself.* Figure 26-33 describes how to identify the right and left working-ends.

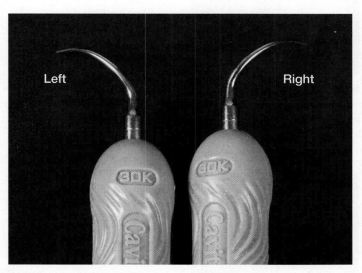

Figure 26-33. Identifying the Right and Left Curved Working-Ends.
- A curved working-end is identified as "right" or "left" by turning the insert so the "point" faces away from the clinician. With the insert in this position, the direction that a working-end bends identifies it as a right or left working-end.
- *The terms "right and left" refer only to the bend in the design, NOT to a location for use in the mouth.*

EFFICIENT SEQUENCE FOR USE OF PAIRED MAGNETO WORKING-ENDS IN A TRANSVERSE ORIENTATION ON THE POSTERIOR TEETH

- The curved slim working-ends can be used with the transverse orientation to remove calculus deposits above and slightly beneath the gingival margin from the mesial and distal surfaces of posterior teeth.
- Instrumentation is accomplished most efficiently by completing all surfaces with the *right* working-end in the transverse orientation (Fig. 26-34) before switching to the *left* working-end (Fig. 26-35).

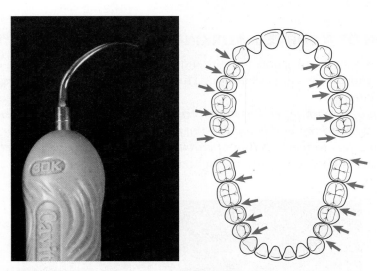

Figure 26-34. Use of the Right Tip in a Transverse Orientation.

- On the illustration, the proximal surfaces indicated by the *red arrows* can be debrided with the right slim-diameter tip using a transverse—curet-like—orientation. In this position the tip can remove calculus deposits located above and slightly below the gingival margin.

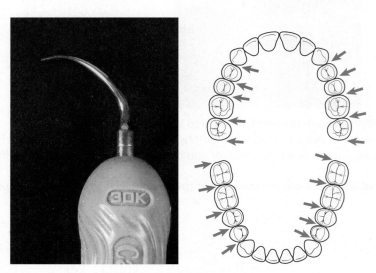

Figure 26-35. Use of the Left Tip in a Transverse Orientation.

- On the illustration, the proximal surfaces indicated by the *teal arrows* can be debrided with the left slim-diameter tip using a transverse—curet-like—orientation. In this position the tip can remove calculus deposits located above and slightly below the gingival margin.

USE OF PAIRED MAGNETO WORKING-ENDS IN A TRANSVERSE ORIENTATION

Figures 26-36 to 26-38 depict use of paired magneto working-ends in the transverse (curet-like) orientation to remove calculus deposits above and slightly beneath the gingival margin from the mesial and distal surfaces of posterior teeth. Curved slim tips can be adapted to the mesial and distal surfaces using a transverse, *curet-like*, orientation.

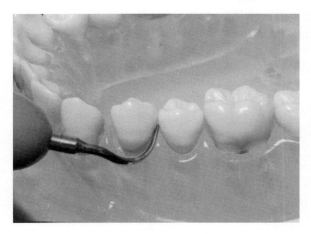

Figure 26-36. Transverse Orientation, Mandibular Left Sextant—Facial Aspect.
- The transverse orientation of the instrument tip is excellent for removing deposits apical to the contact area and deposits in the area of the CEJ.
- The photograph depicts the *right*-curved tip adapted to the mandibular left sextant. (Courtesy of DENTSPLY International.)

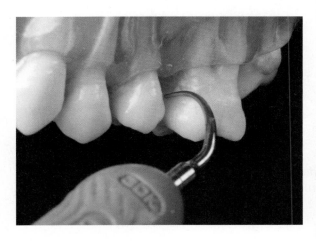

Figure 26-37. Transverse orientation, Maxillary Left Sextant—Facial Aspect. A *left*-curved tip adapted in a transverse orientation to the mesial surface of a maxillary first molar. (Courtesy of DENTSPLY International.)

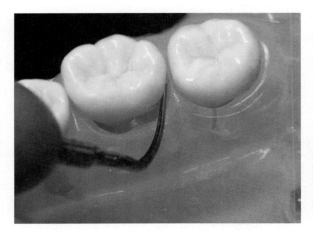

Figure 26-38. Transverse orientation, Mandibular Right Sextant—Lingual Aspect. An example of a *right*-curved tip adapted in a transverse orientation to a distal surface of the mandibular right posterior teeth, lingual aspect. (Courtesy of DENTSPLY International.)

EFFICIENT SEQUENCE FOR USE OF PAIRED MAGNETO WORKING-ENDS IN A VERTICAL ORIENTATION ON THE POSTERIOR TEETH

1. Curved working-ends come in right and left styles and both working-ends are needed to instrument the entire dentition.
2. The right- and left-curved powered working-ends are used in a vertical orientation to instrument root concavities, convexities, and furcation areas.
3. *Instrumentation is accomplished most efficiently by completing all surfaces with the right working-end (Fig. 26-39) before switching to the left working-end (Fig. 26-40).*
   A. For example, the clinician can use the right working-end in a transverse orientation to remove deposits above and slightly below the gingival margin.
   B. Next, the right working-end can be used in a vertical orientation for subgingival debridement of deep periodontal pockets.

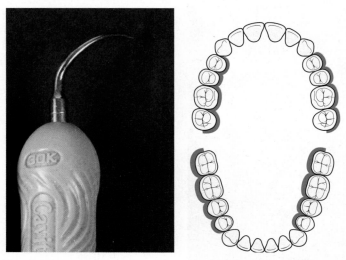

Figure 26-39. Utilization of a Right Curved Tip.
• On the illustration, the red line indicates the tooth surfaces that can be instrumented using the right–slim diameter tip using a vertical—probe-like—orientation.

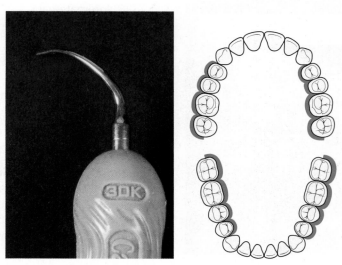

Figure 26-40. Utilization of a Left Curved Tip.
• On the illustration, the teal line indicates the tooth surfaces that can be instrumented using the left–slim diameter tip using a vertical—probe-like—orientation.

USE OF PAIRED MAGNETO WORKING-ENDS IN A VERTICAL ORIENTATION

Figures 26-41 to 26-43 depict use of paired magneto working-ends in a vertical (probe-like) orientation.

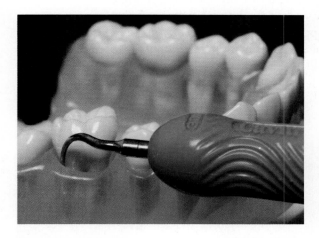

Figure 26-41. Vertical Orientation, Mandibular Right Facial—With Lateral Surface. This photograph shows a *right*-curved tip positioned in a similar manner to a periodontal probe with the lateral surface against the tooth surface being debrided. (Courtesy of DENTSPLY International.)

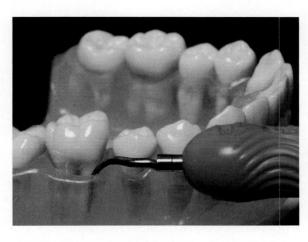

Figure 26-42. Vertical Orientation, Mandibular Right Facial—With Lateral Surface. This photograph shows a *right*-curved tip adapted to the mesiofacial line angle. As the tip moves onto the mesial surface the *back* of the tip will adapt well to the mesial root surface. (Courtesy of DENTSPLY International.)

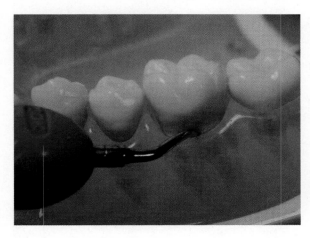

Figure 26-43. Vertical Orientation, Mandibular Left Facial—With Back Surface. This photograph shows the *back* of a *left*-curved tip adapted to the facial root surface. (Courtesy of DENTSPLY International.)

USE OF PAIRED MAGNETO WORKING-ENDS IN A VERTICAL ORIENTATION: CROSS ARCH FINGER REST FOR LINGUAL ASPECTS

The best adaptation to the lingual aspect of the mandibular and maxillary posterior teeth is achieved by adapting the back of a magneto tip to the tooth surface being treated. It can be difficult to adapt the back of the working-end to the lingual surfaces using a standard fulcrum. A cross arch fulcrum on the opposite side of the arch from the treatment area allows adaptation of the back of the instrument tip to the lingual aspects of the mandibular and maxillary arches (Figs. 26-44 to 26-46).

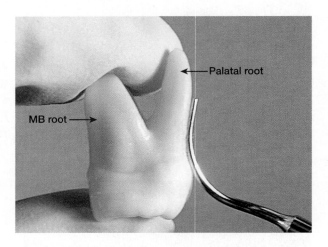

Figure 26-44. Palatal Roots of Maxillary Molars. On maxillary molars, the palatal root curves in a lingual direction. For this reason, the back surface of a curved slim tip adapts well to the palatal root. Use of a cross arch fulcrum facilitates adaptation of the back surface of a powered tip to the lingual aspect of the molar teeth.

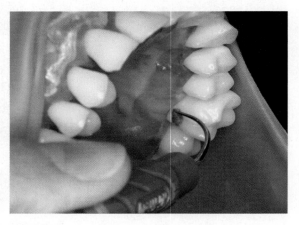

Figure 26-45. Cross Arch Fulcrum for the Lingual Aspects of the Maxillary Arch. The photo shows a cross arch fulcrum with the finger rest on the maxillary right posterior sextant. This cross arch fulcrum facilitates adaptation of the back surface of the tip to the lingual aspect of the maxillary left first molar tooth.

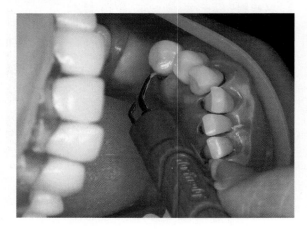

Figure 26-46. Cross Arch Fulcrum for the Lingual Aspects of the Mandibular Arch. In this example, a cross arch fulcrum is established on the mandibular anteriors. The powered tip is adapted in a vertical orientation to the lingual surface of the second premolar tooth.

Section 6
Use of Curved, Paired Piezo Working-Ends

 NOTE: This section discusses use of curved, paired **PIEZO** working-ends. Refer to Section 5 for use of paired **MAGNETO** working-ends.

IDENTIFICATION OF A CURVED WORKING-END AS "RIGHT" OR "LEFT"

- Curved powered working-ends come in right and left styles and both working-ends are needed to instrument the entire dentition. This is similar in concept to using two posterior Gracey curets.
- *The identification of a working-end as either "right" or "left" does NOT refer the location that the working-end is used in the mouth. Rather, the "right" or "left" designation refers to the direction of curvature of the working-end, itself.* Figure 26-47 describes how to identify the right and left working-ends.

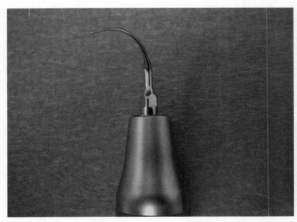 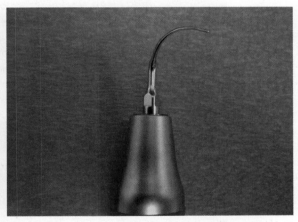

Figure 26-47. Identifying the Right and Left Curved Working-Ends. (A) Left Working-End. (B) Right Working-End.

- A curved working-end is identified as "right" or "left" by turning the insert so the "point" faces away from the clinician. With the insert in this position, the direction that a working-end bends identifies it as a right or left working-end.
- *The terms "right and left" refer only to the bend in the design, NOT to a location for use in the mouth.*

EFFICIENT SEQUENCE FOR USE OF PAIRED PIEZO WORKING-ENDS IN A TRANSVERSE ORIENTATION ON THE POSTERIOR TEETH

- The curved slim working-ends can be used with the transverse orientation to remove calculus deposits above and slightly beneath the gingival margin from the mesial and distal surfaces of posterior teeth.
- Instrumentation is accomplished most efficiently by completing all surfaces with the *right* working-end in the transverse orientation (Fig. 26-48) before switching to the *left* working-end (Fig. 26-49).

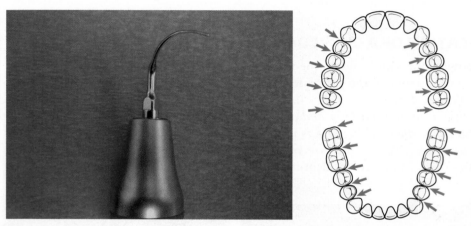

Figure 26-48. Use of the Right Working-End in a Transverse Orientation.
- On the illustration, the proximal surfaces indicated by the *red arrows* can be debrided with the curved right working-end using a transverse orientation. In this position the working-end can remove calculus deposits located above and slightly below the gingival margin.

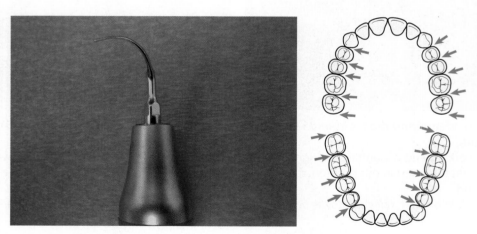

Figure 26-49. Use of the Left Working-End in a Transverse Orientation.
- On the illustration, the proximal surfaces indicated by the *teal arrows* can be debrided with the curved left working-end using a transverse orientation. In this position the working-end can remove calculus deposits located above and slightly below the gingival margin.

USE OF PAIRED PIEZO WORKING-ENDS IN A TRANSVERSE ORIENTATION

Figures 26-50 to 26-52 depict use of paired piezo working-ends in the transverse (curet-like) orientation to remove calculus deposits above and slightly beneath the gingival margin from the mesial and distal surfaces of posterior teeth.

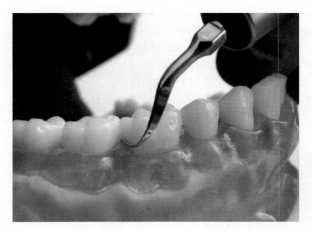

Figure 26-50. Transverse Orientation—Facial Aspect.
- Curved slim working-ends can be adapted to the mesial and distal surfaces using a transverse orientation.
- The transverse orientation of the instrument working-end is excellent for removing deposits apical to the contact area and deposits in the region of the CEJ.

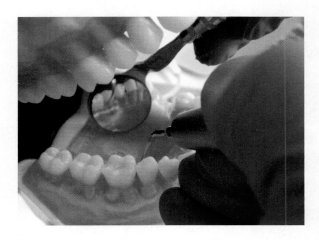

Figure 26-51. Transverse Orientation—Lingual Aspect. An example of a right-curved working-end adapted in a transverse orientation to a proximal surface of the mandibular right posterior teeth, lingual aspect.

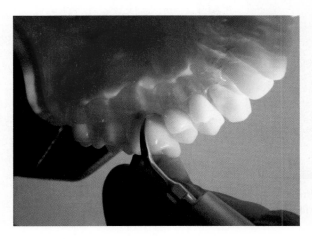

Figure 26-52. Transverse Orientation—Lingual Aspect. A right-curved working-end adapted in a transverse orientation to the mesial surface of a maxillary first molar.

EFFICIENT SEQUENCE FOR USE OF PAIRED PIEZO WORKING-ENDS IN A VERTICAL ORIENTATION ON THE POSTERIOR TEETH

1. Curved working-ends come in right and left styles and both working-ends are needed to instrument the entire dentition.
2. The right- and left-curved powered working-ends are used in a vertical orientation to instrument root concavities, convexities, and furcation areas.
3. *Instrumentation is accomplished most efficiently by completing all surfaces with the right working-end (Fig. 26-53) before switching to the left working-end (Fig. 26-54).*
    A. For example, the clinician can use the right working-end in a transverse orientation to remove deposits above and slightly below the gingival margin.
    B. Next, the right working-end can be used in a vertical orientation for subgingival debridement of deep periodontal pockets.

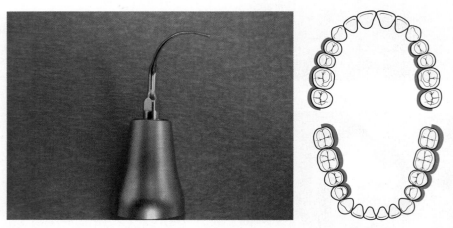

Figure 26-53. Utilization of a Right Curved Working-End.
- On the illustration, the red line indicates the tooth surfaces that can be instrumented using the curved right slim perio working-end in a vertical orientation.

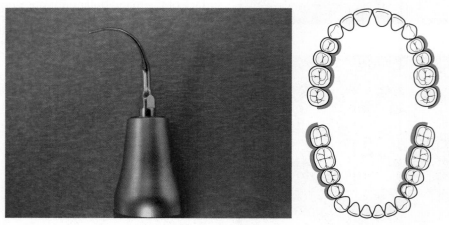

Figure 26-54. Utilization of a Left Curved Working-End.
- On the illustration, the teal line indicates the tooth surfaces that can be instrumented using the curved left slim perio working-end in a vertical orientation.

Section 7
Instrumentation Challenges

REMOVING STUBBORN CALCULUS DEPOSITS

A common misconception among clinicians who are new to powered instrumentation is the belief that a single quick swipe over a deposit will remove it. Powered instruments are very effective at removing calculus deposits, but they are not magic wands. *Adequate time must be spent on any calculus deposit to remove it. A calculus deposit will not vanish in a single stroke, but rather, the deposit will develop micro-fractures as it is exposed to the powered working-end during a series of gentle strokes.*

Effective strategies for removing stubborn calculus deposits include:

1. Select the Proper Working-End For the Task. As with hand instruments, the instrument working-end is selected based on the size and location of the calculus deposit.
   A. Standard Working-Ends. Use standard working-ends to remove moderate to heavy deposits above the gingival margin and in shallow pockets.
   B. Slim Perio Working-Ends. Use slim perio working-ends to remove light to moderate calculus deposits on anterior teeth and on posterior root surfaces.
2. Use a Working-End that Can Withstand Medium Power for Stubborn Deposits. Low power will not be effective in removing tenacious calculus deposits. The working-end selected should be a standard working-end used at a medium-power setting.
3. Maintain Proper Control and Adaptation. It is important to control the movement of the powered working-end so that the 2 to 4 mm active working-end area is adapted to the calculus deposit and many overlapping strokes cover each section of the deposit.
4. Attack a Stubborn Deposit from all Directions. Approach a deposit from a variety of directions. For example, interproximal deposits can be approached from both the facial and lingual aspects. Vertical and oblique strokes are most effective for medium calculus deposits. Horizontal strokes work well for subgingival biofilm removal.
5. Use the Correct Surface of the Powered Working-End. The lateral surfaces of a powered working-end should be used for calculus removal and subgingival biofilm removal.
6. Change to a Different Working-End. Standard working-ends that are round in cross section are less effective in removing stubborn calculus deposits. Standard working-ends with beveled edges or a straight edge with a corner perform better for removing heavy deposits.
7. Begin with a Hand-Activated Periodontal File. Sometimes it is most effective to use a hand-activated periodontal file to fracture a tenacious deposit and follow with a powered instrument working-end.
8. Increase the Power. If all the above strategies fail to remove the deposit, it will be necessary to increase the power setting. In this instance, it would be best to use one of the powered working-ends that are specially designed to withstand a higher-power setting.

SMOOTHING DEFECTIVE MARGINS ON RESTORATIONS

A recontouring procedure is used to correct defective margins of restorations ("overhang") to provide a smooth surface that will deter bacterial accumulation. If a minor amalgam overhang—such as that pictured in Figure 26-55—is acting as a plaque biofilm trap, the excess amalgam can be removed using a specialized powered instrument working-end for this purpose. Figures 26-56 and 26-57 show examples of specialized powered instruments that are effective in smoothing defective amalgam restorations.

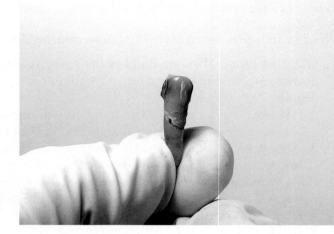

Figure 26-55. Amalgam Overhang. This tooth has an excess of amalgam protruding out from the surface of the tooth. If this tooth were still in the mouth, the amalgam overhang would retain plaque biofilm.

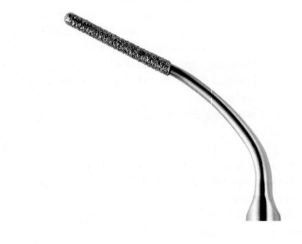

Figure 26-56. A Diamond Coated Working-End. This EMS/Hu-Friedy working-end is an example of diamond-coated working-end used for smoothing defective margins on Dental restorations. (Courtesy of Hu-Friedy Mfg. Co, LLC.)

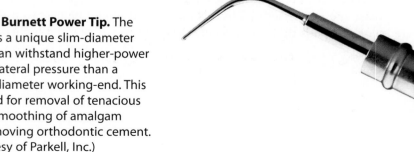

Figure 26-57. The Burnett Power Tip. The Burnett Power Tip is a unique slim-diameter working-end that can withstand higher-power settings and more lateral pressure than a conventional slim-diameter working-end. This tip is recommended for removal of tenacious calculus deposits, smoothing of amalgam overhangs, and removing orthodontic cement. (Photograph courtesy of Parkell, Inc.)

INSTRUMENTING FURCATION AREAS OF MULTI-ROOTED TEETH

Slim perio instrument working-ends are more effective than hand instruments in treating Class II and III furcation areas (12,39,78).

- Standard Gracey curets are too wide to enter the furcation areas of over 50% of all maxillary and mandibular molars (Figs. 26-58 and 26-59).
- The average facial furcation entrance of maxillary and mandibular first molars is from 0.63 to 1.04 mm in width.
- The width of a standard Gracey curet ranges from 0.76 to 1 mm.
- The diameter of a slim perio working-end is 0.55 mm or less in size.

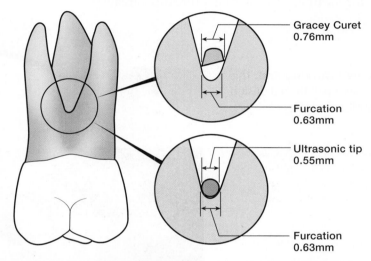

Figure 26-58. Furcation Entrances on a Maxillary First Molar.

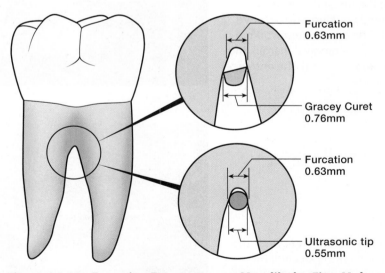

Figure 26-59. Furcation Entrances on a Mandibular First Molar.

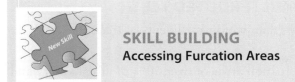

SKILL BUILDING
Accessing Furcation Areas

Certain manufacturers offer specialized powered working-ends with a ball-tipped design for use in the furcation areas of multirooted teeth (Fig. 26-60). The ball-tipped working-end offers a greater surface area for gentle, more thorough debridement of the furcation area. Figures 26-61 and 26-62 depict the technique for locating and entering a furcation area.

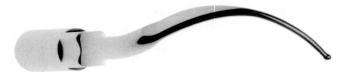

Figure 26-60. Ball-Tipped Working-End. This powered working-end has a ball-tipped design. (Courtesy of Hu-Friedy Mfg. Co, LLC.)

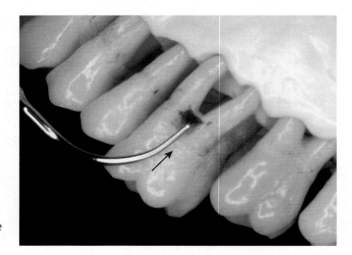

Figure 26-61. Locating a Furcation. The easiest way to locate the furcation area is to **deactivate** the powered working-end (remove foot from foot pedal). The deactivated working-end is inserted beneath the gingival margin and moved in an oblique direction until the entrance to the furcation is detected.

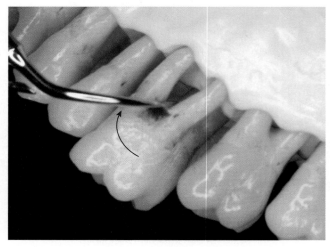

Figure 26-62. Enter Furcation Area. Once the entrance to the furcation area is located, the working-end is turned while rotating the wrist. This twisting motion allows the working-end to access the roof of the furcation. Once the working-end is activated, the ball end is rolled back and forth across the entire roof of the furcation area.

Section 8
Technique Hints for Powered Instrumentation

PATIENT AND CLINICIAN PREPARATION

1. Patient Preparation
   A. As with any treatment procedure, it is important to describe and explain the powered instrumentation procedure to the patient and obtain informed consent for the procedure. The clinician should explain the purpose and functioning of the ultrasonic device, as well as, the water spray and need for evacuation. The patient should be encouraged to ask questions.
   B. A preprocedural rinse for the patient is recommended to reduce the bacterial load in the aerosols generated and released into the surrounding environment during power instrumentation (79–81).
      1. A 1-minute mouthrinse with an antimicrobial mouthwash is recommended for all patients prior to initiation of any type of powered instrumentation.
      2. A preprocedural rinse, however, will not affect blood coming from the operative site or viruses coming from the respiratory tract. A preprocedural rinse should not be relied upon to prevent airborne contamination.
   C. Personal protective gear for the patient is mandatory and should include a plastic or disposable drape, and protective eyewear.
      1. The patient may prefer to cover the nose with a flat-style mask to limit inhalation of aerosols.
      2. Water spray accidentally directed into the eye may cause ocular injury. *During treatment it is strongly recommended that both the clinician and the patient wear eye protection.* Figure 26-63 shows a patient protective mask available from Crosstex.
   D. Nonpetroleum product should be applied to cover the patient's lips for protection from the water spray that may irritate or chap the lips.

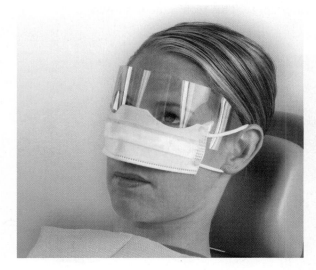

Figure 26-63. Patient Protective Mask. Water spray accidentally directed into the eye may cause ocular injury. During treatment it is strongly recommended that the patient wear eye protection. This patient mask incorporates a flat mask to cover the patient's nose and a face shield to protect the eyes. (Photo courtesy of Crosstex.)

2. Personal Protective Equipment for the Clinician
   A. The clinician should wear a gown with a high neck and long sleeves, mask, protective eyewear and gloves.
   B. A high bacterial filtration efficiency (BFE) mask is recommended for all powered instrumentation procedures (29). By definition, a BFE mask effectively filters out 98% of particles that are three microns or larger in size.
      1. If wearing a face shield, the clinician should also don a facemask, as a face shield does not protect the clinician from breathing in aerosols.
      2. Because of the high level of aerosols generated by powered instrumentation, masks should be changed every 20 minutes, as a damp mask will not provide adequate protection.

FLUID CONTAINMENT DURING INSTRUMENTATION

1. Evacuation for Reduction of Airborne Contamination
   A. During treatment, evacuator working-ends should be used for fluid control. Research on the effectiveness of high-volume evacuator working-ends is conflicting on whether these devices reduce airborne aerosol contamination (82). Additional research is needed on this topic.
   B. It is important to use the *vented* style of evacuator tip for fluid containment. The vent allows the HVE working-end to function without pulling ("suctioning up") soft tissues (cheeks, tongue) into the end of the evacuator working-end.
2. Cupping Techniques for Water Containment. It can be very frustrating for the patient to have his or her face and hair sprayed with the water from the powered tip.
   A. Good water containment can be achieved through a combination of evacuation and use of the patient's lips and cheeks as fluid-deflecting barriers.
   B. When working on the mandibular anterior teeth, pulling the patient's lip up and out away from the teeth allows the lip to act as a barrier to deflect the water back into the mouth and as a "cup" to collect the water for evacuation. Figure 26-64 demonstrates this technique.
   C. A similar technique is used for the posterior teeth, holding the cheek away from the teeth creates a "cheek cup" to catch the water spray. This technique is shown in Figure 26-65.

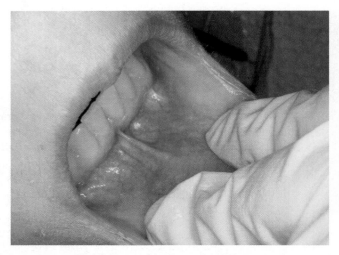 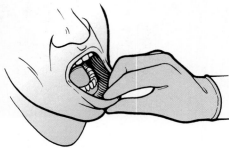

Figure 26-64. Fluid Control in Anterior Sextants. For anterior sextants, the lower and upper lips can be cupped to contain the water spray.

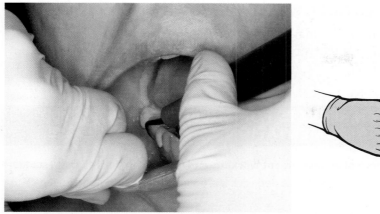
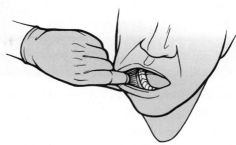

Figure 26-65. Fluid Control in Posterior Treatment Areas. For posterior treatment areas, hold the cheek between the thumb and index finger and pull out and up, or down, to form a cup.

HANDPIECE CORD MANAGEMENT

Some clinicians find that the cord tends to weigh down the end of the handpiece or causes the handpiece to twist during instrumentation. Two techniques that are helpful in reducing the pull of the cord on the handpiece are wrapping the cord around the forearm or resting it in the palm of the hand around the thumb. These techniques are depicted in Figures 26-66 and 26-67.

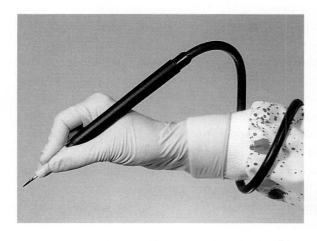

Figure 26-66. Cord Management Strategy #1. One technique for lessening the weight and pull of the handpiece cord is to wrap it around the forearm.

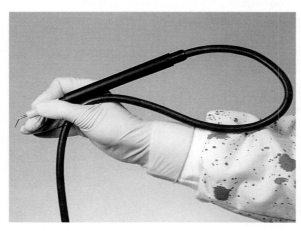

Figure 26-67. Cord Management Strategy #2. Another technique for lessening the pull of the handpiece cord is to rest it in the palm of the hand and loop it around the thumb.

TEN SECRETS FOR SUCCESSFUL POWERED INSTRUMENTATION

Dr. Larry Burnett of Portland, Oregon—a master at powered instrumentation—has developed what he refers to as his "secrets for powered instrumentation". Dr. Burnett's "secrets" are summarized in Table 26-6.

TABLE 26-6. TEN SECRETS FOR SUCCESSFUL POWERED INSTRUMENTATION

1. **Insert Selection. Don't ask more of an instrument working-end than it can deliver.** Use a standard working-end for large- or medium-sized calculus deposits. Use a slim perio working-end for small- to medium-sized deposits.

2. **Power Setting. Set the power setting lower than you think is necessary.** Use medium power settings for calculus removal and low power settings for deplaquing.

3. **Water Flow. Use more water than you think is necessary.** Ensure that the water flow is hitting the active portion of the working-end. Adjust the water until a halo of water surrounds the working-end or until a rapid drip is achieved.

4. **Grasp. Use a lighter grasp than you think is necessary.** Powered instrumentation requires a light, re-laxed grasp similar to that used when probing.

5. **Finger Rest. Use a more stable finger rest than you think is necessary.** Use a stable standard intraoral finger rest or an advanced finger rest.

6. **Angulation. Use less angulation than with a hand instrument.** Approach the deposit from its edge. The lateral surface-to-tooth angulation should be as near to 0 degrees as possible and should never exceed 15 degrees.

7. **Lateral Pressure. Use much less lateral pressure than with hand instrumentation.** Touch the lateral surface of the powered working-end lightly (gently) against the deposit or tooth surface. Moderate or firm pressure decreases the effectiveness of the instrument working-end and can even stop the working-end vibrations all together! Powered instrumentation requires a light touch.

8. **Activation. Use more finger motion than you would with a hand instrument.** Digital (finger) activa-tion is excellent for applying the light stroke pressure needed for powered instrumentation.

9. **Working-End Motion. Never allow the instrument working-end to be idle**. Keep the instrument working-end moving at all times. Never continue to hold the working-end on any one spot.

10. **Stroke Technique. Give each tooth adequate attention.** The powered working-end needs to be moved over a calculus deposit for some time in order to remove it.
    - Slower, repetitive strokes are more effective in removing large or tenacious calculus deposits.
    - Cover every millimeter of a root surface with overlapping, horizontal, vertical, and oblique brush-like strokes.

Section 9
Set-Up of an Ultrasonic Unit

SKILL BUILDING
Steps for Set-Up of a Piezo or Magneto Ultrasonic Unit

Directions: Certain steps should be followed when setting-up an ultrasonic device.

- Clinicians should follow the set-up instructions provided by the manufacturer for the individual ultrasonic device.
- Figures 26-68 through 26-75 depict steps that are common to most ultrasonic devices.

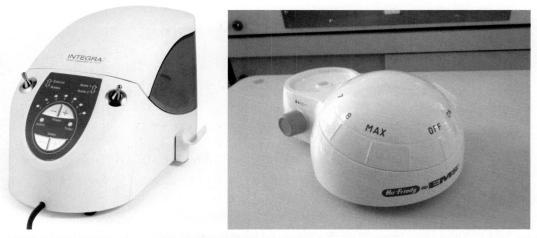

Figure 26-68. Locate the Device on a Stable Work Service. Place the ultrasonic device on a stable countertop or cart so you will have easy access to the device at the dental chair.

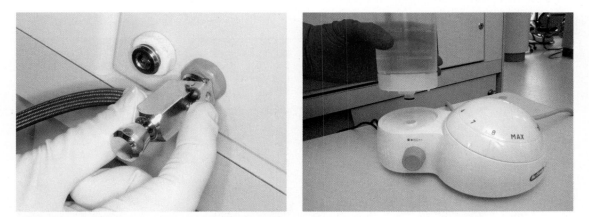

Figure 26-69. Connect the Water/Fluid Supply. As shown in the photo on the left, connect the water supply line from the ultrasonic device to the water outlet on the dental unit. Turn on the dental unit and if necessary, open the dental unit's water control knob. Or, if using a device with an independent fluid reservoir, attach the reservoir to the ultrasonic device, as shown in the right-hand photo.

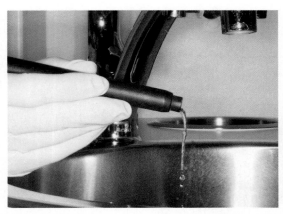
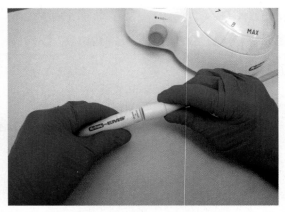

Figure 26-70. Connect Ultrasonic Handpiece and Flush the Water Line Tubing. Attach the handpiece to the ultrasonic cord. Flush the water tubing of stagnant water by holding the handpiece or tubing over a sink and stepping on the foot pedal to activate a steady stream of water. At the start of each day, flush the tubing for a minimum 2 minutes. Between patients, flush the tubing for at least 30 seconds.

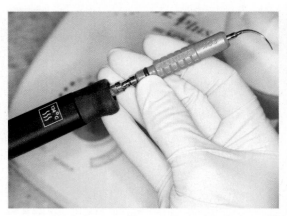
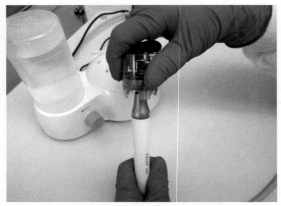

Figure 26-71. Select and Insert/Attach a Powered Working-End. Select an appropriate working-end for the instrumentation. The left-hand photo shows an ultrasonic device that has a metal rod-type insert that is placed into the handpiece. Other ultrasonic devices have tips that are attached to the handpiece with a wrench, as shown above in the right-hand photo.

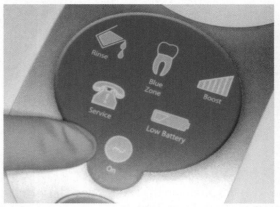
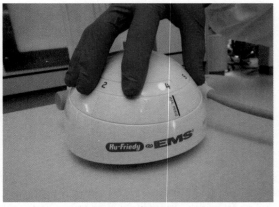

Figure 26-72. Turn on the Ultrasonic Device and Select an Appropriate Power Setting. Set the desired power level for instrumentation. Select an appropriate power setting for the particular working-end (standard-diameter, slim-diameter) and the type of calculus deposit.

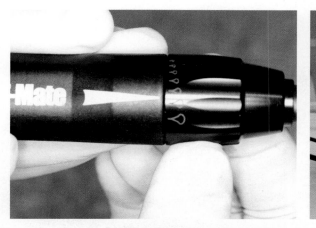
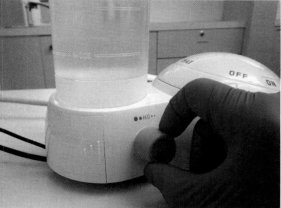

Figure 26-73. Set the Irrigation Flow Rate. Adjust the irrigation flow to create a light mist at the powered working-end.

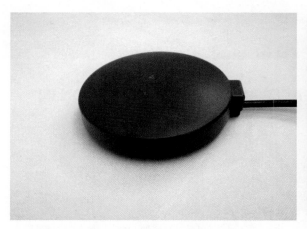
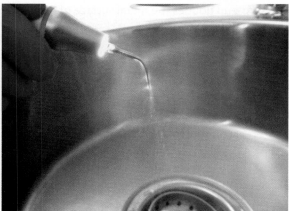

Figure 26-74. Check the Irrigation Spray. Use the foot pedal to activate the handpiece over a sink. Check that the irrigation spray to the working-end is adequate; ultrasonic instrument working-ends must be cooled by fluid to prevent overheating.

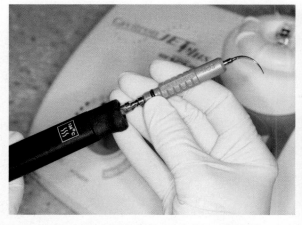
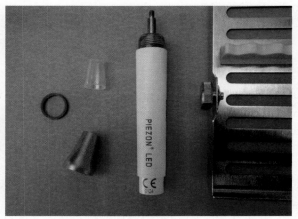

Figure 26-75. End of Treatment: Disassembly and Sterilization. At the end of treatment, disassemble the device. Follow manufacturer's recommendations for sterilization.

Section 10
Skill Application

Directions: Refer to Figures 26-76 to 26-78 to practice ultrasonic technique.

PRACTICAL FOCUS: ADAPTATION OF POWERED WORKING-END

Figure 26-76. Painted Can Practice. Use a painted metal can, such as a decorated cookie tin, to practice correct adaptation of a powered working-end. Practice using the lateral surface to remove the paint from the can using light lateral pressure.

- The lateral surface of the working-end should glide over the surface of the can in a smooth, even manner.
- If the working-end skips off of the surface of the metal (chatters) your technique is incorrect. If the working-end gouges the metal surface of the can, the technique is incorrect.

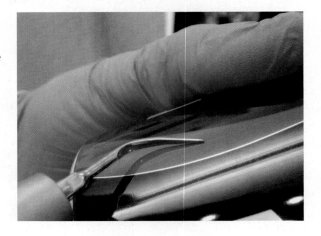

PRACTICAL FOCUS: THE LATERAL SURFACES ARE "WHERE THE ACTION IS!"

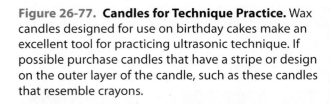

Figure 26-77. Candles for Technique Practice. Wax candles designed for use on birthday cakes make an excellent tool for practicing ultrasonic technique. If possible purchase candles that have a stripe or design on the outer layer of the candle, such as these candles that resemble crayons.

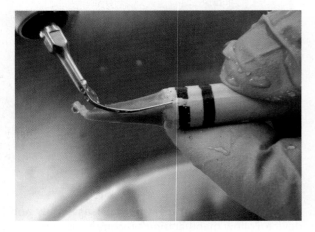
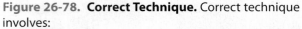
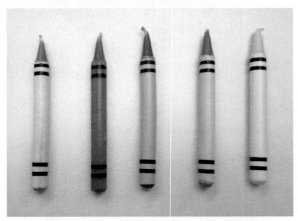

Figure 26-78. Correct Technique. Correct technique involves:
- Adapting a lateral surface of the working-end to the wax candle and using a very light stroke over the surface of the candle.
- Removing the black design from the surface of the candle without gouging the wax.
- Gouging of the candle wax is an indication of too much stroke pressure. Remember the powered working-end does all the work for the clinician.

FICTITIOUS PATIENT CASE: MR. BURLINGTON

Directions: Refer to Figures 26-79A–F for fictitious patient, Mr. Burlington.

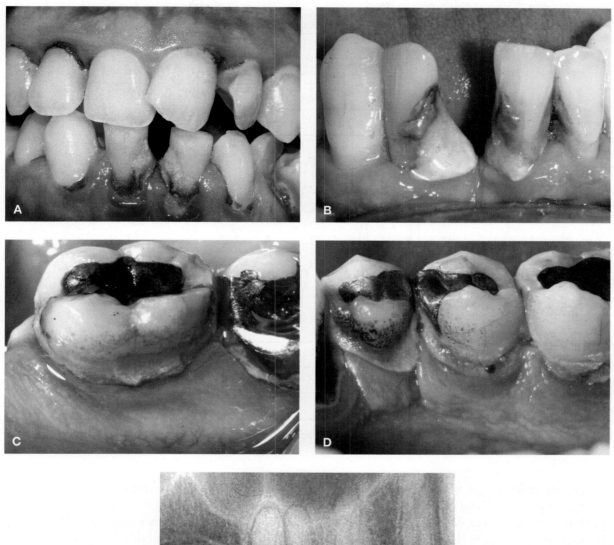

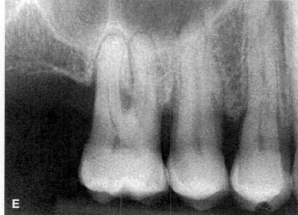

Figures 26-79. **A–E. Intraoral Photos and Periapical Radiograph for Mr. Burlington**

Mr. Burlington: Assessment Data
- Bleeding—generalized heavy bleeding upon probing.
- Subgingival calculus deposits—Medium- to large-sized deposits on all surfaces.
- Subgingival calculus deposits—medium-sized deposits on all surfaces.

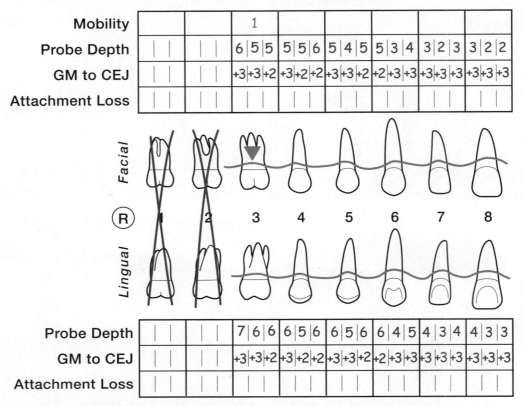

			1																
Mobility			1																
Probe Depth			6|5|5	5|5|6	5|4|5	5|3|4	3|2|3	3|2|2
GM to CEJ			+3|+3|+2	+3|+2|+2	+3|+3|+2	+2|+3|+3	+3|+3|+3	+3|+3|+3
Attachment Loss								

Facial / Lingual — R — 1 2 3 4 5 6 7 8

Probe Depth			7|6|6	6|5|6	6|5|6	6|4|5	4|3|4	4|3|3
GM to CEJ			+3|+3|+2	+3|+2|+2	+3|+3|+2	+2|+3|+3	+3|+3|+3	+3|+3|+3
Attachment Loss								

Figure 26-79. F. Mr. Burlington: Periodontal Chart for Maxillary Right Quadrant

Mr. Burlington: Case Questions
1. *Use the information recorded on Mr. Burlington's chart to calculate the attachment loss on the facial and lingual aspects for teeth #'s 3 to 8.*
2. Does the assessment data indicate normal bone levels or bone loss in this quadrant? Does the assessment data indicate healthy sulci or periodontal pockets in this quadrant? Explain which data you used to make these determinations?
3. Do you expect to instrument any root concavities or furcation areas in this quadrant? If so, indicate which teeth will probably have root concavities and/or furcation areas to be instrumented.
4. Imagine that the three remaining quadrants of the dentition are very similar to the quadrant shown in Figure 26-79F. Based on the assessment information, develop a plan for calculus removal and deplaquing for Mr. Burlington.
   A. Determine how many appointments you will need for calculus removal.
   B. List the treatment area(s) to be completed at each appointment.
   C. List appropriate powered working-ends for use at each appointment. Indicate the sequence the powered working-end use and the size and location of the deposits each powered working-end will remove.

References

1. Arabaci T, Cicek Y, Canakci CF. Sonic and ultrasonic scalers in periodontal treatment: a review. *Int J Dent Hyg.* 2007;5(1):2–12.
2. Flemming TF. Ultrasonics and periodontal pathogens. *Dimens Dent Hyg.* 2007;5(10):14–18.
3. Schenk G, Flemmig TF, Lob S, Ruckdeschel G, Hickel R. Lack of antimicrobial effect on periodontopathic bacteria by ultrasonic and sonic scalers in vitro. *J Clin Periodontol.* 2000;27(2):116–119.
4. Cobb CM. Clinical significance of non-surgical periodontal therapy: an evidence-based perspective of scaling and root planing. *J Clin Periodontol.* 2002;29(Suppl 2):6–16.
5. Hallmon WW, Rees TD. Local anti-infective therapy: mechanical and physical approaches. A systematic review. *Ann Periodontol.* 2003;8(1):99–114.
6. Drisko CL, Cochran DL, Blieden T, et al. Position paper: sonic and ultrasonic scalers in periodontics. Research, Science and Therapy Committee of the American Academy of Periodontology. *J Periodontol.* 2000;71(11):1792–1801.
7. Dragoo MR. A clinical evaluation of hand and ultrasonic instruments on subgingival debridement. 1. With unmodified and modified ultrasonic inserts. *Int J Periodontics Restorative Dent.* 1992;12(4):310–323.
8. Rateitschak-Pluss EM, Schwarz JP, Guggenheim R, Duggelin M, Rateitschak KH. Non-surgical periodontal treatment: where are the limits? An SEM study. *J Clin Periodontol.* 1992;19(4):240–244.
9. Shiloah J, Hovious LA. The role of subgingival irrigations in the treatment of periodontitis. *J Periodontol.* 1993;64(9):835–843.
10. Walmsley AD, Laird WR, Lumley PJ. Ultrasound in dentistry. Part 2–Periodontology and endodontics. *J Dent.* 1992;20(1):11–17.
11. Young NA. Periodontal debridement: re-examining non-surgical instrumentation. Part I: a new perspective on the objectives of instrumentation. *Semin Dent Hyg.* 1994;4(4):1–7.
12. Bower RC. Furcation morphology relative to periodontal treatment. Furcation entrance architecture. *J Periodontol.* 1979;50(1):23–27.
13. Leon LE, Vogel RI. A comparison of the effectiveness of hand scaling and ultrasonic debridement in furcations as evaluated by differential dark-field microscopy. *J Periodontol.* 1987;58(2):86–94.
14. Nosal G, Scheidt MJ, O'Neal R, Van Dyke TE. The penetration of lavage solution into the periodontal pocket during ultrasonic instrumentation. *J Periodontol.* 1991;62(9):554–557.
15. Chapple IL, Walmsley AD, Saxby MS, Moscrop H. Effect of instrument power setting during ultrasonic scaling upon treatment outcome. *J Periodontol.* 1995;66(9):756–760.
16. Tunkel J, Heinecke A, Flemmig TF. A systematic review of efficacy of machine-driven and manual subgingival debridement in the treatment of chronic periodontitis. *J Clin Periodontol.* 2002;29(Suppl 3):72–81; discussion 90–91.
17. Khambay BS, Walmsley AD. Acoustic microstreaming: detection and measurement around ultrasonic scalers. *J Periodontol.* 1999;70(6):626–631.
18. Khosravi M, Bahrami ZS, Atabaki MS, Shokrgozar MA, Shokri F. Comparative effectiveness of hand and ultrasonic instrumentations in root surface planing in vitro. *J Clin Periodontol.* 2004;31(3):160–165.
19. Baehni P, Thilo B, Chapuis B, Pernet D. Effects of ultrasonic and sonic scalers on dental plaque microflora in vitro and in vivo. *J Clin Periodontol.* 1992;19(7):455–459.
20. Jepsen S, Ayna M, Hedderich J, Eberhard J. Significant influence of scaler tip design on root substance loss resulting from ultrasonic scaling: a laserprofilometric in vitro study. *J Clin Periodontol.* 2004;31(11):1003–1006.
21. Gautschi G. *Piezoelectric Sensorics : Force, Strain, Pressure, Acceleration and Acoustic Emission Sensors, Materials and Amplifiers.* Berlin, New York: Springer; 2002. xiii, 264 p.
22. Koster TJ, Timmerman MF, Feilzer AJ, Van der Velden U, Van der Weijden FA. Water coolant supply in relation to different ultrasonic scaler systems, tips and coolant settings. *J Clin Periodontol.* 2009;36(2):127–131.
23. Slots J. Selection of antimicrobial agents in periodontal therapy. *J Periodontal Res.* 2002;37(5):389–398.
24. Costerton JW, Stewart PS, Greenberg EP. Bacterial biofilms: a common cause of persistent infections. *Science.* 1999;284(5418):1318–1322.
25. Gilbert P, Das J, Foley I. Biofilm susceptibility to antimicrobials. *Adv Dent Res.* 1997;11(1):160–167.
26. Nield-Gehrig JS, Willmann DE. *Foundations of Periodontics for the Dental Hygienist.* 3rd ed. Philadelphia, PA: Wolters Kluwer Health/Lippincott Williams & Wilkins; 2011. xvi, 688 p.
27. Daniel SJ, Harfst SA, Wilder RS. *Mosby's Dental Hygiene: Concepts, Cases and Competencies.* 2nd ed. St. Louis, MO: Mosby/Elsevier; 2008. xxii, 1017 p.
28. Wilkins EM. *Clinical Practice of the Dental Hygienist.* 9th ed. Philadelphia, PA: Lippincott Williams & Wilkins; 2005. xxi, 1189 p.
29. Scannapieco FA, Bush RB, Paju S. Associations between periodontal disease and risk for nosocomial bacterial pneumonia and chronic obstructive pulmonary disease. A systematic review. *Ann Periodontol.* 2003;8(1):54–69.
30. Suzuki JB, Delisle AL. Pulmonary actinomycosis of periodontal origin. *J Periodontol.* 1984;55(10):581–584.
31. Lahor-Soler E, Miranda-Rius J, Brunet-Llobet L, Sabate de la Cruz X. Capacity of dental equipment to interfere with cardiac implantable electrical devices. *Eur J Oral Sci.* 2015;123(3):194–201.
32. Garcia JM, Chambers E, 4th, Clark M, Helverson J, Matta Z. Quality of care issues for dysphagia: modifications involving oral fluids. *J Clin Nurs.* 2010;19(11–12):1618–1624.
33. Paramashivaiah R, Prabhuji ML. Mechanized scaling with ultrasonics: perils and proactive measures. *J Indian Soc Periodontol.* 2013;17(4):423–428.
34. Arabaci T, Cicek Y, Ozgoz M, Canakci V, Canakci CF, Eltas A. The comparison of the effects of three types of piezoelectric ultrasonic tips and air polishing system on the filling materials: an in vitro study. *Int J Dent Hyg.* 2007;5(4):205–210.
35. Mann M, Parmar D, Walmsley AD, Lea SC. Effect of plastic-covered ultrasonic scalers on titanium implant surfaces. *Clin Oral Implants Res.* 2012;23(1):76–82.

36. Garg SK, Mittal S, Kaur P. Dental unit waterline management: historical perspectives and current trends. *J Investig Clin Dent*. 2012;3(4):247–252.

37. Guidelines for infection control in dental health-care settings–2003. *MMWR Recomm Rep*. 2003;52(RR-17):1–61.

38. Bennett AM, Fulford MR, Walker JT, Bradshaw DJ, Martin MV, Marsh PD. Microbial aerosols in general dental practice. *Br Dent J*. 2000;189(12):664–667.

39. Holbrook WP, Muir KF, Macphee IT, Ross PW. Bacteriological investigation of the aerosol from ultrasonic scalers. *Br Dent J*. 1978;144(8):245–247.

40. Micik RE, Miller RL, Mazzarella MA, Ryge G. Studies on dental aerobiology. I. Bacterial aerosols generated during dental procedures. *J Dent Res*. 1969;48(1):49–56.

41. Harrel SK. Contaminated dental aerosols: the risks and implications for dental hygienists. *Dimens Dent Hyg*. 2003;1(6):16–20.

42. Harrel SK, Molinari J. Aerosols and splatter in dentistry: a brief review of the literature and infection control implications. *J Am Dent Assoc*. 2004;135(4):429–437.

43. Miller RL, Micik RE. Air pollution and its control in the dental office. *Dent Clin North Am*. 1978;22(3):453–476.

44. Molinari JA, Harte JA, Cottone JA. *Cottone's Practical Infection Control in Dentistry*. 3rd ed. Philadelphia, PA: Wolters Kluwer Health/Lippincott William & Wilkins; 2010. xv, 329 p.

45. Bentley CD, Burkhart NW, Crawford JJ. Evaluating spatter and aerosol contamination during dental procedures. *J Am Dent Assoc*. 1994;125(5):579–584.

46. Gross KB, Overman PR, Cobb C, Brockmann S. Aerosol generation by two ultrasonic scalers and one sonic scaler. A comparative study. *J Dent Hyg*. 1992;66(7):314–318.

47. King TB, Muzzin KB, Berry CW, Anders LM. The effectiveness of an aerosol reduction device for ultrasonic scalers. *J Periodontol*. 1997;68(1):45–49.

48. Legnani P, Checchi L, Pelliccioni GA, D'Achille C. Atmospheric contamination during dental procedures. *Quintessence Int*. 1994;25(6):435–439.

49. Logothetis DD, Gross KB, Eberhart A, Drisko C. Bacterial airborne contamination with an air-polishing device. *Gen Dent*. 1988;36(6):496–499.

50. Muzzin KB, King TB, Berry CW. Assessing the clinical effectiveness of an aerosol reduction device for the air polisher. *J Am Dent Assoc*. 1999;130(9):1354–1359.

51. Rivera-Hidalgo F, Barnes JB, Harrel SK. Aerosol and splatter production by focused spray and standard ultrasonic inserts. *J Periodontol*. 1999;70(5):473–477.

52. Trenter SC, Walmsley AD. Ultrasonic dental scaler: associated hazards. *J Clin Periodontol*. 2003;30(2):95–101.

53. Barnes JB, Harrel SK, Rivera-Hidalgo F. Blood contamination of the aerosols produced by in vivo use of ultrasonic scalers. *J Periodontol*. 1998;69(4):434–438.

54. Harrel SK. Clinical use of an aerosol-reduction device with an ultrasonic scaler. *Compend Contin Educ Dent*. 1996;17(12):1185–1193; quiz 94.

55. Basu MK, Browne RM, Potts AJ, Harrington JM. A survey of aerosol-related symptoms in dental hygienists. *J Soc Occup Med*. 1988;38(1–2):23–25.

56. Cherniack M, Brammer AJ, Nilsson T, et al. Nerve conduction and sensorineural function in dental hygienists using high frequency ultrasound handpieces. *Am J Ind Med*. 2006;49(5):313–326.

57. Hjortsberg U, Rosen I, Orbaek P, Lundborg G, Balogh I. Finger receptor dysfunction in dental technicians exposed to high-frequency vibration. *Scand J Work Environ Health*. 1989;15(5):339–344.

58. Akesson I, Lundborg G, Horstmann V, Skerfving S. Neuropathy in female dental personnel exposed to high frequency vibrations. *Occup Environ Med*. 1995;52(2):116–123.

59. Coles RR, Hoare NW. Noise-induced hearing loss and the dentist. *Br Dent J*. 1985;159(7):209–218.

60. Wilson CE, Vaidyanathan TK, Cinotti WR, Cohen SM, Wang SJ. Hearing-damage risk and communication interference in dental practice. *J Dent Res*. 1990;69(2):489–493.

61. Garner GG, Federman J, Johnson A. A noise induced hearing loss in the dental environment: an audiologist perspective. *J Georgia Dent Assoc*. 2002;15:17–19.

62. Bohay RN, Bencak J, Kavaliers M, Maclean D. A survey of magnetic fields in the dental operatory. *J Can Dent Assoc*. 1994;60(9):835–840.

63. Huang SM, Lin YW, Sung FC, Li CY, Chang MF, Chen PC. Occupational exposure of dentists to extremely-low-frequency magnetic field. *J Occup Health*. 2011;53(2):130–136.

64. Kim DW, Choi JL, Kwon MK, Nam TJ, Lee SJ. Assessment of daily exposure of endodontic personnel to extremely low frequency magnetic fields. *Int Endod J*. 2012;45(8):744–748.

65. Mortazavi SM, Vazife-Doost S, Yaghooti M, Mehdizadeh S, Rajaie-Far A. Occupational exposure of dentists to electromagnetic fields produced by magnetostrictive cavitrons alters the serum cortisol level. *J Nat Sci Biol Med*. 2012;3(1):60–64.

66. Petersilka GJ, Flemmig TF. Periodontal debridement with sonic and ultrasonic scalers. *Periodontal Practices Today*. 2004;1(4):353–362.

67. Sbordone L, Ramaglia L, Gulletta E, Iacono V. Recolonization of the subgingival microflora after scaling and root planing in human periodontitis. *J Periodontol*. 1990;61(9):579–584.

68. Stach D. Powering the calculus away. *Dimens Dent Hyg*. 2005;3(3):18–20.

69. Flemmig TF, Petersilka GJ, Mehl A, Hickel R, Klaiber B. The effect of working parameters on root substance removal using a piezoelectric ultrasonic scaler in vitro. *J Clin Periodontol*. 1998;25(2):158–163.

70. Flemmig TF, Petersilka GJ, Mehl A, Rudiger S, Hickel R, Klaiber B. Working parameters of a sonic scaler influencing root substance removal in vitro. *Clin Oral Investig*. 1997;1(2):55–60.

71. Bailey GM, Gardner JS, Day MH, Kovanda BJ. Implant surface alterations from a nonmetallic ultrasonic tip. *J West Soc Periodontol Periodontal Abstr*. 1998;46(3):69–73.

72. Kawashima H, Sato S, Kishida M, Ito K. A comparison of root surface instrumentation using two piezoelectric ultrasonic scalers and a hand scaler in vivo. *J Periodontal Res*. 2007;42(1):90–95.

73. Kawashima H, Sato S, Kishida M, Yagi H, Matsumoto K, Ito K. Treatment of titanium dental implants with three piezoelectric ultrasonic scalers: an in vivo study. *J Periodontol.* 2007;78(9):1689–1694.

74. Matarasso S, Quaremba G, Coraggio F, Vaia E, Cafiero C, Lang NP. Maintenance of implants: an in vitro study of titanium implant surface modifications subsequent to the application of different prophylaxis procedures. *Clin Oral Implants Res.* 1996;7(1):64–72.

75. Ruhling A, Kocher T, Kreusch J, Plagmann HC. Treatment of subgingival implant surfaces with Teflon-coated sonic and ultrasonic scaler tips and various implant curettes. An in vitro study. *Clin Oral Implants Res.* 1994;5(1):19–29.

76. Sato S, Kishida M, Ito K. The comparative effect of ultrasonic scalers on titanium surfaces: an in vitro study. *J Periodontol.* 2004;75(9):1269–1273.

77. Hodges KO, Calley KH. Optimizing ultrasonic instrumentation. Magnetostrictive ultrasonic insert selection and correct technique in periodontal therapy. *Dimens Dent Hyg.* 2010;8(1):30–35.

78. Hou GL, Chen SF, Wu YM, Tsai CC. The topography of the furcation entrance in Chinese molars. Furcation entrance dimensions. *J Clin Periodontol.* 1994;21(7):451–456.

79. Jacks ME. A laboratory comparison of evacuation devices on aerosol reduction. *J Dent Hyg.* 2002;76(3):202–206.

80. Klyn SL, Cummings DE, Richardson BW, Davis RD. Reduction of bacteria-containing spray produced during ultrasonic scaling. *Gen Dent.* 2001;49(6):648–652.

81. Gupta G, Mitra D, Ashok KP, et al. Efficacy of preprocedural mouth rinsing in reducing aerosol contamination produced by ultrasonic scaler: a pilot study. *J Periodontol.* 2014;85(4):562–568.

82. Desarda H, Gurav A, Dharmadhikari C, Shete A, Gaikwad S. Efficacy of high-volume evacuator in aerosol reduction: truth or myth? A clinical and microbiological study. *J Dent Res Dent Clin Dent Prospects.* 2014;8(3):176–179.

Student Self Evaluation Module 26: Powered Instrumentation

Student: _____   Date: _____

DIRECTIONS FOR STUDENT: Evaluate your skill level as: **S** (satisfactory) or **U** (unsatisfactory).

CRITERIA:		
Equipment Preparation: Connects device to electrical and water sources; disinfects, applies barriers; flushes water line for 2 minutes		
Clinician and Patient Preparation Uses protective attire for self and patient; provides patient with preprocedural rinse		
Explains procedure to the patient including purpose, noise, water spray/evacuation; encourages patient to ask questions and provides appropriate answers; obtains informed consent		
Instrumentation Technique with All Tips: Uses evacuation effectively, positioning patient's head and HVE to collect pooled water		
Adjusts power and water settings as appropriate for powered instrument tip		
Uses a gentle grasp and establishes an appropriate extra- or intraoral fulcrum		
Correctly adapts working-end to the tooth surface being treated		
Keeps the tip in motion using light pressure and slow overlapping, multidirectional, strokes		
Cups patient's lips and cheeks to collect water; deactivates tip occasionally to allow complete evacuation		
Universal or Straight Slim-Diameter Tip: Demonstrates transverse orientation on maxillary anteriors, facial aspect		
Demonstrates vertical orientation on mandibular anteriors, lingual aspect		
Right and Left Curved Slim-Diameter Tips: Identifies right and left tips		
Demonstrates correct tip adaptation with a lateral surface in a transverse orientation		
Demonstrates correct tip adaptation with a lateral surface in a vertical orientation		
Prepares device for next use; packages appropriate items for autoclaving		

Air Polishing for Biofilm Management and Stain Removal

Module Overview

This instructional module describes: (1) the new technology of subgingival air polishing for biofilm management and (2) conventional air polishing for stain removal from enamel surfaces. Subgingival air polishing for the removal of biofilm from root surfaces is a relatively new technology with clinical research supporting its safety and efficacy for biofilm management in nonsurgical periodontal therapy and treatment of peri-implant disease.

Module Outline

Section 1   **The Significance of Biofilm Management**   **717**

Section 2   **Methods of Biofilm Management**   **718**
Traditional Versus Innovative Biofilm Management
Precautions and Contraindications for Air Polishing
Polishing Powder Selection
Preparation for Air Polishing
Integration of Air Polishing into Individualized Patient Care

Section 3   **Clinical Evidence for Subgingival Air Polishing**   **726**

Section 4   **Supragingival Polishing: Using a Standard Nozzle and Conventional Sodium Bicarbonate Powder**   **727**
Dos and Don'ts for Sodium Bicarbonate Polishing
Supragingival Nozzle Placement and Use with Sodium
    Bicarbonate Powder

Section 5   **Subgingival Polishing Using a Standard Metal Nozzle and Glycine-Based Powder**   **729**
Quick Start Guide to the Anterior Sextants Using a Standard Nozzle
    with Glycine-Based Powder
Quick Start Guide to the Posterior Sextants Using a Standard Nozzle
    with Glycine-Based Powder

Section 6

Subgingival Polishing Using a Flexible Plastic Tip and Glycine-Based Powder   **732**

Design Features of Specialized Plastic Subgingival Tip
Insertion and Instrument Stroke with Plastic Tip
Precautions for Use in Periodontal Pockets: Determining Which Teeth to Treat
Quick Start Guide to the Posterior Sextants Using a Plastic Tip with Glycine-Based Powder
Quick Start Guide to the Anterior Sextants Using a Plastic Tip with Glycine-Based Powder

Section 7

Posttreatment Precautions and Instructions   **738**

Posttreatment Precautions and Measures
Posttreatment Instructions

Section 8

Skill Application   **739**

Practical Focus: Use of Supragingival Nozzle
Clinical Focus: Integration of Air Polishing for Care of a Fictitious Patient Case

Online resources:
- ***Module 26B: Cosmetic Polishing Procedures.*** This module covers rubber cup polishing for extrinsic stain removal.
- ***Module 27B: Set-Up Instructions for Hu-Friedy/EMS Air-Flow® Units***
- Available at: http://thepoint.lww.com/GehrigFundamentals8e

Key Terms

Nonsurgical periodontal therapy
Biofilm management
Air polishing technology
Standard metal nozzle
Flexible plastic tip

Conventional air polishing
Subgingival air polishing
Glycine-based powder
Sodium bicarbonate–based powders
Iatrogenic facial emphysema

Aerosol
Mask with a high bacterial filtration efficiency

Learning Objectives

- Explain the importance of professional subgingival biofilm removal from root surfaces as a routine part of nonsurgical periodontal therapy.
- Compare and contrast "*subgingival air polishing with glycine powder for biofilm management*" with "*supragingival air polishing with sodium bicarbonate for stain removal.*"
- Compare the types of air polishing powders available and their appropriate use.
- List medical and dental contraindications of subgingival air polishing for biofilm management and supragingival air polishing for stain removal.
- On a typodont, demonstrate the correct angulation and instrumentation stroke with a standard nozzle for stain removal.
- On a typodont, demonstrate correct insertion and use of the specialized plastic perio tip and glycine-based powder for subgingival biofilm removal.
- In a preclinical or clinical setting, demonstrate correct technique for use of an air polishing device, including treatment room, clinician and patient preparation; armamentarium selection/set-up and infection control; grasp and finger rest; correct technique; and fluid control.
- Discuss the benefits to the patient when supra- and subgingival air polishing is integrated into the treatment plan.

Section 1
The Significance of Biofilm Management

1. What is the significance of biofilm management as part of disease prevention and nonsurgical periodontal therapy?
   A. Nonsurgical periodontal therapy is a term used to describe the many nonsurgical steps used to eliminate inflammation in the periodontium of a patient with periodontitis in an attempt to return the periodontium to a healthy state that can then be maintained by a combination of both professional care and patient self-care.
   B. The goals of nonsurgical periodontal therapy are to:
      1. *Control the bacterial challenge to the patient* (biofilm management).
      2. Minimize the impact of systemic risk factors, to eliminate or control local environmental risk factors.
      3. Stabilize the attachment level.
   C. The formation of plaque biofilm communities on tooth surfaces is the primary cause of gingivitis and periodontitis. Removal of plaque biofilms arrests or slows down the progression of periodontal disease. Toothbrushes, dental floss, or antibacterial rinses cannot reach subgingival biofilms within periodontal pockets (Fig. 27-1).
      1. *Biofilms are resistant to topical chemical control; therefore, frequent mechanical removal of plaque biofilm is an essential component of successful nonsurgical periodontal therapy.*
      2. The thoroughness of biofilm removal can determine the overall success of disease prevention or nonsurgical periodontal therapy in most patients.
         a. Studies indicate that following periodontal instrumentation, the subgingival pathogens return to preinstrumentation levels in approximately 9 to 11 weeks in most patients, though times can vary (1–4).
         b. Research evidence shows that periodontal maintenance—routine care for individuals with periodontal disease—should be performed at least every 3 months or less for the removal and disruption of subgingival periodontal pathogens. *This 3-month interval is the one most frequently recommended, though this interval may need to be adjusted based on clinical observation* (5).

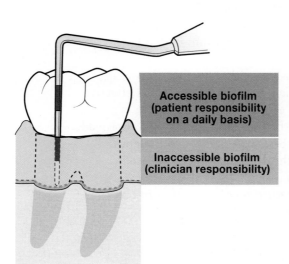

Accessible biofilm (patient responsibility on a daily basis)

Inaccessible biofilm (clinician responsibility)

Figure 27-1. Biofilm Management. Biofilm management is a principal goal of preventive and nonsurgical periodontal therapy. As part of nonsurgical periodontal maintenance, biofilm management requires daily patient self-care combined with frequent professional care for subgingival biofilm removal.

Section 2
Methods of Biofilm Management

TRADITIONAL VERSUS INNOVATIVE BIOFILM MANAGEMENT

1. Traditional Techniques for Professional Biofilm Removal
   A. Traditionally, hand and/or ultrasonic instrumentation has been used for professional biofilm removal.
      1. In the hands of a well-trained clinician, both these techniques are effective in biofilm removal.
      2. The subgingival biofilm removal process using either hand and/or ultrasonic instrumentation, however, is a technically demanding and time-consuming procedure for the clinician and uncomfortable for many patients (6,7). Unpleasant feelings toward dental procedures may have a negative effect on patient compliance.
   B. Biofilm formation occurs rapidly in periodontal pockets following instrumentation. Professional biofilm removal must be performed frequently at regular intervals for subgingival biofilm management.
      1. The main adverse effect of frequent mechanical instrumentation of the root surface is disturbance of the epithelial attachment and cumulative, irreversible root substance removal (8–14) and gingival recession (15,16).
      2. Hard tissue loss is one of the major causes of dentin sensitivity to hot and cold stimuli, as well as sensitivity to toothbrushing (17–20).
      3. Because professional subgingival biofilm removal must be performed as a routine part of nonsurgical periodontal therapy, it is important that removal is accomplished in an efficient manner with minimal hard tissue damage (21).
2. Recent Innovations in Biofilm Management
   A. In the past few years, indications for the use of air polishing technology have been expanded from *supra*gingival use to *sub*gingival air polishing (Fig. 27-2). Air polishing technology uses a combination of an abrasive powder with water and compressed air delivered to the tooth surface through an air polishing nozzle.
   B. Subgingival air polishing for the removal of biofilm from root surfaces is a relatively new technology with clinical research supporting its safety and efficacy for use in nonsurgical periodontal therapy and treatment of peri-implant disease.
      1. Shallow subgingival biofilm removal is accomplished using a standard metal nozzle and a glycine-based powder. Using glycine powder, the standard nozzle is effective for use in sulci or periodontal pockets up to 4 mm in depth (Fig. 27-2A).
      2. Deep subgingival biofilm removal is accomplished with a **flexible plastic tip** shown in Figure 27-2B. Using a glycine powder, the plastic perio tip is effective in pockets greater than 4 mm in depth.
         a. In the United States, the Food and Drug Administration (FDA) has approved the plastic perio tip for use in periodontal pockets up to 5 mm in depth.
         b. In Canada, Health Canada has approved the plastic perio tip for use in periodontal pockets up to 10 mm in depth.
   C. *Prior to using this new technology, clinicians require special training in the proper use of the subgingival air polishing device.*

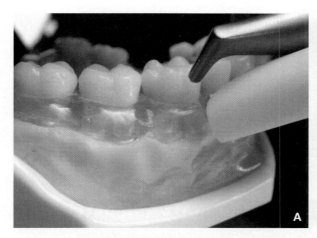
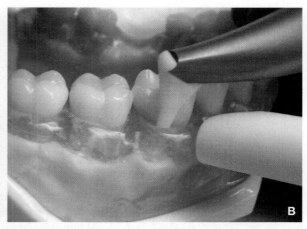

Figure 27-2. Air Polishing Technology. A: Standard Metal Nozzle; shows a standard air polishing nozzle for stain and biofilm removal. **B: Flexible Plastic Tip;** shows a plastic tip for biofilm removal in periodontal pockets 4 mm or greater in depth.

3. Polishing Powders for Conventional versus Subgingival Air Polishing
   A. Conventional Coronal Air Polishing Powders. The most common powder used for conventional air polishing is sodium bicarbonate powder.
      1. Conventional air polishing with sodium bicarbonate powder has been available as an alternative to rubber cup polishing since the late 1970s.
      2. Air polishing is intended for *supragingival* use only.
   B. Subgingival Air Polishing. Subgingival air polishing uses a specially designed low-abrasive powder at a limited pressure.
      1. In the United States, a glycine-based powder is most commonly used for subgingival air polishing. Glycine was first trialed in 2003 and is commonly used in Europe.
      2. In Europe, an erythritol-based powder also is available for subgingival use. In the future, clinicians should expect this powder to be available in the United States and Canada.
4. Sodium Bicarbonate versus Glycine Air Polishing Powders
   A. Sodium Bicarbonate–Based Powders
      1. Sodium bicarbonate–based powders have a large particle size and are recommended for stain removal from enamel surfaces.
      2. Sodium bicarbonate has a salty taste and stinging sensation that some patients find unpleasant.
      3. Sodium bicarbonate–based powders are NOT recommended for use on root surfaces. Five seconds use of sodium bicarbonate powder on root surfaces has been shown to cause considerable damage to cementum (22).
      4. *In patients with exposed root surfaces, cleaning with bicarbonate powder is NOT recommended* (22).
   B. Glycine-Based Powders
      1. Because glycine powder has very fine, round, soft particles, it is an excellent choice for subgingival biofilm removal.
      2. Glycine-based powders are gentle on the soft tissues of the oral cavity and the subgingival epithelium. Glycine powder feels as gentle as the air-water syringe spray on the tissues.

3. Glycine powders are approximately 80% less abrasive than sodium bicarbonate powders (46).
   a. In a study by Sahrmann et al. (22), a 5 second use of sodium bicarbonate produced cemental defect volumes of 0.11 mm^3.
   b. By contrast in the same time period, glycine-based powder produced cemental defect volumes of 0.02 mm^3.
   c. For each time period, abrasion caused by the glycine powder was significantly lower—5- to 20-fold—compared to defects caused by sodium bicarbonate powder.
5. Indications for use of sodium bicarbonate– and glycine-based powders are summarized in Table 27-1.

TABLE 27-1. COMPARISON OF SODIUM BICARBONATE AND GLYCINE AIR POLISHING POWDERS

Indications	Sodium Bicarbonate	Glycine
Removal of plaque biofilm	☺	☺
Removal of extrinsic stain	☺	☺
Use on enamel	☺	☺
Use on cementum	☹	☺
Use on dentin	☹	☺
Use within a sulcus or periodontal pocket	☹	☺
Use on restorative materials	☹	☺
Cleaning of fissures prior to sealant placement	☺	☺
Cleaning of implant surfaces	☹	☺

PRECAUTIONS AND CONTRAINDICATIONS FOR AIR POLISHING

1. **Patient Assessment.** The decision to use air polishing is based on each individual patient's medical and dental histories. A thorough review of the patient's medical history is a must prior to the use of this technology and consultation with the patient's physician may be indicated.
   A. Contraindications for *supra*gingival air polishing with a sodium bicarbonate–based powder include (21,24–27):
      1. Patients on a physician-directed sodium-restricted diet (24,26,28,29). A sodium-restricted diet is considered a contraindication for sodium bicarbonate polishing despite some evidence in the literature that the amount of sodium ingested during air polishing is not sufficient to cause an increase in blood levels of sodium or alkalosis (26,28).
      2. Patients who have respiratory problems such as asthma, bronchitis, chronic obstructive pulmonary disease (COPD), or any condition that interferes with breathing or swallowing. The aerosols created by air polishing may make it difficult for individuals with respiratory problems to breathe and these individuals are vulnerable to the development of pneumonia.

3. Patients who are immunocompromised (*diabetes,* hemophilia, neutropenia, or angranulocytosis). A physician consult should be initiated before performing air polishing on immunocompromised patients.
4. Patients who are pregnant or breastfeeding.
5. Patients who are undergoing certain medical treatments (radiotherapy, chemotherapy).
6. Patients with a communicable infection.
7. Patients with history of allergies may be predisposed to an allergic reaction to the powder. If an allergic reaction is observed, stop the procedure.
8. Patients who have Addison disease, Cushing disease, or metabolic alkalosis.
9. Patients taking medications such as potassium supplements, antidiuretics, or corticoid steroids—all of which can disrupt the body's acid–base balance.
10. Patients with certain restorative materials and luting agents: hybrid, microhybrid, microfilled composites, and glass ionomer restorations. In addition, the margins of amalgam, gold, or porcelain restorations must be avoided due to luting agents (cements) (24,30–33).

B. Contraindications for *sub*gingival air polishing with a glycine-based powder include:
1. Patients who have respiratory problems such as asthma, bronchitis, COPD, or any condition that interferes with breathing or swallowing.
2. Patients who are undergoing certain medical treatments (radiotherapy, chemotherapy).
3. Patients with a communicable infection.
4. Patients with history of allergies may be predisposed to an allergic reaction to the powder. If an allergic reaction is observed, stop the procedure.
5. Since glycine-based powders do not contain sodium, the use of these powders is not contraindicated for conditions such as sodium-restricted diet, hypertension, or renal insufficiency (25).
6. Glycine-based powders are safe for use on all types of restorative materials, including the titanium components of dental implants (34–36).

2. Iatrogenic Facial Emphysema
A. Iatrogenic facial emphysema is a rare condition that results from the accidental introduction and collection of air in the soft tissues of the face from the use of pressurized air in dental procedures.
1. Symptoms of facial emphysemas associated with dental treatments include facial swelling, a crackling feeling of the face and neck area, tenderness, and pain (37,38).
2. It is vital to inform a patient who is experiencing emphysema to seek medical help immediately if he or she experiences difficult or labored breathing, any problems with swallowing, chest pain, or any disturbance of vision or hearing. These may be symptoms of severe health problems such as bilateral pneumothorax, cerebral air embolism, embolism, thrombosis, nerve compression or hypoperfusion of nerve tissue (23,24).
3. *Emergency healthcare providers may be unfamiliar with facial emphysema and may misdiagnose the symptoms as an allergic reaction* (39,40). For this reason, dental professionals must be able to detect the symptoms quickly.
B. Causes of Facial Emphysema
1. Cases of emphysema were reported after the use of high-speed dental handpieces, and air/water syringes, and even after taking impressions (21,41–43).

2. Procedures with supragingival air polishing devices have been associated with emphysema (44,45).
   a. In the Health Device Alerts database, three cases of air embolism were related to the use of air polishing devices between 1977 and 2001 (21,23,46–48). Air emphysema is reported more frequently in the literature after the use of a high-speed dental drill (23).
   b. There have, however, been incidents of facial emphysema resulting from the use of subgingival glycine powder polishing reported in the literature. *Flemmig et al. (49) estimate that the probability of emphysema resulting from subgingival glycine powder polishing is approximately 1 in 666,666.*

POLISHING POWDER SELECTION

1. **Selection of Correct Powder and Powder Chamber.** The particular treatment determines the powder chamber for use.
   • For *supragingival treatment*—stain removal—use sodium bicarbonate–based powders.
   • For *subgingival treatment*—biofilm control—use glycine-based powders. Sodium bicarbonate–based powders should never be used subgingivally. In Europe, an erythritol-based powder also is available for subgingival use. Hygienists should be aware that it is likely that new types of powders will be available in the future.
2. **Powder Exchange or Refill During Treatment.** A common treatment sequence is (1) the use of sodium bicarbonate powder for coronal stain removal (2) followed by glycine powder for subgingival biofilm removal.
   • *This treatment sequence requires the use of one powder chamber filled with sodium bicarbonate powder and a second powder chamber filled with glycine powder.*
   • All sodium bicarbonate powder is purged from the polishing device prior to installing the chamber filled with glycine powder (Fig. 27-3).

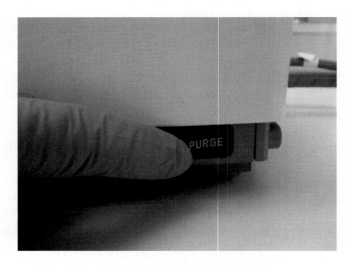

Figure 27-3. Exchanging Power Chambers. When changing from sodium bicarbonate to glycine powder, it is important to purge all the sodium bicarbonate powder from the device. Activate the purge function to remove all powder residues from inside the cord and handpiece.

PREPARATION FOR AIR POLISHING

1. **Aerosol Production and Its Implications for Patient and Occupational Health**
   A. An **aerosol** is defined as a small droplet usually 5 μm (micrometer) or less in diameter, which can remain suspended in air for some time.
      1. The various dental procedures which produce microorganism-laden aerosols include turbine handpieces, sonic and ultrasonic scalers, air polishing devices, polishing cups, and air syringes.
      2. Ultrasonic scalers, dental handpieces and air polishers are the greatest producers of small particle aerosol contamination in dentistry (50,51). These instruments remove material from the operative site that becomes aerosolized by the action of water sprays and compressed air.
      3. Bacterial aerosols are an important consideration for infection control and occupational health in the dental setting, since infective agents can be transmitted via aerosols to patients or dental staff (52,53).
         a. Microorganisms in the mouth and respiratory tract can be transported in the aerosols generated during dental procedures and can contaminate the skin and mucous membranes of the mouth, respiratory passages, and eyes of dental personnel as well as the patients (52,54–56). Small aerosolized particles remain airborne and enter the nasal passage and are capable of penetrating deep into the respiratory tree (57,58).
         b. Several studies show that blood is found routinely in the aerosols produced by powered instrumentation (54,59,60).
   B. **Reduction and Containment of Aerosol Production**
      1. Patients should always be instructed to rinse with an antimicrobial agent prior to treatment to reduce the bacterial load in aerosols that are generated during the air polishing procedure (61).
      2. During treatment, high-volume evacuators should be used to avoid unnecessary contamination of the air in the dental treatment area with aerosols containing potential infectious microorganisms (23,62,63).
         a. The use of a high volume evacuator (HVE) has been shown to universally reduce airborne contamination by 90 to 98% (60,62,64,65). HVE is a mandatory infection control precaution during air polishing.
         b. *It is important to note that a saliva ejector is not an effective means of controlling aerosols during air polishing.* The small diameter of a saliva ejector keeps it from removing enough air to be effective in reducing aerosols.
         c. Use of a high-volume evacuator is vital to aerosol containment.
2. **Patient and Clinician Preparation.** During treatment with an air polishing device, universal precautions should be employed including: (a) barrier protection, (b) high-volume evacuation, and (c) preprocedural rinsing by the patient (26). Each of these precautions adds a layer of protection for the clinician and others in the dental office.
   A. **Patient Preparation**
      1. As with any treatment procedure, it is important to describe and explain the air polishing procedure to the patient and obtain his or her informed consent. The clinician should explain the purpose and functioning of the air polisher, as well as the powder spray, and the need for evacuation. The clinician should discuss the expected successful outcome, as well as the possible risks, unanticipated outcomes, and alternative treatments. The patient should be encouraged to ask questions.

2. A preprocedural rinse for the patient is recommended to reduce the bacterial load in aerosols generated and released into the surrounding.
   a. A 1-minute rinse with an antimicrobial mouthwash is recommended for all patients prior to initiation of any type of powered instrumentation (25,26,64–66).
   b. A preprocedural rinse, however, will not affect blood coming from the operative site or viruses coming from the respiratory tract. Using a preprocedural rinse should not be relied upon to prevent airborne contamination.
3. Personal protective gear for the patient is mandatory and should include a plastic or disposable drape, and protective eyewear. The patient may prefer to cover his or her nose with a flat-style mask to limit inhalation of aerosols.
4. Powder spray accidentally directed into the eye may cause severe ocular injury. ***During treatment, it is strongly recommended that both the clinician and patient wear eye protection.*** It is recommended that the patient remove contact lenses prior to treatment. Figure 27-4 shows an ideal patient protective mask.
5. A nonpetroleum-based lip cover (as petroleum will compromise integrity of latex in gloves, if latex gloves are used) should be applied to cover the patient's lips for protection from the spray that may irritate or chap the lips.

B. Personal Protective Equipment for the Clinician
1. The clinician should wear a gown with a high neck and long sleeves, mask, protective eyewear, and gloves. If wearing a face shield, the clinician should also don a facemask, as the face shield does not protect the clinician from breathing in aerosols.
2. A mask with a high bacterial filtration efficiency (BFE) is recommended for all powered instrumentation procedures (67). By definition, a BFE mask effectively filters out 98% of particles that are three microns or larger in size.

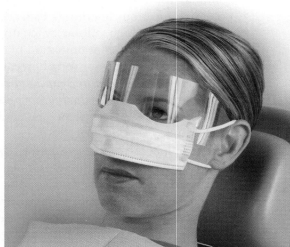

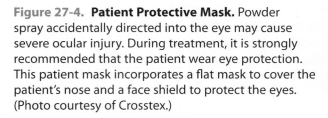

Figure 27-4. Patient Protective Mask. Powder spray accidentally directed into the eye may cause severe ocular injury. During treatment, it is strongly recommended that the patient wear eye protection. This patient mask incorporates a flat mask to cover the patient's nose and a face shield to protect the eyes. (Photo courtesy of Crosstex.)

INTEGRATION OF AIR POLISHING INTO INDIVIDUALIZED PATIENT CARE

Clinicians in Europe—and more recently in North America—who are experienced in the use of subgingival air polishing find that completing air polishing first, before periodontal instrumentation, is the most efficient way to incorporate air polishing into the treatment plan.

1. Many clinicians find periodontal instrumentation easier to accomplish once biofilms are removed from tooth surfaces. Subgingival air polishing is much more efficient in removing subgingival biofilms than a curet or ultrasonic tip (23).
2. Of course, use of the air polisher after instrumentation also is an option when pocket depths are 4 mm or less. (To minimize the risk of air emphysema, air polishing should not be used in pocket depths greater than 4 mm until the epithelium has healed, which takes approximate 14 days.)
3. Clinicians find that once the rationale for air polishing is explained to patients, they are very open to this new treatment sequence.
4. The flow chart in Figure 27-5 provides one example of how a clinician might integrate supra- and subgingival air polishing into a plan of treatment.

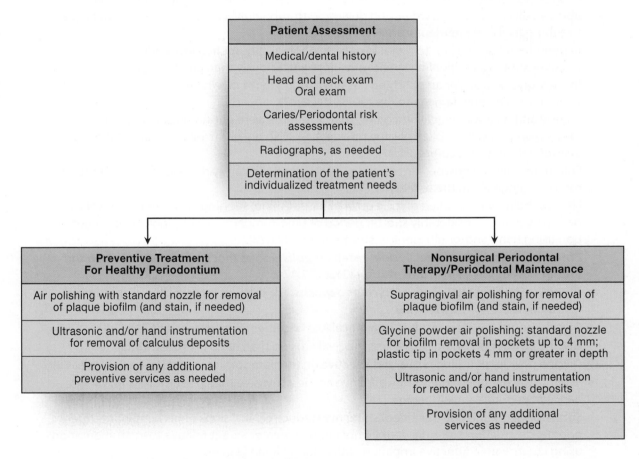

Figure 27-5. Integration of Air Polishing into Treatment Plan. This flow chart gives one example of how a clinician might integrate air polishing into an individualized patient treatment plan.

Section 3
Clinical Evidence for Subgingival Air Polishing

Although subgingival air polishing is an emerging technology in North America, this technology has been used and researched for several years in Europe. In June 2012, during the *Euro-Perio 7 Conference in Vienna* (70), a consensus conference on mechanical biofilm management took place to review the current evidence from the literature on the clinical relevance of subgingival use of air polishing and to make practical recommendations for the clinician. Box 1 summarizes these recommendations, as well as additional current evidence from the research literature on subgingival air polishing for biofilm management.

Box 27-1 | Summary of Current Evidence on Subgingival Air Polishing

- Indications for the use of air polishing devices have been expanded from supragingival to subgingival air polishing in the past few years. In particular, the development of new low-abrasive glycine-based powders and devices with subgingival nozzles provide better access to subgingival and interdental areas (70).

- In periodontal pockets up to 5 mm in depth, subgingivally applied low-abrasive powder removes subgingival biofilm significantly more efficaciously than curets (47,49).

- In vitro, glycine powder air polishing has been found to remove biofilm in 5 to 10 seconds without causing any damage to the root surface (47).

- Clinical and microbiological outcomes up to 2 months were not significantly different following subgingivally applied glycine powder air polishing, ultrasonic instrumentation, or instrumentation with curets (21,27).

- Full-mouth glycine powder air polishing results in a significantly decreased load of Porphyromonas gingivalis in the oral cavity (49).

- Using subgingivally applied glycine powder air polishing, subgingival biofilm removal can be achieved in a considerably shorter period of time compared to subgingival instrumentation using hand and/or ultrasonic instrumentation (21,27).

- ***Patients generally perceive glycine-based air polishing as more comfortable than hand and/or power-driven instrumentation*** (21,23,27,47–69).

- ***Air polishing does NOT remove calculus deposits.*** For calculus removal, hand or ultrasonic instruments are still needed (23).

- Glycine-based powders result in noncritical loss of cemental substance (22,71).

- Glycine powder polishing causes less gingival erosion than hand instrumentation (68).

- Glycine powder polishing is safe and effective on titanium surfaces of dental implants (72,73).

- Glycine powder polishing is more effective and less invasive than plastic curets for maintenance of peri-implant soft tissues (34).

- Subgingival glycine powder air polishing may reduce clinical signs of peri-implantitis (periodontal destruction around a dental implant) to a greater extent relative to instrumentation using curets with adjunctive irrigation with chlorhexidine (35,74).

- Glycine powder is safe on a variety of restorative materials and orthodontic brackets.

- Clinical, microbiologic, and histologic studies have confirmed subgingival glycine powder air polishing is safe, efficient, and comfortable when used as recommended by a trained professional (21,23,25,47–49,70).

Section 4
Supragingival Polishing: Using a Standard Nozzle and Conventional Sodium Bicarbonate Powder

Conventional supragingival air polishing uses a sodium bicarbonate–based powder for stain removal from the enamel tooth surfaces. *As depicted in Figures 27-6 and 27-7, sodium bicarbonate–based powders are used only for supragingival application.* Do not direct the stream of a sodium bicarbonate powder toward the soft tissue, sulcus, restorations, crowns, or fixed bridgework (Figs. 27-8 and 27-9).

DOS AND DON'TS FOR SODIUM BICARBONATE POLISHING

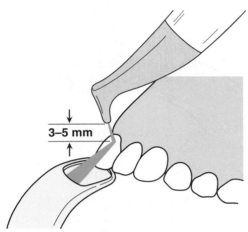

Figure 27-6. Correct Technique: Nozzle to Tooth Distance. The nozzle should be held 3 to 5 mm away from the tooth surface. *Note that the sodium bicarbonate powder spray is directed AWAY from the gingiva.*

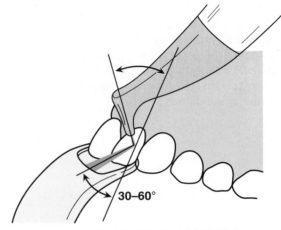

Figure 27-7. Correct Technique: Nozzle Angulation for Anterior Teeth. For anterior teeth, the angle between the nozzle and the tooth can be varied between 30 and 60 degrees.

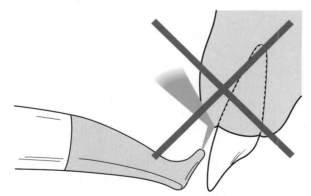

Figure 27-8. Incorrect Technique. Sodium bicarbonate powder spray is powerful and should NEVER be directed into the gingival sulcus or pocket. Directing the powder spray into the gingival sulcus or periodontal pocket can introduce air into the soft tissue spaces causing emphysema.

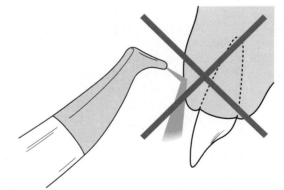

Figure 27-9. Incorrect Technique. Sodium bicarbonate powder spray should NEVER be directed at the gingival tissue. In addition, the nozzle tip should never be directed at the soft tissues of the cheeks, lips, or tongue.

SUPRAGINGIVAL NOZZLE PLACEMENT AND USE WITH SODIUM BICARBONATE POWDER

Figures 27-10 and 27-11 depict correct technique for use of the sodium bicarbonate–based powders for extrinsic stain removal.

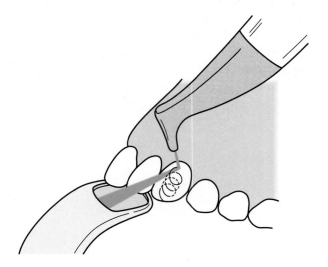

Figure 27-10. Stroke. During treatment, make a constant circular pattern over the coronal tooth surface for 1 to 10 seconds.
- Note the positioning of the nozzle and high-volume evacuator tip for the maxillary teeth.
- Do NOT direct the sodium bicarbonate powder spray toward restorations, crowns, or bridgework, as this could damage these restorations.

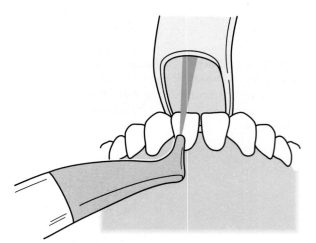

Figure 27-11. Mandibular Teeth. This illustration shows positioning of the nozzle and evacuator tip for mandibular teeth. The illustration shows the view as seen by the clinician seated in the 12:00 position.

Section 5
Subgingival Polishing Using a Standard Metal Nozzle and Glycine-Based Powder

The standard nozzle shown in Figure 27-12 is used with glycine-based powder for removal of light supragingival stain and/or biofilm in sulci or pockets up to 4 mm in depth.

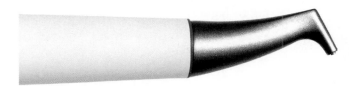

Figure 27-12. Standard Metal Nozzle. The standard nozzle is used with *glycine-based powder* to achieve up to 4 mm of biofilm removal in sulci or shallow pockets. (Courtesy of Hu-Friedy Mfg. Co, LLC.)

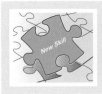

Quick Start Guide to The Anterior Sextants Using a Standard Nozzle With Glycine-Based Powder

Directions: Refer to Figures 27-13 to 27-16 to practice placement of the standard nozzle.

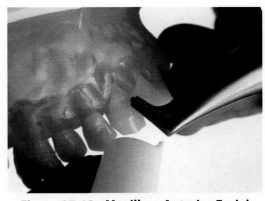

Figure 27-13. Maxillary Anterior Facial.

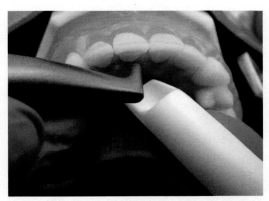

Figure 27-14. Maxillary Anterior Lingual.

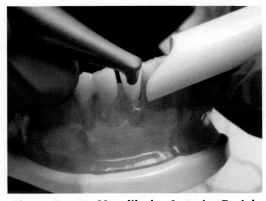

Figure 27-15. Mandibular Anterior Facial.

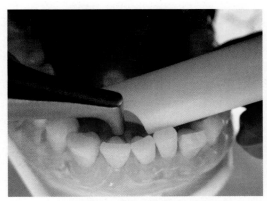

Figure 27-16. Mandibular Anterior Lingual.

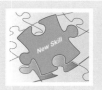

Quick Start Guide to The Posterior Sextants Using a Standard Nozzle With Glycine-Based Powder

Directions: Practice placement of the metal nozzle and evacuator tip for the posterior treatment areas shaded in yellow in Figure 27-17 by referring to Figures 27-18 to 27-21.

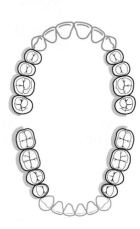

Figure 27-17. While practicing use of the polishing tip on the posterior sextants shaded in *yellow,* right-handed clinicians should sit in the 9:00 position and left-handed clinicians should sit in the 3:00 position.

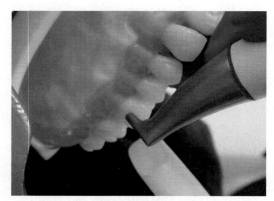

Figure 27-18. **Maxillary Right Facial.**

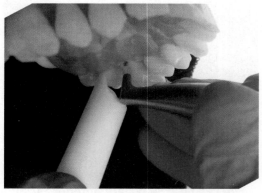

Figure 27-19. **Maxillary Left Lingual.**

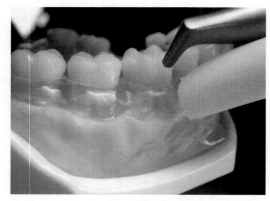

Figure 27-20. **Mandibular Right Facial.**

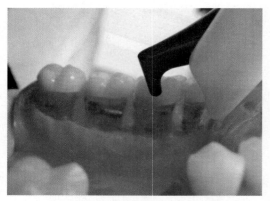

Figure 27-21. **Mandibular Left Lingual.**

Directions: Practice placement of the metal nozzle and evacuator tip for the posterior treatment areas shaded in blue in Figure 27-22 by referring to Figures 27-23 to 27-26.

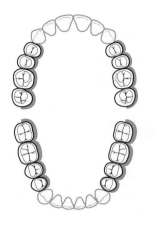

Figure 27-22. Posterior Sextants Facing Away From the Clinician. While practicing use of the polishing tip on the posterior sextants shaded in *blue,* right-handed clinicians should sit in the 10:00 to 11:00 position and left-handed clinicians should sit in the 1:00 to 2:00 position.

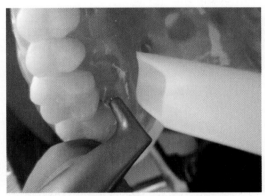

Figure 27-23. Maxillary Right Lingual.

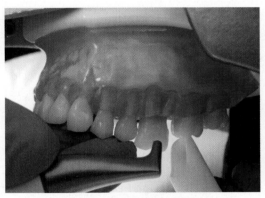

Figure 27-24. Maxillary Left Facial.

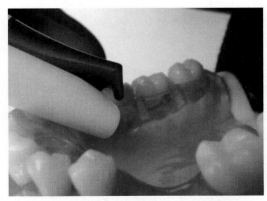

Figure 27-25. Mandibular Right Lingual.

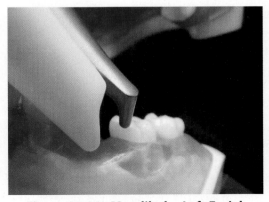

Figure 27-26. Mandibular Left Facial.

Section 6
Subgingival Polishing Using a Flexible Plastic Tip and Glycine-Based Powder

The flexible, plastic air polishing tip shown in Figure 27-27 is used with glycine-based powder for biofilm removal within periodontal pockets.

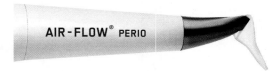

Figure 27-27. Plastic Subgingival Tip. A specialized plastic polishing tip for biofilm control in pockets with depths greater than 4 mm. (Courtesy of Hu-Friedy Mfg. Co, LLC.)

DESIGN FEATURES OF SPECIALIZED PLASTIC SUBGINGIVAL TIP

Figure 27-28 depicts the design of a flexible plastic tip for use with Hu-Friedy/EMS air polishing devices. Note how the glycine powder spray exits the lateral surfaces of the plastic tip as shown in Figure 27-29. This plastic subgingival tip is uniquely designed to protect the soft tissue attachment at the base of the sulcus or periodontal pocket.

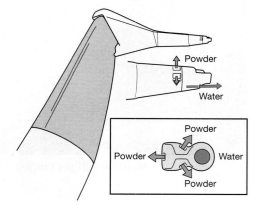

Figure 27-28. Design Features of the Subgingival Plastic Tip. The plastic tip is designed to direct the polishing powder and air mainly toward the root surface—not toward the soft tissue of at the base of the periodontal pocket.

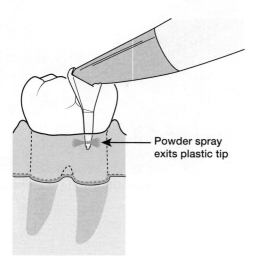

Figure 27-29. Path of Glycine Powder Spray. As depicted, the powder spray exits the lateral surfaces of the plastic tip—not the "point" of the tip. The flexible tip inserts easily into a periodontal pocket.

INSERTION AND INSTRUMENT STROKE WITH PLASTIC TIP

The plastic subgingival tip is activated with a 5-second application per facial, lingual, or interproximal surface to remove subgingival biofilm. The flexible plastic tip is intended for use in pockets greater than 4 mm. Figures 27-30 to 27-32 depict the steps for insertion, positioning, and use of the tip.

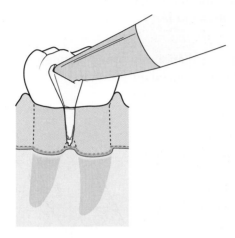

Figure 27-30. Step 1: Insert Plastic Tip. Gently insert the **_unactivated_** plastic tip to the base of the pocket.

- Place the tip in contact with the tooth surface and gently slide it apically (toward the base of the pocket) until it makes light contact with the junctional epithelium at the base of the pocket.
- Never force the tip into a pocket or apply force against the base of a pocket.

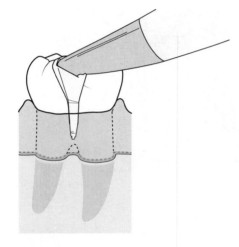

Figure 27-31. Step 2: Position the Tip for Use.

- Position the **_unactivated_** tip by **_withdrawing the tip approximately 1 mm in coronal direction_** (away from the base of the pocket).
- Note that the tip should NOT be touching the base of the pocket.
- The length of the subgingival tip is 10 mm. In the United States, the plastic perio tip is approved by the FDA for use in periodontal pockets up to 5 mm in depth. In Canada, Health Canada has approved the tip for use in periodontal pockets up to 10 mm in depth.

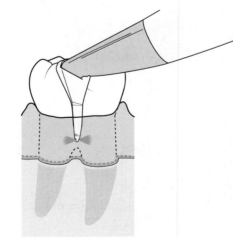

Figure 27-32. Activate Tip. With the tip correctly positioned within the pocket, step on the foot pedal to **_activate_** the powder spray.

- Apply the tip for 5 seconds per facial, lingual, or interproximal aspect of the tooth. Treat each site only once. Do NOT remove the tip from the pocket until completion of the 5-second application. Removing and reinserting the tip can injure the gingival margin.
- Within the pocket space the tip may be moved in overlapping *vertical strokes* over the root surface. **_Do NOT move the tip horizontally in the pocket._**
- Lift the foot off the pedal to **_deactivate_** the powder spray prior to removing the tip from the pocket.

PRECAUTIONS FOR USE IN PERIODONTAL POCKETS: DETERMINING WHICH TEETH TO TREAT

Special precautions should be observed when working in a periodontal pocket that is greater than 4 mm in depth. In the case of a pocket depth greater than 4 mm, the clinician should evaluate the amount of alveolar bone support remaining around the tooth. The plastic subgingival tip is not recommended for use on a tooth that has 3 mm or less of alveolar bone support. *There is a risk of soft tissue emphysema if a tooth site has 3 mm or less of supporting alveolar bone.*

- Figure 27-33 depicts a site within a periodontal pocket that has less than 3 mm of supporting alveolar bone—and thus, the site depicted is not a candidate for subgingival air polishing.
- Figure 27-34 depicts a site within a periodontal pocket that has adequate bone support, thus making this site a good candidate for air polishing.

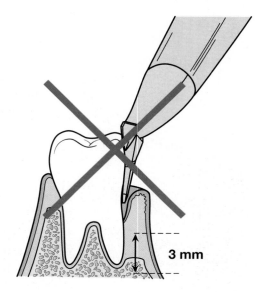

Figure 27-33. Subgingival Polishing NOT Recommended. Subgingival air polishing would NOT be recommended for the tooth in this illustration since it has less than 3 mm of supporting alveolar bone.

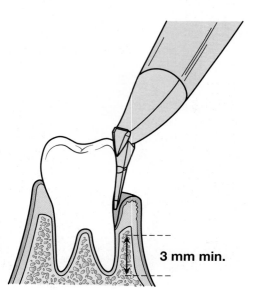

Figure 27-34. Subgingival Polishing Recommended. Subgingival air polishing would be recommended for the tooth in this illustration since it has 3 mm or more of alveolar bone support.

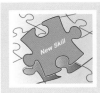

Quick Start Guide to The Posterior Sextants Using a Plastic Tip With Glycine-Based Powder

Directions: Practice placement of the plastic polishing tip and evacuator tip for the posterior treatment areas shaded in yellow in Figure 27-35 by referring to Figures 27-36 to 27-39.

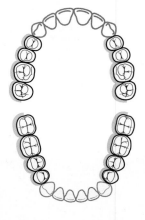

Figure 27-35. Posterior Sextants Facing Toward the Clinician. While practicing use of the polishing tip on the posterior sextants shaded in *yellow,* right-handed clinicians should sit in the 9:00 position and left-handed clinicians should sit in the 3:00 position.

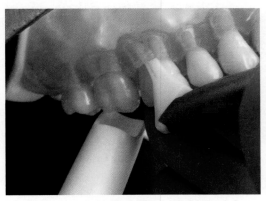

Figure 27-36. Maxillary Right Facial.

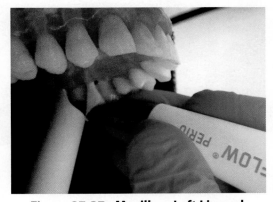

Figure 27-37. Maxillary Left Lingual.

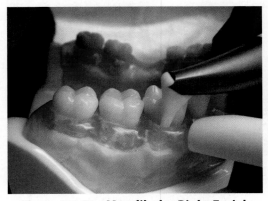

Figure 27-38. Mandibular Right Facial.

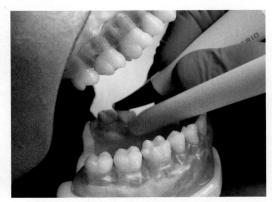

Figure 27-39. Mandibular Left Lingual.

Directions: Practice placement of the plastic polishing tip and evacuator tip for the posterior treatment areas shaded in blue in Figure 27-40 by referring to Figures 27-41 to 27-44.

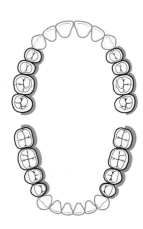

Figure 27-40. Posterior Sextants Facing Away From the Clinician. While practicing use of the polishing tip on the posterior sextants shaded in *blue,* right-handed clinicians should sit in the 10:00 to 11:00 position and left-handed clinicians should sit in the 1:00 to 2:00 position.

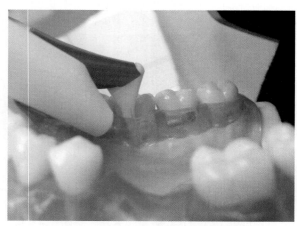

Figure 27-41. Maxillary Right Lingual.

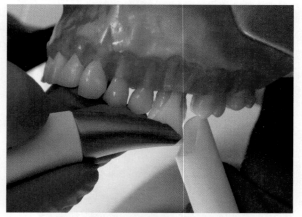

Figure 27-42. Maxillary Left Facial.

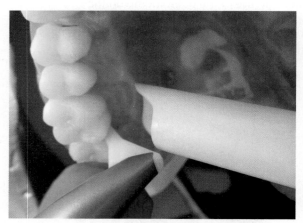

Figure 27-43. Mandibular Right Lingual.

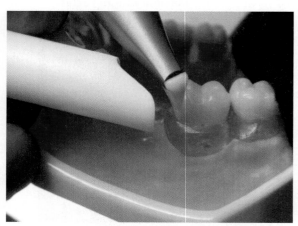

Figure 27-44. Mandibular Left Facial.

Quick Start Guide to The Anterior Sextants Using A Plastic Tip With Glycine-Based Powder

Directions: Refer to Figures 27-45 to 27-48 to practice placement of the plastic polishing tip and evacuator tip in the anterior treatment areas.

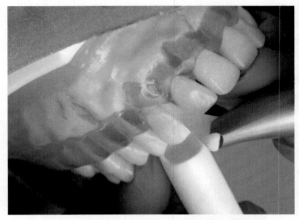

Figure 27-45. Maxillary Anterior Facial.

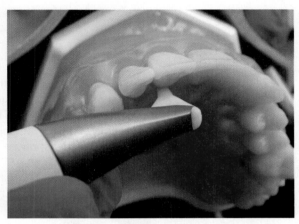

Figure 27-46. Maxillary Anterior Lingual.

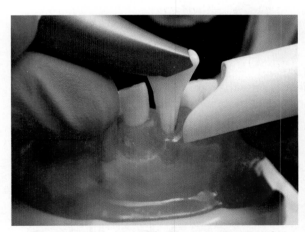

Figure 27-47. Mandibular Anterior Facial.

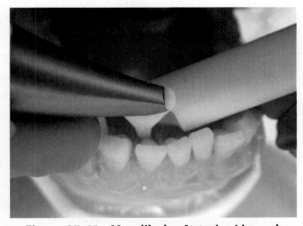

Figure 27-48. Mandibular Anterior Lingual.

Section 7
Posttreatment Precautions and Instructions

Figures 27-49 to 27-51 depict appropriate posttreatment measures and instructions after an air polishing treatment.

POSTTREATMENT PRECAUTIONS AND MEASURES

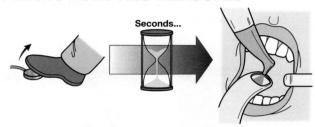

Figure 27-49. Stopping the Flow of the Sodium Bicarbonate Powder. It is important to take into account that the powder spray continues for a few more seconds *after* the clinician removes his or her foot from the foot pedal. During this time period, the nozzle should be introduced into the high-volume evacuator in the patient's mouth. This technique allows time for the polishing unit to decompress with no risk of injuring the soft tissues with the sodium bicarbonate powder spray.

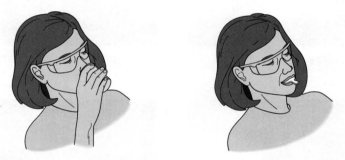

Figure 27-50. Posttreatment Measures. Allow the patient to rinse the mouth with water. After completion of the polishing treatment, it is beneficial to apply a colorless neutral sodium fluoride treatment to the teeth.

POSTTREATMENT INSTRUCTIONS

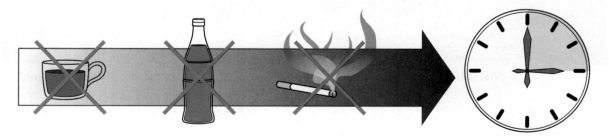

Figure 27-51. Posttreatment Directions for Patient. Treatment with sodium bicarbonate powder completely removes the dental pellicle. Its reconstitution by salivary proteins requires between 2 to 3 hours. During this time, the teeth do not have any natural protection to staining by colored food or drinks. Advise the patient to avoid smoking or consumption of highly colored food or drink for about 3 hours (such as, coffee, wine, blueberries).

MODULE SUMMARY

Mechanical removal of biofilm remains the cornerstone of preventive and periodontal therapy.

Subgingival air polishing with glycine-based powders is more effective and efficient than hand instrumentation and equally effective, but more efficient, than ultrasonic instrumentation in removing biofilm and has the potential to transform professional biofilm management. Research supports that patients are very accepting of air polishing technology and prefer its use to that of ultrasonic instrumentation or rubber cup polishing for biofilm or stain removal. To use air polishing effectively, clinicians need to be trained in the proper technique, the advantages and disadvantages, as well as indications and contraindications for use.

Section 8
Skill Application

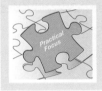

PRACTICAL FOCUS
Use of Supragingival Nozzle

Directions: Practice the technique for supragingival stain removal using sodium bicarbonate powder and a tarnished coin as shown in Figures 27-52 and 27-53.

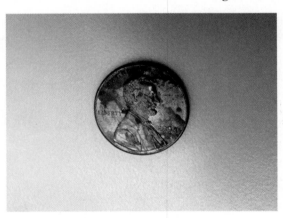

Figure 27-52. Practice Polishing A Coin. Practice supragingival stain removal by polishing a copper penny or other tarnished coin.

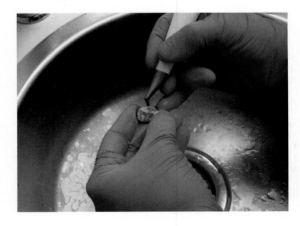

Figure 27-53. Remove the Tarnish. Make back and forth sweeping motions with the powder spray across the surface of the penny to remove the tarnish.

CLINICAL FOCUS: INTEGRATON OF AIR POLISHING FOR CARE OF A FICTITIOUS PATIENT CASE

Directions: Mr. Barnaby is a periodontal maintenance patient (Fig. 27-54) in the periodontics practice in which you are the dental hygienist. Using the clinical photograph and assessment information provided below, integrate air polishing in a treatment plan for Mr. Barnaby.

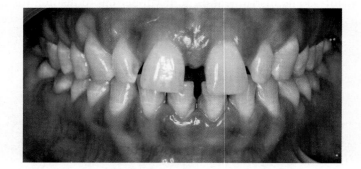

Figure 27-54. Clinical Photo: Mr. Barnaby. (Clinical photograph courtesy of Margaret Lemaster, School of Dental Hygiene, Old Dominion University, Norfolk, VA.)

Patient Assessment Data:

- High cholesterol
- Chronic periodontitis
- Bleeding on probing
- Moderate supragingival calculus deposits on the mandibular anterior sextant
- Light extrinsic stain
- Four sites with 5-mm periodontal pockets (6-mm attachment loss)
- One site with 8-mm loss of attachment (less than 3 mm of supporting bone)
- Five sites with 5-mm periodontal pockets

References

1. Magnusson I, Lindhe J, Yoneyama T, Liljenberg B. Recolonization of a subgingival microbiota following scaling in deep pockets. *J Clin Periodontol.* 1984;11(3):193–207.

2. Sbordone L, Ramaglia L, Amato G, Gulletta E, Valletta G. Bacterial recolonization of deep periodontal lesions after nonsurgical therapy. *Minerva Stomatol.* 1988;37(5):361–371.

3. Shiloah J, Patters MR. Repopulation of periodontal pockets by microbial pathogens in the absence of supportive therapy. *J Periodontol.* 1996;67(2):130–139.

4. Zijnge V, Meijer HF, Lie MA, et al. The recolonization hypothesis in a full-mouth or multiple-session treatment protocol: a blinded, randomized clinical trial. *J Clin Periodontol.* 2010;37(6):518–525.

5. Darcey J, Ashley M. See you in three months! The rationale for the three monthly periodontal recall interval: a risk based approach. *Br Dent J.* 2011;211(8):379–385.

6. Axtelius B, Soderfeldt B, Edwardsson S, Attstrom R. Therapy-resistant periodontitis (II). Compliance and general and dental health experiences. *J Clin Periodontol.* 1997;24(9 Pt 1):646–653.

7. Croft LK, Nunn ME, Crawford LC, et al. Patient preference for ultrasonic or hand instruments in periodontal maintenance. *Int J Periodontics Restorative Dent.* 2003;23(6):567–573.

8. Flemmig TF, Petersilka GJ, Mehl A, Hickel R, Klaiber B. Working parameters of a magnetostrictive ultrasonic scaler influencing root substance removal in vitro. *J Periodontol.* 1998;69(5):547–553.

9. Flemmig TF, Petersilka GJ, Mehl A, Hickel R, Klaiber B. The effect of working parameters on root substance removal using a piezoelectric ultrasonic scaler in vitro. *J Clin Periodontol.* 1998;25(2):158–163.

10. Flemmig TF, Petersilka GJ, Mehl A, Rudiger S, Hickel R, Klaiber B. Working parameters of a sonic scaler influencing root substance removal in vitro. *Clin Oral Investig.* 1997;1(2):55–60.

11. Kocher T, Fanghanel J, Sawaf H, Litz R. Substance loss caused by scaling with different sonic scaler inserts–an in vitro study. *J Clin Periodontol.* 2001;28(1):9–15.

12. Ritz L, Hefti AF, Rateitschak KH. An in vitro investigation on the loss of root substance in scaling with various instruments. *J Clin Periodontol.* 1991;18(9):643–647.

13. Schmidlin PR, Beuchat M, Busslinger A, Lehmann B, Lutz F. Tooth substance loss resulting from mechanical, sonic and ultrasonic root instrumentation assessed by liquid scintillation. *J Clin Periodontol.* 2001;28(11):1058–1066.

14. Zappa U, Smith B, Simona C, Graf H, Case D, Kim W. Root substance removal by scaling and root planing. *J Periodontol.* 1991;62(12):750–754.

15. Badersten A, Nilveus R, Egelberg J. Effect of nonsurgical periodontal therapy. I. Moderately advanced periodontitis. *J Clin Periodontol.* 1981;8(1):57–72.

16. Badersten A, Nilveus R, Egelberg J. Effect of nonsurgical periodontal therapy. II. Severely advanced periodontitis. *J Clin Periodontol.* 1984;11(1):63–76.

17. Chabanski MB, Gillam DG. Aetiology, prevalence and clinical features of cervical dentine sensitivity. *J Oral Rehabil.* 1997;24(1):15–19.

18. Fischer C, Wennberg A, Fischer RG, Attstrom R. Clinical evaluation of pulp and dentine sensitivity after supragingival and subgingival scaling. *Endod Dent Traumatol.* 1991;7(6):259–265.

19. Tammaro S, Wennstrom JL, Bergenholtz G. Root-dentin sensitivity following non-surgical periodontal treatment. *J Clin Periodontol.* 2000;27(9):690–697.

20. von Troil B, Needleman I, Sanz M. A systematic review of the prevalence of root sensitivity following periodontal therapy. *J Clin Periodontol.* 2002;29(Suppl 3):173–177; discussion 95–6.

21. Moene R, Decaillet F, Andersen E, Mombelli A. Subgingival plaque removal using a new air-polishing device. *J Periodontol.* 2010;81(1):79–88.

22. Sahrmann P, Ronay V, Schmidlin PR, Attin T, Paque F. Three-dimensional defect evaluation of air polishing on extracted human roots. *J Periodontol.* 2014;85(8):1107–1114.

23. Petersilka GJ. Subgingival air-polishing in the treatment of periodontal biofilm infections. *Periodontology 2000.* 2011;55(1):124–142.

24. Barnes CM, Covey D, Watanabe H, Simetich B, Schulte JR, Chen H. An in vitro comparison of the effects of various air polishing powders on enamel and selected esthetic restorative materials. *J Clin Dent.* 2014;25(4):76–87.

25. Graumann SJ, Sensat ML, Stoltenberg JL. Air polishing: a review of current literature. *J Dent Hyg.* 2013;87(4):173–180.

26. Gutmann ME. Air polishing: a comprehensive review of the literature. *J Dent Hyg.* 1998;72(3):47–56.

27. Wennstrom JL, Dahlen G, Ramberg P. Subgingival debridement of periodontal pockets by air polishing in comparison with ultrasonic instrumentation during maintenance therapy. *J Clin Periodontol.* 2011;38(9):820–827.

28. Snyder JA, McVay JT, Brown FH, et al. The effect of air abrasive polishing on blood pH and electrolyte concentrations in healthy mongrel dogs. *J Periodontol.* 1990;61(2):81–86.

29. Wilkins EM, Wyche CJ. *Clinical Practice of the Dental Hygienist.* 11th ed. Philadelphia, PA: Wolters Kluwer Health/ Lippincott Williams & Wilkins; 2013:xxiv, 1147 p.

30. Carr MP, Mitchell JC, Seghi RR, Vermilyea SG. The effect of air polishing on contemporary esthetic restorative materials. *Gen Dent.* 2002;50(3):238–241.

31. Gutmann MS, Marker VA, Gutmann JL. Restoration surface roughness after air-powder polishing. *Am J Dent.* 1993;6(2): 99–102.

32. Lubow RM, Cooley RL. Effect of air-powder abrasive instrument on restorative materials. *J Prosthet Dent.* 1986;55(4):462–465.

33. Yap AU, Wu SS, Chelvan S, Tan ES. Effect of hygiene maintenance procedures on surface roughness of composite restoratives. *Oper Dent.* 2005;30(1):99–104.

34. Mussano F, Rovasio S, Schierano G, Baldi I, Carossa S. The effect of glycine-powder airflow and hand instrumentation on peri-implant soft tissues: a split-mouth pilot study. *Int J Prosthodont.* 2013;26(1):42–44.

35. Sahm N, Becker J, Santel T, Schwarz F. Non-surgical treatment of peri-implantitis using an air-abrasive device or mechanical debridement and local application of chlorhexidine: a prospective, randomized, controlled clinical study. *J Clin Periodontol.* 2011;38(9):872–878.

36. Sahrmann P, Ronay V, Sener B, Jung RE, Attin T, Schmidlin PR. Cleaning potential of glycine air-flow application in an in vitro peri-implantitis model. *Clin Oral Implants Res.* 2013;24(6):666–670.

37. Bavinger JV. Subcutaneous and retropharyngeal emphysema following dental restoration: an uncommon complication. *Ann Emerg Med.* 1982;11(7):371–374.
38. Tan WK. Sudden facial swelling: subcutaneous facial emphysema secondary to use of air/water syringe during dental extraction. *Singapore Dent J.* 2000;23(1 Suppl):42–44.
39. Fruhauf J, Weinke R, Pilger U, Kerl H, Mullegger RR. Soft tissue cervicofacial emphysema after dental treatment: report of 2 cases with emphasis on the differential diagnosis of angioedema. *Arch Dermatol.* 2005;141(11):1437–1440.
40. Yang SC, Chiu TH, Lin TJ, Chan HM. Subcutaneous emphysema and pneumomediastinum secondary to dental extraction: a case report and literature review. *Kaohsiung J Med Sci.* 2006;22(12):641–645.
41. Heyman SN, Babayof I. Emphysematous complications in dentistry. *Isr Med Assoc J.* 2005;7(4):278.
42. Karras SC, Sexton JJ. Cervicofacial and mediastinal emphysema as the result of a dental procedure. *J Emerg Med.* 1996;14(1):9–13.
43. Pynn BR, Amato D, Walker DA. Subcutaneous emphysema following dental treatment: a report of two cases and review of the literature. *J Can Dent Assoc.* 1992;58(6):496–499.
44. Finlayson RS, Stevens FD. Subcutaneous facial emphysema secondary to use of the Cavi-Jet. *J Periodontol.* 1988;59(5):315–317.
45. Josephson GD, Wambach BA, Noordzji JP. Subcutaneous cervicofacial and mediastinal emphysema after dental instrumentation. *Otolaryngol Head Neck Surg.* 2001;124(2):170–171.
46. Flemmig TF, Hetzel M, Topoll H, Gerss J, Haeberlein I, Petersilka G. Subgingival debridement efficacy of glycine powder air polishing. *J Periodontol.* 2007;78(6):1002–1010.
47. Petersilka GJ, Steinmann D, Haberlein I, Heinecke A, Flemmig TF. Subgingival plaque removal in buccal and lingual sites using a novel low abrasive air-polishing powder. *J Clin Periodontol.* 2003;30(4):328–333.
48. Petersilka GJ, Tunkel J, Barakos K, Heinecke A, Haberlein I, Flemmig TF. Subgingival plaque removal at interdental sites using a low-abrasive air polishing powder. *J Periodontol.* 2003;74(3):307–311.
49. Flemmig TF, Arushanov D, Daubert D, Rothen M, Mueller G, Leroux BG. Randomized controlled trial assessing efficacy and safety of glycine powder air polishing in moderate-to-deep periodontal pockets. *J Periodontol.* 2012;83(4):444–452.
50. Legnani P, Checchi L, Pelliccioni GA, D'Achille C. Atmospheric contamination during dental procedures. *Quintessence Int.* 1994;25(6):435–439.
51. Logothetis DD, Gross KB, Eberhart A, Drisko C. Bacterial airborne contamination with an air-polishing device. *Gen Dent.* 1988;36(6):496–499.
52. Earnest R, Loesche W. Measuring harmful levels of bacteria in dental aerosols. *J Am Dent Assoc.* 1991;122(12):55–57.
53. Goupil MT. Occupational health and safety emergencies. *Dent Clin North Am.* 1995;39(3):637–647.
54. Barnes JB, Harrel SK, Rivera-Hidalgo F. Blood contamination of the aerosols produced by in vivo use of ultrasonic scalers. *J Periodontol.* 1998;69(4):434–438.
55. Kedjarune U, Kukiattrakoon B, Yapong B, Chowanadisai S, Leggat P. Bacterial aerosols in the dental clinic: effect of time, position and type of treatment. *Int Dent J.* 2000;50(2):103–107.
56. Leggat PA, Kedjarune U. Bacterial aerosols in the dental clinic: a review. *Int Dent J.* 2001;51(1):39–44.
57. Harrel SK, Molinari J. Aerosols and splatter in dentistry: a brief review of the literature and infection control implications. *J Am Dent Assoc.* 2004;135(4):429–437.
58. Molinari JA, Harte JA, Cottone JA, Cottone JA. *Cottone's Practical Infection Control in Dentistry.* 3rd ed. Philadelphia, PA: Wolters Kluwer Health/Lippincott William & Wilkins; 2010:xv, 329 p., 8.
59. Gross KB, Overman PR, Cobb C, Brockmann S. Aerosol generation by two ultrasonic scalers and one sonic scaler. A comparative study. *J Dent Hyg.* 1992;66(7):314–348.
60. Harrel SK. Clinical use of an aerosol-reduction device with an ultrasonic scaler. *Compend Contin Educ Dent.* 1996;17(12):1185–1193; quiz 94.
61. Fine DH, Mendieta C, Barnett ML, et al. Efficacy of preprocedural rinsing with an antiseptic in reducing viable bacteria in dental aerosols. *J Periodontol.* 1992;63(10):821–824.
62. Harrel SK, Barnes JB, Rivera-Hidalgo F. Aerosol reduction during air polishing. *Quintessence Int.* 1999;30(9):623–628.
63. Ishihama K, Koizumi H, Wada T, et al. Evidence of aerosolised floating blood mist during oral surgery. *J Hosp Infect.* 2009;71(4):359–364.
64. Jacks ME. A laboratory comparison of evacuation devices on aerosol reduction. *J Dent Hyg.* 2002;76(3):202–206.
65. Klyn SL, Cummings DE, Richardson BW, Davis RD. Reduction of bacteria-containing spray produced during ultrasonic scaling. *Gen Dent.* 2001;49(6):648–652.
66. Trenter SC, Walmsley AD. Ultrasonic dental scaler: associated hazards. *J Clin Periodontol.* 2003;30(2):95–101.
67. Williams JF, Johnston AM, Johnson B, Huntington MK, Mackenzie CD. Microbial contamination of dental unit waterlines: prevalence, intensity and microbiological characteristics. *J Am Dent Assoc.* 1993;124(10):59–65.
68. Petersilka G, Faggion CM, Jr., Stratmann U, et al. Effect of glycine powder air-polishing on the gingiva. *J Clin Periodontol.* 2008;35(4):324–332.
69. Petersilka GJ, Bell M, Haberlein I, Mehl A, Hickel R, Flemmig TF. In vitro evaluation of novel low abrasive air polishing powders. *J Clin Periodontol.* 2003;30(1):9–13.
70. Sculean A, Bastendorf KD, Becker C, et al. A paradigm shift in mechanical biofilm management? Subgingival air polishing: a new way to improve mechanical biofilm management in the dental practice. *Quintessence Int.* 2013;44(7):475–477.
71. Petersilka GJ, Bell M, Mehl A, Hickel R, Flemmig TF. Root defects following air polishing. *J Clin Periodontol.* 2003;30(2):165–170.
72. Sahrmann P, Ronay V, Hofer D, Attin T, Jung RE, Schmidlin PR. In vitro cleaning potential of three different implant debridement methods. *Clin Oral Implants Res.* 2013;26(3):314–349.
73. Schwarz F, Ferrari D, Popovski K, Hartig B, Becker J. Influence of different air-abrasive powders on cell viability at biologically contaminated titanium dental implants surfaces. *J Biomed Mater Res B Appl Biomater.* 2009;88(1):83–91.
74. Muthukuru M, Zainvi A, Esplugues EO, Flemmig TF. Non-surgical therapy for the management of peri-implantitis: a systematic review. *Clin Oral Implants Res.* 2012;23(Suppl 6):77–83.

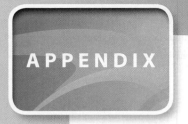

APPENDIX

Problem Identification: Difficulties in Instrumentation

Appendix Overview

This appendix provides solutions for the most common instrumentation problems encountered by beginning clinicians. These problems are divided into seven categories:

| Problem Chart 1 | Can't See the Treatment Area! | 744 |

| Problem Chart 2 | Can't Locate the Calculus! | 745 |

| Problem Chart 3 | Poor Illumination of Treatment Area! | 746 |

| Problem Chart 4 | Can't Adapt Cutting Edge to Tooth Surface! | 746 |

| Problem Chart 5 | Can't Maintain Adaptation! | 747 |

| Problem Chart 6 | Uncontrolled or Weak Calculus Removal Stroke! | 748 |

| Problem Chart 7A–C | Missed Calculus Deposits! | 749 |

7A—Deposits Missed at Midlines of Anterior Teeth
7B—Deposits Missed at Line Angles of Posterior Teeth
7C—Deposits Missed on Proximal Surfaces

Box A-1   Directions for Use of the Problem Charts

1. First select the category *that most closely describes the problem* that you are having. Turn to the problem chart for that category.
2. The "Cause" column lists possible causes of the problem. In each category, the causes are listed in order from the most likely cause to least likely cause.
3. Read the "Solution" column for suggestions on how to correct the problem.

PROBLEM CHART 1: CAN'T SEE THE TREATMENT AREA!

Cause	Solution
Clinician seated in wrong "clock position" for treatment area	Refer to Positioning Summary Sheets.
Patient positioned too high	Lower patient chair until the patient's mouth is below your elbow when you hold your arms against your side.
Patient head position	Mandibular arch = chin-down Maxillary arch = chin-up Aspect toward = turned slightly away Aspect away = turned toward
Not using indirect vision	A combination of direct vision and indirect vision is required in most treatment areas.
Using mirror, but still can't see	Be sure that you are using the mirror to fully retract the tongue or cheek away from the treatment area. If you can't see the treatment area in the mirror's reflecting surface, try rotating the mirror head slightly. Move mirror further away from treatment area. For mandibular lingual aspects, move mirror toward midline of the mouth. For maxillary anteriors, move mirror closer to the mandibular arch.
Finger rest too close to surface to be instrumented	Move rest slightly forward in the mouth so that your finger isn't covering up the surface to be instrumented.
Hand is blocking view	Swivel or pivot your hand and arm until you can see the treatment area.

PROBLEM CHART 2: CAN'T LOCATE THE CALCULUS!

Cause	Solution
Middle finger not resting on shank	You will receive more tactile information if your finger is resting on the shank.
Using middle finger to hold the instrument (index finger is just "going along for the ride" rather than holding the handle)	Using the middle finger to hold the handle prevents it from detecting vibrations. The thumb and index finger should be across from one another. You should be able to lift your middle finger off of the shank and not drop the instrument.
Using "death grasp" on handle	Relax your fingers and grasp the handle as lightly as possible. Try working on a typodont without wearing gloves—if your fingers are blanched, you are holding the handle too tightly.
Not beginning strokes at the junctional epithelium	Be sure to insert the working end to the base of the sulcus or pocket before initiating an assessment stroke. If you can't tell where the base is, get an instructor to help you.
Too few strokes, not overlapping strokes	When working subgingivally, use instrumentation zones and overlapping strokes to cover the entire root surface.
Not detecting calculus at line angles on posterior teeth	Position the working-end distal to the line angle with the explorer tip aimed toward the junctional epithelium (but NOT touching the J.E.) and make short horizontal strokes "around" the line angle toward the front of the mouth.
Not detecting calculus at midlines of anterior teeth	Make small, controlled horizontal strokes at the midline on facial or lingual surfaces.

PROBLEM CHART 3: POOR ILLUMINATION OF TREATMENT AREA!

Cause	Solution
Unit light too close to mouth	Positioning the light close to the patient's mouth creates excessive shadowing and actually makes it harder to see. Light should be an arm's length above or in front of the clinician.
Patient's head positioned incorrectly for treatment area	Mandibular arch = chin-down Maxillary arch = chin-up Aspect toward = turned slightly away Aspect away = turned toward
Not using mirror for indirect illumination	Use mirror to direct light onto the treatment area.

PROBLEM CHART 4: CAN'T ADAPT CUTTING EDGE TO TOOTH SURFACE!

Cause	Solution
Trying to adapt the middle-third of cutting edge	Usually only the tip-third or toe-third of the cutting edge can be adapted.
Using the wrong cutting edge for the tooth surface	Review the visual guidelines for the cutting edge selection for the instrument in question.
Using the wrong instrument for the task or area of the mouth	Review uses and applications of instrument classifications.
Finger rest too far away	Establish a finger rest near to the tooth to be instrumented.
Lower shank not parallel to facial or lingual surface of posterior tooth	On posterior teeth, the lower shank should be parallel to the tooth surface, but not touching it at any point.

PROBLEM CHART 5: CAN'T MAINTAIN ADAPTATION!

Cause	Solution
Incorrect grasp; not rolling instrument handle	Sloppy technique with grasp makes it difficult to control the instrument. As you work around the circumference of the tooth, roll the handle between your index finger and thumb to maintain adaptation.
Split grasp	Keep fingers together in the correct grasp position.
Fulcrum too close or too far away from tooth to be instrumented	Finger rest should be near (but not on) the tooth to be instrumented.
Fulcrum finger lifts off of the tooth as stroke is made	Fulcrum finger should be maintained in a straight, upright position throughout the stroke (acting as a "support beam"). Press down against the tooth with your fulcrum finger so finger can act as a "brake" to stop the stroke.
Tilting the instrument face away from the tooth surface during stroke (so lateral surface or back of working-end contacts tooth)	Maintain correct face-to-tooth surface angulation, as you use a pull stroke to move the working-end in a coronal direction. Handle position should stay parallel to the tooth surface as you make strokes (it should not tilt away from the tooth surface).
Not pivoting on finger rest	On posterior teeth, pivot at line angles to maintain adaptation. In anterior sextants, as you work toward yourself, your hand and arm should gradually pivot closer to your body.

PROBLEM CHART 6: UNCONTROLLED OR WEAK CALCULUS REMOVAL STROKE!

Cause	Solution
Instrument handle is supported solely by index finger and thumb	Handle should rest against the index finger or hand for support.
Split grasp—fingers not in contact	Keep fingers together in correct grasp position for control of strokes.
"Death grip" on handle	Use a firm grasp, but not a choking grasp.
Fulcrum finger lifts off of the tooth as stroke is made	Press down against the tooth with your fulcrum finger so finger can act as a "brake" to stop the stroke.
Fulcrum finger is relaxed and bent	Fulcrum finger should be straight and apply pressure against rest point on tooth (acting as a "support beam").
Stroke not stabilized; no lateral pressure with cutting edge against tooth surface	During a work stroke, the index finger and thumb should apply equal pressure against the instrument handle and the fulcrum finger applies pressure against the tooth surface.
Wrist and arm not in neutral position	Assess patient position, clinician position, and arm position.
Using a push-pull stroke	Apply lateral pressure only when making a stroke away from junctional epithelium; pause and relax grasp at completion of stroke.
Working too rapidly, strokes too fast	Pause briefly after each stroke. Make slow, controlled strokes.
On posterior teeth, lower shank not parallel—shank rocks on height of contour	On posterior teeth, the lower shank should be parallel to the facial or lingual surface, but not touching it at any point.

PROBLEM CHART 7A: MISSED CALCULUS DEPOSITS! DEPOSITS MISSED AT MIDLINES OF ANTERIOR TEETH

Cause	Solution
Not using horizontal strokes at midline of facial or lingual surface	Position the curet to the side of the midline with the toe aiming toward the junctional epithelium (but not touching the J.E.). Make a series of short controlled horizontal strokes.
Not overlapping vertical strokes at midline	Position the working-end so that strokes will overlap for surfaces toward and away.
Not using a specialized instrument when indicated	Use an area-specific curet with a miniature working-end at midlines.

PROBLEM CHART 7B: MISSED CALCULUS DEPOSITS! DEPOSITS MISSED AT LINE ANGLES OF POSTERIOR TEETH

Cause	Solution
Not using horizontal strokes at the line angles	Position the curet distal to the line angle with the toe aiming toward the junctional epithelium (but not touching the J.E.). Make a series of short strokes around the line angle.
Not rolling handle to maintain adaptation to line angle	As you work around a line angle, it is necessary to roll the instrument handle between the index finger and the thumb to maintain adaptation.

PROBLEM CHART 7C: MISSED CALCULUS DEPOSITS! DEPOSITS MISSED ON PROXIMAL SURFACES

Cause	Solution
Not using indirect vision	Beginning clinicians often have trouble learning to use indirect vision and so try to view all surfaces directly. Use of indirect vision is vital for proximal surfaces.
Not rotating reflecting surface to view proximal surfaces	This problem is common on lingual surfaces of anterior teeth. First, angle the mirror to view the surfaces toward you, and then turn the mirror to view the surfaces away from you.
Strokes not extended under contact area	Instrument at least one-half of a proximal surface from the facial and lingual aspects. Place curet between the papilla and the tooth surface. Adapt the working-end to the tooth surface and insert it to the junctional epithelium. (Do not "trace" papilla with working-end.)
Not rolling handle to maintain adaptation	As you work around a line angle and onto the proximal surface, make small, continuous adjustments in adaptation by rolling the handle.
Working-end not "aimed" toward surface to be instrumented	For distal surfaces of posterior teeth, the toe should aim toward the back of the mouth. Don't try to "back the working-end" onto the distal surface.

Index

Page numbers in *italic* designate figures; page numbers followed by "t" designate tables; page numbers followed by "b" designate boxes.

A

Abutment post, online module 20B
Active working-end area, 683
Adaptation, 232–241
 adjacent to papillary gingiva, 347–348, *347–348*
 calculus removal, *683*
 correct adaptation, *682*
 for handle roll, ergonomics of, 237–238, *237–240*
 incorrect, *682*
 of leading-third of working-end, 234, *234*
 probing, 272, *272*
 to proximal surfaces, 345–348, *345–348*
 to root concavities, *524*
 to tooth crown, 235, *235–236*
 two-point contact, 491, *491*
 working-end selection, *240,* 240–241
Advanced fulcrum, 112
Aerosols, production of, 671
AIR-FLOW Handy 3.0 PERIO, set-up of, online module 27B
AIR-FLOW Master Piezon unit, set-up of, online module 27B
Alignment, tooth surface, 229, *229*
Alternate clock positions, online module 21B
Alveolar bone, 417
Amplitude, 665, *665*
Anatomy
 root debridement and, 521, *521*
Angle, online module 1B
Angle of declination, 31
Angulation, 325
 for calculus removal, *325,* 325–326, 378, *378*
 errors in tissue injury or incomplete calculus removal, 326, *326*
 establishment, 332, *332*
 face-to-stone, for sharpening, 616, *616*
 for gingival-margin insertion, 366–369, *366–371*
 for insertion, 366, *366*
 principles of, 225, *225*
 for root debridement, 378
 sharpening stone, 626–627, *626–627*
 sickle scaler
  anterior teeth, 341–344, *341–344*
  posterior teeth, 349–355, *349–355,* 395, *395*
 of teeth in dental arches, 225, *225–226*
 tooth surface orientation, 226, *226–228*
Anterior exploration, working-end for, 297b, 298–299, *298–299*
Anterior sextants
 clock positions for
  left-handed clinician, 58, *58*
  right-handed clinician, 47, *47*
 fulcrum, 112, *112,* 112b, 113t

 mandibular (*See* Mandibular anterior sextants)
 maxillary (*See* Maxillary anterior sextants)
 wrist position, 114–115, 114b, *115*
Anterior sickle scalers, 335
Anterior surfaces away, clock positions for
 left-handed clinician, 60, *60*
 right-handed clinician, 47, *47,* 49, *49*
Anterior surfaces away from clinician, 47, *47,* 58, *58*
Anterior surfaces toward, clock positions for
 left-handed clinician, 59, *59*
 right-handed clinician, 47, 48, *48*
Anterior surfaces toward clinician, 47, *47,* 48, *48,* 58, *58,* 59, *59*
Anterior teeth
 exploration, 293–299, *293–299*
  with Orban-type explorer, 293–295, *293–295*
 probing, 278, *278–280*
 sickle scalers, 341–344, *341–344*
 with 11/12-type explorer, 296–299, *296–299*
Apical direction, instrumentation, online module 1B
Apical migration, 268, *268*
Appointment for re-evaluation, 373
Appointment planning, for calculus removal, 571–573, *572,* 572t, 573b, 573t
Area-specific curets, 451–486
 anterior teeth, 459–462
  applying cutting edge, 460, *460*
  step-by-step technique, *461,* 461–462, *462*
  visual clues, *464*
  working-end selection, 459, *459*
 compared with scalers, 479t
 design, *452, 453,* 453t
 face relation to lower shank, 454, *454*
 functions, *452,* 452
 Gracey series (*See* Gracey curets)
 horizontal stroke, 470, *470*
 lower cutting edge identification, 455 *455,* 455b
 posterior teeth, 463–473
  cutting-edge application, 463, *463*
  mandibular first molar, 465–469, *465–469*
  maxillary first molar, 461–462, *461, 462*
 reference sheet, 453t, 484
 root debridement, 477, *478*
Arthritis, 80
Artificial dental calculus, 344b
Aspect, defined, 50, *50*
Aspects, online module 1B
Assessment instruments, 288
Assessment stroke, 250–251, 291, 291t. *See also* Probe(s); Probing
 pressure forces of, 253

Attached gingiva, 266, 431
Automaticity, 217, 217b

B
Back, of working-end, 204, *204*
Back position, clinician
   masking tape trick, 17, *17*
   neutral, 12, *12*, 17, *17*
   rounded back, 17, *17*
   three curves, 11, *11*
Back position, clinician's neutral, 12, *12*
Balance, instrument, 197, *197*
Bifurcation, 432
Biocompatible, 2, online module 20B
Biofilm disruption, 675b
Bleeding, 423, *423*
Blind zone, 32
Bracket table position, 24
Brain–body coordination, 215b
Burnished calculus deposit, 329, *329*
Burs, metal from sharpening, 629, *629*

C
Calculus recipe, 344b
Calculus removal (scaling), 673
   angulation for, 378, *378*
   application of force for, 327–328, *328*
   appointment planning, 571–573, 572t
   complete, 571
   concepts, *338*, 338–340, 339t, *340*
   fictitious cases, 574–591, *575–577*, *578b*, *579–580*,
      581b, *582–583*, *584b*, *585–586*, *587b*,
      588–590, *589b*, *591b*
   goal, 374b
   insertion for, 366–369, *366–371*
   instrumentation zones, 376–377, *376–377*
   instrument selection, 572, 572t
   instruments for, 206, *206*
   patient cases, 574–591
   planning for, 571–573, *572*, 572t
   stroke pattern, *329*, 329–330, *330*, 375–377, *375–377*
   subgingival deposit removal, 330, *330*, 375–377, *375–377*
   technique, 673
   with universal curet, 390, 390t, *391*
Calculus removal strokes, 251, 674
   preparation for, 379, *379*
   pressure forces of, 253
   production of, 378–382, *378–382*
   sequence of events, 380, *380–382*
   with sickle scaler, 339, 339t, *340*
   steps in, 379b
   with universal curets, *340*
Calculus (tartar)
   deposits, diagramming, 318, *318*
   formation, 309, *309*, 310b
   subgingival
      ledge, *309*, 310b
      restorations, *312*
      spicules, *309*, 310b
   types, characteristics, 309
   undetected, causes, 313, 313t
Capacity for consent, 281, 568
Caries
   detection, 314–316, *314–316*, 315b
   ICDAS codes, 316
   pit and fissure, 315
   subgingival, *311*
Carious lesion, 314, *314*
Carpal tunnel syndrome (CTS), 7, *7*
Cavitated lesion, 314
Cavitation, 664
Chart, periodontal, 270, *270*

Chemotherapeutic agents, 668
Chin-cup technique, 537, *537*
Chin-down position, 20
Chin-up position, 19, 22
Classifications, instruments, 207, *207–208*
Cleaning efficiency, 666, *666*
Clinical attachment level, (CAL), 427
Clinical attachment loss, 427
Clinician's position. *See* Position
Clinician stool selection, 36, 36t
Clock position(s)
   left-handed clinician, *54*, 54–55, *55*
      anterior surfaces away, 60, *60*
      anterior surfaces toward, 59, *59*
      position practice sequence, 56, *56*
      posterior sextants, 61, *61*
         away, 63, *63*
         toward, 62, *62*
      reference sheet, 64, 64t
      textbook use, 57, *57*
   right-handed clinician, *41*, 43–44, *43–44*
      anterior sextants, 47, *47*
      anterior surfaces away, 47, *47*, 49, *49*
      anterior surfaces toward, 47, 48, *48*
      position practice sequence, 45, *45*
      posterior sextants, 50, *50*
         away, 52, *52*
         toward, 51, *51*
      reference sheet, 53, 53t
      textbook use, 46, *46*
Clock positions for instrumentation, 41–42, 42b, 66, *66–67*
Coaxial illumination, dental headlights, 28, *28, 29*
Coaxial illumination source, 28, *28*
Color-coded probes, 265, *265*
Communication with patients, 566–568
Complete calculus removal, 571
Complex shank design, *198*, 198–199, *199*
Comprehensive periodontal assessment, 420
Computer-assisted probes, 264t
Consent for treatment, 568–569, 569b, *570*
Contaminated dental aerosols and powered
   instrumentation, 670–671
Contouring, 615, *615*
Coronal direction, instrumentation, online module 1B
Cowhorn explorer, 290, *290*
Cross arch fulcrum, 533, *533*
Crosshatch pattern, 377
Cross section, 205, online module 1B
CTS. *See* Carpal tunnel syndrome
Cupping techniques, 697
Curet (s), *208*
   adaptation, 234
   for applying horizontal strokes to root surfaces, 532,
      532, 532b
   contouring, 615, *615*
   cross section, *206*
   langer miniature, 497–498, *497–498*, 498t
   modified Gracey, 499–506, *499–506*, 499t, 501t, 506t
   O'Hehir debridement, 509, *509–510*, 509t
   Quétin furcation, 507, *507–508*, *508*, 508t
   sharpening, 620–622, *620–622*
   sharpening position, 625, *625*
   standard vs. modified, 499t, *500*
   vision curvette miniature, 505–506, *505–506*, 506t
Curved cutting edges, 599, *599*, 602
Curved explorer, 290, *290*
Cutting edges, 204, *204*, 613, *613*. *See also* Sharpening

D
Debridement
   advanced root, 518–561
Defogging, 102, 102b

45-degree angle, online module 1B
90-degree angle, online module 1B
Demarco curets, *509*
Dental aerosols, 670
  defined, 670
  overview of, 670
  and powered instrumentation, 671
Dental arches, angulation of teeth, 225, *225–226*
Dental endoscope, 513, *513–514*
Dental headlights, co-axial illumination, 28, *29*
Dental hygienists, ergonomic hazards for, *4, 4–5, 5*
Dental implants, 680, online module 20B
  periodontal instrumentation of, online module 20B
  supported restorations, online module 20B
Dental mirror. *See* Mirror
DentalView, Inc., 513
Distraction technique, 646
Depressions, root debridement and, 522, *522*
Depth
  probing, *269–270, 269–271, 269b*
Depth of field, 31
Design name, 203
Design number, 203
Diagramming calculus deposits, 318, *318*
Diamond-coated instruments, 511, *511–512*
Digital motion activation, 222, *222*
Direct vision, 96
Distal surface(s)
  gingival margin insertion, 369, *369–370*
Double-ended instruments, 202, *202*
Drive finger, 223
Dull cutting edge, *597, 597*
Duration of action of anesthetic, 648
Dynamometer, *81*

E
Electronic probes, 263, 264t
Endoscope, subgingival, 513, *513–514*
Equipment. *See also* specific equipment
  position for mandibular teeth, 19, *20*
  position for maxillary teeth, 19, *19*
  position relative to clinician, *23, 23–24, 24,* 36t
Ergonomic risk factors, musculoskeletal disorders,
      3–8, *4–8*
Ergonomics, 3
Ergonomic seating, evaluation form, 36t
Exercises, for hand strength, 82–84, *82–84*
Exploration
  anterior teeth, 293–299, *293–299*
    with Orban-type, 293–295, *293–295*
    with 11/12-type, 296–299, *296–299*
  horizontal strokes, 307, *307*
  posterior teeth, 300–306, *300–306*
  subgingival conditions interpretation,
      311, *311–312*
  technique alerts, 307–308, *307–308*
Exploratory stroke. *See* Assessment stroke
Explorer(s), 207, *208*
  assessment stroke with, 291, 291t
  Cowhorn, 290, *290*
  curved, 290, *290*
  design of, 289, *289*
  functions of, 288
  lower shank, 289, *289*
  Orban-type, 290, *290,* 293–295, *293–295*
  Pigtail, 290, *290*
  reference sheet for, 319, *319b*
  straight, 290, *290*
  subgingival assessment with, 292, *292*
  tip, 289, *289*
  11/12-type, 290, *290*
  types, 289, *290*

Explorer tip, 289, *289*
Extended lower shank, 200–201, *201*
Extended shanks, 499, *500*
Extensor wad strain, 7, *7*
Extraoral finger rests
  for left-handed clinicians, 552, *552–554*
  for maxillary anterior teeth, 548, *548,* 558, *558*
  for maxillary left posterior sextants, 545, *545–547*
  for maxillary right posterior sextants, 555, *555–557*
  for right-handed clinicians, 542, *542–544*
Extraoral fulcrum, 92, 112
Extraoral fulcruming techniques, 536–541
  benefits and drawbacks of, 536b
  criteria for, 539, *539*
  instrumentation stroke with a finger assist,
      540, *540–541*
  left-handed clinicians, 538, *538*
  right-handed clinicians, 537, *537*
  vs. intraoral fulcrum, 539t

F
Face, of working-end, 204, *204*
Face at 90-degrees to lower shank, 387, 388b,
      394, *394*
Face-to-stone angulation, 616, *616*
Facial aspect, 50, online module 1B
Facial root depression, *527*
Facial surfaces
  gingival insertion on, 369, *370–371*
Feet position, clinician, 18, *18*
Field of view, 32
File(s), 207, *208,* 487–517
  on anterior teeth
    cutting edges, 495–496, *495–496*
  design characteristics, 489, *490,* 490t
  examples, 489
  functions of, 489
  on posterior teeth
    cutting edges, 492–493, *492–494*
  reference sheet, 490t
  selection, 491, 491t
  sharpening, 637, *637*
  two-point contact, 491, *491*
  working-end of, 489
Finger-like formations, of calculus, 309, *309,* 310b
Fingernails, length 81, *81*
Finger-on-finger fulcrum, 534, *534–535*
Finger(s)
  function, 72, 72t
  identification, 72, *72*
  joint hyperextension of, *80*
  joint hypermobility of, *78*
  length, 76, *76*
  placement, 72, *72,* 72t, 75t
Fissures, root debridement and, 522
Flexible shank, 199–200
Fluid lavage, *663,* 664
Fluid reservoirs, 668, *668*
Fogging, 102b, 107b
Force, 5
Forearm position, clinician's neutral, 13, *13*
Foundational skills, building blocks, 9, *9*
  sequencing of, 10
  significance of, 10
Free gingiva, 266
Frequency, 664
Fulcrum(s), 92, 112
  advanced, 112
  establishment, 332, *332*
  extraoral, 92, 112
  intraoral, 92, 112, *112,* 112b, 113t
Functional shank, 200–201, *201*

Furcation(s)
   area, 432
   arrows, 432
   involvement, 432
   probe, 432
   root debridement and, 522, *523*
Furcation involvement, 432, 436
   design characteristics, 437
Furcation probe(s), 437–438, *438*
   design, 437

G
Geometric angles, online module 1B
Get Ready Zone, 367, *367*
Gingiva, 266, *266*
Gingival insertion
   on distal surface, 369, *369–370*
   on facial surface, 369, *370–371*
Gingival margin, 266
   curet beneath, insertion of,
      369, *369–371*
Gingival pocket, 268, *268*
Gingival sulcus, 266, 268, *268*
Gloves fit, 77, *77*
Goldman Fox probe, 263, 264t
Gracey curets, 499–506
   on anterior teeth, 459, *459*
   applications, 457, 457t
   designs, 499–500, *499–500*, 499t
     availability of, 501, 501t
     standard *vs.* modified, 499t, *500*
   with extended shanks, 502, *502*
   with micro-miniature working-ends, 504, *504*
   with miniature working-ends, 503, *503*
   reference sheet, 457t
   vision curvette curet, 505–506, 506t
Gracey design name, 202–203, *203*
Grasp
   arthritis and, 80, *80*
   fine-tuning, 75
   finger function, 72, 72t
   fingernails and, 81, *81*
   finger placement, 72, *72*, 72t, 75t
   gloves fit and, 77, *77*
   hand strength exercises, 82–84, *82–84*
   instrument parts and, 71, *71*
   joint hypermobility and, 78, *78*, 79, *79*
   modified pen, 71, *71, 72*
     left-handed clinician, 74, *74*
     right-handed clinician, 73, *73*
   muscle strength and, 80
   variations, 76, *76*
   with silicone sleeve, 79, *79, 80*

H
Handle, 71, *71*
   instrument, *195*, 195–197, *196*, 196t, *197*
   selection criteria, 196t
Handle roll, 223, *223*
Hand pivot, 224, *224*
Hand position, clinician's neutral, 13, *13*,
     114, 114b
Hand strength exercises, 82–84
Head position, patient's, 21, *21*, 42, *42*
Hearing loss, 671
Hexagonal cross section, online module 1B
Horizontal instrumentation strokes, 248, *250*
Horizontal lines, online module 1B
Horizontal stroke(s). *See also* Strokes
   exploration, 307, *307*
   for left-handed clinicians, 559, *559–561*
   on molar tooth, 307, *307*

   on posterior teeth, 307, *307*
   for right-handed clinicians, 549, *549–551*
Horizontal tooth mobility, 422

I
Identification, instrument, 203, *203*
Illumination, indirect by mirror, 93, *93*
Implied consent, 281, 569
Index and thumb placement, function, 72t
Indirect illumination, 93, *93*
Indirect vision, 92, *92*, 96–97, 97b, 172
Infiltration injection, 643
Informed consent, 568, 569b, *570*
Intrapocket local anesthesia, 652
Informed consent for periodontal instrumentation,
     281–282, 281b, *282*
Informed refusal, 282, 569, *570*
Inner cutting edge, 350, *350*, 393, *393*, 393b
Instrumentation, 215
   airborne contamination, 701, 702
   anatomic descriptors, online module 1B
   challenges, 697
   consent for treatment, 568, 569b, *570*
   forces of
     lateral pressure, 327–328
     pinch pressure, 327
     stabilization, 327
   furcation areas, 699, 700
   mathematical principles, online module 1B
   multirooted teeth with area-specific curets, 529, *529, 530–531*
   of root surfaces, 518–561
     advanced extraoral fulcruming techniques for, 536–541,
       536t, *537–541*, 539t
     advanced intraoral techniques for, 533–535, *533–535*
     anatomical features, 521–528
     extraoral finger rests for left-handed clinicians, 552–558,
       552–558
     extraoral finger rests for right-handed clinicians,
       542–548, *542–548*
     horizontal strokes for left-handed clinicians, 559–561,
       559–561
     horizontal strokes for right-handed clinicians, 549–551,
       549–551
     introduction, 529–532, *529–532*
   sense of touch for subgingival, 364–365, *364–365*
   stroke, 674
     preparation flow chart, *368, 379*
   subgingival, 289
   supragingival, 289
   water containment, 702
   zones, 376–377, *376–377*
Instrumentation strokes
   characteristics of, 248
   direction, 248, *249–250*
   with finger assist, 540, *540–541*
   injuries, strategies for avoiding, 258, 258b
   pressure forces of, 253
   types of, 250–252
Instrumentation stroke with a finger assist, 540, *540–541*
Instrumentation zones, 376–377, *376–377*
Instrument(s), 193–208. *See also* Tip(s); *individual*
     instrument parts
   classifications
     assessment, 207, *207–208*
     calculus removal, 207, *207–208*
   diamond-coated, 511, *511–512*
   face to tooth surface, 324–327, *324–327*
   grasp (*See* Grasp)
   handle, *195*, 195–197, *196*, 196t, *197*
   and hypermobility, 79, *79*
   maintenance, 604, 604t
   parts, 71, *71, 195, 195*

replacement, 602
shank design, *198*, 198–201, *199*, *201*, 201t
sharpening (*See* Sharpening)
single- and double-ended, 202, *202*
working-end design, 202–206, *202–206*
working-end identification, 203, *203*
Instrument tray, 24, *24*
International Caries Detection and Assessment
     System (ICDAS), 316
Intraoral fulcrum, 92, 112
    characteristics, 112b
    summary sheet, 113t
Irrigant solutions, 668

J
Joint hypermobility, 78, *78*
Junctional epithelium, 248, 266, 417

K
Knurling pattern, 197

L
Langer curets (modified)
    application of, *498*, 498t
    availability, 497
    design characteristics, 497, *497*
    miniature, 497, *497*
    use, 497
Lateral pressure, 379
Lateral pressure force, 327–328
Lateral surfaces, of working-end, 204, *204*
Leading-third of working-end, 234, *234*
Ledge calculus, 310b
Light, 23, *23*
    position for mandibular arch, 23, *23*
    position for maxillary arch, 23, *23*
Limited use-life, of instruments, 602
Line angles, online module 1B
Lingual aspect, online module 1B
Little finger placement, function, 72t
Local anesthetic effects, 653
    failure of, 653
    reversal, 653
Loss of attachment (LOA), 417
Loupes, magnification, 30–32, *30–33*, 33b
Lower cutting edge, 451
Lower (terminal) shank, 200–201, *201*
    explorer, 289, *289*
    universal curet, working-end of, 392, *392*, 392b
Lubricant, 606, *607*
Lubrication, of sharpening stone, 606, *607*

M
Magnification loupes, 30–32, *30–33*, 33b
Magnetic fields, 671
Magnetostrictive ("magneto") devices, 661
Maintenance of instruments, 604, 604t
Mandibular anterior sextants
    left-handed clinician
        lingual aspect: surfaces away, 106, *106*
        lingual aspect: surfaces toward, 106, *106*
    right-handed clinician
        lingual aspect: surfaces away, 101, *101*
        lingual aspect: surfaces toward, 101, *101*
Mandibular anterior teeth
    handle positions for, 118b, 121b, 131b, 134b
    left-handed clinician
        facial aspect: surfaces away, 135, *135*
        facial aspect: surfaces toward, 132, *132*
        lingual aspect: surfaces away, 136, *136*
        lingual aspect: surfaces toward, 133, *133*
        surfaces away, 134, *134*

surfaces toward, 131, *131*
    right-handed clinician
        facial aspect: surfaces away, 122, *122*
        facial aspect: surfaces toward, 119, *119*
        lingual aspect: surfaces away, 123, *123*
        lingual aspect: surfaces toward, 120, *120*
        reference sheet, 130, 130t
        surfaces away, 121, *121*
        surfaces toward, 118, *118*
Mandibular arch
    light position, 23, *23*
    patient head tilt, 22, 22t
    patient position for, 19, 20t
Mandibular posterior sextants
    left-handed clinician
        alternate clock positions, online module 21B
        facial aspect: surfaces away, 161, *161*, 161b
        facial aspect: surfaces toward, 158, *158*, 158b
        left sextant: facial aspect, 106, *106*, 159, *159*
        left sextant: lingual aspect, 107, *107*, 163, *163*
        right sextant: facial aspect, 107, *107*, 162, *162*
        right sextant: lingual aspect, 107, *107*, 160, *160*
    mirror and finger rests, 147–164
        building blocks, 149, *149*
        finger length on grasp, 150, *150*
        practicing, directions for, 150b
    reference sheet for, 130t, 157, 157t, 164, 164t
    right-handed clinician
        alternate clock positions, online module 21B
        clock position, facing away, 154, *154*, 154b
        clock position, facing toward, 151, *151*, 151b
        left sextant: facial aspect, 155, *155*
        left sextant: lingual aspect, 102, *102*, 153, *153*
        lingual aspect: surfaces away, 101, *101*
        lingual aspect: surfaces toward, 101, *101*
        right sextant: facial aspect, 101, *101*, 102, *102*, 152, *152*
        right sextant: lingual aspect, 102, *102*, 156, *156*
Mandibular teeth, *101–102*
    angulation, 226, *226*
    mirror uses, 101–102, *101–102*, 106–107, *106–107*
    patient position for, 19, 20t
Masking tape trick, 17, *17*
Mathematical principles, instrumentation,
     online module 1B
Maxillary anterior sextants
    left-handed clinician
        lingual, surfaces away, 104, *104*
        lingual, surfaces toward, 104, *104*
    right-handed clinician
        lingual, surfaces away, 99, *99*
        lingual, surfaces toward, 99, *99*
Maxillary anterior teeth
    handle positions for, 124b, 127b, 137b, 140b
    left-handed clinician
        facial aspect: surfaces away, 141, *141*
        facial aspect: surfaces toward, 138, *138*
        lingual aspect: surfaces away, 142, *142*
        lingual aspect: surfaces toward, 139, *139*
        reference sheet, 143, *143*
        surfaces away, 140, *140*
        surfaces toward, 137, *137*
    right-handed clinician
        facial aspect: surfaces away, 128, *128*
        facial aspect: surfaces toward, 125, *125*
        lingual aspect: surfaces away, 129, *129*
        lingual aspect: surfaces toward, 126, *126*
        reference sheet, 130, 130t
        surfaces away, 127, *127*
        surfaces toward, 124, *124*
Maxillary arch
    light position, 23, *23*
    patient position for, 19, 19t

Maxillary posterior sextants
  left-handed clinician
    clock position, facing away, 183, *183*
    clock position, facing toward, 180, *180*
    left sextant: facial aspect, 104, *104*, 181, *181*
    left sextant: lingual aspect, 105, *105, 185, 185*
    reference sheet, 186, 186t
    right sextant: facial aspect, 105, *105*, 184, *184*
    right sextant: lingual aspect, 105, *105*, 182, *182*
  mirror and finger rests, 169–188
    building blocks, 171, *171*
    musculoskeletal strain, indirect vision and prevention
      of, 172
    practicing, directions for, 172b
    stretches for, 187, 187b, *188*
  right-handed clinician
    clock position, facing away, 176, *176*, 176b
    clock position, facing toward, 173, *173*, 173b
    left sextant: facial aspect, 99, *99*, 102, *102*, 177, *177*
    left sextant: lingual aspect, 100, *100*, 175, *175*
    reference sheet, 179, 179t
    right sextant: facial aspect, 100, *100*, 174, *174*
    right sextant: lingual aspect, *100*, 178, *178*
Maxillary teeth, 99–100, *99–100*
  angulation, 225, *225*
  handle positions for, 173b, 176b, 180b, 183b
  mirror uses, 99–100, *99–100*, 104–105, *104–105*
Metal burs, from sharpening, 629, *629*
Micro-miniature curets, 504, *504*
Micro-miniature working-ends, 499, *500*
Middle finger placement, function, 72t
Midline, online module 1B
Millimeter markings, 265, *265*
Millimeter measurements, online module 1B
Miniature curets
  Langer, 497–498, *497–498*, 498t
  vision curvette, 505–506, *505–506*, 506t
Miniature working-ends, 499, *500*
Mirror
  functions of, 92–94, *92–94*
  for retraction, 98–100, *98–100*
    left-handed clinician, 103–105, *103–105*
  surface types, 91t
  transillumination, *93, 93, 94*
  types, 91, *91*, 91t
  uses, 91–94, *91–94*, 91t
    mandibular teeth, 101–102, *101–102*, 106–107,
      106–107
    maxillary teeth, 99–100, *99–100*, 104–105,
      104–105
Modified curets, 499–506. *See also* Gracey curets
Modified pen grasp, 71, *71*, 72
  left-handed clinician, 74, *74*
  right-handed clinician, 73, *73*
  variations in, *76*
Module skill evaluations (online), 37, *37*
Molar(s)
  horizontal stroke on, 307, *307*
  maxillary
    probing, 272, *272*
Mobility, 422
Mobility-rating scales, 422
Motion activation, 219–222
  digital, 222, *222*
  introduction, 219
  wrist, 220–221, *220–221*
Mouth mirror, 91, *91*
Moving instrument technique, 612. *See also* Sharpening
Moving stone technique, 612. *See also* Sharpening
Multidirectional strokes, 248, 377
Muscle strength, 80
Musculoskeletal damage, 671

Musculoskeletal disorder(s)
  causes of, 3–4
  hazards to, 4–5, *5*
  prevalence of, 3
  risk factors, 3–8, *4–8*
Musculoskeletal risk assessment, 190, 190t
Myelination, 216, 217

N
Neck position, clinician's neutral, 12, *12*
Neutral position
  clinician, seated, *11*, 11–13, *12, 13*, 14–18, *14–18*
  clinician's back, 12, *12*, 17, *17*
  clinician's forearm, 13, *13*
  clinician's hand, 13, *13*
  clinician's neck, 12, *12*
  clinician's shoulder, 12, *12*
  clinician's torso, 12, *12*
  clinician's upper arms, 13, *13*
Neutral posture, 4
Neutral wrist position, 115, *115*
Nitrous oxide/oxygen inhalation sedation, 645
Nodule calculus, *309*, 310b
Noncavitated lesion, 314
Nonresponsive disease sites, 373
Novatech probe, 263, 264t
Number, design, 203

O
Oblique instrumentation strokes, 248, *249*
Oblique lines, online module 1B
Occupational risks
  musculoskeletal disorders, 3–8, *4–8*
O'Hehir debridement curets, 509, *509–510*, 509t
Online module skill evaluations, 37, *37*
Opposite arch fulcrum, 533, *533*
Orban-type explorer, 290, *290*, 293–295, *293–295*
Orientation, to tooth surface, 226, *226–228*
Osseointegration, online module 20B
Outer cutting edge, 350, *350*, 393, *393*, 393b
Out of the line of fire, 113t, 255, 369
Overhead dental light, 23, *23*

P
Pain control, 642–654
  allaying fear, strategies for, 644–646
  distraction techniques, 646
  in hygiene care, 642–643
  nitrous oxide and oxygen inhalation sedation, 645
  local anesthesia, 647–650
    action duration, 648
    agents, selection, 648–649, 649b, 650t
    C-CLAD, 654
    failure of, 653
    infiltration anesthesia, 650
    intrapocket local anesthesia, 652
    potency, 648
    regional nerve block anesthesia, 650, 651
    reversal of effects, 653
    topical anesthesia, 652
    transmucosal patches, 653
    types, 650–651, 651, 651t
    vasoconstrictors, 648, 648t
    vasodilation, 648
  modalities, 647–650
  patient anxiety and, 646
  relaxation techniques, 646
  transmucosal anesthesia patches, 653
Paired working-ends, 202, *202*
Palatal root depression, *527*
Palm facing out technique, 537, *537*
Parallel lines, online module 1B

Patient
    cases, for calculus removal, 574–591, 575–577, 578b,
        579–580, 581b, 582–583, 584b, 585–586, 587b,
        588–590, 589b, 591b
    treatment consent, 568–569, 569b, 570
Patients, communication with, 566–568
Patient's position
    chair height, 27, 27
    chin-down, 20t, 23, 27, 53t, 64t
    chin-up, 19t, 22, 23, 27, 53t, 64t
    head, 21, 22, 22
    head adjustment, optimal visibility, 22, 22
    for mandibular teeth, 19, 20t
    for maxillary arch, 19, 19t
    neutral hand, 114, 114b
    neutral seated, 25, 25b, 26
    neutral wrist, 115, 115
    relative to seated clinician, 25–26, 25b, 26
    supine vs. semi-supine, 19–20, 19t, 20t
Pen grasp, modified, 71, 71
Peri-implant tissues, online module 20B
Periodontal attachment system
    alveolar bone, 417
    calibrated probes, 420
    clinical attachment level, 427–430, 429
    in disease, 417, 417, 418t
    gingiva fibers, 417
    in health, 417, 417, 418t
    junctional epithelium, 417
    ligament fibers, 417
    oral deviations measurement, 421, 421
Periodontal chart, 270, 270
Periodontal files, 207, 208, 487–517
    application of, 491t
    design characteristics, 489, 490, 490t
    examples, 489
    functions of, 489
    reference sheet, 490t
    two-point contact, 491, 491
    working-end of, 489
Periodontal instrumentation, 372
    dental hygiene care and, 384
    healing, 374, 374
    informed consent for, 568–569, 569b, 570
    objective of, 566
    rationale for, 566
    word choice, with patient, 566–568
Periodontal ligament fibers, 417
Periodontal maintenance, 566
Periodontal pockets, 266–268, 267–268, 268, 268
    formation, 268, 268
Peri-implant tissues, online module 20B
Periodontal probes, 202, 260, 262
    design, 262, 262
    functions, 262
Periodontal typodonts, 368
Periodontitis, 267
Periodontium, 324, 324, 365, 365
Perioscopy Incorporated, 513
Perpendicular lines, online module 1B
Piezoelectric ("piezo") devices, 661
Pigtail explorer, 290, 290
Pinch pressure forces, 327
Pit and fissure caries, 315
Pivot, 224
Pivoting, on fulcrum, 224, 224
Planning
    for calculus removal, 571–573
    for multiple appointments, 571–573
Plaque retentive, 309
Plastic probe, 263, 264t
Point-of-use filter, 670

Polishing, 8
Position, equipment
    bracket table, 24
    dental headlights, coaxial illumination, 28, 29
    instrument tray, 24, 24
    magnification loupes, 30–32, 30–33, 33b
    overhead dental light, 23, 23
Positioning principles, 1–33
Posterior aspects facing away from clinician, 50, 61
Posterior aspects facing toward clinician, 50, 61
Posterior exploration, working-end for, 300, 300, 301b
Posterior sextants
    clock positions for
        left-handed clinician, 61, 61–63, 62, 63
        right-handed clinician, 50, 50–52, 51, 52
Posterior sickle scalers, 335
Posterior teeth
    exploration, 300–306, 300–306
    universal curet, working-end for, 392–395, 392–395, 392b
Posture, 4. See also Neutral posture; Static posture
Potency of anesthetic agent, 648
Powered instrumentation devices, 660, 660
    adaptation of working-end, 682–683, 682, 683
    calculus removal with, 673, 673
    cleaning efficiency of, 666, 666
    contraindications for, 669, 669t
    curved working-end as right or left, 687, 687
    evolution of, 661t
    fluid reservoirs and, 668
    fundamental skills and techniques, 672
        adaptation, 672
        assessment/end point of instrumentation, 672
        finger rests, 672
        grasp, 672
        lateral pressure, 672
        position, 672
    health concerns for
        dental aerosols, 670–671
        hearing loss, 671
        magnetic fields, 671
        musculoskeletal damage, 671
        occupational risks, 671
        water tubing contamination, 670, 670
    limitations of, 662
    mechanisms of action of, 664–665
        amplitude, 665, 665
        frequency, 664, 664
    modes of action, 664
    orientation of working-end to tooth surface, 683
        transverse working-end orientation, 683, 684, 685, 685b,
            685
        vertical working-end orientation, 684, 684, 686,
            686b, 686
    paired magneto working-ends in transverse orientation,
        689, 689
        efficient sequence for use of, 688, 688
    paired magneto working-ends in vertical orientation, 691,
        691
        cross arch finger rest for lingual aspects, 692, 692
        efficient sequence for use of, 690, 690
    pattern of working-end movement, 666
    powered working-end design, 676
        dental implants, 680, 680
        slim perio tips, 679
        wear and replacement, 681, 681
        working-end selection and sequence for instrumentation,
            676–678
    sonic powered devices, 661
    strengths of, 662, 663
    strokes
        for calculus removal, 674
        for subgingival biofilm removal, 674–675

Powered instrumentation devices, *(continued)*
  types of, 661, *661*
  ultrasonic devices, 661
    classification of, 661, *661*
    effectiveness of, 662
    hand instrumentation and, 662, 663t
    water/irrigant flow to powered working-end, 667,
      667, 668
  working-end in action, 660, *660*
Power Putty, 82
Practicing position sequence, 45, *45*
  clock positions
    left-handed clinician, 56, *56*
    right-handed clinician, 45, *45*
Premolar(s)
  root debridement, 525, *525*
Pressure forces, of instrumentation stroke, 253
Primary teeth, 356–357, *356–357*
Probe(s), 207, *207. See also* Probing
  calibrations, *265*
  color-coded, 265, *265*
  computer-assisted, 264t
  design, 262, *262,* 263t–264t
  functions, 262
  millimeter markings, 265, *265*
  millimeter measurements, online module 1B
  in periodontal pocket, 267, *267*
  in sulcus, 267, *267*
Probing
  adaptation in, 272, *272*
  anterior teeth, 278, *278–280*
  depth measurements, 269, *269,* 269b
  maxillary molars, 272
  measurement limitations, 271, *271*
  posterior teeth, 275, *275–277*
  proximal root surfaces, 273, *273*
  walking stroke, 274, *274*
Probing depth, 269, *269,* 269b
Pronator syndrome, 6, *6*
Proprioception, 78
Pseudo-pocket, *268*
Psychomotor skills, 215
  and brain, 216
  development of, 215
  learning strategies, 218t
  stages of, 215, 216t

Q
Quality of practice, 217
Quétin furcation curets, 507–508, *507–508,* 508t
Quick start guides, clock positions
  left-handed clinician, 58, *58,* 61, *61*
  right-handed clinician, 47, *47,* 50, *50*

R
Recontouring, 615, *615,* 622, *622*
Regional nerve block injection, 643, 650
Relaxation technique 646
Repetitive task, as injury risk factor, 5
Residual calculus deposits, 251, 309, 373
Restorations
  deficient margin, *312*
  overhanging margin, *312*
Retraction, by mirror, 93, *93*
Right angle, online module 1B
Rigid shank, 199
Ring calculus, 309, *309,* 310b
Ring finger placement, function, 72t
Rolling the instrument handle, 223, *223*
Root concavities, 522, *522–523*
  adaptation to, *524*
  in cross section, *524*

exploration of, *525*
  working-end to, *524*
Root debridement
  advanced root surface, 518–561
  anatomical features complicating, 521, *521*
  angulation for, 378
  depressions and, 522, *522*
  exploration, 525–528
    mandibular first molar, 526, *526*
    maxillary first molar, 527, *527–528*
    maxillary first premolar, proximal concavity,
      525, *525*
  Gracey curets for, 499–506
  Langer miniature curets for, 497–498, *497–498,* 498t
  O'Hehir debridement curets, 509, *509–510,* 509t
  Quétin furcation curets, 507–508, *507–508,* 508t
  root surface anatomy, 521–528
Root debridement stroke, 251–252
  angulation, 474, 475t
  pressure forces of, 253
Root depression, 522, *522*
Root fissures, 522
Root grooves, 522, *522*
Root instrumentation, 521–528, *521–528. See also*
    Root debridement
Root surfaces, instrumentation of, 518–561
  advanced extraoral fulcruming techniques for, 536–541,
    536t, *537–541,* 539t
  advanced intraoral techniques for, 533–535, *533–535*
  anatomical features, 521–528
    exploration, 525–528, *525–528*
    furcation areas, 522, *523*
    grooves, 522
    missed deposits in concavities, *524–525*
    root concavity, 521, *521,* 522, *522–523,* 525
  extraoral finger rests for left-handed clinicians, 552–558,
    552–558
  extraoral finger rests for right-handed clinicians, 542–548
  horizontal strokes for left-handed clinicians, 559–561,
    559–561
  horizontal strokes for right-handed clinicians, 549–551,
    549–551
  introduction, 529–532, *529–532*
Rotator cuff tendinitis, 6, *6*
Rounded back position, clinician, 17, *17*

S
Seated position
  clinician's neutral, *11,* 11–13, *12, 13,* 14–18, *14–18*
  importance, 18, *18*
Self-angulated curet, 451
Semi-supine patient position, 19, 20t
Sextants, online module 1B
  anterior, clock positions for, 47, *47,* 58, *58*
  posterior, clock positions for, *50, 50–52, 51, 52, 61,*
    61–63, 62, 63
Shank design, *198,* 198–201, *199,* 201, 201t
  extended lower, 200–201, *201*
  flexibility, 199–200
  functional, 200–201, *201*
  lower, 200–201, *201*
  as related to use, 201t
  rigid, 199
  simple and complex, *198,* 198–199, *199*
  terminal, 200
Shanks, 71, *71*
  position, *4*
Sharp cutting edge, 595, *595*
Sharpening, 592–609, 610–637
  advantages of sharp instruments, 594
  broken instrument tips, 603, 603b
  common errors in, 601, *601–602*